D1202101

The Neuropsychology of Cortical Dementias

Chad A. Noggle, PhD, ABN, is an associate professor of clinical psychiatry and chief of the division of behavioral and psychosocial oncology at Southern Illinois University–School of Medicine. He previously served as an assistant professor at Southern Illinois University–School of Medicine and both Ball State University and Middle Tennessee State University. Dr. Noggle holds a BA in psychology from the University of Illinois at Springfield and completed his MA and PhD at Ball State University with specialization in clinical neuropsychology. He completed a 2-year postdoctoral residency at the Indiana Neuroscience Institute at St. Vincent's Hospital with specialization in pediatric and adult/geriatric neuropsychology. To date, Dr. Noggle has published more than 300 articles, book chapters, encyclopedia entries, and research abstracts and has made over 100 presentations at national and international conferences in neuropsychology. He served as the lead editor of *The Encyclopedia of Neuropsychological Disorders, The Neuropsychology of Psychopathology, The Neuropsychology of Cancer and Oncology,* and *Neuropsychological Rehabilitation,* the latter three representing additional volumes of the Contemporary Neuropsychology series. He currently serves as a reviewer for a number of neuropsychology journals and is a member of the editorial board for *Applied Neuropsychology: Adult* and *Applied Neuropsychology: Child.* Dr. Noggle is a diplomate of the American Board of Professional Neuropsychology and a professional member of the American Psychological Association (divisions 5, 22, 38, 40), the National Academy of Neuropsychology, and the International Neuropsychological Society. For his contributions to the field of neuropsychology, Dr. Noggle was named a fellow of the National Academy of Neuropsychology. He is also a fellow of the American College of Professional Neuropsychology. Dr. Noggle is a licensed psychologist in both Illinois and Indiana. His research interests focus on both adult and pediatric populations, spanning psychiatric illnesses, dementia, pervasive developmental disorders, and neuromedical disorders.

Raymond S. Dean, PhD, ABPP, ABN, ABPdN, holds a BA in psychology (magna cum laude) and an MS in research and psychometrics from the State University of New York at Albany. As a Parachek–Frazier Research Fellow, he completed a PhD in school/child clinical psychology at Arizona State University in 1978. Dr. Dean completed an internship focused on neuropsychology at the Arizona Neuropsychiatric Hospital and postdoctoral work at the University of Wisconsin at Madison. Since his doctoral degree, he has served in a number of positions and has been recognized for his work. From 1978 to 1980, Dr. Dean was an assistant professor and director of the Child Clinic at the University of Wisconsin at Madison. During this time, he was awarded the Lightner Witmer Award by the school psychology division of the American Psychological Association (APA). From 1980 to 1981, he served as assistant professor of psychological services at the University of North Carolina at Chapel Hill. From 1981 to 1984, Dr. Dean served as assistant professor of medical psychology and director of the neuropsychology internship at Washington University School of Medicine in St. Louis. During this same time, Dr. Dean received both the Outstanding Contribution Award from the National Academy of Neuropsychology and the Early Contribution Award by division 15 of the APA. He was named the George and Frances Ball distinguished professor of neuropsychology and director of the neuropsychology laboratory at Ball State University and has served in this position since 1984. In addition, Dr. Dean served as distinguished visiting faculty at the Staff College of the National Institute of Mental Health. Dr. Dean is a diplomate of the American Board of Professional Psychology, the American Board of Professional Neuropsychology, and the American Board of Pediatric Neuropsychology. He is a fellow of the APA (divisions: clinical, educational, school, and clinical neuropsychology), the National Academy of Neuropsychology, and the American Psychopathological Association. Dr. Dean is a past president of the clinical neuropsychology division of the APA and the National Academy of Neuropsychology. He also served as editor of the *Archives of Clinical Neuropsychology, Journal of School Psychology,* and the *Bulletin of the National Academy of Neuropsychology.* Dr. Dean has published some 600 research articles, books, chapters, and tests. For his work, he has been recognized by awards from the National Academy of Neuropsychology, the *Journal of School Psychology,* and the Clinical Neuropsychology Division of the APA.

CONTEMPORARY NEUROPSYCHOLOGY SERIES

The Neuropsychology of Cortical Dementias

EDITORS

Chad A. Noggle, PhD, ABN
Raymond S. Dean, PhD, ABPP, ABN, ABPdN

ASSOCIATE EDITORS

Shane S. Bush, PhD, ABPP (CN, RP, CL)
Steven W. Anderson, PhD, ABPP (CN)

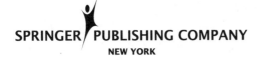
SPRINGER PUBLISHING COMPANY
NEW YORK

Springer Publishing Company, LLC
11 West 42nd Street
New York, NY 10036
www.springerpub.com

Acquisitions Editor: Nancy S. Hale
Production Editor: Shelby Peak
Composition: Newgen Knowledge Works

ISBN: 978-0-8261-0726-8
e-book ISBN: 978-0-8261-0727-5

14 15 16 17 / 5 4 3 2 1

The author and the publisher of this Work have made every effort to use sources believed to be reliable to provide information that is accurate and compatible with the standards generally accepted at the time of publication. The author and publisher shall not be liable for any special, consequential, or exemplary damages resulting, in whole or in part, from the readers' use of, or reliance on, the information contained in this book. The publisher has no responsibility for the persistence or accuracy of URLs for external or third-party Internet websites referred to in this publication and does not guarantee that any content on such websites is, or will remain, accurate or appropriate.

Library of Congress Cataloging-in-Publication Data

The neuropsychology of cortical dementias / editors, Chad A. Noggle, Raymond S. Dean ; associate editors, Shane S. Bush, Steven W. Anderson.
    p. ; cm. — (Contemporary neuropsychology series)
  Includes bibliographical references.
  ISBN 978-0-8261-0726-8 — ISBN 978-0-8261-0727-5
  I. Noggle, Chad A., editor. II. Dean, Raymond S., editor. III. Bush, Shane S., 1965- , editor. IV. Anderson, Steven W., editor. V. Series: Contemporary neuropsychology series.
  [DNLM: 1. Dementia. 2. Cerebral Cortex—physiopathology. 3. Neuropsychology. WM 220]
  RC521
  616.8'3—dc23   2014028536

Printed in the United States of America by Bang Printing.

I dedicate this to my grandparents, Forrest and Ruth Noggle. Like many other families, mine came face-to-face with the realities of dementia when my grandmother was diagnosed with Alzheimer's disease—CAN

To my children with all my heart—RSD

Contents

Contributors

Steven W. Anderson, PhD, ABPP (CN)
Associate Professor
Departments of Neurology, Neurosurgery,
  and Radiation Oncology
Carver College of Medicine
University of Iowa
Iowa City, Iowa

Brian S. Appleby, MD
Associate Professor
Departments of Neurology and Psychiatry
Case Western University School of Medicine
  and University Hospitals
Cleveland, Ohio

Valerie Hobson Balldin, PhD
Assistant Professor
Department of Neurology
University of Texas Health Science Center
  San Antonio
San Antonio, Texas

Mark T. Barisa, PhD, ABPP (CN)
Director, Neurological Services
Department of Neuropsychology
Baylor Institute of Rehabilitation
Dallas, Texas

Mark W. Bondi, PhD
Professor
Department of Psychiatry
University of California, San Diego
Psychology Service
VA San Diego Healthcare System
San Diego, California

Shane S. Bush, PhD, ABPP (CN, RP, CL)
Neuropsychologist
Long Island Neuropsychology, PC
Lake Ronkonkoma, New York
Department of Psychology
VA New York Harbor Healthcare System
St. Albans, New York

Stefano F. Cappa, MD
Professor
IUSS Pavia and San Raffaele Scientific
  Institute
Milan, Italy

Dominic A. Carone, PhD, ABPP (CN)
Clinical Associate Professor
Physical Medicine and Rehabilitation
SUNY Upstate Medical University
Syracuse, New York

Martin D. Cassell, PhD
Professor
Department of Anatomy and Cell Biology
Carver College of Medicine
University of Iowa
Iowa City, Iowa

Chiara Cerami, MD
Research Fellow
Division of Neuroscience
San Raffaele Scientific Institute and
  Vita-Salute
San Raffaele University
Department of Clinical Neuroscience
San Raffaele Hospital
Milan, Italy

Jennifer Duncan Davis, PhD
Associate Professor
Department of Psychiatry and Human
   Behavior
Warren Alpert Medical School of Brown
   University and Rhode Island Hospital
Providence, Rhode Island

Kevin Duff, PhD, ABPP (CN)
Center for Alzheimer's Care, Imaging,
   and Research
Department of Neurology
University of Utah
Salt Lake City, Utah

Melissa L. Edwards, MA
Doctoral Student
Department of Psychology
University of North Texas
Denton, Texas

Rhonda Friedman, PhD
Professor
Director, Center for Aphasia Research
   and Rehabilitation (CARR)
Director, Cognitive Neuropsychology
   Laboratory at GUMC
Georgetown University School
   of Medicine
Washington, DC

Tania Giovannetti, PhD
Associate Professor
Department of Psychology
Temple University
Philadelphia, Pennsylvania

Dong (Dan) Y. Han, PsyD
Assistant Professor
Departments of Neurology, Neurosurgery,
   and Physical Medicine & Rehabilitation
University of Kentucky Medical Center
Lexington, Kentucky

Robert H. Howland, MD
Associate Professor of Psychiatry
University of Pittsburgh School
   of Medicine
Western Psychiatric Institute and Clinic
Pittsburgh, Pennsylvania

Daniel Krauss, JD, PhD, ABPP (FP)
Professor and Chair
Department of Psychology
Claremont McKenna College
Claremont, California

Melissa Lamar, PhD
Associate Professor of Psychology
   and Psychiatry
Director of Cognitive Aging
   and Vascular Health
Department of Psychiatry
University of Illinois College of Medicine
Chicago, Illinois

David J. Libon, PhD
Professor
Department of Neurology
Drexel University
Philadelphia, Pennsylvania

Sally Long, PhD
Assistant Professor
Department of Neurology
Georgetown University
   School of Medicine
Washington, DC

Oscar L. López, MD
Professor of Neurology
Department of Neurology
University of Pittsburgh School
   of Medicine
Pittsburgh, Pennsylvania

Daniel A. Nation, PhD
Assistant Professor
Department of Psychology
Dana and David Dorsife College
   of Arts and Letters
University of Southern California
Los Angeles, California

Chad A. Noggle, PhD, ABN
Associate Professor
Department of Psychiatry
Chief, Behavioral and Psychosocial
   Oncology
Southern Illinois University School
   of Medicine
Springfield, Illinois

Sid E. O'Bryant, PhD
Associate Professor
Department of Internal Medicine
University of North Texas Health Science
   Center
Fort Worth, Texas

Catherine C. Price, PhD
Assistant Professor
Department of Clinical and Health
 Psychology
Department of Anesthesiology
University of Florida
Gainesville, Florida

Benjamin A. Pyykkonen, PhD
Assistant Professor
Department of Psychology
Wheaton College
Wheaton, Illinois

Daniel Rexroth, PsyD
Director, Neuropsychology Clinic in
 Psychiatry
Associate Clinical Professor
Indiana University School of Medicine
Departments of Psychiatry and Neurology
Indianapolis, Indiana

Mario Riverol, MD
Professor
Department of Neurology
University of Pittsburgh School
 of Medicine
Pittsburgh, Pennsylvania
Department of Neurology
Clínica Universidad de Navarra
Pamplona, Spain

Melanie Rylander, MD
Assistant Professor of Psychiatry
University of Colorado School of Medicine
Denver, Colorado

David P. Salmon, PhD
Professor in Residence
Department of Neurosciences
University of California San Diego
La Jolla, California

Frederick A. Schmitt, PhD
Professor
Department of Neurology
University of Kentucky Medical Center
Lexington, Kentucky

Lokesh Shahani, MD
Fellow
Baylor College of Medicine
Houston, Texas

Anne L. Shandera-Ochsner, PhD
Neuropsychology Fellow
Mayo Clinic
Jacksonville, Florida

Julie Sheffler, BA
Student
Department of Psychiatry
Southern Illinois University School of
 Medicine
Springfield, Illinois

Rod Swenson, PhD, ABN
Clinical Professor
Department of Clinical Neuroscience
University of North Dakota Medical School
Associate Member, Graduate Faculty
Department of Psychology
North Dakota State University
Fargo, North Dakota
Clinical Professor
Graduate School of Psychology
Touro College
New York, New York

Jon C. Thompson, PsyD, ABPP (CN)
Director, Neuropsychology Division
St. Vincent's Hospital
Indiana Neuroscience Institute
Indianapolis, Indiana

Geoffrey Tremont, PhD
Associate Professor
Department of Psychiatry
 and Human Behavior
Warren Alpert Medical School of Brown
 University and Rhode Island Hospital
Providence, Rhode Island

R. Scott Turner, MD, PhD
Professor
Department of Neurology
Director, Memory Disorders Program
Georgetown University School of Medicine
Georgetown University Hospital
Pasquerilla Healthcare Center
Washington, DC

Stacey Wood, PhD
Associate Professor
Department of Psychology
Scripps College
Claremont, California

Preface

Today the fastest-growing segment of our population is persons aged 65 and older. With advances in medical technologies and interventions, the average human life span has increased dramatically over the past several decades. We have seen a subsequent increase in the number of individuals developing dementia in some form as the risk for almost every primary dementing process increases with increasing age. *Dementia*, itself, does not describe a specific disease entity; rather, the term refers to a clinical syndrome that negatively affects an individual's ability to participate in normal activities and relationships due to impaired cognitive functioning. The underlying cause and/or point of anatomical origin oftentimes dictates the specific clinical constellation observed.

Given the growing number of individuals developing dementia, scientific and clinical advances are constantly in demand. Neuropsychology has taken its place at the forefront of this movement. Professional neuropsychologists as well as those in training must remain up to date with the changing landscape that is the practice and science of assessing, diagnosing, and treating dementia.

The goal of *The Neuropsychology of Cortical Dementias* is to discuss the most recent advances in our understanding of this group of disorders and disease processes. Intended to advance clinical skills of professionals and trainees alike, this text covers the most advanced practices and techniques in early differential diagnosis, assessment, and treatment. The book focuses on cortical dementias as opposed to also discussing subcortical dementias. This permits a more in-depth discussion of individual types of cortical dementia, allowing for coverage of the most contemporary findings on the subject matter. This text discusses the foundations of neuropsychology in the assessment, diagnosis, and treatment of cortical dementias. Individual dementing processes are discussed in detail, from traditional presentations such as Alzheimer's disease and Lewy body dementia to less commonly discussed entities such as primary progressive aphasia and chronic traumatic encephalopathy. Advances in neuroimaging and the utilization of biomarkers in early detection are discussed. Additional chapters are dedicated to related topics including the role of caregivers and determination of capacity. In all, the text offers a contemporary and comprehensive coverage of the subject matter that will be immediately applicable to scientists and clinicians alike, regardless of their level of training.

Acknowledgments

We want to acknowledge the work put forth by the assistant editors of this book, including Dr. Amy R. Steiner, who served as the lead assistant editor; Dr. Michelle Pagoria; Dr. John Joshua Hall; and Dr. Javan Horwitz.

A book such as this is only made possible through the contributions of various authors. We acknowledge their willingness to volunteer their time and knowledge to this work. As always, we want to acknowledge the support of our colleagues and associated institutions, without whom this project would not have been possible. Finally, we would like to express our sincerest gratitude to our publisher and those with whom we have worked very closely to complete this book, especially Nancy S. Hale and Shelby Peak.

SERIES EDITORS
Chad A. Noggle, PhD, ABN
Raymond S. Dean, PhD, ABPP, ABN, ABPdN

The Neuropsychology of Psychopathology

The Neuropsychology of Cancer and Oncology

Neuropsychological Rehabilitation

The Neuropsychology of Cortical Dementias

The Neuropsychology of Pervasive Developmental Disorders

The Neuropsychology of Psychopharmacology

Foundations and Principles

The Neuroscience of Cortical Dementias: Linking Neuroanatomy, Neurophysiology, and Neuropsychology

Daniel A. Nation, David P. Salmon, and Mark W. Bondi

Dementia is a clinical syndrome characterized by the impairment of multiple cognitive domains that is severe enough to interfere with one's usual social and occupational functioning. The impairment must represent a decline from a previously higher level of functioning and not occur exclusively during the course of delirium. According to widely applied diagnostic schemes (e.g., *Diagnostic and Statistical Manual of Mental Disorders, Fourth Edition—Text Revision [DSM-IV-TR]*; American Psychiatric Association, 2000), the cognitive impairment must include decline in memory and one or more of the following: aphasia, apraxia, agnosia, or executive dysfunction. Although these criteria are widely used in clinical and research settings, they have been criticized for being weighted toward the clinical features of dementia due to Alzheimer's disease (AD), particularly because they require decline in memory and lack emphasis on neurobehavioral symptoms. This weighting can make it difficult to diagnose dementia in non-AD neurodegenerative disorders that cause profound losses of functional capacity due primarily to personality changes and behavioral deficits without decline in memory and, in some cases, only minimal decline in other cognitive domains. These limitations have led to the recent development of broader conceptualizations of dementia that account for the heterogeneous nature of clinical presentations (Ganguli & Rodriguez, 2011).

The clinical heterogeneity of dementia is a reflection of the variety of neurodegenerative diseases and neuropathological substrates that can give rise to the syndrome. Neuropsychological research that has taken a comparative approach to the study of various dementing disorders has shown that etiologically and neuropathologically distinct neurodegenerative diseases engender different patterns of relatively preserved and impaired cognitive abilities. This has been most clearly shown through the comparison of dementia syndromes associated with neurodegenerative diseases that primarily involve regions of the cerebral cortex (e.g., AD, frontotemporal dementia [FTD]) and those that have their primary locus in subcortical brain structures (e.g., Huntington's disease [HD], Parkinson's disease [PD], progressive supranuclear palsy [PSP]). Although it is well known that pathological changes in these various disorders are not limited to either cortical or subcortical brain regions, the cortical-subcortical dementia distinction serves as a heuristically useful model for describing the pattern of neuropsychological deficits that are observed in these patient groups.

Our chapter describes the neuropsychological, neuroanatomical, and neurophysiological features of several of the more common "cortical dementias." These conditions primarily impact the association cortices and related limbic system structures (e.g., hippocampus, amygdala, cingulate cortex). We will first review AD, the most common form of dementia, and then compare and contrast the features of AD with those of other disorders that involve significant cortical pathology including dementia with Lewy bodies (DLB), FTD, and cortical vascular dementia (VaD). All of these disorders involve the selective targeting of "large-scale" cortical neuroanatomical networks, but they present with distinct neuropsychological profiles that are consistent with the anatomical locus of cortical neuropathology (Seeley, Crawford, Zhou, Miller, & Greicius, 2009; Weintraub & Mesulam, 1993, 2009; Weintraub & Mesulam, 1996). For quick reference, a table is provided near the end of this chapter containing shorthand descriptions of the typical disease onset, course, neuropsychology, neuroimaging, and neuropathology associated with each cortical dementia syndrome (see Table 1.1).

ALZHEIMER'S DISEASE

AD is an age-related neurodegenerative disease characterized by the abnormal extracellular accumulation of amyloid in diffuse and senile plaques, the abnormal formation of tau-protein positive neurofibrillary tangles in neurons, cortical atrophy with associated neuron and synapse loss, and alterations in neurogenesis (Crews & Masliah, 2010; Masliah & Salmon, 1999). These neuropathological changes usually occur first in medial temporal lobe (MTL) structures such as the entorhinal cortex and hippocampus, and then advance to anterior and lateral cortical areas such as the basal forebrain and frontal and temporal lobe association cortices. Eventually, the pathology occurs in association cortices in the parietal and occipital lobes (Braak & Braak, 1991). The primary sensory and motor cortex usually remains free of AD pathology, with the exception of the olfactory cortex (Pearson, Esiri, Hiorns, Wilcock, & Powell, 1985). Subcortical structures (e.g., thalamus, basal ganglia) and cerebellum are also relatively spared, making AD a classic form of diffuse cortical dementia.

The development of cognitive deterioration associated with AD mirrors this temporal sequence of neuropathological changes. In the earliest stages of AD, patients often exhibit short-term memory loss and subtle executive dysfunction and semantic memory deficits (i.e., anomia and agnosia; Mickes et al., 2007) consistent with early MTL damage and marginal involvement of frontal and temporal cortices. As the disease progresses through frontal and temporal areas, memory deficits become severe and executive and language impairment becomes more prominent. Parietal areas may begin to be affected, leading to mild constructional deficits (i.e., apraxia) fairly early in the disease (Bondi et al., 2008). Patients may exhibit additional deficits in basic attention, abstract reasoning, and visuospatial abilities even during the relatively early stages of the disease (Salmon & Bondi, 2009). By the time moderate to severe stages of the disease are reached, all cortical association areas are substantially affected. These cognitive deficits may become profound.

Research focusing on the nature of the cognitive deficits found in patients with AD has improved our understanding of brain–behavior relationships by relating cognitive functions to the specific forms of neuropathology found in AD. This research has also provided a means of diagnosing the disease in the absence of any sufficiently sensitive and specific biomarkers. By examining the pattern and course of cognitive impairment that are characteristic of AD, neuropsychologists have provided a method for differentiating AD from other causes of dementia. Early diagnosis may have important clinical implications as disease-modifying therapies become available, and can be important for providing a prognosis, selecting symptom-based treatments, and planning for future care. This is particularly important given that AD is the most common cause of dementia, particularly in those older than 65 years, with an age of onset typically in the seventh and eighth decades of life. The incidence of AD increases with age and approximately 25% of individuals will have the disease by 85 years of age (Brookmeyer, Johnson, Ziegler-Graham, & Arrighi, 2007).

The following sections review cognitive and neurophysiological research centered on understanding the brain–behavior mechanics involved in the cognitive deterioration associated with AD.

Episodic Memory

The most prominent and early clinical feature of AD is short-term episodic memory loss, characterized by a deficit in the ability to learn, store, and retrieve information that is newly acquired through personal experience. The learning and memory deficit present in AD patients involves both verbal and nonverbal (i.e., visual) memory and is characterized by "rapid forgetting" of recently acquired information (Salmon & Bondi, 2009). This deficit occurs in the context of normal attentional processes. AD patients show a failure to retain newly acquired information after a delay even when retrieval demands are reduced by use of a recognition format (Welsh, Butters, Hughes, Mohs, & Heyman, 1991).

The pattern of memory loss in AD stands in contrast to that of patients with subcortical neurodegeneration such as in HD. HD is an autosomal dominant genetic disorder characterized by degeneration of the neostriatum (caudate and putamen) with relative sparing of cortical tissues. HD patients develop a movement disorder (chorea), behavioral changes (e.g., depression, apathy), and progressive dementia (Vonsattel & DiFiglia, 1998). In contrast to AD, patients with HD exhibit learning and memory deficits on tests of free recall but show improved performance on recognition testing (Delis et al., 1991). This suggests that the memory deficit in HD patients may reflect retrieval dysfunction (Butters, Wolfe, Granholm, & Martone, 1986). This suggestion is consistent with research implicating frontostriatal circuits that are damaged in HD in working memory and the organization and retrieval of information from long-term storage. In contrast, the memory deficit observed in AD patients appears to reflect a failure to consolidate new information so that the information is never transferred from immediate working memory to a more permanent long-term storage (Tröster et al., 1993). Thus, the rapid forgetting of new information, together with the inability to retrieve that information despite the provision of a more structured recognition format, is characteristic of the episodic memory loss observed in AD.

Another important aspect of memory loss in patients with AD is retrograde amnesia (i.e., the inability to remember events that occurred prior to the onset of disease). The retrograde amnesia of AD is characterized by a temporal gradient in which recently acquired memories show greater impairment than more remotely acquired memories. For example, Hodges, Salmon, and Butters (1993) showed that AD patients have a temporal gradient in terms of their ability to recognize famous people sampled from each decade of the patients' lives, with famous people from earlier in their lives being better preserved than those from their more recent history.

This prominent episodic memory loss in AD is consistent with the early deterioration of MTL structures known to underlie the ability to form new memories (Squire, 1987). Specifically, patients in the early stages of AD show substantial neuropathological changes in the hippocampus, parahippocampal cortex, perirhinal cortex, entorhinal cortex, and related cortical association areas that are responsible for the formation and consolidation of new memories (Squire, 1998). Degeneration begins in the entorhinal cortex, disconnecting the perforant pathway from the entorhinal cortex to the dentate gyrus of the hippocampus, and then includes intrahippocampal pathways connecting the dentate granular cells and CA3, CA1, and the subiculum (Hyman, Van Hoesen, & Damasio, 1987). These circuits integrating MTL structures are critical for the formation of new memories. In vivo evidence of MTL deafferentation can be visualized by structural neuroimaging studies, which have found that AD patients show hippocampal atrophy early in the course of disease and that these hippocampal changes are associated with memory disturbance (Deweer et al., 1995). Functional neuroimaging studies in AD patients and those at risk of AD have also demonstrated alterations in hippocampal cerebral blood flow and blood oxygen level dependent (BOLD) signal, both at rest and during new memory formation (Dai et al., 2009; Fleisher et al., 2005). Individuals with circumscribed lesions within these MTL structures display memory deficits that are similar to those found in AD, further implicating these structures in the episodic memory loss seen in AD patients (Albert, Butters, & Levin, 1979; Squire, 1998).

Reciprocal connections between the MTL structures and neocortical association areas throughout the brain are thought to underlie the process of new memory formation and consolidation (Dickerson & Eichenbaum, 2010). Specifically, neocortical areas send projections to the parahippocampal area, which sends projections back to these neocortical areas, and to other hippocampal sectors. These hippocampal projections follow a serial, unidirectional pathway from the dentate gyrus to CA3 and then on to CA1 and the subiculum, both of which then project back to the parahippocampal cortex (Eichenbaum, 2000). Plastic change of synaptic connections within the neocortical association areas is thought to be ultimately responsible for the storage of new information in long-term memory. The MTL structures are different from other cortical areas in that they have a selectively dedicated function to facilitate this memory consolidation process. Converging evidence from human and animal research suggests that after experience with a stimulus, specialized neurons within MTL structures play a role in matching a memory cue to a stored template of the stimulus in cortical association areas (Eichenbaum, 2004). Although the exact details of how the MTL forms new memories and retrieves them through coordination with cortical areas remain unclear, these highly specialized structures are critical to memory function.

Alzheimer's pathology tends to most severely impact large glutaminergic pyramidal neurons in the entorhinal cortex and the CA1 and CA2 regions of the hippocampus (Masliah & Salmon, 1999). Damage to these large projecting neurons may profoundly impact signaling between MTL structures and disrupt the ability of these structures to coordinate signals with neocortical areas. Interruption of communication between MTL and neocortical areas necessary for the long-term synaptic change that underlies memory formation is likely to play a large role in the profound episodic memory loss observed in AD patients.

Semantic Memory

Semantic memory is distinct from episodic memory in that it is knowledge that is culturally shared, usually overlearned, and not temporally specific, whereas episodic memory is based on personal experiences that are time and place specific. Retrieval of semantic memories is less dependent on MTL function, as patients with circumscribed MTL lesions with profound episodic memory loss exhibit relatively intact semantic memory (Squire, 1998). In AD, there is substantial evidence for deficits in semantic memory that are distinct from their episodic memory deficits. For example, AD patients exhibit early deficits in semantic fluency (i.e., rapidly naming exemplars from a given category; Monsch et al., 1992) and confrontation naming (Mickes et al., 2007). In AD patients, spontaneous speech is often vague, empty of content words, and filled with indefinite phrases and circumlocutions (Nicholas, Obler, Albert, & Helm-Estabrooks, 1985). This breakdown in semantic memory is progressive, with the loss being more prominent in the later stages of the disease when a frank agnosia is present (Nebes, 1989). In fact, studies have shown that on tests of general semantic knowledge (e.g., the Number Information Test), which ask questions such as "How many days are in a year?" AD patient performance declines over the course of the disease (Norton, Bondi, Salmon, & Goodglass, 1997). Furthermore, patients are highly consistent in the items that they miss from year to year, suggesting a true loss of knowledge rather than a retrieval deficit. Loss of knowledge is also indicated by other studies that have found that when AD patients appear to have lost a concept (e.g., "horse") on one particular test, this deficit is present across many tests and modes of access including spontaneous verbal production, confrontation naming, and the ability to properly sort the concept into the correct semantic category (e.g., "domestic animal"; Hodges, Salmon, & Butters, 1992).

Semantic memory is thought to be a cortical function that is not dependent on subcortical or limbic structures. In support of this notion, patients with subcortical forms of dementia, such as HD, do not exhibit deficits in semantic memory. Patients with HD may have generalized slowing that can reduce their verbal output on fluency tests, but they do not have disproportionate impairment (relative to normal controls) on fluency tasks that depend on semantic knowledge (i.e., produce as many animal names as possible in 1 minute) relative to those that do not (i.e., producing as many words that begin with the letter "F" as possible in 1 minute). In contrast, AD patients are significantly more impaired (relative to normal controls) on semantic fluency than phonemic fluency tasks (Henry, Crawford, & Phillips, 2004). These deficits may reflect the loss of semantic knowledge (i.e., general knowledge of facts, concepts, and the meanings or words) for particular items or concepts (Hodges & Patterson, 1995).

The semantic memory loss associated with AD is thought to be related to the degeneration of neocortical association areas of the temporal, frontal, and parietal lobes (Masliah, Miller, & Terry, 1993). Functional MRI (fMRI) and EEG studies have advanced our understanding of how semantic processing occurs in both normal and AD patients. Evidence from studying brain-damaged patients indicates that the organization, storage, and retrieval of semantic information involves a distributed network of neocortical and limbic areas, with particular reliance on posterior inferior parietal and inferotemporal regions (Damasio, Tranel, Grabowski, Adolphs, & Damasio, 2004). A recent meta-analysis of fMRI studies in normal individuals concluded that semantic processing involves a variety of left-lateralizing cortical regions across all four brain lobes, but particularly the middle temporal gyrus, posterior inferior parietal lobe, dorsomedial prefrontal cortex, inferior frontal gyrus, ventromedial frontal cortex, fusiform gyrus, cingulate gyrus, and the parahippocampal gyrus (Binder, Desai, Graves, & Conant, 2009). These studies attempt to parcel out the purely semantic aspects of language from simple lexical, syntactic, and phonological processes by contrasting the processing of meaningful words from nonwords. However, these methods are difficult to interpret given evidence from EEG and magnetoencephalography (MEG) experiments, indicating that the different components of language, including phonological, lexical, syntactic, and semantic processes, are performed in both serial and parallel circuits within temporal, parietal, and frontal regions (Pulvermüller, Shtyrov, & Hauk, 2009). There is also ongoing debate as to whether semantic information is stored in a modular fashion, with specific brain areas being dedicated to specific conceptual categories (e.g., living things vs. nonliving things), or in a distributed fashion based on attributes (e.g., furry vs. smooth; Done & Hajilou, 2005). Nevertheless, converging evidence implicates a variety of cortical areas, with special emphasis on parietal and temporal regions, both modular and distributed storage of attributes and categories, and both serial and parallel processing of semantic information in normal adults.

Fewer imaging studies have contrasted normal and AD participants on semantic processing tasks. In a recent study, Wierenga et al. used an fMRI-based semantic processing paradigm that allowed for examination of both modular (living vs. nonliving) and attribute (global vs. local) based semantic processing in normal older adults and AD patients (Wierenga et al., 2011). AD patients exhibited altered brain responses throughout a wide variety of frontal, temporal, and parietal brain regions irrespective of whether processing was modular or attribute based. These alterations suggest that semantic memory deficits in AD may be the result of generally abnormal and disorganized semantic processing throughout the distributed network of brain regions involved in storage of semantic information. Additional findings indicated that, during the task, AD patients recruited frontal regions within the right hemisphere that were not active in normal older adults. This observation suggests that AD patients may recruit additional brain regions not typically involved in semantic processing in order to compensate for their deficits, or that a failure to inhibit these unrelated brain regions may contribute to their processing deficits. Thus, the loss of semantic knowledge is thought to be related to the degradation of semantic network function represented within the higher cortical association areas that tend to be affected by AD.

Semantic memory involves integration of modular- and attribute-based representations across a variety of cortical areas through a cascade of serial and parallel circuits. This suggests that a high level of coordinated cortical activity may be required to effectively maintain and access semantic knowledge. Alzheimer's pathology causes neuronal damage within neocortical layers that is partially selective for large glutamatergic pyramidal neurons (Masliah & Salmon, 1999). Clustering of neurofibrillary tangles in neurons within neocortical layers II and III is thought to result in disconnection of cortico-cortical fibers, which may lead to disruption of circuits responsible for communication both between and within cortical areas important for semantic processing (Esiri & Chance, 2006). Tangle clustering also occurs extensively within layer V neurons, potentially disrupting cortico-subcortical fibers that may indirectly sustain coordination of cortical activity through thalamic relay nuclei (Pearson et al., 1985). Together these findings support the cortico-cortical disconnectivity hypothesis of AD, which posits that neurofibrillary tangle and neuritic plaque formation causes neuronal dysfunction within cortical layers responsible for cellular communication across cortical regions (De Lacoste & White, 1993). The disconnection of cortical regions would impair functions that rely on distributed networks, integration of storage modalities, and the ability to bind information obtained through parallel processing circuits, all of which appear to be involved in semantic memory. This is analogous but distinct from the disconnectivity that occurs early in the disease process between MTL structures and the neocortex, which results in loss of episodic memory.

Executive Functions and Attention

Deficits in executive and attentional abilities known to be related to frontal lobe function are observed in patients with AD (Collette, Schmidt, Scherrer, Adam, & Salmon, 2009). Executive deficits include difficulties with mental manipulation of information, concept formation, problem solving, and cue-directed behavior (Perry & Hodges, 1999; Perry, Watson, & Hodges, 2000). Specifically, AD patients are impaired on tasks requiring set-shifting, self-monitoring, and sequencing but not cue-directed attention or verbal problem solving. They show deficits on more difficult problem-solving tests, tests of relational integration, nonverbal abstract reasoning, and timed tests involving executive functions (Grady et al., 1988; Lange, Sahakian, Quinn, Marsden, & Robbins, 1995; Waltz et al., 2004). Deficits on specific tests of executive function such as those involving inhibition and switching have also been predictive of more global cognitive declines (Clark et al., 2012) or progression to dementia from mild cognitive impairment states in nondemented older adults (Brandt et al., 2009), although in general they may not be as sensitive to progression as episodic or semantic memory tasks (Aretouli, Okonkwo, Samek, & Brandt, 2011; Mickes et al., 2007).

Deficits in complex executive functioning tasks may be due to neuronal damage within frontal lobe structures, as AD pathology spreads to these areas relatively early in the disease (Masliah et al., 1993). Another possible explanation for executive dysfunction is damage to forebrain areas supporting the acetylcholine diffuse activating system (Perry, Irving, & Perry, 1991). Forebrain regions, including the nucleus basalis of Meynert and the diagonal band of Broca, contain cholinergic neurons that project to a variety of cortical areas, including frontal regions known to be important in supporting higher executive abilities (e.g., prefrontal cortex; Schliebs & Arendt, 2006). The acetylcholine supplied by these diffuse activating systems is partly responsible for tonic activation of these regions during wakefulness. Thus, damage to forebrain regions should result in decreased activation of frontal regions and reduced ability to perform executive tasks. Acetylcholinesterase inhibitors (e.g., donepezil) are frequently prescribed during the early stages of AD to increase acetylcholine bioavailability through inhibition of the acetylcholine degrading enzyme (Cummings, 2000). If the acetylcholine depletion that results from basal forebrain damage is responsible for the executive function deficits observed early in the course of AD, then increased acetylcholine bioavailability should improve executive functions. In support of this hypothesis, a recent study found that the degree of acetylcholinesterase inhibition provided by donepezil treatment correlated with performance on attentional and executive tasks but not memory tasks in patients with mild AD (Bohnen et al., 2005). However, neuropathological studies have also separately linked tangle load within the basal forebrain to memory dysfunction in AD (Samuel, Terry, DeTeresa, Butters, & Masliah, 1994). Additionally, cholinergic receptor activity within frontal and anterior cingulate regions was predictive of future decline in executive function in AD patients (Colloby et al., 2010).

Other studies have found that decreased gray matter volume within the prefrontal and posterior inferior parietal cortex correlates with poor performance on executive function tasks in AD (Pa et al., 2010). These atrophic changes are likely related to the underlying AD pathology, as neuropathological studies found that the loss of large pyramidal neurons within midfrontal regions correlates with performance on tests of global cognition (Masliah & Salmon, 1999). This association suggests that both neurodegenerative and neurochemical abnormalities within the prefrontal cortex may contribute to the executive dysfunction found in AD patients.

Visuospatial Abilities

Beyond the deficits in episodic memory, semantic memory, and executive function discussed previously, AD patients ultimately develop visuospatial processing deficits that are thought to be related to the encroachment of AD pathology on parietal, occipital, and ventral posterior temporal association areas. These deficits are not always present during the earliest stages of the disease but are present by the moderate stage of disease. This later appearance is consistent with neurofibrillary tangle and neuritic plaque progression that spares occipital and parietal regions in the early stages of disease, but ultimately engages all cortical association areas (Braak & Braak, 1991).

Visuospatial deficits in patients with AD are frequently apparent on visuoconstructional tasks such as the block design test (Padovani et al., 1995) and figure copy tests (Locascio, Growdon, & Corkin, 1995). Several studies have compared the visuospatial deficits found in AD to those found in subcortical dementia (e.g., HD). Patients with AD may be particularly impaired on tests that require processing of information presented in an extrapersonal orientation (Brouwers, Cox, Martin, Chase, & Fedio, 1984). This was shown on a task that examined the ability of AD and HD patients to perform mental rotation of visual stimuli (Lineweaver, Salmon, Bondi, & Corey-Bloom, 2005). Patients with AD were impaired at performing the mental rotation but did not show a reduction in speed when they were successful. In contrast, HD patients could perform mental rotation accurately, but showed a deficit in speed of processing consistent with bradyphrenia. The deficit in mental rotation exhibited by patients with AD suggests that they have dysfunction of cortical regions involved in processing visual motion. One such area, the middle temporal gyrus, typically has a heavy burden of AD pathology. On the other hand, it could be that deficits in extrapersonal orientation are due to disconnection between multiple cortical areas consistent with cortico-cortical disconnectivity.

Further evidence for cortico-cortical disconnectivity as the source of visuospatial impairment in AD comes from another study comparing AD and HD patients on a visual sensory integration task (Festa et al., 2005). In this task, subjects were required to detect the direction of coherently moving dots that could be distinguished from randomly moving distracter dots by color (red vs. green) or by luminance (light gray vs. dark gray). Both normal control subjects and HD patients were able to utilize color or luminance information to enhance their ability to detect the direction of motion of coherently moving dots. AD patients were able to utilize luminance information, but not color information to detect the direction of motion. This impairment suggests a deficit in the ability to bind motion and color information, which are processed in distinct cortical visual systems: the dorsal (magnocellular) visual processing stream for motion and the ventral (parvocellular) visual processing stream for color (Macko et al., 1982). In contrast, motion and luminance are both processed within the same dorsal visual processing stream. These findings suggest that the inability to bind information processed in distinct cortical pathways may underlie the visuospatial deficits observed in AD. This is consistent with the cortico-cortical disconnectivity hypothesis and points to a general inability to bind information gathered from multiple cortical processing streams in AD.

More pronounced visuospatial deficits may be observed early in the posterior variant of AD, termed *posterior cortical atrophy* (PCA). PCA is a rare clinical dementia syndrome characterized by preserved memory, language, and insight with prominent visual agnosia (sometimes with prosopagnosia) and constructional apraxia. Patients may also exhibit many or all of the features of Balint's syndrome, including optic ataxia, gaze apraxia, and simultanagnosia (i.e., can detect visual details of an object but cannot organize them into a meaningful whole). They may also exhibit many or all of the components of Gerstmann's syndrome, including acalculia, right-left disorientation, finger agnosia, and agraphia (Caine, 2004). The condition is associated with atrophy and decreased blood flow to the occipital and posterior parietal cortex. PET studies have demonstrated metabolic derangement in posterior cortical areas, which may particularly impact the dorsal visual stream or "where" pathway (Nestor, Caine, Fryer, Clarke, & Hodges, 2003). The underlying neuropathology associated with this syndrome is frequently AD (i.e., neuritic plaques and neurofibrillary tangles), but may also occur with other neurodegenerative diseases. In cases where AD neuropathology is present, it exhibits the same laminar distribution within the cortex, suggesting the same mechanism of cortical damage as seen in the typical AD case (Hof, Vogt, Bouras, & Morrison, 1997).

DEMENTIA WITH LEWY BODIES

DLB is the second most common neurodegenerative cause of dementia (McKeith et al., 2004). This clinicopathological condition is characterized by a dementia syndrome that occurs in the presence of cell loss and the deposition of Lewy bodies in the brain. Lewy bodies are abnormal intracytoplasmic eosinophilic neuronal inclusion bodies that are comprised of alpha-synuclein- and ubiquitin-containing fibrillary aggregates (McKeith et al., 2005). In DLB, Lewy body pathology (including Lewy neurites) is distributed in a subcortical pattern similar to that of PD (e.g., in brain stem nuclei including the substantia nigra, locus ceruleus, dorsal motor nucleus of the vagus, and substantia innominata) and is also found diffusely distributed throughout the limbic system (e.g., cingulate, insula, amygdala, hippocampus, entorhinal cortex, and transentorhinal cortex) and neocortex. In limbic and neocortical regions, Lewy bodies typically involve the small neurons of the cortical layer V (Spillantini et al., 1997). In most cases, there is also AD pathology (i.e., neuritic plaques, neurofibrillary tangles) that occurs in the same general distribution throughout the brain as in "pure" AD (Gómez-Tortosa, Irizarry, Gómez-Isla, & Hyman, 2000).

The clinical presentation of DLB can be distinguished from that of PD based on the type of extrapyramidal signs and the course of these motor signs relative to cognitive decline. DLB patients tend to show cognitive deterioration at or before the onset of motor symptoms and show a more rapid cognitive decline, whereas PD patients typically present with motor signs of the disease for some number of years prior to the onset of cognitive decline if it occurs at all. Additionally, DLB patients are more likely to show axial signs, such as rigidity, masked facies, gait abnormalities, or postural instability, rather than lateral signs, such as resting tremor (McKeith et al., 2004). DLB may be distinguished from AD on the basis of the pattern of cognitive decline. DLB is characterized by a pattern of early severe executive and visuospatial impairment that is disproportionate to mild, retrieval-based memory impairment. This sharply contrasts with the typical AD presentation, which is characterized by early severe episodic memory impairment with milder executive dysfunction and relatively preserved visuospatial abilities early in the disease (Simard, van Reekum, & Cohen, 2000). Other features that may help distinguish DLB from AD are its increased frequency of vivid well-formed visual hallucinations, rapid eye movement sleep behavior disorder, and fluctuations in cognition with pronounced variation in attention and alertness (McKeith et al., 2005).

Structural MRI studies often show diffuse cerebral cortical atrophy in DLB similar to that found in other forms of dementia (e.g., PD and AD; Watson, Blamire, & O'Brien, 2009), but a few studies suggest greater atrophy of frontal, parietal, and left occipital regions in DLB relative to AD or PD patients (Beyer, Larsen, & Aarsland, 2007; Whitwell et al., 2007). One challenge facing neuroimaging studies in DLB is selection of an adequate control group. Typically, DLB patients are compared with AD patients, PD patients with dementia, PD patients without dementia, normal controls, or all of these participant groups. This is because DLB patients may have both AD and Lewy body pathology; however, it is not possible to distinguish between DLB patients with and without comorbid AD pathology for these in vivo comparisons. This complicates interpretation of study findings.

It is a potentially important clinical problem to distinguish DLB from AD because they represent the two most common causes of neurodegenerative dementia, neither condition has a reliable biomarker, and they are known to have a different disease course and response to treatment that could alter quality of life and mortality. For instance, DLB patients are more likely than AD patients to show improved cognition in response to treatment with acetylcholinesterase inhibitors, but are also more likely to experience neuroleptic malignant syndrome, a potentially life-threatening condition, in response to antipsychotic medication (McKeith et al., 2005). Given the frequency with which treatment decisions are made concerning these medications in these highly prevalent forms of dementia, the differential diagnosis of DLB from AD is an important area of research. The present review focuses on cortically mediated cognitive deficits in visuospatial abilities, executive functions, and memory that may be most salient in differentiating DLB from AD.

Visuospatial Abilities

Although there are a number of clinical features that distinguish DLB from AD, the presence of visuospatial impairment has been found to be the best predictor of DLB pathology in autopsy-based studies (83% positive predictive value and 90% negative predictive value; Tiraboschi et al., 2006). The early and disproportionately severe visuospatial dysfunction found in patients with DLB may be detected on tests of basic visuoperceptual abilities (Calderon et al., 2001), visual search (Cormack, Aarsland, Ballard, & Tovée, 2004), and visuoconstruction (Aarsland et al., 2003). DLB patients with severe visuospatial deficits are more likely than those with mild deficits to develop visual hallucinations during the course of disease, and the severity of visuospatial impairment may predict the rate of subsequent global cognitive decline (Hamilton et al., 2008).

Consistent with disproportionately severe deficits in visuospatial processes, PET studies have shown hypometabolism, and single-photon emission computed tomography (SPECT) studies have shown hypoperfusion, within the primary visual cortex and visual association cortex in DLB but not in AD (Ishii et al., 1999; Minoshima et al., 2001). These studies found greater deficits in metabolism and blood flow to lateral occipitotemporal areas than medial and ventral areas. Other studies have found hypometabolism within posterior association areas that include parieto-occipital (Colloby et al., 2002; Ishii et al., 2007) and temporo-parietal cortex (Ishii et al., 2007). An fMRI study found reduced BOLD signal in DLB compared to AD within the lateral occipito-temporal cortex during a visual motion detection task, and within the ventral occip-itotemporal cortex during a face recognition task (Sauer, ffytche, Ballard, Brown, & Howard, 2006).

Pathological studies have found white matter spongiform change with coex-isting gliosis (Higuchi et al., 2000) and Lewy bodies (Gómez-Tortosa et al., 1999) within the occipital cortex of DLB patients. These neuropathological findings may help explain the visuospatial dysfunction observed in DLB. However, the pattern of neuropathology typically found in DLB brains is more frequently located within limbic structures, particularly the anterior cingulate cortex; entorhinal cortex; amygdala; and frontal, parietal, and temporal association areas (Kövari, Horvath, & Bouras, 2009). Lewy body pathology itself does not consistently correlate with cognitive dysfunction, suggesting that other pathophysiological events not neces-sarily related to Lewy bodies may be responsible for the cognitive deterioration associated with DLB. Some investigators maintain that synapse loss occurs even in the absence of Lewy bodies and shows more robust correlations with clinical symptoms (Duda, 2004). This may account for the apparent lack of occipital Lewy bodies in a substantial portion of DLB patients with visuospatial impairment. An additional complication of correlating neuropathological measures with cogni-tive symptoms is that Lewy bodies may be present at lower levels in the most advanced stages of the disease due to widespread neuronal loss. Thus, there may be a curvilinear relationship between the degree of Lewy body pathology and the severity of the disease with low levels in the beginning stages, highest levels during the middle stage when Lewy bodies are present but neuronal loss is not widespread, and low levels again during the most advanced stage with extensive neuronal loss.

The prominent visuospatial deficit and visual hallucinations associated with DLB could be related to neurotransmitter dysfunction (Lippa, Smith, & Perry, 1999). Among the brain regions particularly affected by Lewy body pathology are fore-brain areas that make up the cholinergic diffuse activating system, specifically the nucleus basalis of Meynert and the interstitial nucleus of the diagonal band (Lippa et al., 1999). Although these changes are analogous to those seen in AD, there is much more extensive pathological involvement and neuronal loss of the nucleus basalis in DLB than in AD. Choline acetyltransferase, the enzyme responsible for the synthesis of the neurotransmitter acetylcholine, is manufactured within the cell bodies of the nucleus basalis and transported to axonal terminals diffusely spread throughout the neocortex. Levels of this enzyme represent a stable marker of acetylcholine activ-ity at the synapse and have been found to be depleted even during the early stages of DLB and to a much greater degree than in AD (Lippa et al., 1999). Although AD patients exhibit a compensatory upregulation of cholinergic activity within limbic and neocortical regions after damage to the basal forebrain, DLB patients show a lack of compensatory response.

Similar to clinical symptomatology, neurotransmitter changes in DLB do not necessarily correlate with neuropathological measures of Lewy body disease (Perry et al., 1995). In contrast, measures of neurotransmitter dysfunction do correlate with cognitive and other clinical symptoms in DLB. For instance, DLB patients with visual hallucinations show greater cholinergic deficits than those without hallucinations within the temporal cortex with a known role in visual recognition (e.g., Brodman area 36; Ballard et al., 2000). Cholinergic deficits are found throughout the entire neocortex in DLB to a greater extent than in AD. DLB and AD patients both show deficits in expression of the M1 muscarinic receptor in the hippocampus, but DLB patients exhibit a relative preservation of neocortical M1 receptor expression while AD patients do not. This may account for the greater clinical response to cholinest-erase inhibitor therapy observed in DLB patients (McKeith et al., 2000). Additional cholinergic deficits observed in DLB include decreased expression of high-affinity nicotinic receptors within the substantia nigra and temporal cortex (Duda, 2004). Low-affinity nicotinic receptors are also underexpressed in DLB. Underexpression of low-affinity nicotinic receptors within temporal areas important for visual pro-cessing (i.e., Brodman areas 20 and 36) and high-affinity receptors within occipi-tal areas has been associated with visual hallucinations in DLB (Court et al., 2001; O'Brien et al., 2008).

Executive Functions

In addition to prominent visuospatial deficits, DLB patients exhibit disproportionate executive dysfunction relative to AD patients. These deficits are evident on tests of attention (Hansen et al., 1990), initiation and perseveration (Aarsland et al., 2003), verbal fluency (Galasko, Katzman, Salmon, & Hansen, 1996), and abstract reasoning (Shimomura et al., 1998). Other attentional and executive abilities disproportionately impaired in DLB relative to AD include visual attention (Sahgal et al., 1992) and spa-tial working memory (Sahgal, McKeith, Galloway, Tasker, & Steckler, 1995). These findings are consistent with the presence of Lewy bodies within the frontal lobes of DLB patients and with evidence of cholinergic dysfunction, hypometabolism, and hypoperfusion of the frontal cortex that is more prominent in DLB than in AD (Fong, Inouye, Dai, Press, & Alsop, 2011). Cholinergic nicotinic receptor activity is associ-ated with the progression of executive dysfunction in both AD and DLB (Colloby et al., 2010).

Memory

One robust finding distinguishing DLB from AD is the relative preservation of MTL structures such as the hippocampus, entorhinal cortex, and parahippocampal gyrus in DLB compared to AD (Sabattoli et al., 2008; Watson et al., 2009). This distinction is consistent with milder memory impairment in DLB than in AD, despite similar levels of global cognitive dysfunction (Hamilton et al., 2004). The mild memory impairment of DLB patients is often characterized by difficulty learning new infor-mation, a relatively preserved ability to retain what is learned, and enhanced per-formance with cuing or recognition testing compared to free recall (Salmon et al., 1996). This contrasts with the memory impairment of AD, which is characterized by impaired learning, poor retention over time, and little or no enhancement of performance with recognition testing (Calderon et al., 2001). The relatively good retention and improvement in performance when retrieval demands are reduced with recognition testing suggests that a deficit in retrieval plays a greater role in the memory impairment of DLB than AD. This is likely because subcortical and/ or frontal lobe dysfunction contributes more to the memory deficit in DLB than in AD. In addition, there is a different pattern of atrophy and cholinergic receptor expression in the hippocampus in DLB and AD (Watson et al., 2009). Pathological findings indicate that MTL atrophy in DLB is associated with senile plaques and neurofibrillary tangles, but not Lewy body pathology (Burton et al., 2009). Thus, the relative preservation of memory in DLB may be related to the relative lack of concomitant AD pathology.

FRONTOTEMORAL DEMENTIA

Frontotemporal dementia (FTD) is a clinicopathological condition characterized by deterioration of personality and cognition associated with prominent frontal and temporal lobar atrophy. Although FTD is relatively uncommon in older adults, its prevalence rivals that of AD in individuals younger than 65 years (Ratnavalli, Brayne, Dawson, & Hodges, 2002). Frontotemporal lobar degenerative disorders manifest as three separate clinical syndromes that may be distinguished by early prominent symptoms: (a) behavioral variant FTD (bvFTD) characterized by early change in personality, behavior, and cognition associated with frontal lobe atrophy; (b) semantic dementia (SD) characterized by early progressive loss of word meanings associated with anterior temporal degeneration; and (c) progressive nonfluent aphasia (PNFA) characterized by an early progressive anomic aphasia associated with deterioration of perisylvian cortical areas (Snowden, Neary, & Mann, 2007). Although these specific clinical syndromes can be distinguished early in the course of the disease, more advanced presentations often involve more generalized cognitive decline and combinations of features. Neuropathological findings in FTD include predominantly tau-positive (FTD-TAU) inclusions in PNFA, ubiquitinated TAR DNA-binding protein 43 (TDP-43)-positive (FTD-TDP) inclusion bodies in SD, and an equal proportion of both pathologies in bvFTD (Hodges et al., 2004; Seelaar et al., 2010; Shi et al., 2005; Snowden et al., 2007). The minority of remaining cases contain either RNA-binding protein fused in sarcoma (FUS)-positive bodies, other FUS- and TDP-negative but ubiquitin-positive bodies, or no distinctive histopathology (Seelaar et al., 2010).

The clinical and neuropathological features of FTD overlap with several other distinct conditions, including corticobasal degeneration, PSP, and amyotrophic lateral sclerosis (Josephs, 2008). Gene mutations identified in familial variants of FTD account for between 5% and 11% of cases and include microtubule-associated protein tau (*MAPT*) associated with FTD-TAU and progranulin (*PGRN*) associated with FTD-TDP (Rohrer et al., 2009). In a major recent discovery, the expansion of a non-coding GGGGCC sequence linked to chromosome 9p21 was found to be the most common genetic abnormality in familial FTD, accounting for 11.7% of cases in one sample (DeJesus-Hernandez et al., 2011).

Behavioral Variant

bvFTD begins with an insidiously progressive alteration in personality and behavior that may include inappropriate social conduct, inertia and apathy, disinhibition, perseverative behavior, loss of insight, hyperorality, or decreased speech output (Grossman, 2002). These alterations in behavior and personality have been linked to atrophy and neuropathological changes within the rostral limbic system, including the anterior cingulate, anterior insular, amygdala, orbitofrontal, ventrolateral frontal, ventromedial frontal, and ventral neostriatal areas (Snowden et al., 2007). These regions are thought to underlie processing and output related to socially appropriate behavior, which may include evaluating motivational and emotional content of internal and external stimuli, decision making, and error detection (Boccardi et al., 2005; Rolls, 2000). Recent histopathological and neuroimaging (e.g., MRI and SPECT) studies have specifically implicated the selective vulnerability of bipolar von Economo neurons located in layer V of the anterior cingulate, orbitofrontal, medial frontal, and insular areas in the early pathogenesis of bvFTD (Seeley, 2008). These neurons play a critical role in the integration of visceral-autonomic inputs that guide social-emotional behavior (Craig, 2002). Early disruption of the pathways involving these neurons within the rostral limbic system is consistent with the initial behavioral manifestations of bvFTD.

There may also be cognitive deficits in bvFTD that include alterations in judgment, problem solving, concept formation, and executive functions, with a relative sparing of visuospatial and memory abilities (Libon et al., 2009). Although aspects of the personality changes found in bvFTD differ from those typically found in other neurodegenerative conditions, many of these features overlap significantly with behavioral changes associated with AD (Varma et al., 1999). Many of the cognitive deficits found in these patients also overlap with those found in AD, particularly with regard to language impairment and executive dysfunction. Comparison with other forms of dementia is necessary to establish the cognitive profile specific to FTD; however, these studies are challenged by a number of methodological difficulties (Wittenberg et al., 2008). First, studies must match FTD patients to patients with other forms of dementia, particularly AD, in terms of dementia severity in order to compare their pattern of neuropsychological test performance. Second, many studies label participants generically as FTD without specifying participants by one of the three initial clinical presentations (i.e., bvFTD, SD, and PNFA). Finally, studies require clinico-neuropathological confirmation of bvFTD to assure the diagnosis and the lack of AD pathology that could contaminate the results of cognitive analyses.

Although these limitations have led to mixed findings concerning the cognitive signature of bvFTD, some general statements can be made regarding the pattern of test performance between FTD patients and those with AD. For example, FTD patients exhibit more severe deficits in executive functions than in other cognitive abilities, whereas AD patients have executive dysfunction that is proportional to their deficits in language and visuospatial abilities and less prominent than their episodic memory deficit (Förstl et al., 1996; Starkstein et al., 1994). Patients with mild-to-moderate FTD display greater impairment on word generation tasks (i.e., letter and category fluency tasks) but less impairment on tests of memory and visuospatial abilities compared to patients with AD (Rascovsky et al., 2002). These findings are consistent with greater frontal and anterior and lateral temporal lobe involvement in FTD than in AD, with relative sparing of medial temporal and parietal association areas only in FTD (Grossman et al., 2007; Libon et al., 2007). It is interesting to note that in terms of verbal fluency, FTD patients were equally impaired on all word generation tasks while AD patients showed greater impairment on semantic fluency than phonemic fluency tasks. This suggests that FTD patients' deficits were primarily driven by poor effortful retrieval and diminished active strategic search that may depend on frontal lobe function, whereas the impairment of patients with AD was at least partially driven by semantic deficits related to temporal lobe neocortical dysfunction. Importantly, FTD patients presenting with PNFA or SD show greater impairment on semantic fluency than letter fluency tasks, similar to AD patients, presumably due to temporal lobe neocortex damage in those FTD subtypes. Thus, greater impairment (relative to normal controls) of letter fluency than semantic fluency may represent a pattern of cognitive impairment that is somewhat specific to bvFTD (Mesulam, 1982).

Some studies have failed to find significant differences in visuospatial-constructional abilities between bvFTD and AD patients when using the Rey–Osterrieth Complex Figure copying task (Lindau, Almkvist, Johansson, & Wahlund, 1998). However, this task is known to not only require intact visuospatial abilities, but also may be influenced by attentional and strategic-organizational requirements dependent upon the frontal lobes (Varma et al., 1999). In support of this distinction, a recent neuroimaging study found that poor performance on this complex figure task was correlated with right parietal cortex atrophy in AD and right prefrontal cortex atrophy in bvFTD (Possin, Laluz, Alcantar, Miller, & Kramer, 2011).

As the studies reviewed in the previous pages suggest, the cognitive deficits associated with bvFTD are related to neuropathological changes within frontal and temporal cortices. Histopathological studies of FTD have revealed loss of project-ing pyramidal cells with glutamatergic activity and local-circuit inhibitory neurons within the upper cortical layers of the frontal cortex (Ferrer, 1999). Other findings indi-cate loss of postsynaptic sites within the remaining neurons of these upper cortical layers (Kersaitis, Halliday, & Kril, 2004). Cognitive changes typically follow changes in personality and behavior in bvFTD, suggesting that the temporal manifestation of cognitive dysfunction may be related to the progression of neuropathology. Studies examining the time course of frontotemporal neuropathology suggest that there is early mild atrophy of orbital and superior medial frontal cortices and hippocam-pus, followed by anterior frontal, temporal, and basal ganglia atrophy, and finally involvement of all remaining frontotemporal areas (Broe et al., 2003). Although it remains unclear what specific brain regions are responsible for various aspects of cognitive impairment in bvFTD, more severe and widespread atrophy may correlate with the extent of cognitive symptoms.

Progressive Nonfluent Aphasia

Patients presenting with a protracted period of aphasia often lasting years prior to the onset of more generalized cognitive decline represent a minority of FTD patients. These individuals exhibit two to three forms of aphasia, including nonflu-ent, semantic, and logopenic. Neuroimaging and postmortem autopsy studies have indicated that patients with FTD-PNFA show greater temporal lobe than frontal lobe pathology.

PNFA (also termed primary progressive aphasia) is characterized by hesitant speech production (i.e., apraxia of speech), agrammatism, deficits in processing syntac-tically complex sentences, anomia, and enhanced commission of phonemic paraphasic errors with relative preservation of word comprehension (Grossman, 2002). Measures of grammatical impairment, such as sentence comprehension tasks (Hodges & Patterson, 1996), are particularly sensitive to PNFA. Grammatical impairment may be particularly important in the language deficits observed in these patients, as they show greater deficits on sentence-picture matching tasks requiring an appreciation of grammatical relationships than word–picture matching and word-reading ability (Hodges & Patterson, 1996).

Functional neuroimaging studies using PET, SPECT, and fMRI suggest decreased cortical activity within the inferior and dorsolateral prefrontal cortex and the superior temporal cortex, possibly extending into the inferior parietal cor-tex, of the left hemisphere (Grossman, 2010). Some studies further indicate that during grammatical comprehension tasks, particularly for complex sentences, these patients exhibit reduced cortical activity that is poorly correlated with task performance (Cooke et al., 2003; Grossman et al., 1998). These findings correspond well with findings from structural neuroimaging studies. The earliest areas to be affected structurally are the anterior perisylvian regions, including the inferior, opercular, and insular areas of the frontal lobe (Gorno-Tempini, Murray, Rankin, Weiner, & Miller, 2004). With disease progression, atrophy spreads to the dorsolat-eral prefrontal cortex, orbital and anterior cingulate regions, and superior temporal cortex (Grossman, 2010).

Semantic Dementia

The SD subtype of FTD presents with a "fluent" aphasia characterized by empty speech, prominent anomia, circumlocution, frequent semantic paraphasic errors, and difficulty understanding the meaning of words with relatively preserved syntax and phonology (Hodges, Patterson, Oxbury, & Funnell, 1992). This pattern of language deficits is thought to be due to deterioration of representational or semantic knowledge. In support of this hypothesis, studies have found that when a particular concept becomes degraded in SD, it cannot be accessed by any modality (e.g., auditory recognition, confrontation naming, word–picture matching; Hodges, Patterson, et al., 1992). Furthermore, the loss of semantic knowledge occurs from the "bottom-up" direction in that the subordinate features of a concept (e.g., knowing that a horse is domestic) are lost before the superordinate features (e.g., knowing that a horse is an animal). Most other cognitive abilities remain relatively intact during the early stages, including episodic memory, nonverbal problem solving, working memory, and visuospatial abilities (Snowden, 1999).

This circumscribed semantic deficit is consistent with findings from neuroimaging studies that indicate prominent and relatively circumscribed left temporal lobe atrophy in patients with SD. Specifically, the left anterior temporal lobe is heavily affected with relative preservation of MTL structures (Hodges & Patterson, 1996). Functional neuroimaging with PET or SPECT reveals cortical hypometabolism within the left temporal lobe extending into the inferior frontal lobe (Grossman, 2002). Some studies have also found decreased recruitment of the left posterior inferior temporal cortex during a semantic decision task (Mummery et al., 1999).

On tests of remote semantic memory (e.g., the famous faces test) patients with SD show a pattern of memory impairment characterized by severe retrograde amnesia with memories from the recent past better retained than memories from the distant past (Graham, Becker, & Hodges, 1997). This is the opposite pattern of that seen in AD where the remote memory deficit shows a temporal gradient with memories from the more distant past better retained than those from the recent past (Beatty, Salmon, Butters, Heindel, & Granholm, 1988). This double dissociation is thought to be indicative of the distinction between the hippocampally based memory impairment seen in AD and the cortically based impairment seen in SD (Hodges & Graham, 1998). While AD is associated with prominent disease within MTL structures (e.g., the hippocampus), SD is associated with prominent disease within the left perisylvian cortex (Hodges & Patterson, 1996). This distinction is evident early in the course of these conditions, but may become less salient as patients with AD experience a gradual shift from hippocampally based impairment to cortically based impairment (Masliah & Salmon, 1999).

VASCULAR DEMENTIA

VaD refers to a cumulative decline in cognitive functioning secondary to parenchymal damage of vascular origin that is sufficient to cause impairment in activities of daily living. There are a number of difficulties in the definition of VaD due to the heterogeneity of its underlying etiology and clinical presentation. There is a wide range of vascular etiologies that may lead to the brain injury and resulting cognitive impairment responsible for VaD. These include but are not limited to multiple large infarctions, strategically placed infarctions, multiple small ischemic injuries, hemorrhagic lesions, and degenerative changes secondary to ischemia (e.g., hippocampal sclerosis or gliosis; Ince, 2005). Due to the heterogeneous nature of these different forms of neuropathology, there is no accepted neuropathological scheme for quantifying cerebrovascular disease as a whole with a "vascular pathology score" analogous to the Braak and Braak score for AD pathology (Braak, Braak, & Bohl, 1993; Jellinger, 2007b). The clinical presentation of VaD is also quite variable because the nature of a given patient's cognitive impairment will be determined by such a broad range of etiologies. Consequently, there is no singular or specific neuropsychological profile for VaD in general. For example, even within the subgroup of patients with VaD due to multiple large infarctions, the clinical presentation may vary dramatically according to the location of the infarctions. The necessity of memory impairment for *DSM-IV-TR* criteria for dementia is particularly problematic for VaD since patients may have profound deficits in multiple cognitive domains without memory impairment if their lesions are limited to cortical regions that are not critical for memory function (Wetterling, Kanitz, & Borgis, 1996).

As a result of these and other nosological difficulties, there is no single set of criteria for the clinical diagnosis of VaD that is generally accepted; consequently, prevalence estimates and other generalizations regarding the condition remain controversial (Chui, 2006; Jellinger, 2007b). Nevertheless, various attempts have been made to break the diagnosis into several subcategories, some of which may be more specifically characterized neuropsychologically. These conditions generally fall into at least three large categories: multi-infarct dementia (MID) associated with multiple large cortical infarctions (usually affecting 10 mL or more of brain tissue), dementia due to a single strategically placed infarction, and subcortical ischemic vascular dementia due to subcortical small-vessel disease that results from multiple lacunar strokes, leukoaraiosis (Binswanger's disease), or diffuse white matter pathology (Kalaria et al., 2004).

Specific research criteria for the broadly defined diagnosis of VaD have been proposed (Chui et al., 1992). In general, these guidelines require that multiple cognitive deficits (i.e., dementia) occur in the presence of focal neurological signs and symptoms and/or laboratory (e.g., CT or MRI scan) evidence of cerebrovascular disease that is thought to be etiologically related to the cognitive impairment. A relationship between dementia and cerebrovascular disease is often indicated if the onset of dementia occurs within several months of a recognized stroke, there is an abrupt deterioration in cognitive functioning, or the course of cognitive deterioration is fluctuating or stepwise. In one set of diagnostic criteria, VaD can be subcategorized on the basis of the suspected type of vascular pathology (as determined by clinical, radiological, and neuropathological features), and possible or probable VaD may be assigned depending on the certainty of the contribution of cerebrovascular disease to the dementia syndrome. Definite VaD is diagnosed only on the basis of histopathological evidence of cerebrovascular disease that occurs in the absence of neurofibrillary tangles and neuritic plaques exceeding those expected for age (i.e., AD) and without clinical evidence of any other disorder capable of producing dementia (e.g., Pick's disease, diffuse Lewy body disease).

A recent statement from the American Heart Association and the American Stroke Association made an attempt to redefine VaD in light of the many problems with current conceptualizations (Gorelick et al., 2011). The term *vascular cognitive impairment* was used to indicate any cognitive impairment thought to be due to any form of vascular disease. The use of this broader term is favored because it improves the recognition of individuals with cognitive impairment that has not yet reached the severity of dementia, which may allow for earlier identification and treatment of high-risk patients (Hachinski, 1992). Vascular cognitive impairment is then broken down into VaD and vascular mild cognitive impairment, which anticipates the likelihood that the *DSM-5* will break dementia into major neurocognitive disorder and minor neurocognitive disorder (www.dsm5.org). Memory is no longer required for the diagnosis of VaD and the emphasis is placed on executive dysfunction. These criteria also de-emphasize the presence of neurological signs, biomarkers, and stepwise decline since research has consistently failed to demonstrate their sensitivity to VaD (Erkinjuntti & Gauthier, 2002). Imaging remains an important component of the diagnosis because it is required to show evidence of cerebrovascular disease unless there is a history of clinical stroke. There is also increased recognition of the substantial overlap between AD and ischemia (Schneider, 2009), which cannot be readily disentangled by current imaging or biomarker technologies (Chui et al., 2006; Jellinger, 2007a). These new criteria represent a major advancement in the diagnosis of VaD, and the importance of neuropsychological testing is featured prominently. This makes cognitive function in VaD and vascular mild cognitive impairment an attractive area for future research in neuropsychology.

The most likely VaD etiologies to produce a cortical dementia that requires memory impairment are MID and a strategic infarct. MID usually occurs due to cortical lesions arising from occlusions of the main branches of the anterior, middle, or posterior cerebral arteries. Depending on the specific site and size of the cortical lesions, MID is characterized by memory impairment, aphasia, agnosia, and/or apraxia. The cognitive deficits of MID usually have a sudden onset and progress in a stepwise fashion as successive occlusions occur. A single strategically placed infarct can also lead to a cortical dementia syndrome if it involves brain areas important for memory, language, or visuospatial abilities. For example, an anterior cerebral or middle cerebral artery infarct that affects the angular gyrus can cause poor memory, alexia with agraphia, constructional apraxia, and anomia. Studies have shown that strokes within the posterior cerebral artery territory are particularly likely to result in dementia, including lesions affecting the dorsal paramedian areas of the thalamus, which can cause a diencephalic amnestic disorder, and lesions involving mesial temporal areas causing AD-like amnesia (Castaigne et al., 1981; Glees & Griffith, 1952). Ischemic lesions within the orbitofrontal, medial frontal, and cingulate areas supplied by the anterior cerebral artery, and caudate nucleus lesions involving the lateral lenticulostriatal arteries of the middle cerebral artery, also cause behavioral disturbances resulting in dementia (Mendez, Adams, & Lewandowski, 1989; Zekry et al., 2003). Other causes of VaD, such as a subarachnoid hemorrhage, can cause memory impairment, frontal lobe dysfunction, and language deficits that are usually associated with the cortical dementia syndrome (Jellinger, 2007b). It is interesting to consider what brain regions may emerge as "strategic infarct zones" with the new VaD criteria that no longer require memory impairment for the diagnosis. This subtype of VaD may be more common under the new criteria and is likely to involve a much greater variety of brain areas because the diagnosis of VaD simply requires impairment in two or more cognitive domains with substantial decline in activities of daily living (Gorelick et al., 2011).

A particularly important area of research in the neuropsychology of VaD involves the cognitive characterization of subcortical ischemic small vessel disease (Pantoni, 2010). This VaD subtype, formerly referred to as Binswanger's disease (Libon, Price, Davis Garrett, & Giovannetti, 2004), is characterized by extensive subcortical white matter lesions with no cortical infarcts observed on MRI. The relatively circumscribed damage to the white matter suggests that there may be an identifiable neuropsychological syndrome or profile associated with the disease, which would make this form of VaD more readily definable by operationalized research criteria. One challenge to this field is the high rates of subcortical white matter disease in VaD, AD, mixed dementia, and normal adults (O'Brien et al., 2002). Studies comparing the neuropsychological deficits associated with this subcortical form of VaD and AD largely show that patients with VaD are more impaired than those with AD on tests of executive functions, whereas patients with AD are more impaired than those with VaD on tests of episodic memory (particularly delayed recall). In addition, these studies suggest that the executive dysfunction associated with VaD is its most prominent deficit, perhaps because white matter pathology interrupts fronto-subcortical circuits that mediate this aspect of cognition. One study showed that VaD patients with a significant volume of white matter abnormality on imaging exhibited a profile of greater executive dysfunction and visuoconstructional impairment than impairment of memory and language abilities (Mathias & Burke, 2009; Price, Jefferson, Merino, Heilman, & Libon, 2005). These findings have been generally confirmed in a recent meta-analysis that included studies that used neuropsychological test performance to differentiate between VaD and AD (Mathias & Burke, 2009). Although this analysis showed that cognitive measures were limited in their ability to discriminate between the two disorders, patients with VaD were more impaired than patients with AD on tests that required recognition of emotions in pictured faces, whereas patients with AD were more impaired than those with VaD on tests of episodic memory that required delayed recall.

Neuropsychological studies provide consistent evidence for distinct cognitive profiles in VaD and AD, yet almost all of these studies employed clinically diagnosed patients without autopsy confirmation of diagnosis. This may have led to some degree of misclassification of patients across groups because AD and VaD are quite heterogeneous and can overlap in their clinical presentations. To avoid this potential confound, a recent study compared the profiles of neuropsychological deficits exhibited by patients with autopsy-confirmed VaD (primarily subcortical vascular pathology) or AD (Reed et al., 2007). Consistent with previous studies of clinically diagnosed patients, patients with AD had a deficit in episodic memory (both verbal and nonverbal memory) that was significantly greater than their executive function deficit. In contrast, patients with VaD had a deficit in executive functions that was greater than their deficit in verbal (but not nonverbal) episodic memory, but this difference was not significant. To further explore these differences, an analysis of individual patient profiles was carried out. This analysis showed that 71% of AD patients exhibited a profile with memory impairment more prominent than executive dysfunction, whereas only 45% of patients with VaD exhibited a profile with more prominent executive dysfunction than memory impairment. Interestingly, relatively severe cerebrovascular disease at autopsy was often not associated with clinically significant cognitive decline. When the profile analysis was restricted to those patients who exhibited significant cognitive impairment at their clinical assessment, the distinction between VaD and AD patients was more pronounced with 79% of AD patients exhibiting a low memory profile (5% with a low executive profile) and 67% of VaD patients exhibiting a low executive profile (0% with a low memory profile). The results of this study suggest that relatively distinct cognitive deficit profiles might be clinically useful in differentiating between VaD and AD, but additional research with autopsy diagnosed patients is needed to further characterize the deficit profile that will best differentiate between these disorders.

The distinction between AD and VaD on the basis of dysexecutive versus memory impairment is likely due to the more prominent involvement of subcortical dysfunction in VaD than in AD (Pantoni, 2010). Thus, VaD patients with subcortical vascular disease may be more readily characterized than other forms of VaD as neuropsychologically distinct from AD. It should be noted, however, that a dysexecutive syndrome can also occur as the result of cortical pathology that directly affects the frontal cortex (e.g., as in FTD).

Patients with VaD due to MID or strategic infarcts may mimic a variety of cortical syndromes including frontal lobe associated behavioral and cognitive deficits of bvFTD, prominent episodic memory deficit of AD, or aphasia associated with PNFA or SD. This is due to the fact that cortical infarction may occur in nearly any cortical region and result in the total ablation of the associated cognitive ability. For example, all forms of aphasia may result from strokes within a variety of frontal and temporal regions perfused by the middle cerebral artery (e.g., Broca's area, Wernicke's area). Behavioral syndromes found in bvFTD and AD (e.g., disinhibition, inertia) may result from orbitofrontal or medial frontal lobe infarction. Forms of visual agnosia (e.g., Balint's syndrome, object recognition deficits) found in PCA (i.e., visual variant of AD) may result from posterior cerebral artery infarction. There are certain cortical syndromes, however, that are relatively specific to vascular disease. For example, left hemispatial neglect may result from right middle cerebral artery infarction, but is rarely caused by a nonvascular neurodegenerative disease.

Heterogeneity of presentation is a feature of VaD that is difficult to quantify or apply to the "average" case, or to incorporate into research criteria. However, it is frequently helpful to note the "spotty" presentation of cognitive deficits when making a clinical differential diagnosis of VaD because that characteristic differs from the fairly typical presentation and course of most other cortical neurodegenerative diseases. One promising approach involves the use of intra- and inter-test variability measures to quantify the degree of performance variability within and across test domains (Crawford, Garthwaite, Howell, & Venneri, 2003; Schretlen, Munro, Anthony, & Pearlson, 2003). Measurement of variability in test performance may quantify the "spotty" nature of cognitive deficits that is observed in some patients with VaD, but more research is needed before this approach becomes clinically useful.

SUMMARY

The dementias are a clinically heterogeneous group of syndromes whose variations stem from their differences on a neuropathological level. That is, the etiological and neuropathological differences between such neurodegenerative diseases correspond to the relatively distinct neurocognitive profiles of each presentation. This is most obvious when comparing neurodegenerative diseases that primarily involve the cerebral cortex versus those that primarily involve subcortical regions. Although this distinction is not pure (i.e., pathological changes are not limited to either cortical or subcortical regions), the cortical–subcortical dementia distinction serves as a heuristically useful model for describing the pattern of neuropsychological deficits that are observed in these patient groups. Knowledge of the functional link between neuroanatomy and neurophysiology of neurodegenerative processes and neuropsychological outcomes is critical for clinical practice. By understanding this pathology–functional relationship, clinical review and objective assessment can make precise judgments about the etiology and, thus, type of neurodegenerative process.

TABLE 1.1 Cortical Dementias: Characteristics of Disease Onset, Course, Neurocognition, Neuroimaging, and Neuropathology

ONSET AND COURSE	NEUROCOGNITION	NEUROIMAGING	NEUROPATHOLOGY
Alzheimer's Dementia			
Insidious onset with steady decline. Cognitive dysfunction precedes changes in personality and motor function.	• Attention—Basic attention may be preserved early, with deficits in complex attention and working memory. • Memory—Rapid forgetting of episodic memories. Minimal improvement in structured format. • Executive Function—Mild deficits early in disease course. • Language—Early deficits in semantic fluency progress to anomia and agnosia. • Visuospatial—Deficits emerge during moderate stages of the disease.	• Hippocampal atrophy on MRI. • Amyloid positive on PET-Pittsburgh compound B (PiB)	• Amyloid plaques • Neurofibrillary tangles • Cortical and hippocampal atrophy • Cerebral amyloid angiopathy
Dementia With Lewy Bodies			
Cognitive deficit occurs with or before motor signs (no or mild tremor). Vivid visual hallucinations, REM behavior disorder, and fluctuating cognition may be present.	• Memory—Mild retrieval-based memory deficit. • Visuospatial function—Prominent early deficits disproportionate to memory deficits. • Executive function—Prominent early deficits disproportionate to memory deficits.	• Reduced posterior metabolism on PET. • Cortical atrophy.	• Cortical and subcortical Lewy bodies
Frontotemporal Dementia			
Early age of onset. Insidious onset with steady decline. Preservation of episodic memory.	• Behavioral variant (BV)—Early prominent personality changes prior to cognitive decline. Reduced verbal output and/or executive dysfunction may be present. • Progressive nonfluent aphasia (PNFA)—Early prominent nonfluent aphasia with intact comprehension. • Semantic dementia (SD)—Early prominent semantic memory loss with fluent speech.	• BV—Atrophy of frontal regions. • PNFA—Atrophy of perisylvian regions. • SD—Atrophy of anterior temporal regions.	• Atrophy of frontotemporal regions • FTD-TAU bodies or … • FTD-TDP bodies or … • FUS bodies
Vascular Dementia			
Abrupt onset with stepwise decline. May show striking contrast between areas of preservation versus impairment.	• Memory—Mild retrieval-based memory impairment. • Executive function—Impairment is equal to or greater than memory deficits. • Increased variability across cognitive domains.	• Severe subcortical white matter disease or … • Multiple large infarcts or … • Strategic infarct on MRI	• Infarctions • Hemorrhages • White and gray matter rarefaction • Atherosclerosis • Arteriosclerosis

FTD-TAU, frontotemporal dementia predominantly tau-positive; FTD-TDP, ubiquitinated TAR DNA-binding protein 43 (TDP-43)-positive; PET, positron emission tomography; REM, rapid eye movement.

REFERENCES

Aarsland, D., Litvan, I., Salmon, D., Galasko, D., Wentzel-Larsen, T., & Larsen, J. P. (2003). Performance on the dementia rating scale in Parkinson's disease with dementia and dementia with Lewy bodies: Comparison with progressive supranuclear palsy and Alzheimer's disease. *Journal of Neurology, Neurosurgery, and Psychiatry, 74*(9), 1215–1220.

Albert, M. S., Butters, N., & Levin, J. (1979). Temporal gradients in the retrograde amnesia of patients with alcoholic Korsakoff's disease. *Archives of Neurology, 36*(4), 211–216.

American Psychiatric Association. (2000). *Diagnostic and statistical manual of mental disorders IV-R.* Arlington, VA: American Psychiatric Publishing.

Aretouli, E., Okonkwo, O. C., Samek, J., & Brandt, J. (2011). The fate of the 0.5s: Predictors of 2-year outcome in mild cognitive impairment. *Journal of the International Neuropsychological Society, 17*(2), 277–288.

Ballard, C., Piggott, M., Johnson, M., Cairns, N., Perry, R., McKeith, I.,...Perry, E. (2000). Delusions associated with elevated muscarinic binding in dementia with Lewy bodies. *Annals of Neurology, 48*(6), 868–876.

Beatty, W. W., Salmon, D. P., Butters, N., Heindel, W. C., & Granholm, E. L. (1988). Retrograde amnesia in patients with Alzheimer's disease or Huntington's disease. *Neurobiology of Aging, 9*(2), 181–186.

Beyer, M. K., Larsen, J. P., & Aarsland, D. (2007). Gray matter atrophy in Parkinson disease with dementia and dementia with Lewy bodies. *Neurology, 69*(8), 747–754.

Binder, J. R., Desai, R. H., Graves, W. W., & Conant, L. L. (2009). Where is the semantic system? A critical review and meta-analysis of 120 functional neuroimaging studies. *Cerebral Cortex, 19*(12), 2767–2796.

Boccardi, M., Sabattoli, F., Laakso, M. P., Testa, C., Rossi, R., Beltramello, A.,...Frisoni, G. B. (2005). Frontotemporal dementia as a neural system disease. *Neurobiology of Aging, 26*(1), 37–44.

Bohnen, N. I., Kaufer, D. I., Hendrickson, R., Ivanco, L. S., Lopresti, B. J., Koeppe, R. A.,...Moore, R. Y. (2005). Degree of inhibition of cortical acetylcholinesterase activity and cognitive effects by donepezil treatment in Alzheimer's disease. *Journal of Neurology, Neurosurgery, and Psychiatry, 76*(3), 315–319.

Bondi, M. W., Jak, A. J., Delano-Wood, L., Jacobson, M. W., Delis, D. C., & Salmon, D. P. (2008). Neuropsychological contributions to the early identification of Alzheimer's disease. *Neuropsychology Review, 18*(1), 73–90.

Braak, H., & Braak, E. (1991). Neuropathological staging of Alzheimer-related changes. *Acta Neuropathologica, 82*(4), 239–259.

Braak, H., Braak, E., & Bohl, J. (1993). Staging of Alzheimer-related cortical destruction. *European Neurology, 33*(6), 403–408.

Brandt, J., Aretouli, E., Neijstrom, E., Samek, J., Manning, K., Albert, M. S., & Bandeen-Roche, K. (2009). Selectivity of executive function deficits in mild cognitive impairment. *Neuropsychology, 23*(5), 607–618.

Broe, M., Hodges, J. R., Schofield, E., Shepherd, C. E., Kril, J. J., & Halliday, G. M. (2003). Staging disease severity in pathologically confirmed cases of frontotemporal dementia. *Neurology, 60*(6), 1005–1011.

Brookmeyer, R., Johnson, E., Ziegler-Graham, K., & Arrighi, H. M. (2007). Forecasting the global burden of Alzheimer's disease. *Alzheimer's & Dementia, 3*(3), 186–191.

Brouwers, P., Cox, C., Martin, A., Chase, T., & Fedio, P. (1984). Differential perceptual-spatial impairment in Huntington's and Alzheimer's dementias. *Archives of Neurology, 41*(10), 1073–1076.

Burton, E. J., Barber, R., Mukaetova-Ladinska, E. B., Robson, J., Perry, R. H., Jaros, E., ... O'Brien, J. T. (2009). Medial temporal lobe atrophy on MRI differentiates Alzheimer's disease from dementia with Lewy bodies and vascular cognitive impairment: A prospective study with pathological verification of diagnosis. *Brain: A Journal of Neurology, 132*(Pt 1), 195–203.

Butters, N., Wolfe, J., Granholm, E., & Martone, M. (1986). An assessment of verbal recall, recognition and fluency abilities in patients with Huntington's disease. *Cortex, 22*(1), 11–32.

Caine, D. (2004). Posterior cortical atrophy: A review of the literature. *Neurocase, 10*(5), 382–385.

Calderon, J., Perry, R. J., Erzinclioglu, S. W., Berrios, G. E., Dening, T. R., & Hodges, J. R. (2001). Perception, attention, and working memory are disproportionately impaired in dementia with Lewy bodies compared with Alzheimer's disease. *Journal of Neurology, Neurosurgery, and Psychiatry, 70*(2), 157–164.

Castaigne, P., Lhermitte, F., Buge, A., Escourolle, R., Hauw, J. J., & Lyon-Caen, O. (1981). Paramedian thalamic and midbrain infarct: Clinical and neuropathological study. *Annals of Neurology, 10*(2), 127–148.

Chui, H. C. (2006). Vascular cognitive impairment: Today and tomorrow. *Alzheimer's & Dementia, 2*(3), 185–194.

Chui, H. C., Victoroff, J. I., Margolin, D., Jagust, W., Shankle, R., & Katzman, R. (1992). Criteria for the diagnosis of ischemic vascular dementia proposed by the State of California Alzheimer's Disease Diagnostic and Treatment Centers. *Neurology, 42*(3 Pt 1), 473–480.

Chui, H. C., Zarow, C., Mack, W. J., Ellis, W. G., Zheng, L., Jagust, W. J., ... Vinters, H. V. (2006). Cognitive impact of subcortical vascular and Alzheimer's disease pathology. *Annals of Neurology, 60*(6), 677–687.

Clark, L. R., Schiehser, D. M., Weissberger, G. H., Salmon, D. P., Delis, D. C., & Bondi, M. W. (2012). Specific measures of executive function predict cognitive decline in older adults. *Journal of the International Neuropsychological Society, 18*(1), 118–127.

Collette, F., Schmidt, C., Scherrer, C., Adam, S., & Salmon, E. (2009). Specificity of inhibitory deficits in normal aging and Alzheimer's disease. *Neurobiology of Aging, 30*(6), 875–889.

Colloby, S. J., Fenwick, J. D., Williams, E. D., Paling, S. M., Lobotesis, K., Ballard, C., ... O'Brien, J. T. (2002). A comparison of (99m)Tc-HMPAO SPET changes in dementia with Lewy bodies and Alzheimer's disease using statistical parametric mapping. *European Journal of Nuclear Medicine and Molecular Imaging, 29*(5), 615–622.

Colloby, S. J., Perry, E. K., Pakrasi, S., Pimlott, S. L., Wyper, D. J., McKeith, I. G., ... O'Brien, J. T. (2010). Nicotinic 123I-5IA-85380 single photon emission computed tomography as a predictor of cognitive progression in Alzheimer's disease and dementia with Lewy bodies. *The American Journal of Geriatric Psychiatry, 18*(1), 86–90.

Cooke, A., DeVita, C., Gee, J., Alsop, D., Detre, J., Chen, W., & Grossman, M. (2003). Neural basis for sentence comprehension deficits in frontotemporal dementia. *Brain and Language, 85*(2), 211–221.

Cormack, F., Aarsland, D., Ballard, C., & Tovée, M. J. (2004). Pentagon drawing and neuropsychological performance in Dementia with Lewy Bodies, Alzheimer's disease, Parkinson's disease and Parkinson's disease with dementia. *International Journal of Geriatric Psychiatry, 19*(4), 371–377.

Court, J. A., Ballard, C. G., Piggott, M. A., Johnson, M., O'Brien, J. T., Holmes, C., ... Perry, E. K. (2001). Visual hallucinations are associated with lower alpha bungarotoxin binding in dementia with Lewy bodies. *Pharmacology, Biochemistry, and Behavior, 70*(4), 571–579.

Craig, A. D. (2002). How do you feel? Interoception: The sense of the physiological condition of the body. *Nature Reviews. Neuroscience, 3*(8), 655–666.

Crawford, J. R., Garthwaite, P. H., Howell, D. C., & Venneri, A. (2003). Intra-individual measures of association in neuropsychology: Inferential methods for comparing a single case with a control or normative sample. *Journal of the International Neuropsychological Society, 9*(7), 989–1000.

Crews, L., & Masliah, E. (2010). Molecular mechanisms of neurodegeneration in Alzheimer's disease. *Human Molecular Genetics, 19*(R1), R12–R20.

Cummings, J. L. (2000). Cholinesterase inhibitors: A new class of psychotropic compounds. *The American Journal of Psychiatry, 157*(1), 4–15.

Dai, W., Lopez, O. L., Carmichael, O. T., Becker, J. T., Kuller, L. H., & Gach, H. M. (2009). Mild cognitive impairment and Alzheimer disease: Patterns of altered cerebral blood flow at MR imaging. *Radiology, 250*(3), 856–866.

Damasio, H., Tranel, D., Grabowski, T., Adolphs, R., & Damasio, A. (2004). Neural systems behind word and concept retrieval. *Cognition, 92*(1–2), 179–229.

De Lacoste, M. C., & White, C. L. (1993). The role of cortical connectivity in Alzheimer's disease pathogenesis: A review and model system. *Neurobiology of Aging, 14*(1), 1–16.

DeJesus-Hernandez, M., Mackenzie, I. R., Boeve, B. F., Boxer, A. L., Baker, M., Rutherford, N. J.,…Rademakers, R. (2011). Expanded GGGGCC hexanucleotide repeat in noncoding region of C9ORF72 causes chromosome 9p-linked FTD and ALS. *Neuron, 72*(2), 245–256.

Delis, D. C., Massman, P. J., Butters, N., Salmon, D. P., Cermak, L. S., & Kramer, J. H. (1991). Profiles of demented and amnesic patients on the California verbal learning test: Implications for the assessment of memory disorders. *Psychological Assessment, 3*, 19–26.

Deweer, B., Lehéricy, S., Pillon, B., Baulac, M., Chiras, J., Marsault, C.,…Dubois, B. (1995). Memory disorders in probable Alzheimer's disease: The role of hippocampal atrophy as shown with MRI. *Journal of Neurology, Neurosurgery, and Psychiatry, 58*(5), 590–597.

Dickerson, B. C., & Eichenbaum, H. (2010). The episodic memory system: Neurocircuitry and disorders. *Neuropsychopharmacology, 35*(1), 86–104.

Done, D. J., & Hajilou, B. B. (2005). Loss of high-level perceptual knowledge of object structure in DAT. *Neuropsychologia, 43*(1), 60–68.

Duda, J. E. (2004). Pathology and neurotransmitter abnormalities of dementia with Lewy bodies. *Dementia and Geriatric Cognitive Disorders, 17*(Suppl 1), 3–14.

Eichenbaum, H. (2000). A cortical-hippocampal system for declarative memory. *Nature Reviews. Neuroscience, 1*(1), 41–50.

Eichenbaum, H. (2004). Hippocampus: Cognitive processes and neural representations that underlie declarative memory. *Neuron, 44*(1), 109–120.

Erkinjuntti, T., & Gauthier, S. (Eds.). (2002). *Vascular cognitive impairment*. London, UK: Martin Dunitz Ltd.

Esiri, M. M., & Chance, S. A. (2006). Vulnerability to Alzheimer's pathology in neocortex: The roles of plasticity and columnar organization. *Journal of Alzheimer's Disease, 9*(3 Suppl), 79–89.

Ferrer, I. (1999). Neurons and their dendrites in frontotemporal dementia. *Dementia and Geriatric Cognitive Disorders, 10*(Suppl 1), 55–60.

Festa, E. K., Insler, R. Z., Salmon, D. P., Paxton, J., Hamilton, J. M., & Heindel, W. C. (2005). Neocortical disconnectivity disrupts sensory integration in Alzheimer's disease. *Neuropsychology, 19*(6), 728–738.

Fleisher, A. S., Houston, W. S., Eyler, L. T., Frye, S., Jenkins, C., Thal, L. J., & Bondi, M. W. (2005). Identification of Alzheimer disease risk by functional magnetic resonance imaging. *Archives of Neurology, 62*(12), 1881–1888.

Fong, T. G., Inouye, S. K., Dai, W., Press, D. Z., & Alsop, D. C. (2011). Association cortex hypoperfusion in mild dementia with Lewy bodies: A potential indicator of cholinergic dysfunction? *Brain Imaging and Behavior, 5*(1), 25–35.

Förstl, H., Besthorn, C., Hentschel, F., Geiger-Kabisch, C., Sattel, H., & Schreiter-Gasser, U. (1996). Frontal lobe degeneration and Alzheimer's disease: A controlled study on clinical findings, volumetric brain changes and quantitative electroencephalography data. *Dementia, 7*(1), 27–34.

Galasko, D., Katzman, R., Salmon, D. P., & Hansen, L. (1996). Clinical and neuropathological findings in Lewy body dementias. *Brain and Cognition, 31*(2), 166–175.

Ganguli, M., & Rodriguez, E. (2011). Age, Alzheimer's disease, and the big picture. *International Psychogeriatrics/IPA, 23*(10), 1531–1534.

Glees, P., & Griffith, H. B. (1952). Bilateral destruction of the hippocampus (cornu ammonis) in a case of dementia. *Monatsschrift für Psychiatrie und Neurologie, 123*(4–5), 193–204.

Gómez-Tortosa, E., Irizarry, M. C., Gómez-Isla, T., & Hyman, B. T. (2000). Clinical and neuropathological correlates of dementia with Lewy bodies. *Annals of the New York Academy of Sciences, 920,* 9–15.

Gómez-Tortosa, E., Newell, K., Irizarry, M. C., Albert, M., Growdon, J. H., & Hyman, B. T. (1999). Clinical and quantitative pathologic correlates of dementia with Lewy bodies. *Neurology, 53*(6), 1284–1291.

Gorelick, P. B., Scuteri, A., Black, S. E., Decarli, C., Greenberg, S. M., Iadecola, C., . . . Seshadri, S.; American Heart Association Stroke Council, Council on Epidemiology and Prevention, Council on Cardiovascular Nursing, Council on Cardiovascular Radiology and Intervention, and Council on Cardiovascular Surgery and Anesthesia. (2011). Vascular contributions to cognitive impairment and dementia: A statement for healthcare professionals from the American Heart Association/American Stroke Association. *Stroke, 42*(9), 2672–2713.

Gorno-Tempini, M. L., Murray, R. C., Rankin, K. P., Weiner, M. W., & Miller, B. L. (2004). Clinical, cognitive and anatomical evolution from nonfluent progressive aphasia to corticobasal syndrome: A case report. *Neurocase, 10*(6), 426–436.

Grady, C. L., Haxby, J. V., Horwitz, B., Sundaram, M., Berg, G., Schapiro, M., . . . Rapoport, S. I. (1988). Longitudinal study of the early neuropsychological and cerebral metabolic changes in dementia of the Alzheimer type. *Journal of Clinical and Experimental Neuropsychology, 10*(5), 576–596.

Graham, K. S., Becker, J. T., & Hodges, J. R. (1997). On the relationship between knowledge and memory for pictures: Evidence from the study of patients with semantic dementia and Alzheimer's disease. *Journal of the International Neuropsychological Society, 3*(6), 534–544.

Grossman, M. (2002). Frontotemporal dementia: A review. *Journal of the International Neuropsychological Society, 8*(4), 566–583.

Grossman, M. (2010). Primary progressive aphasia: Clinicopathological correlations. *Nature Reviews. Neurology, 6*(2), 88–97.

Grossman, M., Libon, D. J., Forman, M. S., Massimo, L., Wood, E., Moore, P., . . . Trojanowski, J. Q. (2007). Distinct antemortem profiles in patients with pathologically defined frontotemporal dementia. *Archives of Neurology, 64*(11), 1601–1609.

Grossman, M., Payer, F., Onishi, K., D'Esposito, M., Morrison, D., Sadek, A., & Alavi, A. (1998). Language comprehension and regional cerebral defects in frontotemporal degeneration and Alzheimer's disease. *Neurology, 50*(1), 157–163.

Hachinski, V. (1992). Preventable senility: A call for action against the vascular dementias. *Lancet, 340*(8820), 645–648.

Hamilton, J. M., Salmon, D. P., Galasko, D., Delis, D. C., Hansen, L. A., Masliah, E.,...Thal, L. J. (2004). A comparison of episodic memory deficits in neuropathologically-confirmed dementia with Lewy bodies and Alzheimer's disease. *Journal of the International Neuropsychological Society, 10*(5), 689–697.

Hamilton, J. M., Salmon, D. P., Galasko, D., Raman, R., Emond, J., Hansen, L. A.,...Thal, L. J. (2008). Visuospatial deficits predict rate of cognitive decline in autopsy-verified dementia with Lewy bodies. *Neuropsychology, 22*(6), 729–737.

Hansen, L., Salmon, D., Galasko, D., Masliah, E., Katzman, R., DeTeresa, R.,...Klauber, M. (1990). The Lewy body variant of Alzheimer's disease: A clinical and pathologic entity. *Neurology, 40*(1), 1–8.

Henry, J. D., Crawford, J. R., & Phillips, L. H. (2004). Verbal fluency performance in dementia of the Alzheimer's type: A meta-analysis. *Neuropsychologia, 42*(9), 1212–1222.

Higuchi, M., Tashiro, M., Arai, H., Okamura, N., Hara, S., Higuchi, S.,...Sasaki, H. (2000). Glucose hypometabolism and neuropathological correlates in brains of dementia with Lewy bodies. *Experimental Neurology, 162*(2), 247–256.

Hodges, J. R., Davies, R. R., Xuereb, J. H., Casey, B., Broe, M., Bak, T. H.,...Halliday, G. M. (2004). Clinicopathological correlates in frontotemporal dementia. *Annals of Neurology, 56*(3), 399–406.

Hodges, J. R., & Graham, K. S. (1998). A reversal of the temporal gradient for famous person knowledge in semantic dementia: Implications for the neural organisation of long-term memory. *Neuropsychologia, 36*(8), 803–825.

Hodges, J. R., & Patterson, K. (1995). Is semantic memory consistently impaired early in the course of Alzheimer's disease? Neuroanatomical and diagnostic implications. *Neuropsychologia, 33*(4), 441–459.

Hodges, J. R., & Patterson, K. (1996). Nonfluent progressive aphasia and semantic dementia: A comparative neuropsychological study. *Journal of the International Neuropsychological Society, 2*(6), 511–524.

Hodges, J. R., Patterson, K., Oxbury, S., & Funnell, E. (1992). Semantic dementia. Progressive fluent aphasia with temporal lobe atrophy. *Brain: A Journal of Neurology, 115 (Pt 6)*, 1783–1806.

Hodges, J. R., Salmon, D. P., & Butters, N. (1992). Semantic memory impairment in Alzheimer's disease: Failure of access or degraded knowledge? *Neuropsychologia, 30*(4), 301–314.

Hodges, J. R., Salmon, D. P., & Butters, N. (1993). Recognition and naming of famous faces in Alzheimer's disease: A cognitive analysis. *Neuropsychologia, 31*(8), 775–788.

Hof, P. R., Vogt, B. A., Bouras, C., & Morrison, J. H. (1997). Atypical form of Alzheimer's disease with prominent posterior cortical atrophy: A review of lesion distribution and circuit disconnection in cortical visual pathways. *Vision Research, 37*(24), 3609–3625.

Hyman, B. T., Van Hoesen, G. W., & Damasio, A. R. (1987). Alzheimer's disease: Glutamate depletion in the hippocampal perforant pathway zone. *Annals of Neurology, 22*(1), 37–40.

Ince, P. (2005). Acquired forms of vascular dementia. In H. Kalimo (Ed.), *Cerebrovascular diseases* (pp. 316–323). Basel: ISN Neuropath Press.

Ishii, K., Soma, T., Kono, A. K., Sofue, K., Miyamoto, N., Yoshikawa, T.,...Murase, K. (2007). Comparison of regional brain volume and glucose metabolism between patients with mild dementia with lewy bodies and those with mild Alzheimer's disease. *Journal of Nuclear Medicine, 48*(5), 704–711.

Ishii, K., Yamaji, S., Kitagaki, H., Imamura, T., Hirono, N., & Mori, E. (1999). Regional cerebral blood flow difference between dementia with Lewy bodies and AD. *Neurology, 53*(2), 413–416.

Jellinger, K. A. (2007a). The enigma of mixed dementia. *Alzheimer's & Dementia, 3*(1), 40–53.

Jellinger, K. A. (2007b). The enigma of vascular cognitive disorder and vascular dementia. *Acta Neuropathologica, 113*(4), 349–388.

Josephs, K. A. (2008). Frontotemporal dementia and related disorders: Deciphering the enigma. *Annals of Neurology, 64*(1), 4–14.

Kalaria, R. N., Kenny, R. A., Ballard, C. G., Perry, R., Ince, P., & Polvikoski, T. (2004). Towards defining the neuropathological substrates of vascular dementia. *Journal of the Neurological Sciences, 226*(1–2), 75–80.

Kersaitis, C., Halliday, G. M., & Kril, J. J. (2004). Regional and cellular pathology in frontotemporal dementia: Relationship to stage of disease in cases with and without Pick bodies. *Acta Neuropathologica, 108*(6), 515–523.

Kövari, E., Horvath, J., & Bouras, C. (2009). Neuropathology of Lewy body disorders. *Brain Research Bulletin, 80*(4–5), 203–210.

Lange, K. W., Sahakian, B. J., Quinn, N. P., Marsden, C. D., & Robbins, T. W. (1995). Comparison of executive and visuospatial memory function in Huntington's disease and dementia of Alzheimer type matched for degree of dementia. *Journal of Neurology, Neurosurgery, and Psychiatry, 58*(5), 598–606.

Libon, D. J., Price, C. C., Davis Garrett, K., & Giovannetti, T. (2004). From Binswanger's disease to leuokoaraiosis: What we have learned about subcortical vascular dementia. *The Clinical Neuropsychologist, 18*(1), 83–100.

Libon, D. J., Xie, S. X., Moore, P., Farmer, J., Antani, S., McCawley, G., …Grossman, M. (2007). Patterns of neuropsychological impairment in frontotemporal dementia. *Neurology, 68*(5), 369–375.

Libon, D. J., Xie, S. X., Wang, X., Massimo, L., Moore, P., Vesely, L., …Grossman, M. (2009). Neuropsychological decline in frontotemporal lobar degeneration: A longitudinal analysis. *Neuropsychology, 23*(3), 337–346.

Lindau, M., Almkvist, O., Johansson, S. E., & Wahlund, L. O. (1998). Cognitive and behavioral differentiation of frontal lobe degeneration of the non-Alzheimer type and Alzheimer's disease. *Dementia and Geriatric Cognitive Disorders, 9*(4), 205–213.

Lineweaver, T. T., Salmon, D. P., Bondi, M. W., & Corey-Bloom, J. (2005). Differential effects of Alzheimer's disease and Huntington's disease on the performance of mental rotation. *Journal of the International Neuropsychological Society, 11*(1), 30–39.

Lippa, C. F., Smith, T. W., & Perry, E. (1999). Dementia with Lewy bodies: Choline acetyltransferase parallels nucleus basalis pathology. *Journal of Neural Transmission, 106*(5–6), 525–535.

Locascio, J. J., Growdon, J. H., & Corkin, S. (1995). Cognitive test performance in detecting, staging, and tracking Alzheimer's disease. *Archives of Neurology, 52*(11), 1087–1099.

Macko, K. A., Jarvis, C. D., Kennedy, C., Miyaoka, M., Shinohara, M., Sololoff, L., & Mishkin, M. (1982). Mapping the primate visual system with [2–14C]deoxyglucose. *Science, 218*(4570), 394–397.

Masliah, E., Miller, A., & Terry, R. D. (1993). The synaptic organization of the neocortex in Alzheimer's disease. *Medical Hypotheses, 41*(4), 334–340.

Masliah, E., & Salmon, D. (1999). Neuropathological correlates of demantia in Alzheimer's disease. In A. Peters & J. H. Morrison (Eds.), *Cerebral cortex* (Vol. 14). New York: Kluwer Academic/Plenium Publishers.

Mathias, J. L., & Burke, J. (2009). Cognitive functioning in Alzheimer's and vascular dementia: A meta-analysis. *Neuropsychology, 23*(4), 411–423.

McKeith, I., Del Ser, T., Spano, P., Emre, M., Wesnes, K., Anand, R., ... Spiegel, R. (2000). Efficacy of rivastigmine in dementia with Lewy bodies: A randomised, double-blind, placebo-controlled international study. *Lancet, 356*(9247), 2031–2036.

McKeith, I., Mintzer, J., Aarsland, D., Burn, D., Chiu, H., Cohen-Mansfield, J., ... Reid, W.; International Psychogeriatric Association Expert Meeting on DLB. (2004). Dementia with Lewy bodies. *Lancet Neurology, 3*(1), 19–28.

McKeith, I. G., Dickson, D. W., Lowe, J., Emre, M., O'Brien, J. T., Feldman, H., ... Yamada, M.; Consortium on DLB. (2005). Diagnosis and management of dementia with Lewy bodies: Third report of the DLB Consortium. *Neurology, 65*(12), 1863–1872.

Mendez, M. F., Adams, N. L., & Lewandowski, K. S. (1989). Neurobehavioral changes associated with caudate lesions. *Neurology, 39*(3), 349–354.

Mesulam, M. M. (1982). Slowly progressive aphasia without generalized dementia. *Annals of Neurology, 11*(6), 592–598.

Mickes, L., Wixted, J. T., Fennema-Notestine, C., Galasko, D., Bondi, M. W., Thal, L. J., & Salmon, D. P. (2007). Progressive impairment on neuropsychological tasks in a longitudinal study of preclinical Alzheimer's disease. *Neuropsychology, 21*(6), 696–705.

Minoshima, S., Foster, N. L., Sima, A. A., Frey, K. A., Albin, R. L., & Kuhl, D. E. (2001). Alzheimer's disease versus dementia with Lewy bodies: Cerebral metabolic distinction with autopsy confirmation. *Annals of Neurology, 50*(3), 358–365.

Monsch, A. U., Bondi, M. W., Butters, N., Salmon, D. P., Katzman, R., & Thal, L. J. (1992). Comparisons of verbal fluency tasks in the detection of dementia of the Alzheimer type. *Archives of Neurology, 49*(12), 1253–1258.

Mummery, C. J., Patterson, K., Wise, R. J., Vandenberghe, R., Vandenbergh, R., Price, C. J., & Hodges, J. R. (1999). Disrupted temporal lobe connections in semantic dementia. *Brain: A Journal of Neurology, 122*(Pt 1), 61–73.

Nebes, R. D. (1989). Semantic memory in Alzheimer's disease. *Psychological Bulletin, 106*(3), 377–394.

Nestor, P. J., Caine, D., Fryer, T. D., Clarke, J., & Hodges, J. R. (2003). The topography of metabolic deficits in posterior cortical atrophy (the visual variant of Alzheimer's disease) with FDG-PET. *Journal of Neurology, Neurosurgery, and Psychiatry, 74*(11), 1521–1529.

Nicholas, M., Obler, L. K., Albert, M. L., & Helm-Estabrooks, N. (1985). Empty speech in Alzheimer's disease and fluent aphasia. *Journal of Speech and Hearing Research, 28*(3), 405–410.

Norton, L. E., Bondi, M. W., Salmon, D. P., & Goodglass, H. (1997). Deterioration of generic knowledge in patients with Alzheimer's disease: Evidence from the Number Information Test. *Journal of Clinical and Experimental Neuropsychology, 19*(6), 857–866.

O'Brien, J. T., Colloby, S. J., Pakrasi, S., Perry, E. K., Pimlott, S. L., Wyper, D. J., ... Williams, E. D. (2008). Nicotinic alpha4beta2 receptor binding in dementia with Lewy bodies using 123I-5IA-85380 SPECT demonstrates a link between occipital changes and visual hallucinations. *NeuroImage, 40*(3), 1056–1063.

O'Brien, J. T., Wiseman, R., Burton, E. J., Barber, B., Wesnes, K., Saxby, B., & Ford, G. A. (2002). Cognitive associations of subcortical white matter lesions in older people. *Annals of the New York Academy of Sciences, 977*, 436–444.

Pa, J., Possin, K. L., Wilson, S. M., Quitania, L. C., Kramer, J. H., Boxer, A. L., ... Johnson, J. K. (2010). Gray matter correlates of set-shifting among neurodegenerative disease, mild cognitive impairment, and healthy older adults. *Journal of the International Neuropsychological Society, 16*(4), 640–650.

Padovani, A., Di Piero, V., Bragoni, M., Iacoboni, M., Gualdi, G. F., & Lenzi, G. L. (1995). Patterns of neuropsychological impairment in mild dementia: A comparison between Alzheimer's disease and multi-infarct dementia. *Acta Neurologica Scandinavica, 92*(6), 433–442.

Pantoni, L. (2010). Cerebral small vessel disease: From pathogenesis and clinical characteristics to therapeutic challenges. *Lancet Neurology, 9*(7), 689–701.

Pearson, R. C., Esiri, M. M., Hiorns, R. W., Wilcock, G. K., & Powell, T. P. (1985). Anatomical correlates of the distribution of the pathological changes in the neocortex in Alzheimer disease. *Proceedings of the National Academy of Sciences of the United States of America, 82*(13), 4531–4534.

Perry, E. K., Irving, D., & Perry, R. H. (1991). Cholinergic controversies. *Trends in Neurosciences, 14*(11), 483–484; author reply 485.

Perry, E. K., Morris, C. M., Court, J. A., Cheng, A., Fairbairn, A. F., McKeith, I. G., ... Perry, R. H. (1995). Alteration in nicotine binding sites in Parkinson's disease, Lewy body dementia and Alzheimer's disease: Possible index of early neuropathology. *Neuroscience, 64*(2), 385–395.

Perry, R. J., & Hodges, J. R. (1999). Attention and executive deficits in Alzheimer's disease. A critical review. *Brain: A Journal of Neurology, 122*(Pt 3), 383–404.

Perry, R. J., Watson, P., & Hodges, J. R. (2000). The nature and staging of attention dysfunction in early (minimal and mild) Alzheimer's disease: Relationship to episodic and semantic memory impairment. *Neuropsychologia, 38*(3), 252–271.

Possin, K. L., Laluz, V. R., Alcantar, O. Z., Miller, B. L., & Kramer, J. H. (2011). Distinct neuroanatomical substrates and cognitive mechanisms of figure copy performance in Alzheimer's disease and behavioral variant frontotemporal dementia. *Neuropsychologia, 49*(1), 43–48.

Price, C. C., Jefferson, A. L., Merino, J. G., Heilman, K. M., & Libon, D. J. (2005). Subcortical vascular dementia: Integrating neuropsychological and neuroradiologic data. *Neurology, 65*(3), 376–382.

Pulvermüller, F., Shtyrov, Y., & Hauk, O. (2009). Understanding in an instant: Neurophysiological evidence for mechanistic language circuits in the brain. *Brain and Language, 110*(2), 81–94.

Rascovsky, K., Salmon, D. P., Ho, G. J., Galasko, D., Peavy, G. M., Hansen, L. A., & Thal, L. J. (2002). Cognitive profiles differ in autopsy-confirmed frontotemporal dementia and AD. *Neurology, 58*(12), 1801–1808.

Ratnavalli, E., Brayne, C., Dawson, K., & Hodges, J. R. (2002). The prevalence of frontotemporal dementia. *Neurology, 58*(11), 1615–1621.

Reed, B. R., Mungas, D. M., Kramer, J. H., Ellis, W., Vinters, H. V., Zarow, C., ... Chui, H. C. (2007). Profiles of neuropsychological impairment in autopsy-defined Alzheimer's disease and cerebrovascular disease. *Brain: A Journal of Neurology, 130*(Pt 3), 731–739.

Rohrer, J. D., Guerreiro, R., Vandrovcova, J., Uphill, J., Reiman, D., Beck, J., ... Rossor, M. N. (2009). The heritability and genetics of frontotemporal lobar degeneration. *Neurology, 73*(18), 1451–1456.

Rolls, E. T. (2000). The orbitofrontal cortex and reward. *Cerebral Cortex, 10*(3), 284–294.

Sabattoli, F., Boccardi, M., Galluzzi, S., Treves, A., Thompson, P. M., & Frisoni, G. B. (2008). Hippocampal shape differences in dementia with Lewy bodies. *NeuroImage, 41*(3), 699–705.

Sahgal, A., Galloway, P. H., McKeith, I. G., Lloyd, S., Cook, J. H., Ferrier, I. N., & Edwardson, J. A. (1992). Matching-to-sample deficits in patients with senile dementias of the Alzheimer and Lewy body types. *Archives of Neurology, 49*(10), 1043–1046.

Sahgal, A., McKeith, I. G., Galloway, P. H., Tasker, N., & Steckler, T. (1995). Do differences in visuospatial ability between senile dementias of the Alzheimer and Lewy body types reflect differences solely in mnemonic function? *Journal of Clinical and Experimental Neuropsychology, 17*(1), 35–43.

Salmon, D. P., & Bondi, M. W. (2009). Neuropsychological assessment of dementia. *Annual Review of Psychology, 60,* 257–282.

Salmon, D. P., Galasko, D., Hansen, L. A., Masliah, E., Butters, N., Thal, L. J., & Katzman, R. (1996). Neuropsychological deficits associated with diffuse Lewy body disease. *Brain and Cognition, 31*(2), 148–165.

Samuel, W., Terry, R. D., DeTeresa, R., Butters, N., & Masliah, E. (1994). Clinical correlates of cortical and nucleus basalis pathology in Alzheimer dementia. *Archives of Neurology, 51*(8), 772–778.

Sauer, J., ffytche, D. H., Ballard, C., Brown, R. G., & Howard, R. (2006). Differences between Alzheimer's disease and dementia with Lewy bodies: An fMRI study of task-related brain activity. *Brain: A Journal of Neurology, 129*(Pt 7), 1780–1788.

Schliebs, R., & Arendt, T. (2006). The significance of the cholinergic system in the brain during aging and in Alzheimer's disease. *Journal of Neural Transmission, 113*(11), 1625–1644.

Schneider, J. A. (2009). High blood pressure and microinfarcts: A link between vascular risk factors, dementia, and clinical Alzheimer's disease. *Journal of the American Geriatrics Society, 57*(11), 2146–2147.

Schretlen, D. J., Munro, C. A., Anthony, J. C., & Pearlson, G. D. (2003). Examining the range of normal intraindividual variability in neuropsychological test performance. *Journal of the International Neuropsychological Society, 9*(6), 864–870.

Seelaar, H., Klijnsma, K. Y., de Koning, I., van der Lugt, A., Chiu, W. Z., Azmani, A.,...van Swieten, J. C. (2010). Frequency of ubiquitin and FUS-positive, TDP-43-negative fronto-temporal lobar degeneration. *Journal of Neurology, 257*(5), 747–753.

Seeley, W. W. (2008). Selective functional, regional, and neuronal vulnerability in frontotemporal dementia. *Current Opinion in Neurology, 21*(6), 701–707.

Seeley, W. W., Crawford, R. K., Zhou, J., Miller, B. L., & Greicius, M. D. (2009). Neurodegenerative diseases target large-scale human brain networks. *Neuron, 62*(1), 42–52.

Shi, J., Shaw, C. L., Du Plessis, D., Richardson, A. M., Bailey, K. L., Julien, C.,...Mann, D. M. (2005). Histopathological changes underlying frontotemporal lobar degeneration with clinicopathological correlation. *Acta Neuropathologica, 110*(5), 501–512.

Shimomura, T., Mori, E., Yamashita, H., Imamura, T., Hirono, N., Hashimoto, M.,...Hanihara, T. (1998). Cognitive loss in dementia with Lewy bodies and Alzheimer disease. *Archives of Neurology, 55*(12), 1547–1552.

Simard, M., van Reekum, R., & Cohen, T. (2000). A review of the cognitive and behavioral symptoms in dementia with Lewy bodies. *The Journal of Neuropsychiatry and Clinical Neurosciences, 12*(4), 425–450.

Snowden, J., Neary, D., & Mann, D. (2007). Frontotemporal lobar degeneration: Clinical and pathological relationships. *Acta Neuropathologica, 114*(1), 31–38.

Snowden, J. S. (1999). Semantic dysfunction in frontotemporal lobar degeneration. *Dementia and Geriatric Cognitive Disorders, 10*(Suppl 1), 33–36.

Spillantini, M. G., Schmidt, M. L., Lee, V. M., Trojanowski, J. Q., Jakes, R., & Goedert, M. (1997). Alpha-synuclein in Lewy bodies. *Nature, 388*(6645), 839–840.

Squire, L. R. (1987). The organization and neural substrates of human memory. *International Journal of Neurology, 21–22,* 218–222.

Squire, L. R. (1998). Memory systems. *Comptes Rendus de l'Académie Des Sciences. Série III, Sciences de la vie, 321*(2–3), 153–156.

Starkstein, S. E., Migliorelli, R., Tesón, A., Sabe, L., Vázquez, S., Turjanski, M., . . . Leiguarda, R. (1994). Specificity of changes in cerebral blood flow in patients with frontal lobe dementia. *Journal of Neurology, Neurosurgery, and Psychiatry, 57*(7), 790–796.

Tiraboschi, P., Salmon, D. P., Hansen, L. A., Hofstetter, R. C., Thal, L. J., & Corey-Bloom, J. (2006). What best differentiates Lewy body from Alzheimer's disease in early-stage dementia? *Brain: A Journal of Neurology, 129*(Pt 3), 729–735.

Tröster, A. I., Butters, N., Salmon, D. P., Cullum, C. M., Jacobs, D., Brandt, J., & White, R. F. (1993). The diagnostic utility of savings scores: Differentiating Alzheimer's and Huntington's diseases with the logical memory and visual reproduction tests. *Journal of Clinical and Experimental Neuropsychology, 15*(5), 773–788.

Varma, A. R., Snowden, J. S., Lloyd, J. J., Talbot, P. R., Mann, D. M., & Neary, D. (1999). Evaluation of the NINCDS-ADRDA criteria in the differentiation of Alzheimer's disease and frontotemporal dementia. *Journal of Neurology, Neurosurgery, and Psychiatry, 66*(2), 184–188.

Vonsattel, J. P., & DiFiglia, M. (1998). Huntington disease. *Journal of Neuropathology and Experimental Neurology, 57*(5), 369–384.

Waltz, J. A., Knowlton, B. J., Holyoak, K. J., Boone, K. B., Back-Madruga, C., McPherson, S., . . . Miller, B. L. (2004). Relational integration and executive function in Alzheimer's disease. *Neuropsychology, 18*(2), 296–305.

Watson, R., Blamire, A. M., & O'Brien, J. T. (2009). Magnetic resonance imaging in lewy body dementias. *Dementia and Geriatric Cognitive Disorders, 28*(6), 493–506.

Weintraub, S., & Mesulam, M. -M. (1996). From neuronal networks to dementia: Four clinical profiles. In F. Fôret, Y. Christen, & F. Boller (Eds.), *La demence: Pourquoi?* (pp. 75–97). Paris: Foundation Nationale de Gerontologie.

Weintraub, S., & Mesulam, M. (1993). Four neuropsychological profiles of dementia. In F. Boller & J. Grafman (Eds.), *Handbook of neuropsychology* (Vol. 8). Amsterdam: Elsevier.

Weintraub, S., & Mesulam, M. (2009). With or without FUS, it is the anatomy that dictates the dementia phenotype. *Brain: A Journal of Neurology, 132*(Pt 11), 2906–2908.

Welsh, K., Butters, N., Hughes, J., Mohs, R., & Heyman, A. (1991). Detection of abnormal memory decline in mild cases of Alzheimer's disease using CERAD neuropsychological measures. *Archives of Neurology, 48*(3), 278–281.

Wetterling, T., Kanitz, R. D., & Borgis, K. J. (1996). Comparison of different diagnostic criteria for vascular dementia (ADDTC, DSM-IV, ICD-10, NINDS-AIREN). *Stroke, 27*(1), 30–36.

Whitwell, J. L., Weigand, S. D., Shiung, M. M., Boeve, B. F., Ferman, T. J., Smith, G. E., . . . Jack, C. R. (2007). Focal atrophy in dementia with Lewy bodies on MRI: A distinct pattern from Alzheimer's disease. *Brain: A Journal of Neurology, 130*(Pt 3), 708–719.

Wierenga, C. E., Stricker, N. H., McCauley, A., Simmons, A., Jak, A. J., Chang, Y. L., . . . Bondi, M. W. (2011). Altered brain response for semantic knowledge in Alzheimer's disease. *Neuropsychologia, 49*(3), 392–404.

Wittenberg, D., Possin, K. L., Rascovsky, K., Rankin, K. P., Miller, B. L., & Kramer, J. H. (2008). The early neuropsychological and behavioral characteristics of frontotemporal dementia. *Neuropsychology Review, 18*(1), 91–102.

Zekry, D., Duyckaerts, C., Belmin, J., Geoffre, C., Moulias, R., & Hauw, J. J. (2003). Cerebral amyloid angiopathy in the elderly: Vessel walls changes and relationship with dementia. *Acta Neuropathologica, 106*(4), 367–373.

CHAPTER 2

Integration of Imaging in Cortical Dementia Diagnosis

Chiara Cerami and Stefano F. Cappa

Cortical dementias belong to a heterogeneous group of disorders, sharing a common natural history, characterized by a chronic course following a variable preclinical phase, and reflecting progressive neuronal cell loss. The prototype of cortical dementia is Alzheimer's disease (AD). Although diagnosis of dementia is still made based on clinical judgment, current research criteria (Dubois et al., 2007; McKhann et al., 2011) emphasize the potential role of biomarkers in early and, possibly, even presymptomatic diagnosis. Among the candidate biomarkers, neuroimaging techniques are gaining increasing importance, in particular in supporting and guiding differential diagnosis. Traditionally, standard structural brain imaging investigation techniques, such as CT and MRI, have been considered to play a preliminary critical role in discriminating neurodegenerative diseases from other treatable and reversible disorders (i.e., brain tumors or central nervous system infections; see, for example, the practice parameter of the American Academy of Neurology—Knopman et al., 2001). "Negative" structural imaging findings therefore represent a considerable part of the routine clinical assessment of dementias. In addition, standard structural neuroimaging may show global volumetric changes, typical of neurodegenerative diseases, as well as localized decreases in gyral size (global and/or selective atrophy), associated with increased sulci, reflecting specific degeneration of brain systems or networks. These changes, however, occur much later than neuronal loss and synaptic density reduction. Quantitative assessment of structural changes allows for early identification of localized gray matter density and/or concentration changes with techniques such as voxel-based morphometry (VBM; http://dbm.neuro.uni-jena.de/vbm), which is based on statistical parametric mapping (SPM), a software package designed for the analysis of brain imaging data sequences such as a series of images from different cohorts or time-series from the same subject (http://www.fil.ion.ucl.ac.uk/spm).

In addition, functional neuroimaging techniques allow for increased understanding of the pathophysiology of neurodegenerative disorders. It has become progressively possible to identify in vivo evidence of the specific neuropathology of primary dementias using validated and disease-specific biomarkers. Validated topographical markers such as fluorodeoxyglucose (FDG) for PET, used to assess the downstream brain changes induced by the neurodegenerative processes, are becoming progressively more available in clinical practice. New pathophysiological biomarkers have also been developed for PET, such as tracers for amyloid, [^{11}C] Pittsburgh Compound-B (PiB) ligand, or for activated microglia, [^{11}C]PK, which may in the near future improve clinicians' ability to differentiate neurodegenerative dementias.

To summarize, structural and functional imaging techniques are increasing the possibility of identifying disease-specific topographical patterns of degeneration, extending the diagnosis to the very early, presymptomatic disease phase. The potential clinical implications include the possibility of introducing subjects to therapy earlier and monitoring disease progression as well as treatment response. Given the probable future availability of disease-modifying treatments targeted at specific etiopathologies, such as the beta-amyloid deposition in AD or the aggregation of pathological proteins in tauopathies (i.e., corticobasal degeneration [CBD] or progressive supranuclear palsy [PSP]) or TDP-43 proteinopathies (i.e., semantic variant of frontotemporal dementia), it becomes of utmost importance to develop accurate diagnostic markers, allowing an early identification of these neurodegenerative disorders.

In this chapter, we provide a brief guide to the main brain imaging techniques from the point of view of their usefulness in differentiating the principal forms of cortical dementias, that is, AD, posterior cortical atrophy (PCA), frontotemporal lobar degeneration (FTLD), and dementia with Lewy bodies (DLB), which have relatively specific imaging findings. We also consider mild cognitive impairment (MCI) because it is a clinical condition that is often prodromal to cortical dementias, in particular AD. We discuss in detail other dementias associated with movement disorders, that is, the CBD and PSP, because they belong to the FTLD spectrum, and vascular dementia (VaD), which is frequently considered in differential diagnosis of cortical dementias. We also supply a quick look at future directions in neuroimaging, which will most likely be based on the combination of different techniques of structural, molecular, and functional imaging.

ALZHEIMER'S DISEASE

AD is a clinical–pathological entity, which usually presents as a distinctive phenotype characterized by episodic memory impairment, and is accompanied by specific neuropathological changes. To date, a specific diagnostic test capable of identifying this kind of dementia is still not available; thus, the definite diagnosis remains pathological. The contemporary research effort aims at the identification of in vivo biomarkers for the early and reliable detection of AD pathology (for a review, see Ballard et al., 2011).

In clinical practice, the routine use of neuroimaging in neurodegenerative dementias is based on visual inspection of structural or functional imaging scans. Nevertheless, it is well-known that quantitative analyses increase the sensitivity and specificity of imaging methods and may lead to an earlier and more accurate diagnosis. In AD, clinical diagnosis is often made at a relatively late stage in the course of the disease, when symptoms appear and cerebral functions are already affected. Neuroimaging is an essential part of the diagnostic algorithm aiming to recognize a typical pattern of neurodegeneration and to exclude the presence of other causes of cognitive deterioration. Structural imaging methods, particularly MRI, often allow, even on visual inspection, detection of the typical pattern of medial temporal lobe atrophy. The evaluation of hippocampal volume is suggested as a marker of medial temporal lobe atrophy because its boundaries are rather easy to recognize, especially on coronal T1-weighted scans (Figure 2.1). Nevertheless, these structural changes occur relatively late in the course of the disease.

As shown by the neuropathological findings (Braak & Braak, 1991), the earliest sites of tau deposition in AD are typically along the perforant hippocampal pathway, fitting with the clinical manifestation of predominant memory impairment. This topographical distribution of neurobiological changes in AD subjects is consistently mirrored by regional atrophy; it is usually assessed on visual inspection of high-resolution T1-weighted MRI, which starts from parahippocampal and hippocampal structures, and then spreads over the neocortex, typically with temporoparietal predominance (for a review, see Frisoni, Fox, Jack, Scheltens, & Thompson, 2010). Microscopic alterations thus drive the macroscopic structure changes. Minimal regional structural changes, which seem to occur early in the disease course, can be better assessed with volumetric MRI, as documented in a recent meta-analysis of MRI volumetric studies (Shi, Liu, Zhou, Yu, & Jiang, 2009), reporting a reduction of hippocampal volume compared to matched controls of 20% in mild AD and 10% in MCI.

All these findings support the importance of evaluating regional atrophy, in particular medial temporal lobe changes, in the suspicion of AD. MRI can help in the diagnosis of AD even in the preclinical phase, according to the new research criteria (Dubois et al., 2007). In spite of all this evidence, as medial temporal lobe atrophy can also be present in non-AD dementias or in healthy elderly people (Barkhof et al., 2007), it is mandatory for clinicians to combine clinical information with imaging data in order to minimize false positives. Other pathophysiological (i.e., cerebrospinal fluid [CSF] measures of amyloid and tau proteins or positive [¹¹C]PiB-PET scans) and topographical (i.e., FDG-PET temporoparietal hypometabolism) biomarkers may also reliably detect AD and can be used in addition to structural imaging to

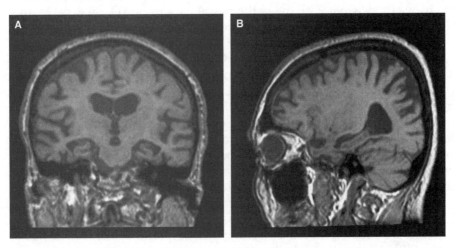

FIGURE 2.1 Bilateral atrophy of the medial temporal lobe in a 75-year-old AD patient as seen on T1-weighted coronal (A) and sagittal (B) MRI scans. The imaging was done at 5 years from the clinical onset. You can notice the loss of hippocampus and parietal neocortex volume, the third and lateral ventricle expansion, and the widening of the sylvian fissure. Image B is displayed orientated on the hippocampal axis.

AD, Alzheimer's disease.

Images courtesy of Prof. A. Falini, Neuroradiology—CERMAC, Vita-Salute University and San Raffaele Scientific Institute, Milan, Italy.

improve the diagnostic accuracy. It can be assumed that in the very near future all these biomarkers will most likely play a vital role in the clinical practice of detecting and managing AD.

A non-amnestic, focal cortical syndrome is a less common presentation of AD pathology. Almost a third of pathologically verified AD subjects present with clinical syndromes that are described further on in this chapter: PCA, corticobasal syndrome (CBS), primary progressive aphasia (PPA), or behavioral manifestations similar to the behavioral variant of FTLD (bvFTD; Alladi et al., 2007). In all these cases, exclusive reliance on medial temporal lobe MRI atrophy as an AD biomarker is largely ineffective. It is therefore very important to evaluate global and regional atrophy in order to recognize atypical MRI patterns with involvement of nontemporal regions. Early-onset AD cases often have atypical initial presentation with behavioral, language, or visuospatial disorders. They may thus present with MRI patterns differing from the medial temporal lobe involvement, typical of late-onset cases. This is supported by some volumetric comparison studies between early- and late-onset AD (Frisoni et al., 2007; Ishii et al., 2005; Karas et al., 2007), which have highlighted, in the first group, a predominance of parietotemporal, posterior cingulate, and precuneus gray matter loss. This makes distinguishing atypical AD from other cortical dementias with posterior onset (i.e., DLB) extremely hard, though the use of a quantitative evaluation method can prove beneficial. At the same time, early-onset AD can also exhibit prevalent behavioral or language deficits, leading clinicians to hypothesize that the features are indicative of a presentation such as FTLD. In this case, the co-occurrence of posterior cingulate cortex atrophy may be helpful in distinguishing AD from FTLD pathology (Lehmann et al., 2010).

In fact, even the use of precise volumetric evaluation of structural MRI is often not sufficient, especially in atypical AD presentation or in the earliest phases of the disease. On the contrary, at the beginning, functional neuroimaging (i.e., FDG-PET and single photon emission computed tomography [SPECT]) can highlight regional brain changes consistent with the pathological pattern of AD. Bilateral temporoparietal hypometabolism or hypoperfusion are characteristics of AD, though they are not always easy to detect on visual inspection. Multiple studies, mainly conducted in the last decade, have demonstrated with FDG-PET an impairment of glucose metabolism in parietal or superior/posterior temporal regions, posterior cingulate cortex, and precuneus (for a review, see Herholz, 2003), which extend to anterior regions in late phases of the disease (Choo et al., 2007). This method represents a reliable indicator of synaptic dysfunction associated with neurodegeneration; thus, it is a high-level diagnostic tool, useful in clinical practice. The pattern of hypometabolism usually reflects clinical symptoms and neuropsychological findings. In contrast to other degenerative dementias (i.e., FTLD or DLB), the basal ganglia and the primary motor and visual cortex are typically spared.

The visual inspection of FDG-PET images has a good specificity and sensitivity for identifying neurodegenerative processes, particularly AD (Hoffman et al., 2000). Nevertheless, as demonstrated by a clinical–neuropathological study (Jagust, Reed, Mungas, Ellis, & Decarli, 2007), the implementation of quantitative analyses on single-subject FDG-PET scan evaluation certainly increases the ability of clinicians to make the correct diagnosis. As previously reported for MRI, voxel-based analysis helps to recognize the typical hypometabolic pattern earlier than visual inspection, showing changes also at an early disease stage (Minoshima et al., 1997). Therefore, it is always advisable to base the interpretation of PET studies on quantitative mapping with reference to an appropriate normal sample. A positive FDG-PET AD pattern can be evident even in the very early stages (Anchisi et al., 2005; Morbelli et al., 2010), when the baseline clinical and neuropsychological evaluation do not allow a diagnosis of AD (see the Mild Cognitive Impairment section). FDG-PET might aid in differential diagnosis of AD as well, showing a different pattern of hypometabolism compared to other cortical dementias, such as FTLD (Foster et al., 2007). The inclusion of this neuroimaging method in current clinical evaluations can increase diagnostic accuracy and confidence for AD, adding important information on the topographical localization of the pathological process, even in the single subject. The severity and extent of hypometabolism could also be helpful in predicting the possible prognosis of AD. Longitudinal studies have demonstrated that the extent of metabolic impairment increases in medial temporal structures and spreads over the associative cortex as the disease progresses (for a review, see Herholz, Carter, & Jones, 2007).

Regional SPECT hypoperfusion mirrors the FDG-PET findings; however, direct comparisons between these two methods have shown superior accuracy of PET. In a sample of more than 200 mild-to-moderate AD patients, parietotemporal and posterior cingulate cortex involvement is more frequently present in FDG-PET scans (93.1% of cases) than in SPECT studies (81.6% of cases; Morinaga et al., 2010).

More recently, the usage of protein-specific radiolabeled ligands such as [11C]PiB for amyloid load or [11C]PK for activated microglia showed very promising results. Measuring the amyloid load even in the single subject, [11C]PiB-PET has a high potential to discriminate amyloid-related disorders from other neurodegenerative dementias (Rabinovici et al., 2007). Although the routine use of these PET techniques remains to be established, their clinical application could be particularly useful in recognizing atypical presentation of AD, as in the case of the frontal variant of AD or the logopenic variant of PPA (LPA; see below).

MILD COGNITIVE IMPAIRMENT

MCI is a condition characterized by cognitive deficits that are not sufficient to impair activities of daily living. It is a complex clinical syndrome, which can affect memory as well as other cognitive functions and may represent a prodromal form of different dementias (Petersen, 2004).

As in the case of dementia in general, clinicians must follow a diagnostic flowchart, including clinical–instrumental investigation, which allows exclusion of potentially treatable causes of cognitive decline. Structural imaging is routinely used in MCI diagnosis, in particular with the aim to predict the progression to dementia. Patients affected by amnestic MCI have a higher rate of conversion to dementia, and particularly to AD, than normal aging people (Petersen, 2004). Therefore, the volumetric measurements of specific brain regions, such as the hippocampus or entorhinal cortex, typically affected by AD neuropathology, have been reported as useful predictors of progression to AD (Chételat et al., 2005; Killiany et al., 2000). Although structural markers seem to be more sensitive than markers for amyloid deposition (i.e., molecular imaging or CSF analysis) to detect MCI conversion (Jack et al., 2009; Sluimer et al., 2010), the combined positivity of different biomarkers has a higher predictive power (Sluimer et al., 2010).

In present practice, positive finding of hippocampal atrophy in MRI scans of MCI subjects must alert the clinician and lead to a close follow-up of the case because of the high possibility of progression to AD dementia. A recent longitudinal qualitative MRI study, carried out within 3 years in a sample of 190 amnestic MCI, documented a significant correlation between the rate of progression of medial temporal atrophy, evaluated by a visual rating scale, and the risk of developing dementia, suggesting that obtaining an MRI during the earliest phases of the neurodegenerative disorder adds relevant information about the risk of progression to dementia (DeCarli et al., 2007). In addition, as shown by van der Flier et al. (2005) in a large group of nondisabled elderly people, the presence of a combination of hippocampal volume reduction with vascular pathology, documented in MRI by white matter hyperintensities, results in a fourfold increase in the presence of mild cognitive deficits.

Several studies have consistently indicated functional imaging as a valid tool to evaluate the underlying neurodegenerative process in patients with memory impairment, thus predicting the development of AD in MCI cohorts. As reported in a recent meta-analysis (Yuan, Gu, & Wei, 2009), FDG-PET has a high sensitivity for predicting rapid conversion of subjects with MCI to AD. A normal FDG-PET scan in an MCI at baseline indicates a low chance of progression within 1 year (Anchisi et al., 2005). Posterior cingulate and precuneus hypometabolism is also an early sign of memory impairment in mild cognitive-impaired subjects, while hypometabolism in the left temporal cortex seems to mark the conversion to AD (Morbelli et al., 2010). It is important to note that hippocampal or entorhinal hypometabolism is difficult to assess visually on a PET scan, because of the small size of the area and of partial volume effects.

It is also known that approximately 60% of amnestic MCI subjects are likely to have evidence of increased [^{11}C]PiB retention and a high possibility of conversion to AD (around 50% over a 1-year follow-up period; Okello et al., 2009). In the same study, [^{11}C]PiB-positive MCI subjects were significantly more likely to convert than [^{11}C]PiB-negative patients, and faster converters had higher [^{11}C]PiB retention levels at baseline than slower converters. Other findings, documented in a cohort of patients affected by MCI and early AD studied with [^{11}C]PiB-PET, indicate it to be an excellent tool for early AD detection, even in the prodromal phase (Forsberg et al., 2008; for a review, see Nordberg, 2008). [^{11}C]PiB-PET was also found to be able to significantly discriminate between nonamnestic and amnestic MCI. This finding provides further suggestion that the amnestic subtype of MCI is an amyloid-related disorder; thus, it is a prodromal phase of AD.

POSTERIOR CORTICAL ATROPHY

PCA refers to a clinical syndrome characterized by high-order visual processing impairments, consistent with predominant damage to visual processing streams (Benson, Davis, & Snyder, 1988). Alexia, agraphia, and transcortical sensory aphasia are also frequent and an early onset is common. Neuropathologically, the syndrome is mainly associated with AD, and is thus considered an atypical, posterior, or visual variant of AD. Nevertheless, other degenerative causes, such as tauopathy (i.e., CBD) or α-synucleinopathy (i.e., DLB), may be responsible for this syndrome (McMonagle, Deering, Berliner, & Kertesz, 2006; Tang-Wai et al., 2004).

Predominant parieto-occipital atrophy has already been demonstrated on routine structural imaging in the two cases originally reported by Benson, Davis, and Snyder (1988). MRI mainly demonstrates bilateral parietal associative cortex atrophy (Goethals & Santens, 2001), even in early phases of the disease. Structural MRI findings can be highly variable among different cases and can asymmetrically also involve temporal, occipital, and frontal lobes (Schmidtke, Hüll, & Talazko, 2005). Subcortical gliosis of posterior white matter has also been described, in a clinical–neuropathological study, as a typical finding (Schmidtke et al., 2005). Two major clinical syndromes reflecting involvement of the occipito-temporal (ventral) and biparietal (dorsal) cortical areas have been proposed by Ross et al. (1996), in association with PCA. The first is characterized by difficulties in object recognition, agnosia, and alexia, and reflects the involvement of the primary visual cortex or the occipito-temporal stream. The other syndrome presents with visuospatial problems, agraphia, and dyspraxia, and reflects a parietal or occipito-parietal disruption. The dorsal presentation seems, however, to be more common (McMonagle et al., 2006). Although MRI may support a PCA diagnosis, it is not always sufficient to make a correct differential diagnosis. A recent quantitative voxel-based MRI analysis (Migliaccio et al., 2009) comparing AD with PCA and LPA demonstrated large areas of overlapping atrophy (bilateral parietal, occipital, precuneus, posterior cingulate, posterior temporal, and hippocampal regions) among the three clinical conditions, thus suggesting that both PCA and LPA are atypical clinical manifestations of the AD pathology. Nevertheless, the same study identified specific regional atrophy localizations for each group, which may help in the differential diagnosis, in particular the right ventral-occipital and superior parietal regions in PCA and the left middle and superior temporal gyri in LPA. The application of advanced imaging techniques, such as voxel-based or diffusion tensor imaging (DTI), may be helpful, also in the single subject, in the early detection of typical neurodegenerative patterns and in monitoring disease progression, which can in PCA syndrome show a final common pathway with AD pathology (Duning et al., 2009).

Brain SPECT and FDG-PET imaging of PCA subjects demonstrate bilateral parieto-occipital hypoperfusion and hypometabolism (Figure 2.2), involving frontal lobe structures only later in the course of the disease (Aharon-Peretz, Israel, Goldsher, & Peretz, 1999; Goethals & Santens, 2001). Quantitative FDG-PET studies show a selective hypometabolism primarily affecting the posterior cerebral hemispheres, bilaterally or asymmetrically (Bokde et al., 2001; Nestor et al., 2003; Schmidtke et al., 2005). Compared to AD, SPM group analysis of PCA demonstrates occipito-parietal hypometabolism (Nestor et al., 2003) and variable superior temporal area involvement (Bokde et al., 2001). The comparison of PCA subjects with healthy controls shows predominant hypometabolism of the convexity and medial surface of the associative parietal cortex, which extends to the adjacent occipital and temporal associative cortex (Schmidtke et al., 2005). A symmetric involvement of the frontal lobes is present in a minority of cases (Nestor et al., 2003; Schmidtke et al., 2005), involving the region of the frontal eye fields, secondary to deafferentation from the occipitoparietal region (Cerami et al., 2014). As in AD, subcortical structures seem mostly spared, except for the rare findings of basal ganglia hypometabolism due to ipsilateral prefrontal cortex deafferentation (Schmidtke et al., 2005).

FRONTOTEMPORAL LOBAR DEGENERATION

The FTLD spectrum of disorders is a relatively common group of early-onset primary dementias, which includes two major clinical presentations (Rabinovici & Miller, 2010): a behavioral variant (bvFTD) and a language variant, known as PPA. The main feature of PPA is a prominent, isolated language deficit, which usually can be categorized into three clinical profiles (Gorno-Tempini, Dronkers, et al., 2004): nonfluent/agrammatic (PNFA), semantic (SD), and logopenic (LPA). The latter variant often is not due to FTLD, but represents an atypical presentation of AD (see the following text). This spectrum of disorders is due to different neurodegenerative conditions, which are histopathologically not homogeneous but share (with the exception of LPA) the characteristic of being associated with selective damage of frontal and temporal lobes.

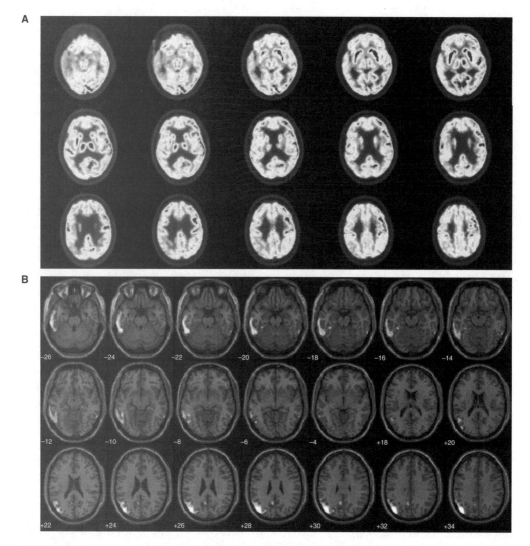

FIGURE 2.2 (*See color insert*.) [18]FDG-PET imaging (A) and the relative SPM analysis at *p* < .001 threshold (B) of a 58-year-old man affected by amnestic MCI. The images show hypometabolism of the left medial and inferior temporal cortex and inferior parietal lobule. The patient clinically converted to AD after 18 months, as seen from PET acquisition.

AD, Alzheimer's disease; FDG, fluorodeoxyglucose; MCI, mild cognitive impairment.

Images courtesy of Prof. D. Perani, Nuclear Medicine, Vita-Salute University and San Raffaele Scientific Institute, Milan, Italy.

Although not included in the current clinical diagnostic criteria (Neary et al., 1998), imaging is considered a basic element of the diagnostic process in FTLD. Currently, an international consortium of researchers has been working on the revision of present criteria in order to improve diagnostic accuracy (Gorno-Tempini et al., 2011; Rascovsky et al., 2007). Thus, a probable bvFTD diagnosis requires specific clinical features with evidence of progression and unequivocal positive neuroimaging finding, while definite diagnosis is reserved for those with neuropathological confirmation or with a pathogenic gene mutation. These new bvFTD criteria are currently undergoing validation against neuropathological changes. The role of neuroimaging is crucial also in the recent PPA classification. Structural and functional data are highly supportive of the diagnosis of different variants, because the site of maximal damage within the language network is responsible for the different clinical presentations of PPA (Gorno-Tempini et al., 2011).

FTLD is characterized by high familiar aggregation, with a direct mendelian heritability in almost 10% of the cases. Microtubule-associated protein tau (*MAPT*) and progranulin (*GRN*) genes, both linked to 17q21 loci, are the most frequent causes of autosomal dominant FTLD, accounting for a high proportion of familiar cases (Piguet, Hornberger, Mioshi, & Hodges, 2011). Mutated subjects usually present peculiar atrophy patterns. Many *MAPT* mutated subjects have severe temporal lobe atrophy (medial and lateral regions and temporal pole), mostly right lateralized (Josephs et al., 2009), while *GRN* mutated carriers could present an atypical neuroradiological profile, mainly characterized by asymmetric cortical atrophy with right predominance as well as with parietal involvement (Beck et al., 2008; Le Ber et al., 2008; Figure 2.3).

Behavioral Variant of Frontotemporal Dementia

BvFTD patients initially show a focal degeneration of frontal mesial and orbital cortices, followed by dorsolateral cortex and anterior temporal regions. These regions, earlier atrophied in bvFTD, are basic components of the emotional processing networks, which are already impaired in this disorder near the beginning. Hippocampus and subcortical structures (caudate, striatum, putamen, thalamus, and hypothalamus) can also be affected. This pattern is mirrored by the progression of atrophy of cortical–subcortical structures and neuronal loss seen from MRI findings (Kril, Macdonald, Patel, Png, & Halliday, 2005). In addition, as shown in a neuropathological study, severe amygdala atrophy is an efficient discriminator between bvFTD and AD, in contrast to hippocampal atrophy that does not seem to be specific (Barnes et al., 2006).

Four anatomically definite bvFTD subtypes have been described using a hierarchical clustering approach (Whitwell et al., 2009). The frontal dominant subtype is defined by the presence of medial and lateral frontal lobe atrophy, the frontotemporal subtype by atrophy of frontal and temporal lobes, the temporal subtype by predominant involvement of medial and lateral temporal lobes, and the temporofrontoparietal subtype by temporal lobe atrophy associated with frontal and parietal region involvement. The anatomical subtype seems to be a strong predictor of functional decline over time, even more than clinical–neuropsychological measures, and frontal dominant and frontotemporal subtypes are the two variants with the most severe prognosis (Josephs et al., 2011).

In the early phase of the disease, MRI findings can also be negative on visual inspection. A negative scan in the first stage of the disease does not however exclude the diagnosis of bvFTD. Near the disease beginning, bvFTD diagnosis is not always easy, and subtle behavioral changes are often overlooked or ascribed to psychiatric disorders, thus delaying the diagnosis. As the disease progresses, more signs of degeneration appear, as demonstrated by the serial volumetric MRI study by Chan et al. (2001), which shows a higher annual rate of whole-brain atrophy in FTLD compared to that documented for AD patients, and a greater spread of atrophy in the frontal variant of FTLD compared to the temporal one.

It is also increasingly evident that a subset of patients with clinical symptoms consistent with a behavioral variant diagnosis does not progress over time and remains stable over many years. These nonprogressing subjects, or phenocopies, are

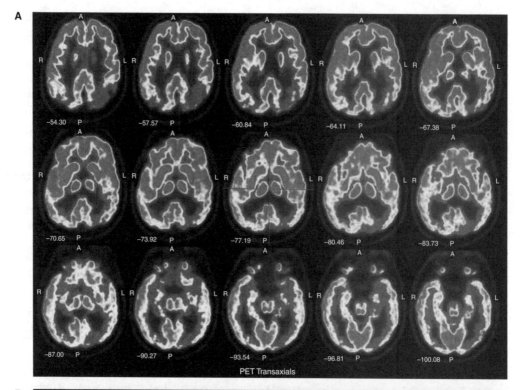

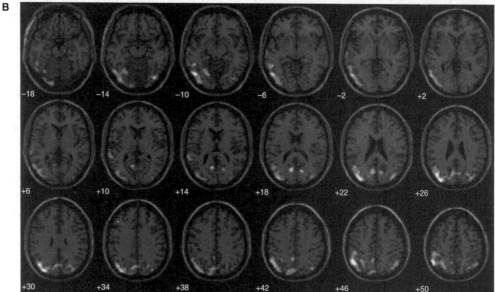

FIGURE 2.3 (*See color insert.*) [18]FDG-PET imaging (A) and the relative SPM analysis at *p* < .001 threshold (B) of a 67-year-old man affected by PCA. The image shows prominent hypometabolism of the posterior brain regions bilaterally, involving the temporoparietal and occipital cortex bilaterally, mostly on the left side.

FDG, fluorodeoxyglucose; PCA, posterior cortical atrophy; SPM, statistical parametric mapping.

Images courtesy of Prof. D. Perani, Nuclear Medicine, Vita-Salute University and San Raffaele Scientific Institute, Milan, Italy.

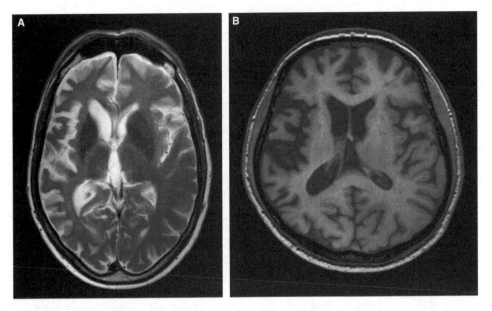

FIGURE 2.4 (A) T2-weighted axial MRI scan of a 57-year-old man and (B) T1-weighted axial scan of a 65-year-old woman affected by bvFTD and carrying a *GRN* mutation. Both images show severe cortico-subcortical atrophy, predominantly affecting the right side and the frontal and temporoparietal areas. The T2-weighted image also shows a shaded hyperintensity of white matter on the right side. Both images are in radiologic orientation.

bvFTD, behavioral variant of frontotemporal dementia; *GRN*, progranulin.

Images courtesy of Prof. A. Falini, Neuroradiology—CERMAC, Vita-Salute University and San Raffaele Scientific Institute, Milan, Italy.

basically distinguished from true bvFTD patients because they present with normal cognitive performance and display a lack of evident atrophy and hypometabolism on MRI and PET imaging (Davies et al., 2006; Kipps, Hodges, Fryer, & Nestor, 2009). Thus, the baseline anatomical characteristics have a significant diagnostic value and are very useful for evaluating the disease progression, especially combined with clinical and neuropsychological measures.

Quantitative MRI methods, such as VBM, are useful in revealing focal atrophy of orbitobasal, anterior cingulate, or insular cortices already in the earliest stages, with a selective pattern distinct from those of AD and other dementias (Boccardi et al., 2005; Seeley et al., 2008; Figure 2.4). Automated cortical thickness measurement also demonstrated differences in regional atrophy distribution between AD and bvFTD (Du et al., 2007). Compared to bvFTD patients, AD patients had a thinner cortex in the parietal and precuneus regions bilaterally, with a pattern similar to that described by the VBM method. Task-free functional MRI (fMRI) is also helpful in discriminating between bvFTD and other dementias. Recent findings suggest that bvFTD and AD subjects present with different network connectivity disruption patterns—anterior "salience" and posterior "default mode" networks, respectively—consistent with the clinical–neuropsychological features of the two disorders (Zhou et al., 2010). Thus, these methods could also provide simple disease signatures and offer noninvasive biomarkers for differential diagnosis in early phases.

Changes of white matter next to atrophied gyri and expanding into deep white matter reflect the gray matter loss. Increased subcortical signal intensity in

T2- and proton density-weighted images could be helpful in discriminating focal cortical dementia subtypes. White matter atrophy corresponds to the adjacent neuronal loss in the frontal and temporal lobes, with a different pattern in the behavioral and semantic variant of frontotemporal dementia (Chao et al., 2007). The anterior portion of corpus callosum may also be more atrophic in bvFTD than in AD (Yamauchi et al., 2000), even though more recent findings that used computerized voxel-based analysis did not confirm this evidence (Hensel et al., 2004). DTI, which allows clinicians to evaluate white matter microstructural changes mostly due to the axonal degeneration associated with cell body death, shows different patterns of white matter degradation in bvFTD, compared with AD, particularly in white matter tracts within the frontal lobe or connecting frontal and temporal brain regions (Zhang et al., 2009). Moreover, the bvFTD DTI pattern also seems different from that of a language variant. SD presents with predominant left temporal lobe involvement, with tract abnormalities in the inferior longitudinal and uncinate fasciculi, while PNFA reveals damage of the left inferior frontal lobe, insula, and supplemental motor areas, with tract abnormalities in the superior longitudinal fasciculus (Whitwell, Avula, et al., 2010). These findings, however, are not precise enough to represent a diagnostic marker of each subtype.

Functional neuroimaging may also represent a sensitive biomarker for the diagnosis of early, even preclinical, stages of dementia. Cerebral glucose metabolism in bvFTD subjects is mainly impaired in mesial or dorsolateral frontal cortices, and differs from the impairment observed in AD, which is predominant in temporoparietal and posterior cingulate cortices (Kanda et al., 2008). The same pattern of hypoperfusion can be observed in SPECT imaging. FDG-PET could also be useful in identifying bvFTD phenocopies, as they show no significant hypometabolism (Kipps et al., 2009). In summary, functional neuroimaging investigation techniques in bvFTD are powerful tools that can be reliably used in differential diagnosis and prognostic evaluations.

Semantic Variant of PPA

Each PPA variant is associated with characteristic linguistic features, usually corresponding to distinct patterns of brain atrophy. The recent PPA variant classification (Gorno-Tempini et al., 2011) proposes an imaging-supported diagnostic level as more accurate than mere clinical diagnosis. The core features of the semantic variant of PPA are anomia and single-word comprehension deficit, both essential for diagnosis. It is anatomically characterized by a selective pattern of atrophy in the anterior temporal lobe, mainly on the left side (Gorno-Tempini, Dronkers, et al., 2004; Figure 2.5). As demonstrated by quantitative studies, the cortical left hemisphere atrophy predominantly involves the infero-lateral temporal lobe, fusiform gyrus, temporal pole, and amygdala (Mummery et al., 2000). The degree of semantic memory impairment significantly correlates with the atrophy of ventral and lateral portions of the temporal lobe, while amygdala atrophy is related to emotional processing impairment (Rosen et al., 2006). Imaging findings are often pronounced, showing a severe "knife-edge"-type atrophy, thus making this clinical syndrome easier to disclose. However, at the very beginning of the disease, its diagnosis could be challenging; so the use of coronal MRI acquisitions might help to better detect the size changes of the left anterior temporal lobe.

Although SD is mainly associated with a distinctive pattern of temporal brain atrophy, it shares common regions of gray matter tissue loss with other FTLD subtypes. SD subjects may present with atrophy in the ventromedial and posterior

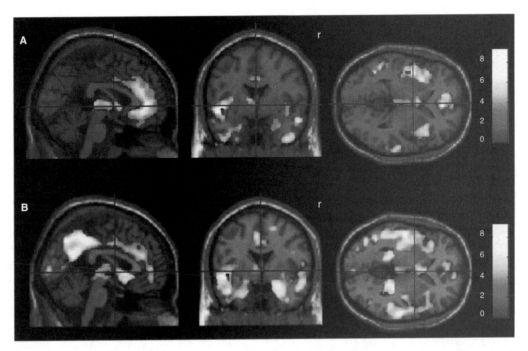

FIGURE 2.5 *(See color insert.)* VBM analysis on bvFTD (A) and AD (B) samples, compared to healthy matched subjects, showing different patterns of gray matter density loss. (A) bvFTD: anterior cingulated cortex, medial and orbitobasal frontal cortex, temporal poles, and amygdala and insula bilaterally; (B) AD: hippocampus, parahippocampal regions, amygdala bilaterally, and parietal and lateral posterior superior temporal regions. All images are displayed at $p < .005$ corrected threshold.

AD, Alzheimer's disease; bvFTD, behavioral variant of frontotemporal dementia; r, right; VBM, voxel-based morphometry.

Images courtesy of Dr. A. Canessa, Vita-Salute University, Milan, Italy.

orbital frontal cortices, in the insula bilaterally, and in the left anterior cingulate cortex, overlapping with those of bvFTD patients (Rosen et al., 2002). These changes are correlated with the presence of behavioral alteration. Nevertheless, it is important to remember that in these two FTLD subtypes there are also different patterns of gray matter loss, characterized by atrophy of dorsolateral frontal and premotor cortices in bvFTD, as well as the temporopolar cortex and anterior hippocampal region in SD (Rosen et al., 2002), which might help in differential diagnosis. The hippocampus can also be affected, but its atrophy is not specific for the disease (Galton et al., 2001).

Sometimes, SD patients can present with a predominant right-sided lateralization of atrophy. As demonstrated by a recent quantitative MRI study carried out in a sample of about one hundred FTLD cases, almost 20% of the subjects showed a right temporal dominant atrophy pattern (Josephs et al., 2009). Although the majority of these subjects (12 of 20 cases) present initial clinical diagnosis of bvFTD, 8 subjects were SD. Some of these cases were also associated with underlying TDP-43 pathology.

Nonfluent/Agrammatic Variant of PPA

The main features of PNFA are effortful and halting speech with sound errors and distortions, and/or agrammatism in language production. It presents a gray matter loss pattern, typically characterized on neuroimaging by focal left-sided perisylvian region involvement, particularly of the posterior frontal lobe and insula (Gorno-Tempini, Dronkers, et al., 2004). The diagnosis of an imaging-supported nonfluent variant of PPA requires inferior posterior frontal gyrus and insular atrophy (Gorno-Tempini et al., 2011). Premotor and supplemental motor areas can also be affected and are related to clinical manifestation of apraxia of speech (Josephs et al., 2006). Functional neuroimaging shows reduced cerebral activity mostly in left anterior brain cortex areas (Turner, Kenyon, Trojanowski, Gonatas, & Grossman, 1996).

PNFA can be considered the most heterogeneous PPA variant; it shows highly variable clinical–instrumental findings during the disease evolution and is related to different neuropathological conditions (Cappa, Perani, Messa, Miozzo, & Fazio, 1996). Some PNFA cases clinically and pathologically overlap with CBD, which is mainly characterized by asymmetric extrapyramidal syndrome, myoclonus, dystonia, and limb apraxia with alien limb phenomenon. There is a clinical continuum between these two conditions; thus, the same patient can present signs of PNFA and CBD, either subsequently or co-occurring during the disease course (Figure 2.6). A longitudinal voxel-based single case study of a subject with a PNFA clinical onset who then developed the classical signs of CBD demonstrated a progression of anatomical damage from the inferior posterior frontal gyrus to the left insula and later the medial frontal lobes (Gorno-Tempini, Murray, et al., 2004). However, the opposite sequence has also been reported (Kertesz, Martinez-Lage, Davidson, & Munoz, 2000).

Logopenic Variant of PPA

LPA is the most recently described PPA subtype (Gorno-Tempini, Dronkers, et al., 2004). Its main features are word retrieval and sentence repetition deficits. Spontaneous speech is slow in rate and full of pauses. Consistent with the hypothesis of a phonologic short-term memory impairment as the main feature of this subtype, left temporoparietal atrophy is an imaging mark of the disease (Gorno-Tempini, Dronkers, et al., 2004; Figure 2.7). Recent findings show that AD is probably the most common underlying pathology of LPA (Rabinovici et al., 2008). In this [^{11}C]PiB-PET study, LPA subjects presented higher cortical uptake of a radioligand than PNFA and SD patients. In addition, the distribution pattern of [^{11}C] PiB-positive PPA was diffuse and comparable to those of the AD-matched subjects. FDG-PET imaging in LPA shows a selective pattern of cortical hypometabolism with significant left asymmetric atrophy (Figure 2.7).

DEMENTIA WITH MOVEMENT DISORDERS

Cognitive impairment can be associated with signs of motor involvement, in particular with an extrapyramidal syndrome. Lewy body pathology is the most common cause of progressive cognitive decline with parkinsonism, and the typical feature is α-synuclein-positive Lewy body neuronal inclusions in the cortex, brainstem, and substantia nigra. DLB and Parkinson's disease (PD) dementia are common types of dementia associated with parkinsonism, considered as part of a unique spectrum of disorders and representing the most prevalent neurodegenerative dementias after AD. Because, in these dementia types, acetylcholinesterase inhibitors can be useful in reducing clinical symptoms and antipsychotic drugs are badly tolerated, it is extremely important to make the correct diagnosis. Neuroimaging is considered very important for the clinical characterization of both diseases, and particularly for the clinical-diagnostic classification of DLB (McKeith et al., 2005).

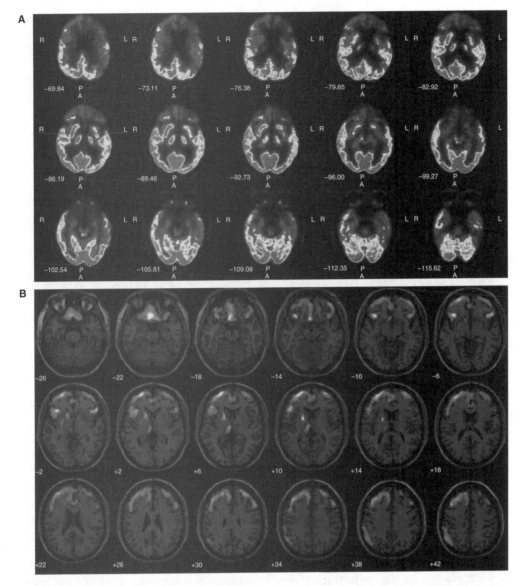

FIGURE 2.6 (*See color insert.*) [18]FDG-PET imaging (A) and the relative SPM analysis at *p* < .001 threshold (B) of a 53-year-old woman affected by bvFTD. The image shows bilateral cortico-subcortical hypometabolism, more pronounced on the left side and mostly involving the orbitobasal, dorsolateral, medial frontal, and inferior parietal cortices.

bvFTD, behavioral variant of frontotemporal dementia; FDG, fluorodeoxyglucose; SPM, statistical parametric mapping.

Images courtesy of Prof. D. Perani, Nuclear Medicine, Vita-Salute University and San Raffaele Scientific Institute, Milan, Italy.

CBD and PSP are other subtypes of atypical parkinsonism, showing peculiar clinical and anatomical features. Neuropathologically, they both belong to the group of tauopathies, within the FTLD spectrum of disorders. Therefore, they must be considered in the possible differential diagnosis of other parkinsonism or FTLD subtypes. Near the beginning of the disease, the differential diagnosis might be very difficult,

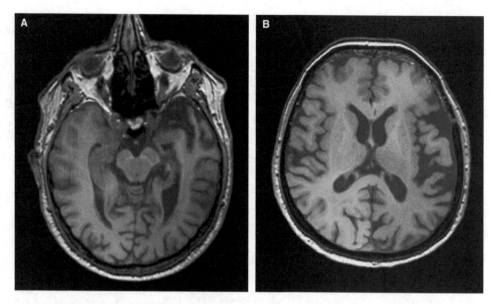

FIGURE 2.7 [¹¹C]PiB-PET study showing left temporoparietal atrophy in an patient with LPA.

because of the extreme heterogeneity in clinical presentation. Therefore, neuroimaging is an essential tool helping to discriminate them from other dementias.

Dementia With Lewy Bodies

DLB is clinically characterized by progressive memory and visuospatial ability decline, visual hallucinations, and fluctuation of cognition (McKeith et al., 2005). It mainly presents with a diffuse, unspecific atrophic pattern on MRI, which usually does not help in differential diagnosis. Functional imaging can raise the diagnostic accuracy. In DLB subjects, FDG-PET usually demonstrates a predominant occipital hypometabolism, in addition to temporal, parietal, and lesser frontal involvement commonly indistinguishable from AD (Ishii et al., 1998). On the contrary, ¹²³I-FP-CIT SPECT may be helpful in diagnosing DLB, detecting nigrostriatal dopaminergic system degeneration, thus offering a potential biological diagnostic marker. Presynaptic dopaminergic dysfunction correlates well with the neuropathological findings, confirming the high sensitivity and specificity of the procedure in DLB (for a review, see Tatsch, 2008). Several studies confirm the accuracy of the technique, showing a high correlation between the low binding activity of presynaptic dopamine transporter measured with ¹²³I-FP-CIT SPECT and the clinical diagnosis of DLB (McKeith et al., 2007; O'Brien et al., 2009). Reduced dopaminergic activity in the basal ganglia, documented in a SPECT or PET scan, is then considered relevant for diagnostic purposes, and is thus included in the clinical revised criteria as a highly suggestive characteristic of the disease (McKeith et al., 2005). Other supportive features of DLB diagnosis, commonly present but not proven to have any diagnostic specificity, are relatively preserved medial–temporal-lobe structures on MRI scan, occipital FDG-PET or SPECT hypoperfusion, and abnormal MIBG myocardial scintigraphy. All the evidence suggests a useful role of imaging to increase diagnostic accuracy, even in early phases when cognitive symptoms are prevalent and extrapyramidal signs are barely definite.

Corticobasal Degeneration

CBD is classically characterized by a predominant asymmetric frontal and/or parietal atrophy, and basal ganglia changes on MRI (Savoiardo, Grisoli, & Girotti, 2000) corresponding to the main cortical symptoms (contralateral limb apraxia, visuospatial disorders, and aphasia) and the extrapyramidal signs (Figure 2.6). An involvement of the temporal lobe is possible but not frequent.

In quantitative MRI studies, CBD subjects, compared to healthy subjects, showed an asymmetric pattern of brain atrophy, predominant on the left side, involving bilateral premotor cortex, superior parietal lobules, and striatum, while the same analysis in PSP cases displayed a prevalent atrophy of midbrain, pontine tegmentum, thalamus, and striatum (Boxer et al., 2006). Therefore, in clinically uncertain cases, a prevalent dorsal, frontal, parietal, or midbrain involvement leads to considering either a CBD or PSP diagnosis. DTI carried out in the early phase of CBD reveals a frontoparietal fiber damage (long frontoparietal connecting tracts, intraparietal associative fibers, and corpus callosum), clinically correlated with apraxia (Borroni et al., 2008).

While CBD is typically associated with underlying tauopathy, CBS can also be related to other aetiopathogenesis, such as AD pathology. A recent neuropathological and quantitative MRI study proved that a specific pattern of atrophy in CBS subjects can help in predicting the underlying pathology (Whitwell, Jack, et al., 2010). Although the VBM analysis showed overall gray matter loss in all subjects in premotor cortices, supplemental motor area, and insula, widespread patterns of frontotemporal and temporoparietal loss were documented, respectively, in TDP-43- and AD-associated pathological cases.

Functional imaging mirrors structural imaging findings, with involvement of prefrontal, premotor, and sensorimotor areas; cingulate cortex; and parietal and superior temporal regions (Brooks, 2000; Juh et al., 2005; Kreisler et al., 2005).

Progressive Supranuclear Palsy

PSP is characterized by an akinetic–rigid parkinsonism with postural instability and frequent falls, which are associated with an impairment of vertical eye movement. Structural imaging features can be helpful in the clinical diagnosis. On visual assessment, MRI highlights third ventricle dilatation and dorsal midbrain atrophy, with a significant reduction of the anteroposterior diameter. The measurement of anteroposterior midbrain diameter from axial T2-weighted MR images has been shown to be a reliable tool to differentiate PSP subjects from other typical or atypical parkinsonisms (Warmuth-Metz, Naumann, Csoti, & Solymosi, 2001). On sagittal MRI scans, a typical finding due to the atrophy of rostral midbrain tegmentum is the "hummingbird" sign (Figure 2.8). The evaluation of the area of midbrain tegmentum and pons on sagittal MRI can also offer useful information to differentiate PSP from multisystem atrophy of the Parkinson type (MSA-P), even if the midbrain sizes of MSA-P cases sometimes overlap with those of PSP (Oba et al., 2005). The reduction of the midbrain–pons ratio is another MRI characteristic feature, called "penguin sign," caused by the thinning of the quadrigeminal plate, the third ventricle dilatation, dorsal pontine tegmental atrophy, and an increased periaqueductal signal (Figure 2.8). Another peculiar MRI finding has been described as the "morning glory sign" (Figure 2.8). More elaborate measurements of brainstem structures confirm the diagnostic value of the presence of midbrain atrophy and superior cerebellar peduncle width reduction in PSP subjects (Quattrone et al., 2008). Nevertheless, the same authors also confirm a possible

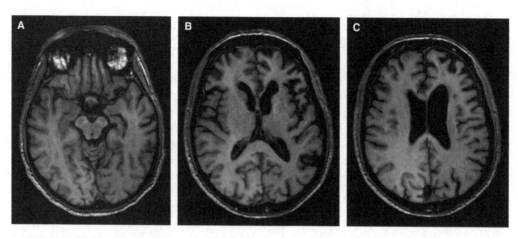

FIGURE 2.8 T1-weighted axial MRI scans of a CBD–PNFA subject, showing a severe left cortico-subcortical atrophy. You can notice the reduced midbrain volume and thinned left superior cerebellar peduncle (A), and a basal ganglia and left frontoparietal atrophy (B and C).

CBD–PNFA, corticobasal degeneration–progressive nonfluent aphasia.

Images courtesy of Prof. A. Falini, Neuroradiology—CERMAC, Vita-Salute University and San Raffaele Scientific Institute, Milan, Italy.

overlap between affected and nonaffected subjects at the single-subject level. Hence, in the early phases of the disease, with mild clinical signs and/or symptoms, a correct differential diagnosis may be very difficult.

In PSP subjects, FDG-PET imaging can display a reduction of glucose metabolism in the caudate, putamen, thalamus, pons, and frontal cortex (Foster et al., 1988). However, this finding is too generic to be useful in the diagnostic process. Advanced imaging analyses, such as automated image-based classification (Tang et al., 2010), have a higher specificity in distinguishing among parkinsonian disorders. In a diffusion-weighted MRI study (Rizzo et al., 2008), the region of interest-based analyses showed significantly greater putaminal apparent diffusion coefficient (ADC) values in PSP and CBD compared to those of PD subjects, confirming that early putaminal ADC evaluation provides a good discrimination between PD and atypical parkinsonism. This method may be helpful in the characterization and differentiation of these two diseases, as it can detect additional brain microstructural alterations correlated with the typical signs and symptoms of PSP and CBD.

VASCULAR DEMENTIA

The occurrence of cognitive deficits, in particular of memory function, associated with the presence of neuroimaging of a vascular lesion load sufficient to determine cognitive impairment represents a fundamental criterion for VaD (Román et al., 1993). However, the high variability of clinical manifestations and topographical vascular lesion distribution makes it extremely difficult to delineate a distinct clinical–instrumental pattern typical of cognitive impairment of vascular origin (for a review, see Román, 2004).

Repeated vascular injuries cause brusque and gradual lowering of cognitive performances directly related to the occurrence of new vascular lesions, particularly with cortical involvement. Cognitive impairment of vascular origin includes "global" cognitive impairment as well as focal neurological deficits of cognitive functions, which may reach a critical threshold for the onset of dementia. Multiple risk factors have been associated with the development of dementia in stroke patients. Advanced age, past history of other strokes, strokes in cortical territories, left hemispheric location, and middle cerebral artery involvement have been recognized as the most important risk factors for VaD (Censori et al., 1996; Pohjasvaara et al., 1998).

Standard neuroimaging is an essential tool in the diagnosis of VaD, which includes several subtypes. The most common subtypes are multi-infarct dementia (MID), whose clinical manifestation is related to the localization of specific cortical/subcortical vascular lesions (Hachinski, Lassen, & Marshall, 1974); small-vessel pathology; and dementia due to a single strategic ischemic lesion (Román et al., 1993).

The clinical hallmark of MID is the presence of focal neurologic symptoms and signs associated with imaging evidence of vascular lesions and a temporal relationship between cognitive impairment and cerebrovascular injuries.

T2-weighted and fluid-attenuation inversion recovery (FLAIR) MR images are very sensitive to ischemic injury related to small- and large-vessel disease. On the contrary, pure neurodegenerative dementia (i.e., AD or FTLD) does not usually present major changes on T2/FLAIR scans. Large-vessel disease usually causes wide cortico-subcortical infarcts with specific patterns mirroring the vascularization distribution. In contrast, small-vessel disease causes complete or incomplete subcortical infarcts, mostly in the capsular territory involving gray matter nuclei and large white matter fibers running in the internal capsule. In FLAIR images, incomplete ischemic infarcts appear as hyperintensities, whereas complete ones present as lacunes of tissue loss, hypointense to the brain. Subcortical vascular injuries affect cognitive functions and cause mainly disexecutive disorders, due to the involvement of frontal-striatal circuits (Kramer et al., 2002). In contrast to classic MID, this pattern of subcortical injury results in a set of symptoms usually comparable to that seen in primary neurodegenerative dementias. What can be considered as the critical vascular load, which can be associated with cognitive impairment, remains an unsettled issue. On SPECT/PET imaging, MID patients show a typical pattern of cortical and/or subcortical gray matter hypometabolism/hypoperfusion, correlating with the vascular lesions detectable on standard structural imaging.

Many MID subjects also have microhemorrhages, highlighted on T2/FLAIR imaging as hypointensities, corresponding to hemosiderin deposition. Microbleeds are particularly frequent in hypertensive subjects and are usually localized in the cortical–subcortical junctions, as in the case of lacunes (Lee et al., 2004). Axial MRI sequences are most commonly used to detect these kinds of vascular lesions. MID patients typically present not only with white matter changes, but also with focal strokes or lacunes and secondary focal atrophy and diffuse ventricular system dilatation. Nevertheless, the extent of atrophy is generally less selective and pronounced than in primary neurodegenerative dementia.

A difficult diagnostic challenge is represented by patients with imaging findings compatible with both AD and VaD. These patients, usually diagnosed as affected by "mixed" dementia, represent a considerable proportion of dementia cases, especially among the very old population. The evaluation of the respective contribution of AD versus vascular pathology in the individual patient is often impossible on clinical grounds.

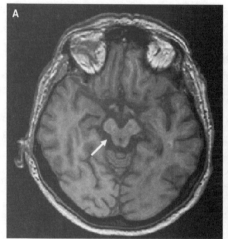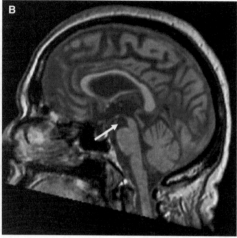

FIGURE 2.9 Typical MRI findings of PSP of a 72-year-old subject 36 months from the clinical onset. Both images are T1-weighted, axial (A) and sagittal (B), and in radiologic orientation. The white arrow in image A shows the "morning glory sign" (the concave appearance of the lateral margin of the tegmentum of the midbrain resembles the lateral margin of the morning glory flower), while the arrow on image B highlights the "penguin sign" (a small midbrain to pons ratio resembles a penguin shape) and the "hummingbird" sign (due to the atrophy of the midbrain tegmentum and relative increase in the length of the anteroposterior midbrain tegmentum diameter).

PSP, progressive supranuclear paralysis.

Images courtesy of Prof. A. Falini, Neuroradiology—CERMAC, Vita-Salute University and San Raffaele Scientific Institute, Milan, Italy.

CREUTZFELDT–JAKOB DISEASE

Neuroimaging also plays a role in the diagnosis of Creutzfeldt–Jakob disease (CJD). MRI has high sensitivity and specificity for the premortem diagnosis of sporadic CJD (Zerr et al., 2009). In particular, FLAIR and diffusion-weighted imaging (DWI) show typical findings (Tian, Zhang, Lang, & Wang, 2010). In the case of clinical suspicion of CJD, symmetric hyperintensities of cortical gyri and striatum, and sometimes thalamus, on DWI or FLAIR scans are highly suggestive of the diagnosis of sporadic or genetic prion disease. Cortical involvement is usually widespread and concerns frontal or occipital lobes; however, isolated cortical involvement could also occur (Figure 2.9). DWI is the most sensitive MRI technique for the early diagnosis of sporadic CJD, showing a cortical–subcortical involvement in the majority of cases (Shiga et al., 2004; Young et al., 2005). Instead, T2-weighted imaging could be useful in detecting variant CJD, in which it is present as the "pulvinar sign," a bilateral hyperintensity of the thalamic pulvinar nucleus; it is greater than the hyperintensity in the caudate and putamen nuclei, which also could be evident in FLAIR and DWI sequences (Figure 2.10; Zeidler et al., 2000). Furthermore, variant CJD shows no cortical involvement. Nevertheless, bilateral pulvinar hyperintensity has also been described in sporadic CJD or other neurological disorders (de la Torre Laviana, 2009; Mihara et al., 2005). These typical gray matter hyperintensities in DWI and FLAIR images, specifically not involving limbic regions, are also useful in differentiating CJD from other subacute dementias, such as limbic encephalitis (Vitali et al., 2011).

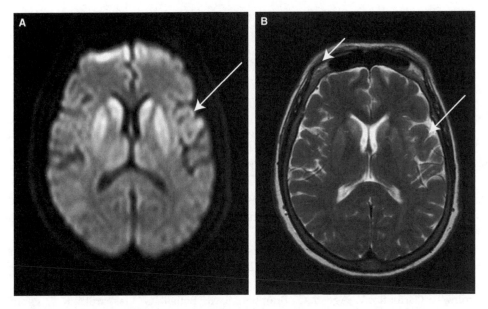

FIGURE 2.10 DWI (A) and T2-weighted (B) MRI scans of a 49-year-old woman affected by pathologically proven sporadic CJD. The images show hyperintensity of the left lateral frontal cortex (arrow), and caudate, putamen (with an anteroposterior gradient), and pulvinar nuclei bilaterally.

CJD, Creutzfeldt–Jakob disease; DWI, diffusion-weighted imaging.

Images courtesy of Prof. A. Falini, Neuroradiology—CERMAC, Vita-Salute University and San Raffaele Scientific Institute, Milan, Italy.

SUMMARY

Neuroimaging plays a crucial role in the differential diagnosis of cortical dementia. CT and MRI are helpful in detecting intracranial alterations responsible for (i.e., regional cortical brain atrophy, brain tumor, or hydrocephalus) or contributing to (i.e., cerebrovascular lesions) dementia syndromes. Quantitative structural and functional analyses comparing patients' groups with age-matched controls have been successfully used to define imaging patterns specific to the different dementia subtypes, providing useful information for differential diagnosis.

REFERENCES

Aharon-Peretz, J., Israel, O., Goldsher, D., & Peretz, A. (1999). Posterior cortical atrophy variants of Alzheimer's disease. *Dementia and Geriatric Cognitive Disorders, 10*(6), 483–487.

Alladi, S., Xuereb, J., Bak, T., Nestor, P., Knibb, J., Patterson, K., & Hodges, J. R. (2007). Focal cortical presentations of Alzheimer's disease. *Brain: A Journal of Neurology, 130*(Pt 10), 2636–2645.

Anchisi, D., Borroni, B., Franceschi, M., Kerrouche, N., Kalbe, E., Beuthien-Beumann, B.,…Perani, D. (2005). Heterogeneity of brain glucose metabolism in mild cognitive impairment and clinical progression to Alzheimer disease. *Archives of Neurology, 62*(11), 1728–1733.

Ballard, C., Gauthier, S., Corbett, A., Brayne, C., Aarsland, D., & Jones, E. (2011). Alzheimer's disease. *Lancet, 19;377*(9770), 1019–1031.

Barkhof, F., Polvikoski, T. M., van Straaten, E. C., Kalaria, R. N., Sulkava, R., Aronen, H. J.,...
Erkinjuntti, T. (2007). The significance of medial temporal lobe atrophy: A postmortem
MRI study in the very old. *Neurology, 69*(15), 1521–1527.

Barnes, J., Whitwell, J. L., Frost, C., Josephs, K. A., Rossor, M., & Fox, N. C. (2006). Measurements
of the amygdala and hippocampus in pathologically confirmed Alzheimer disease and
frontotemporal lobar degeneration. *Archives of Neurology, 63*(10), 1434–1439.

Beck, J., Rohrer, J. D., Campbell, T., Isaacs, A., Morrison, K. E., Goodall, E. F., ... Mead, S.
(2008). A distinct clinical, neuropsychological and radiological phenotype is associated
with progranulin gene mutations in a large UK series. *Brain, 131*(Pt 3), 706–720.

Benson, D. F., Davis, R. J., & Snyder, B. D. (1988). Posterior cortical atrophy. *Archives of
Neurology, 45*(7), 789–793.

Boccardi, M., Sabattoli, F., Laakso, M. P., Testa, C., Rossi, R., Beltramello, A.,...Frisoni, G. B.
(2005). Frontotemporal dementia as a neural system disease. *Neurobiology of Aging, 26*(1),
37–44.

Bokde, A. L., Pietrini, P., Ibáñez, V., Furey, M. L., Alexander, G. E., Graff-Radford, N.
R.,...Horwitz, B. (2001). The effect of brain atrophy on cerebral hypometabolism in the
visual variant of Alzheimer disease. *Archives of Neurology, 58*(3), 480–486.

Borroni, B., Garibotto, V., Agosti, C., Brambati, S. M., Bellelli, G., Gasparotti, R.,...Perani, D.
(2008). White matter changes in corticobasal degeneration syndrome and correlation
with limb apraxia. *Archives of Neurology, 65*(6), 796–801.

Boxer, A. L., Geschwind, M. D., Belfor, N., Gorno-Tempini, M. L., Schauer, G. F., Miller, B.
L.,...Rosen, H. J. (2006). Patterns of brain atrophy that differentiate corticobasal degeneration syndrome from progressive supranuclear palsy. *Archives of Neurology, 63*(1),
81–86.

Braak, H., & Braak, E. (1991). Neuropathological staging of Alzheimer-related changes. *Acta
Neuropathologica, 82*(4), 239–259.

Brooks, D. J. (2000). Functional imaging studies in corticobasal degeneration. *Advances in
Neurology, 82*, 209–215.

Cappa, S. F., Perani, D., Messa, C., Miozzo, A., & Fazio, F. (1996). Varieties of progressive nonfluent aphasia. *Annals of the New York Academy of Sciences, 777*, 243–248.

Censori, B., Manara, O., Agostinis, C., Camerlingo, M., Casto, L., Galavotti, B.,...Mamoli,
A. (1996). Dementia after first stroke. *Stroke; A Journal of Cerebral Circulation, 27*(7),
1205–1210.

Cerami, C., Crespi, C., Della Rosa, P. A., Dodich, A., Marcone, A., Magnani, G . . . Perani, D.
(2014, August 11). Brain changes within the visuo-spatial attentional network in posterior cortical atrophy. *Journal of Alzheimer's Disease.* Advance online publication.

Chan, D., Fox, N. C., Jenkins, R., Scahill, R. I., Crum, W. R., & Rossor, M. N. (2001). Rates of
global and regional cerebral atrophy in AD and frontotemporal dementia. *Neurology,
57*(10), 1756–1763.

Chao, L. L., Schuff, N., Clevenger, E. M., Mueller, S. G., Rosen, H. J., Gorno-Tempini, M. L.,...
Weiner, M. W. (2007). Patterns of white matter atrophy in frontotemporal lobar degeneration. *Archives of Neurology, 64*(11), 1619–1624.

Chételat, G., Landeau, B., Eustache, F., Mézenge, F., Viader, F., de la Sayette, V.,...Baron, J. C.
(2005). Using voxel-based morphometry to map the structural changes associated with
rapid conversion in MCI: A longitudinal MRI study. *NeuroImage, 27*(4), 934–946.

Choo, I. H., Lee, D. Y., Youn, J. C., Jhoo, J. H., Kim, K. W., Lee, D. S.,...Woo, J. I. (2007).
Topographic patterns of brain functional impairment progression according to clinical
severity staging in 116 Alzheimer disease patients: FDG-PET study. *Alzheimer Disease
and Associated Disorders, 21*(2), 77–84.

Davies, R. R., Kipps, C. M., Mitchell, J., Kril, J. J., Halliday, G. M., & Hodges, J. R. (2006). Progression in frontotemporal dementia: Identifying a benign behavioral variant by magnetic resonance imaging. *Archives of Neurology, 63*(11), 1627–1631.

DeCarli, C., Frisoni, G. B., Clark, C. M., Harvey, D., Grundman, M., Petersen, R. C., … Scheltens, P.; Alzheimer's Disease Cooperative Study Group. (2007). Qualitative estimates of medial temporal atrophy as a predictor of progression from mild cognitive impairment to dementia. *Archives of Neurology, 64*(1), 108–115.

de la Torre Laviana, F. J. (2009). Bilateral hyperintensity of the pulvinar in sporadic Creutzfeldt-Jakob disease. *Neurologia, 24*(3), 202–208.

Du, A. T., Schuff, N., Kramer, J. H., Rosen, H. J., Gorno-Tempini, M. L., Rankin, K., … Weiner, M. W. (2007). Different regional patterns of cortical thinning in Alzheimer's disease and frontotemporal dementia. *Brain: A Journal of Neurology, 130*(Pt 4), 1159–1166.

Dubois, B., Feldman, H. H., Jacova, C., Dekosky, S. T., Barberger-Gateau, P., Cummings, J., … Scheltens, P. (2007). Research criteria for the diagnosis of Alzheimer's disease: Revising the NINCDS-ADRDA criteria. *Lancet Neurology, 6*(8), 734–746.

Duning, T., Warnecke, T., Mohammadi, S., Lohmann, H., Schiffbauer, H., Kugel, H., … Deppe, M. (2009). Pattern and progression of white-matter changes in a case of posterior cortical atrophy using diffusion tensor imaging. *Journal of Neurology, Neurosurgery, and Psychiatry, 80*(4), 432–436.

Forsberg, A., Engler, H., Almkvist, O., Blomquist, G., Hagman, G., Wall, A., … Nordberg, A. (2008). PET imaging of amyloid deposition in patients with mild cognitive impairment. *Neurobiology of Aging, 29*(10), 1456–1465.

Foster, N. L., Gilman, S., Berent, S., Morin, E. M., Brown, M. B., & Koeppe, R. A. (1988). Cerebral hypometabolism in progressive supranuclear palsy studied with positron emission tomography. *Annals of Neurology, 24*(3), 399–406.

Foster, N. L., Heidebrink, J. L., Clark, C. M., Jagust, W. J., Arnold, S. E., Barbas, N. R., … Minoshima, S. (2007). FDG-PET improves accuracy in distinguishing frontotemporal dementia and Alzheimer's disease. *Brain: A Journal of Neurology, 130*(Pt 10), 2616–2635.

Frisoni, G. B., Fox, N. C., Jack, C. R., Scheltens, P., & Thompson, P. M. (2010). The clinical use of structural MRI in Alzheimer disease. *Nature Reviews. Neurology, 6*(2), 67–77.

Frisoni, G. B., Pievani, M., Testa, C., Sabattoli, F., Bresciani, L., Bonetti, M., … Thompson, P. M. (2007). The topography of grey matter involvement in early and late onset Alzheimer's disease. *Brain: A Journal of Neurology, 130*(Pt 3), 720–730.

Galton, C. J., Patterson, K., Graham, K., Lambon-Ralph, M. A., Williams, G., Antoun, N., … Hodges, J. R. (2001). Differing patterns of temporal atrophy in Alzheimer's disease and semantic dementia. *Neurology, 57*(2), 216–225.

Goethals, M., & Santens, P. (2001). Posterior cortical atrophy. Two case reports and a review of the literature. *Clinical Neurology and Neurosurgery, 103*(2), 115–119.

Gorno-Tempini, M. L., Dronkers, N. F., Rankin, K. P., Ogar, J. M., Phengrasamy, L., Rosen, H. J., … Miller, B. L. (2004). Cognition and anatomy in three variants of primary progressive aphasia. *Annals of Neurology, 55*(3), 335–346.

Gorno-Tempini, M. L., Murray, R. C., Rankin, K. P., Weiner, M. W., & Miller, B. L. (2004). Clinical, cognitive and anatomical evolution from nonfluent progressive aphasia to corticobasal syndrome: A case report. *Neurocase, 10*(6), 426–436.

Gorno-Tempini, M. L., Hillis, A. E., Weintraub, S., Kertesz, A., Mendez, M., Cappa, S. F., … Grossman, M. (2011). Classification of primary progressive aphasia and its variants. *Neurology, 76*(11), 1006–1014.

Hachinski, V. C., Lassen, N. A., & Marshall, J. (1974). Multi-infarct dementia. A cause of mental deterioration in the elderly. *Lancet, 2*(7874), 207–210.

Hensel, A., Ibach, B., Muller, U., Kruggel, F., Kiefer, M., & Gertz, H. J. (2004). Does the pattern of atrophy of the Corpus callosum differ between patients with frontotemporal dementia and patients with Alzheimer's disease? *Dementia and Geriatric Cognitive Disorders, 18*(1), 44–49.

Herholz, K. (2003). PET studies in dementia. *Annals of Nuclear Medicine, 17*(2), 79–89.

Herholz, K., Carter, S. F., & Jones, M. (2007). Positron emission tomography imaging in dementia. *The British Journal of Radiology, 80*(Spec No 2), S160–S167.

Hoffman, J. M., Welsh-Bohmer, K. A., Hanson, M., Crain, B., Hulette, C., Earl, N., & Coleman, R. E. (2000). FDG PET imaging in patients with pathologically verified dementia. *Journal of Nuclear Medicine, 41*(11), 1920–1928.

Ishii, K., Imamura, T., Sasaki, M., Yamaji, S., Sakamoto, S., Kitagaki, H.,…Mori, E. (1998). Regional cerebral glucose metabolism in dementia with Lewy bodies and Alzheimer's disease. *Neurology, 51*(1), 125–130.

Ishii, K., Kawachi, T., Sasaki, H., Kono, A. K., Fukuda, T., Kojima, Y., & Mori, E. (2005). Voxel-based morphometric comparison between early- and late-onset mild Alzheimer's disease and assessment of diagnostic performance of z score images. *American Journal of Neuroradiology, 26*(2), 333–340.

Jack, C. R. Jr., Lowe, V. J., Weigand, S. D., Wiste, H. J., Senjem, M. L., Knopman, D. S., … Petersen, R. C; Alzheimer's Disease Neuroimaging Initiative. (2009). Serial PIB and MRI in normal, mild cognitive impairment and Alzheimer's disease: Implications for sequence of pathological events in Alzheimer's disease. *Brain, 132*(Pt 5), 1355–1365.

Jagust, W., Reed, B., Mungas, D., Ellis, W., & Decarli, C. (2007). What does fluorodeoxyglucose PET imaging add to a clinical diagnosis of dementia? *Neurology, 69*(9), 871–877.

Josephs, K. A., Duffy, J. R., Strand, E. A., Whitwell, J. L., Layton, K. F., Parisi, J. E.,…Petersen, R. C. (2006). Clinicopathological and imaging correlates of progressive aphasia and apraxia of speech. *Brain: A Journal of Neurology, 129*(Pt 6), 1385–1398.

Josephs, K. A., Whitwell, J. L., Knopman, D. S., Boeve, B. F., Vemuri, P., Senjem, M. L.,…Jack, C. R. (2009). Two distinct subtypes of right temporal variant frontotemporal dementia. *Neurology, 73*(18), 1443–1450.

Josephs, K. A. Jr., Whitwell, J. L., Weigand, S. D., Senjem, M. L., Boeve, B. F., Knopman, D. S., … Petersen, R. C. (2011). Predicting functional decline in behavioural variant frontotemporal dementia. *Brain, 134*(Pt 2), 432–448.

Juh, R., Pae, C. U., Kim, T. S., Lee, C. U., Choe, B., & Suh, T. (2005). Cerebral glucose metabolism in corticobasal degeneration comparison with progressive supranuclear palsy using statistical mapping analysis. *Neuroscience Letters, 383*(1–2), 22–27.

Kanda, T., Ishii, K., Uemura, T., Miyamoto, N., Yoshikawa, T., Kono, A. K., & Mori, E. (2008). Comparison of grey matter and metabolic reductions in frontotemporal dementia using FDG-PET and voxel-based morphometric MR studies. *European Journal of Nuclear Medicine and Molecular Imaging, 35*(12), 2227–2234.

Karas, G., Scheltens, P., Rombouts, S., van Schijndel, R., Klein, M., Jones, B.,…Barkhof, F. (2007). Precuneus atrophy in early-onset Alzheimer's disease: A morphometric structural MRI study. *Neuroradiology, 49*(12), 967–976.

Kertesz, A., Martinez-Lage, P., Davidson, W., & Munoz, D. G. (2000). The corticobasal degeneration syndrome overlaps progressive aphasia and frontotemporal dementia. *Neurology, 55*(9), 1368–1375.

Killiany, R. J., Gomez-Isla, T., Moss, M., Kikinis, R., Sandor, T., Jolesz, F.,…Albert, M. S. (2000). Use of structural magnetic resonance imaging to predict who will get Alzheimer's disease. *Annals of Neurology, 47*(4), 430–439.

Kipps, C. M., Hodges, J. R., Fryer, T. D., & Nestor, P. J. (2009). Combined magnetic resonance imaging and positron emission tomography brain imaging in behavioural variant frontotemporal degeneration: Refining the clinical phenotype. *Brain: A Journal of Neurology, 132*(Pt 9), 2566–2578.

Knopman, D. S., DeKosky, S. T., Cummings, J. L., Chui, H., Corey-Bloom, J., Relkin, N.,… Stevens, J. C. (2001). Practice parameter: Diagnosis of dementia (an evidence-based review). Report of the Quality Standards Subcommittee of the American Academy of Neurology. *Neurology, 56*(9), 1143–1153.

Kramer, J. H., Reed, B. R., Mungas, D., Weiner, M. W., & Chui, H. C. (2002). Executive dysfunction in subcortical ischaemic vascular disease. *Journal of Neurology, Neurosurgery, and Psychiatry, 72*(2), 217–220.

Kreisler, A., Defebvre, L., Lecouffe, P., Duhamel, A., Charpentier, P., Steinling, M., & Destée, A. (2005). Corticobasal degeneration and Parkinson's disease assessed by HmPaO SPECT: The utility of factorial discriminant analysis. *Movement Disorders: Official Journal of the Movement Disorder Society, 20*(11), 1431–1438.

Kril, J. J., Macdonald, V., Patel, S., Png, F., & Halliday, G. M. (2005). Distribution of brain atrophy in behavioral variant frontotemporal dementia. *Journal of the Neurological Sciences, 232*(1–2), 83–90.

Le Ber, I., Camuzat, A., Hannequin, D., Pasquier, F., Guedj, E., Rovelet-Lecrux, A.,…Brice, A.; French research network on FTD/FTD-MND. (2008). Phenotype variability in progranulin mutation carriers: A clinical, neuropsychological, imaging and genetic study. *Brain: A Journal of Neurology, 131*(Pt 3), 732–746.

Lee, S. H., Bae, H. J., Ko, S. B., Kim, H., Yoon, B. W., & Roh, J. K. (2004). Comparative analysis of the spatial distribution and severity of cerebral microbleeds and old lacunes. *Journal of Neurology, Neurosurgery, and Psychiatry, 75*(3), 423–427.

Lehmann, M., Rohrer, J. D., Clarkson, M. J., Ridgway, G. R., Scahill, R. I., Modat, M.,…Fox, N. C. (2010). Reduced cortical thickness in the posterior cingulate gyrus is characteristic of both typical and atypical Alzheimer's disease. *Journal of Alzheimer's Disease, 20*(2), 587–598.

McKeith, I., O'Brien, J., Walker, Z., Tatsch, K., Booij, J., Darcourt, J., Padovani, A.,…Reininger, C.; DLB Study Group. (2007). Sensitivity and specificity of dopamine transporter imaging with 123I-FP-CIT SPECT in dementia with Lewy bodies: A phase III, multicentre study. *Lancet Neurology, 6*(4), 305–313.

McKeith, I. G., Dickson, D. W., Lowe, J., Emre, M., O'Brien, J. T., Feldman, H.,…Yamada, M.; Consortium on DLB. (2005). Diagnosis and management of dementia with Lewy bodies: Third report of the DLB Consortium. *Neurology, 65*(12), 1863–1872.

McKhann, G. M., Knopman, D. S., Chertkow, H., Hyman, B. T., Jack, C. R., Kawas, C. H.,… Phelps, C. H. (2011). The diagnosis of dementia due to Alzheimer's disease: Recommendations from the National Institute on Aging-Alzheimer's Association workgroups on diagnostic guidelines for Alzheimer's disease. *Alzheimer's & Dementia: The Journal of the Alzheimer's Association, 7*(3), 263–269.

McMonagle, P., Deering, F., Berliner, Y., & Kertesz, A. (2006). The cognitive profile of posterior cortical atrophy. *Neurology, 66*(3), 331–338.

Migliaccio, R., Agosta, F., Rascovsky, K., Karydas, A., Bonasera, S., Rabinovici, G. D.,…Gorno-Tempini, M. L. (2009). Clinical syndromes associated with posterior atrophy: Early age at onset AD spectrum. *Neurology, 73*(19), 1571–1578.

Mihara, M., Sugase, S., Konaka, K., Sugai, F., Sato, T., Yamamoto, Y.,…Sakoda, S. (2005). The "pulvinar sign" in a case of paraneoplastic limbic encephalitis associated with non-Hodgkin's lymphoma. *Journal of Neurology, Neurosurgery, and Psychiatry, 76*(6), 882–884.

Minoshima, S., Giordani, B., Berent, S., Frey, K. A., Foster, N. L., & Kuhl, D. E. (1997). Metabolic reduction in the posterior cingulate cortex in very early Alzheimer's disease. *Annals of Neurology, 42*(1), 85–94.

Morbelli, S., Piccardo, A., Villavecchia, G., Dessi, B., Brugnolo, A., Piccini, A.,…Nobili, F. (2010). Mapping brain morphological and functional conversion patterns in amnestic MCI: A voxel-based MRI and FDG-PET study. *European Journal of Nuclear Medicine and Molecular Imaging, 37*(1), 36–45.

Morinaga, A., Ono, K., Ikeda, T., Ikeda, Y., Shima, K., Noguchi-Shinohara, M.,…Yamada, M. (2010). A comparison of the diagnostic sensitivity of MRI, CBF-SPECT, FDG-PET and cerebrospinal fluid biomarkers for detecting Alzheimer's disease in a memory clinic. *Dementia and Geriatric Cognitive Disorders, 30*(4), 285–292.

Mummery, C. J., Patterson, K., Price, C. J., Ashburner, J., Frackowiak, R. S., & Hodges, J. R. (2000). A voxel-based morphometry study of semantic dementia: Relationship between temporal lobe atrophy and semantic memory. *Annals of Neurology, 47*(1), 36–45.

Neary, D., Snowden, J. S., Gustafson, L., Passant, U., Stuss, D., Black, S.,…Benson, D. F. (1998). Frontotemporal lobar degeneration: A consensus on clinical diagnostic criteria. *Neurology, 51*(6), 1546–1554.

Nestor, P. J., Caine, D., Fryer, T. D., Clarke, J., & Hodges, J. R. (2003). The topography of metabolic deficits in posterior cortical atrophy (the visual variant of Alzheimer's disease) with FDG-PET. *Journal of Neurology, Neurosurgery, and Psychiatry, 74*(11), 1521–1529.

Nordberg, A. (2008). Amyloid plaque imaging in vivo: Current achievement and future prospects. *European Journal of Nuclear Medicine and Molecular Imaging, 35*(Suppl 1), S46–S50.

Oba, H., Yagishita, A., Terada, H., Barkovich, A. J., Kutomi, K., Yamauchi, T.,…Suzuki, S. (2005). New and reliable MRI diagnosis for progressive supranuclear palsy. *Neurology, 64*(12), 2050–2055.

O'Brien, J. T., McKeith, I. G., Walker, Z., Tatsch, K., Booij, J., Darcourt, J.,…Reininger, C.; DLB Study Group. (2009). Diagnostic accuracy of 123I-FP-CIT SPECT in possible dementia with Lewy bodies. *The British Journal of Psychiatry: The Journal of Mental Science, 194*(1), 34–39.

Okello, A., Koivunen, J., Edison, P., Archer, H. A., Turkheimer, F. E., Någren, K.,…Brooks, D. J. (2009). Conversion of amyloid positive and negative MCI to AD over 3 years: An 11C-PIB PET study. *Neurology, 73*(10), 754–760.

Petersen, R. C. (2004). Mild cognitive impairment as a diagnostic entity. *Journal of Internal Medicine, 256*(3), 183–194.

Piguet, O., Hornberger, M., Mioshi, E., & Hodges, J. R. (2011). Behavioural-variant frontotemporal dementia: Diagnosis, clinical staging, and management. *Lancet Neurology, 10*(2), 162–172.

Pohjasvaara, T., Erkinjuntti, T., Ylikoski, R., Hietanen, M., Vataja, R., & Kaste, M. (1998). Clinical determinants of poststroke dementia. *Stroke; A Journal of Cerebral Circulation, 29*(1), 75–81.

Quattrone, A., Nicoletti, G., Messina, D., Fera, F., Condino, F., Pugliese, P.,…Gallo, O. (2008). MR imaging index for differentiation of progressive supranuclear palsy from Parkinson disease and the Parkinson variant of multiple system atrophy. *Radiology, 246*(1), 214–221.

Rabinovici, G. D., Furst, A. J., O'Neil, J. P., Racine, C. A., Mormino, E. C., Baker, S. L., . . . Jagust, W. J. (2007). 11C-PIB PET imaging in Alzheimer disease and frontotemporal lobar degeneration. *Neurology, 68*(15), 1205–1212.

Rabinovici, G. D., Jagust, W. J., Furst, A. J., Ogar, J. M., Racine, C. A., Mormino, E. C., . . . Gorno-Tempini, M. L. (2008). Abeta amyloid and glucose metabolism in three variants of primary progressive aphasia. *Annals of Neurology, 64*(4), 388–401.

Rabinovici, G. D., & Miller, B. L. (2010). Frontotemporal lobar degeneration: Epidemiology, pathophysiology, diagnosis and management. *CNS Drugs, 24*(5), 375–398.

Rascovsky, K., Hodges, J. R., Kipps, C. M., Johnson, J. K., Seeley, W. W., Mendez, M. F., . . . Miller, B. M. (2007). Diagnostic criteria for the behavioral variant of frontotemporal dementia (bvFTD): Current limitations and future directions. *Alzheimer Disease and Associated Disorders, 21*(4), S14–S18.

Rizzo, G., Martinelli, P., Manners, D., Scaglione, C., Tonon, C., Cortelli, P., . . . Lodi, R. (2008). Diffusion-weighted brain imaging study of patients with clinical diagnosis of corticobasal degeneration, progressive supranuclear palsy and Parkinson's disease. *Brain: A Journal of Neurology, 131*(Pt 10), 2690–2700.

Román, G. C. (2004). Facts, myths, and controversies in vascular dementia. *Journal of the Neurological Sciences, 226*(1–2), 49–52.

Román, G. C., Tatemichi, T. K., Erkinjuntti, T., Cummings, J. L., Masdeu, J. C., Garcia, J. H., . . . Hofman, A. (1993). Vascular dementia: Diagnostic criteria for research studies. Report of the NINDS-AIREN International Workshop. *Neurology, 43*(2), 250–260.

Rosen, H. J., Gorno-Tempini, M. L., Goldman, W. P., Perry, R. J., Schuff, N., Weiner, M., . . . Miller, B. L. (2002). Patterns of brain atrophy in frontotemporal dementia and semantic dementia. *Neurology, 58*(2), 198–208.

Rosen, H. J., Wilson, M. R., Schauer, G. F., Allison, S., Gorno-Tempini, M. L., Pace-Savitsky, C., . . . Miller, B. L. (2006). Neuroanatomical correlates of impaired recognition of emotion in dementia. *Neuropsychologia, 44*(3), 365–373.

Ross, S. J., Graham, N., Stuart-Green, L., Prins, M., Xuereb, J., Patterson, K., & Hodges, J. R. (1996). Progressive biparietal atrophy: An atypical presentation of Alzheimer's disease. *Journal of Neurology, Neurosurgery, and Psychiatry, 61*(4), 388–395.

Savoiardo, M., Grisoli, M., & Girotti, F. (2000). Magnetic resonance imaging in CBD, related atypical parkinsonian disorders, and dementias. *Advances in Neurology, 82*, 197–208.

Schmidtke, K., Hüll, M., & Talazko, J. (2005). Posterior cortical atrophy: Variant of Alzheimer's disease? A case series with PET findings. *Journal of Neurology, 252*(1), 27–35.

Seeley, W. W., Crawford, R., Rascovsky, K., Kramer, J. H., Weiner, M., Miller, B. L., & Gorno-Tempini, M. L. (2008). Frontal paralimbic network atrophy in very mild behavioral variant frontotemporal dementia. *Archives of Neurology, 65*(2), 249–255.

Shi, F., Liu, B., Zhou, Y., Yu, C., & Jiang, T. (2009). Hippocampal volume and asymmetry in mild cognitive impairment and Alzheimer's disease: Meta-analyses of MRI studies. *Hippocampus, 19*(11), 1055–1064.

Shiga, Y., Miyazawa, K., Sato, S., Fukushima, R., Shibuya, S., Sato, Y., . . . Itoyama, Y. (2004). Diffusion-weighted MRI abnormalities as an early diagnostic marker for Creutzfeldt-Jakob disease. *Neurology, 63*(3), 443–449.

Sluimer, J. D., Bouwman, F. H., Vrenken, H., Blankenstein, M. A., Barkhof, F., van der Flier, W. M., & Scheltens, P. (2010). Whole-brain atrophy rate and CSF biomarker levels in MCI and AD: A longitudinal study. *Neurobiology of Aging, 31*(5), 758–764.

Tang, C. C., Poston, K. L., Eckert, T., Feigin, A., Frucht, S., Gudesblatt, M., . . . Eidelberg, D. (2010). Differential diagnosis of parkinsonism: A metabolic imaging study using pattern analysis. *Lancet Neurology, 9*(2), 149–158.

Tang-Wai, D. F., Graff-Radford, N. R., Boeve, B. F., Dickson, D. W., Parisi, J. E., Crook, R.,...
Petersen, R. C. (2004). Clinical, genetic, and neuropathologic characteristics of posterior
cortical atrophy. *Neurology, 63*(7), 1168–1174.

Tatsch, K. (2008). Imaging of the dopaminergic system in differential diagnosis of
dementia. *European Journal of Nuclear Medicine and Molecular Imaging, 35*(Suppl 1),
S51–S57.

Tian, H. J., Zhang, J. T., Lang, S. Y., & Wang, X. Q. (2010). MRI sequence findings in sporadic
Creutzfeldt-Jakob disease. *Journal of Clinical Neuroscience, 17*(11), 1378–1380.

Turner, R. S., Kenyon, L. C., Trojanowski, J. Q., Gonatas, N., & Grossman, M. (1996). Clinical,
neuroimaging, and pathologic features of progressive nonfluent aphasia. *Annals of
Neurology, 39*(2), 166–173.

van der Flier, W. M., van Straaten, E. C., Barkhof, F., Ferro, J. M., Pantoni, L., Basile, A.
M.,...Scheltens, P.; LADIS Study Group. (2005). Medial temporal lobe atrophy and
white matter hyperintensities are associated with mild cognitive deficits in non-disabled
elderly people: The LADIS study. *Journal of Neurology, Neurosurgery, and Psychiatry,
76*(11), 1497–1500.

Vitali, P., Maccagnano, E., Caverzasi, E., Henry, R. G., Haman, A., Torres-Chae, C.,...
Geschwind, M. D. (2011). Diffusion-weighted MRI hyperintensity patterns differentiate
CJD from other rapid dementias. *Neurology, 76*(20), 1711–1719.

Warmuth-Metz, M., Naumann, M., Csoti, I., & Solymosi, L. (2001). Measurement of the midbrain diameter on routine magnetic resonance imaging: A simple and accurate method of
differentiating between Parkinson disease and progressive supranuclear palsy. *Archives
of Neurology, 58*(7), 1076–1079.

Whitwell, J. L., Avula, R., Senjem, M. L., Kantarci, K., Weigand, S. D., Samikoglu, A.,...
Jack, C. R. (2010). Gray and white matter water diffusion in the syndromic variants of
frontotemporal dementia. *Neurology, 74*(16), 1279–1287.

Whitwell, J. L., Jack, C. R., Boeve, B. F., Parisi, J. E., Ahlskog, J. E., Drubach, D. A.,...
Josephs, K. A. (2010). Imaging correlates of pathology in corticobasal syndrome.
Neurology, 75(21), 1879–1887.

Whitwell, J. L., Przybelski, S. A., Weigand, S. D., Ivnik, R. J., Vemuri, P., Gunter, J. L.,...
Josephs, K. A. (2009). Distinct anatomical subtypes of the behavioural variant of frontotemporal dementia: A cluster analysis study. *Brain: A Journal of Neurology, 132*(Pt 11),
2932–2946.

Yamauchi, H., Fukuyama, H., Nagahama, Y., Katsumi, Y., Hayashi, T., Oyanagi, C.,...
Shio, H. (2000). Comparison of the pattern of atrophy of the corpus callosum in fronto-
temporal dementia, progressive supranuclear palsy, and Alzheimer's disease. *Journal of
Neurology, Neurosurgery, and Psychiatry, 69*(5), 623–629.

Young, G. S., Geschwind, M. D., Fischbein, N. J., Martindale, J. L., Henry, R. G., Liu, S.,...
Dillon, W. P. (2005). Diffusion-weighted and fluid-attenuated inversion recovery imag-
ing in Creutzfeldt-Jakob disease: High sensitivity and specificity for diagnosis. *American
Journal of Neuroradiology, 26*(6), 1551–1562.

Yuan, Y., Gu, Z. X., & Wei, W. S. (2009). Fluorodeoxyglucose-positron-emission tomography,
single-photon emission tomography, and structural MR imaging for prediction of rapid
conversion to Alzheimer disease in patients with mild cognitive impairment: A meta-
analysis. *American Journal of Neuroradiology, 30*(2), 404–410.

Zeidler, M., Sellar, R. J., Collie, D. A., Knight, R., Stewart, G., Macleod, M. A.,...
Colchester, A. F. (2000). The pulvinar sign on magnetic resonance imaging in variant
Creutzfeldt-Jakob disease. *Lancet, 355*(9213), 1412–1418.

Zerr, I., Kallenberg, K., Summers, D. M., Romero, C., Taratuto, A., Heinemann, U.,... Sanchez-Juan, P. (2009). Updated clinical diagnostic criteria for sporadic Creutzfeldt-Jakob disease. *Brain: A Journal of Neurology, 132*(Pt 10), 2659–2668.

Zhang, Y., Schuff, N., Du, A. T., Rosen, H. J., Kramer, J. H., Gorno-Tempini, M. L.,... Weiner, M. W. (2009). White matter damage in frontotemporal dementia and Alzheimer's disease measured by diffusion MRI. *Brain: A Journal of Neurology, 132*(Pt 9), 2579–2592.

Zhou, J., Greicius, M. D., Gennatas, E. D., Growdon, M. E., Jang, J. Y., Rabinovici, G. D.,... Seeley, W. W. (2010). Divergent network connectivity changes in behavioural variant frontotemporal dementia and Alzheimer's disease. *Brain: A Journal of Neurology, 133*(Pt 5), 1352–1367.

CHAPTER 3

Neuropsychological Assessment and Differential Diagnosis of Cortical Dementias

Melissa L. Edwards, Valerie Hobson Balldin, and Sid E. O'Bryant

With the elderly population rapidly increasing worldwide, neuropsychologists are often called upon to conduct assessments of possible neurodegenerative disorders. As such, a fundamental understanding of these conditions is key for practitioners and scientists alike. Neuropsychological testing plays a critical role in the assessment of neurodegenerative dementias for a wide range of reasons including differential diagnosis, treatment planning, progress monitoring, selection for entry into thera- peutic trials, as well as detecting efficacy of novel treatments. This chapter will pro- vide an overview of the differential diagnostics via neuropsychological methods of cortical dementia syndromes.

Over the last several decades, clinicians have seen significant changes with regard to daily practice in interprofessional settings, which are becoming more com- monplace for practicing neuropsychologists. As such, practitioners have become integral parts of teams and are regularly asked to put their evaluation into the con- text of a broader medical evaluation. Therefore, this chapter is intended to provide guidance/input/assistance for practitioners working in such settings. While the debate of "fixed versus flexible" batteries is somewhat relevant to this context, this will not be discussed. However, the length of examination is a significant point for consideration with the current climate calling for "briefer" examinations in many clinical settings. One consideration is the fact that many payment parties will restrict the number of allowable hours for examinations. The working relationship with the broader team or referring physician is another consideration. Last, and most important, is patient burden. In particular, the clinician must balance obtaining suf- ficient information without overwhelming the patient. Geriatric patients regularly are unable to complete full-day evaluations due to fatigue, and multiple visits are oftentimes impractical.

When considering specific tests to utilize in the assessment of possible neuro- degenerative syndromes, it is important to note the literature on the tests. There is a large amount of literature on neurodegenerative diseases that is growing every day. However, there are neuropsychological instruments that are commonly utilized in dementia batteries (clinical and research); utilization of these measures will allow the clinician to directly compare findings from his or her patients to the literature published by the leading research groups on these diseases. Each of the measures outlined in the following text has been utilized substantially in dementia research, clinic based and/or population based. Additionally, the current authors are in the process of generating normative data on many of the tests outlined in this chapter, specifically for English- and Spanish-speaking Mexican American elders in a project entitled the "Texas Mexican American Normative Studies."

OVERVIEW OF COMMONLY UTILIZED INSTRUMENTS IN DEMENTIA BATTERIES

Of note, this is not an exhaustive list of neuropsychological instruments, but only a review of some of the more frequently utilized instruments in dementia protocols.

Global Cognition

Mini-Mental State Examination (MMSE; Folstein, Folstein, & McHugh, 1975) is the most commonly administered psychometric screening assessment of global cognitive functioning. The MMSE assesses working memory, recall, orientation, naming, ability to follow commands, reading, and writing, and is used to screen for global cognitive impairment, track changes in cognitive functioning over time, and oftentimes to assess the effects of therapeutic agents on cognitive function (Strauss, Sherman, & Spreen, 2006). Since its development, there has been a wealth of literature published on the MMSE, demonstrating it to be a relatively sensitive marker of dementia (Harvan & Cotter, 2006). The MMSE has demonstrated high reliability, sensitivity, and characterization of cognitive decline in dementia patients over time. Research has also shown that the MMSE is reliable in predicting functional abilities (Razani et al., 2009). The MMSE has been adapted to more than a dozen languages, and is used with diverse ethnicities and individuals from different socioeconomic status groups. In addition, the MMSE has been shown to be useful in individuals with low education as well as with highly educated individuals when the cut-off score is adjusted (O'Bryant et al., 2008; Spering et al., 2012). Although not a neuropsychological instrument, the MMSE is regularly administered in dementia clinics and research settings alike and may be useful for comparison purposes.

The Montreal Cognitive Assessment (MoCA) was developed as a tool to screen patients with mild cognitive complaints who generally perform in the normal range on the MMSE. It is a one-page 30-point test that can be administered in 10 minutes. This assessment tests short-term memory recall, visuospatial abilities, executive functioning, phonemic fluency, verbal abstraction, attention, concentration, working memory, and orientation to time and place (Nasreddine et al., 2005).

Saint Louis University Mental Status Examination (SLUMS) is a 30-point, 11-item clinician-administered scale similar in format to the MMSE. The SLUMS supplements the MMSE with enhanced tasks. The SLUMS is similar to the MMSE in sensitivity and specificity; however, the SLUMS was slightly better than the MMSE in differentiating a mild neurocognitive disorder from normal cognitive functioning (Tariq, Tumosa, Chibnall, Perry, & Morley, 2006).

Dementia Severity

The Clinical Dementia Rating scale (CDR) is a widely used rating scale for measuring dementia severity. The CDR assesses memory, temporal orientation, judgment and problem solving, community activities, and home activities and hobbies (Lezak, 2004). The CDR yields both a global (CDR-GS) and a sum of boxes (CDR-SB) score. The CDR-GS is typically used for staging purposes, while the CDR-SB is more of a detailed quantitative general index. O'Bryant et al. demonstrated that the CDR-SB scores could be used to stage dementia, and the CDR-SB reliably discriminated between mild cognitive impairment (MCI) and very early Alzheimer's disease (AD; O'Bryant et al., 2008, 2010).

Attention

Digit Span is a component of the Wechsler Memory Scale-IV (or WMS-IV; Weschler, 2009), which is a task used for measuring simple attention (digit span forward) and working memory (digits backward).

Trails Making Test (TMTA and TMTB) is a neuropsychological instrument that measures attention, processing speed, and mental flexibility, and is considered to be a sensitive marker of cognitive dysfunction and decline (Strauss et al., 2006).

Memory

The WMS-IV (Wechsler, 2009) is a memory battery that assesses a range of memory skills with the most commonly utilized being tasks of immediate and delayed verbal and visual memory through a range of story, figure, and list-learning tasks. The WMS-III Logical Memory (LM-I and LM-II) subtest is the most common story-memory task; in fact, Story 1 is currently included as part of the National Alzheimer's Coordinating Center (NACC) Uniform Data Set (UDS). Visual Reproduction (VR-I and VR-II) is commonly utilized to tap visual memory capacity.

The California Verbal Learning Test (CVLT; Delis & Kramer, 2000) is a 16-item word-learning test presented over five trials. Immediately after the last learning trial, a second list of 16 words is presented as an interference trial, followed by a short (a few minutes) and a long (20 minutes) delayed free and cued recall of the original list, and a recognition memory trial. The CVLT-Short Form (CVLT-SF; Delis & Kramer, 2000) is a measure of verbal learning and memory where a list of 9 words is given repeatedly over 4 trials and delayed recall is obtained after a short 10-minute delay. This test provides information on immediate and delayed memory.

The Rey Auditory-Verbal Learning Test (AVLT; Rey, 1964; Schmidt, 1996) is a measure comprised of verbal exposure to 15 words (list A) over 5 trials, a presentation of an interference list (list B), one immediate recall followed by a 30-minute delayed recall, and a recognition trial.

The Rey-Osterrieth Complex Figure (ROCF; Knight & Kaplan, 2003) measures delayed memory and consists of requiring that an individual recall a design from memory that was presented 30 minutes prior to the recall task.

Executive Functioning

Wisconsin Card Sorting Test (WCST; Heaton, 2008) is a complex measure of cognitive reasoning. Participants are instructed to match the 64 stimulus cards to 4 key cards; however, the cards can only be matched based on the principles of color, shape, or number.

The Executive Interview (EXIT25; Royall, Mahurin, & Gray, 1992) is a global measure of executive control that covers a range of tasks including sequencing, fluency, anomalous sentence repetition, thematic perception, automatic behaviors, and go–no-go tasks. EXIT25 scores are significantly correlated with other validated measures of executive functioning. Scores range from 0 to 50, with higher scores suggestive of greater impairment; a score of 15 or greater best discriminates nondemented elderly controls from those with dementing illnesses.

The Clocks Drawing Tests (CLOX-1 and CLOX-2; Royall, Cordes, & Polk, 1998) is a brief instrument that assesses executive functioning by requiring the participant to draw the figure of a clock from memory. The CLOX affords the opportunity to the clinician to take into account visuo-construction abilities when examining executive abilities.

The Stroop Color-Word Test (Jensen & Rohwer, 1966; Stroop, 1935) requires participants to read a list of words and correctly identify the color of the words or the color notated by the word, depending on the trial.

Language

Boston Naming Test (BNT; Kaplan, Goodglass, & Weintraub, 1983) is a 60-item measure that assesses language fluency, both semantic and phonemic. Participants are shown 60 pictures and are instructed to indicate the name of the object, if known.

Controlled Oral Word Association (Strauss et al., 2006) assesses both phonemic (FAS) and categorical (Animal Naming) fluency tasks, which are both standard neuropsychological assessment techniques that are sensitive indicators of cognitive dysfunction and dementia (Strauss et al., 2006).

Screening Batteries

Alzheimer's Disease Assessment Scale-Cognitive Subscale (ADAS-Cog; Rosen, Mohs, & Davis, 1984) contains 11 subtests, which include word recall, naming, following commands, construction, ideational praxis, orientation, word recognition, recall of test instructions, spoken language ability, word-finding difficulty, comprehension of spoken language, memory, praxis, and language. The ADAS-Cog is the most commonly utilized cognitive assessment tool in pharmaceutical trials of AD.

The Consortium to Establish a Registry for Alzheimer's Disease (CERAD; Morris, Heyman, et al., 1989; Morris, Edland, et al., 1993; Rosen et al., 1984) is a neuropsychological assessment battery that includes a verbal fluency test, BNT, MMSE, word-list memory, constructional praxis, word-list recall, and word-list recognition.

The Repeatable Battery for the Assessment of Neuropsychological Status (RBANS; Duff et al., 2005; Randolph, 1998) is a brief neuropsychological instrument that assesses multiple cognitive domains (Duff et al., 2005). It contains 12 subtests that combine to create five indices: Attention, Language, Visuospatial/ Constructional abilities, Immediate recall, and Delayed recall. The RBANS has accumulated a large amount of normative data (Aupperle, Beatty, Shelton, & Gontkovsky, 2002) and has well-established psychometric properties (Larson, Kirschner, Bode, Heinemann, & Goodman, 2005). The RBANS has been shown to have acceptable diagnostic accuracy in detecting AD (Clark, Hobson, & O'Bryant, 2010; Duff et al., 2008).

ALZHEIMER'S DISEASE

Overview

AD is the most common of the neurodegenerative dementias, with approximately 5.4 million Americans suffering from AD according to the 2011 Alzheimer's Disease Facts and Figures (Thies & Bleiler, 2011). AD is characteristic of a progressive decline in memory, executive functioning, visuospatial abilities, language, and behaviors as a result of neurodegeneration in the brain. There are multiple diagnostic criteria in use for AD, the most common being that of the *Diagnostic and Statistical Manual of Mental Disorders, Fifth Edition* (*DSM-5*; American Psychiatric Association, 2013) and the National Institute on Aging and Alzheimer's Association Workgroup (McKhann et al., 2011). The cognitive portion of the *DSM-5* criteria for AD is memory or learning impairment plus impairment in at least one other cognitive domain. The revised National Institute on Aging-Alzheimer's Association (NIA-AA) criteria require meeting the diagnosis of all-cause core criteria for dementia, which includes functional impairment, a change in cognition from prior levels of functioning; symptoms are not due to delirium or major psychiatric condition, and objective evidence of impairment is obtained through both (a) history provided by the patient and (b) objective assessment, which can be a "bedside" mental status evaluation or detailed neuropsychological assessment. For a diagnosis of probable AD dementia, one must meet the clinical core criteria for dementia as well as present with an insidious onset and cognitive disturbances that are classified as amnestic (memory disturbances) or nonamnestic (i.e., executive functioning, language, or visuospatial). It is noteworthy that memory impairment is no longer required as was the case prior to the National Institute of Neurological and Communicative Disorders and Stroke and the Alzheimer's Disease and Related Disorders Association (NINCDS–ADRDA) criteria for probable AD, and the current *DSM-5* criteria. The revised criteria provide information regarding known genetic mutations causing AD. Lastly, biomarkers (neuroimaging and cerebrospinal fluid [SCF]) are incorporated for increasing or decreasing the confidence of a diagnosis due to AD with pathophysiological evidence of AD. The introduction of AD-specific biomarkers is of importance and may be novel for many practitioners. While a review of these biomarkers is beyond the scope of this chapter, a brief mentioning of them is warranted and the reader is encouraged to review the new NIA-AA criteria along with reviews/literature provided in that manuscript. The first classes of biomarkers introduced are those related to brain amyloid-beta (Aβ): low CSF $A\beta_{1-42}$ and PET amyloid imaging (now Food and Drug Administration [FDA] approved for AD diagnostics). The second class of markers introduced was markers of "downstream neuronal degeneration or injury," which included CSF markers of tau (p-tau and total-tau) as well as changes in structural imaging and functional imaging (FDG [fluorodeoxyglucose]-PET). It was suggested that these markers will increase confidence in diagnosis of those who meet core clinical criteria, but they are not yet implemented in standard diagnostic processes due largely to lack of uniform standards. However, the clinicians should be aware of this change as they will be utilized more regularly as these assessments become more readily available. Revised criteria for possible AD as well as for pathophysiologically proved AD are also provided (i.e., meets clinical and neuropathological criteria).

Cognitive Symptoms

With AD, the most commonly reported initial symptom is a decline in semantic memory abilities, with additional deficits in executive functioning and language being common early symptoms. In rare cases, visual memory may be selectively impaired first, which is reflective of the posterior nature of the neuropathological progression. In terms of the differential diagnosis, it is important to keep in mind that the development of cognitive dysfunction among AD cases is insidious and the progression is slow, which must be queried with a valid informant during the interview process. Unfortunately, this insidious, slow nature also makes it quite difficult for loved ones to detect subtle changes early in the course of the disease though they oftentimes will acknowledge changes far beyond their initial disclosure upon detailed questioning.

Behavioral Symptoms

AD cases oftentimes experience behavioral, emotional, and personality changes. Depression and social withdrawal can be among the earliest manifestations of AD (Starkstein, Mizrahi, & Power, 2008). Although some patients experience such symptoms owing to insight into their declining mental status, anosognosia (lack of insight) is also common (Kashiwa et al., 2005). As with the cognitive presentation, these changes are typically insidious and may progress with some patients becoming violent and combative, while others may become more docile. Unfortunately, there is no current means for predicting what, if any, behavioral symptoms a particular AD patient will develop. However, what is clear from the literature is that the behavioral symptoms are the most distressing aspect of AD for family members (Robinson, Adkisson, & Weinrich, 2001).

Clinical Interview

As with any neuropsychological assessment, a key component is the clinical interview. In the case of AD, there are several topics that are particularly useful in making a differential diagnosis. In addition to obtaining a broader medical history, it is important to obtain a detailed history regarding the presentation and progression of cognitive symptoms, which requires a knowledgeable informant. One useful technique for obtaining a more precise estimate of the initial onset is the provision of an anchoring event/time. Specifically, on elicitation of initial symptoms and estimated duration, it can be helpful to then link that to an event and/or time near this time frame. If the patient reportedly began having problems "two years ago" and the evaluation is being conducted in December, the clinician may ask the informant "How was [insert patient's name] around Christmas time two years ago?" It is also important to know the results of the patient's medical evaluations. If neuroimaging has not been conducted, this should be completed to rule out other neurological illnesses that can lead to cognitive decline (e.g., normal pressure hydrocephalus, cerebrovascular disease). Clinicians should be aware that the FDA has now approved Aβ for diagnostic utility. Clinical labs (e.g., B_{12}, thyroid levels) and current medications also need to be taken into account as these can have significant impact on cognition. In order to determine if the patient fulfills criteria for dementia more broadly, the clinician must get a detailed report on the patient's activities of daily living (basic and instrumental). The CDR scale (outlined previously) can be useful in this process and there are functional assessment instruments available. The clinical distinction is whether the cognitive dysfunction has progressed sufficiently to cause impairment in the patient's daily life; without such impairment, the patient cannot be diagnosed with dementia.

Neuropsychological Assessment

Given the prototypical presentation common to most early AD cases, neuropsychological assessments of AD should include measures of memory (verbal and visual), executive functioning, and language at a minimum. While there is a visual variant of AD (Lee & Martin, 2004), early semantic memory problems are typical. Classic memory measures in AD batteries (brief or longer) are story and list-learning measures. AD patients oftentimes have greater difficulty with semantic fluency as compared to phonemic fluency, although this is not a rule. Simple attention (e.g., digit span) is typically retained in AD.

Differential Diagnosis

With the ever-growing public awareness, and fear, of AD, clinicians are examining an increased number of elderly patients who are experiencing earlier stages of disease progression. First and foremost is to determine if in fact the patient has objective impairments. A pattern of semantic memory along with semantic fluency impairment is commonly seen. With regards to memory, a pattern of poor learning followed by rapid decay of previously learned material is typical. Additionally, AD cases typically perform poorly on the recognition format. Deficits in executive functioning are also common. When in the context of a slow progression of disease by history, AD is highly suspect. If other medical illnesses are ruled out, AD is the likely conclusion. Early motor disturbances (e.g., rigidity, shuffling gait), hallucinations, rapid progression, and decline suggest against an AD diagnosis.

Biomarkers/Genetics

There are known genetic mutations that cause familial early-onset AD, which are mutations to the amyloid precursor protein (*APP*), presenilin 1 (*PSEN1*), and presenilin 2 (*PSEN2*) genes, which are autosomal and dominantly inherited. There are no definitive genetic markers of nonfamilial AD although many genes have been linked to this disease. The most powerful genetic risk factor for nonfamilial AD is the apolipoprotein E (*APOE*) gene with the e4 allele conveying the increased risk (Roses et al., 1994; Silverman et al., 2008). There has also been recent growth in blood-based biomarkers that have diagnostic utility in AD (O'Bryant et al., 2008, 2010).

Neuroimaging

MRI

AD is associated with neurodegenerative properties in the cerebral cortex, which are detectable by means of MRI (Dickerson et al., 2009). Neuroimaging has become increasingly utilized for assessing brain atrophy (Callen, Black, Gao, Caldwell, & Szalai, 2001; De Santi et al., 2001; Soininen et al., 1994) and has been shown to be a useful factor in determining "temporal progression in the neuropathology of Alzheimer's disease" (Driscoll et al., 2009; Fox, Cousens, Scahill, Harvey, & Rossor, 2000; Jack et al., 2004; Misra, Fan, & Davatzikos, 2009; Thambisetty et al., 2010). It has been suggested that thinning in the cortical regions is associated with symptom severity; in addition, it has been thought that this cortical thinning has the possibility of being utilized as an imaging biomarker for AD (Dickerson et al., 2009). As mentioned earlier, Aβ imaging via PET scan has now received FDA approval for diagnosis of AD.

FRONTOTEMPORAL DEMENTIA

Overview

Frontotemporal dementia (FTD) is a neurodegenerative disorder that commonly impacts individuals in midlife and is often mistaken for other disorders such as AD (McKhann et al., 2001; Pasquier, Lebert, Grymonprez, & Petit, 1995; Snowden, Neary, & Mann, 2002; Yamauchi et al., 2000). Prevalence rates indicate that FTD occurs in up to 20% of the presenile dementia cases, thereby making it the third most common primary form of neurodegenerative dementia, after AD (Scarmeas & Honig, 2004; Snowden et al., 2002). The onset of symptoms is reported to occur most commonly between the ages of 45 and 65 years; however, diagnosis can be made as early as at 30 years of age as well as in those older than 65 years (Snowden et al., 2002). It is reported that there is an equal rate of occurrence in both men and women across age ranges (Snowden et al., 2002). The mean duration of the disorder is 8 years, with the range of occurrence spanning anywhere from 2 to 20 years (Snowden et al., 2002). Additionally, the family history of the disease is only seen in about half of all diagnosed cases (Snowden et al., 2002).

FTD, which is often interchanged with the term *Pick's disease*, is known to be an all-encompassing term for several clinical dementia syndromes including semantic dementia (SD), primary progressive aphasia (PPA), cortical basal degeneration, and motor neuron disease of the FTD type (Snowden et al., 2002), which all are discussed later in this chapter. The clinical syndromes of FTD can be broken into groupings based on frontal or temporal variants of the disease. The syndromes associated with the temporal variant encompass symptoms regarding behavioral problems, whereas the syndromes associated with the frontal variant include symptoms related to deficits in language and executive functioning (Snowden et al., 2002). The most common presentation of FTD is related to behavioral dysfunction, specifically social and personal misconduct (Snowden et al., 2002).

Diagnosis

Diagnosis of FTD is based on two sets of proposed criteria; one proposed by Neary et al. (1998) and the other by the Lund and Manchester group (Englund et al., 1994). The Lund and Manchester group criterion focuses on a more behavioral description, whereas the criteria of Neary et al. (1998) focus largely on language-based descriptions.

Neuropsychological Assessment

FTD impacts cognition, specifically facets of attention and executive functioning. Deficits related to abstract constructs, set shifting, information processing, and verbal fluency, in addition to planning, are commonly observed among those with FTD (Scarmeas & Honig, 2004). Neuropsychological tests recommended for assessment of FTD include the WCST (Heaton, 2008), the Stroop Color-Word Test (Jensen & Rohwer, 1966; Stroop, 1935), and the Trails Making Tests (TMTA and TMTB; Strauss et al., 2006). Those with FTD experience greater difficulty with regard to tasks that require free recall in contrast to those requiring recognition. Therefore, recognition trials can often be useful in discriminating FTD from AD when memory decline begins to manifest (see the section on AD for review of memory tests). When compared with AD, those with FTD are shown to perform worse on tasks that require phonemic and semantic fluency (Elfgren, Passant, & Risberg, 1993; Miller et al., 1991;

Pasquier et al., 1995; Rascovsky et al., 2002; Scarmeas & Honig, 2004). Frequently administered neuropsychological tests of verbal fluency include those of phonemic (letter) and semantic (categorical) fluency (e.g., Controlled Oral Word Association; Strauss et al., 2006). Both FAS and Animal Naming have been shown to be sensitive indicators of cognitive dysfunction and dementia (Strauss et al., 2006). However, individuals with FTD often perform well on tasks that require the naming of pictures and word–picture matching (Hodges et al., 1999; Perry & Hodges, 2000) and therefore the BNT (Kaplan et al., 1983) is frequently useful in the differential diagnostic process. A commonly identified key neuropsychological difference between AD and FTD is early impairment of visuospatial abilities among FTD cases (Hodges, 2001; Neary, Snowden, Northen, & Goulding, 1988; Pasquier et al., 1995; Rascovsky et al., 2002; Rosen et al., 2002; Scarmeas & Honig, 2004).

Differential Diagnosis

Methods for distinguishing FTD from other cortical dementias should incorporate a comprehensive neuropsychological assessment that specifically incorporates language-based tasks. Because FTD presents with speech deficits, such as echolalia and perseverations, assessments should focus on this area in addition to phonemic and semantic fluency. Furthermore, FTD has a significant behavioral component that distinguishes it from other cortical dementias such as AD. Addressing behavioral factors such as personal and social awareness is important given that FTD is considered to impact the early loss of awareness of self and others. Additionally, it can be important when trying to diagnosis FTD to assess for signs of disinhibition or emotional unconcern. There are also affective changes that can be shown to occur with FTD including depression or anxiety. However, affective changes should be addressed carefully as they have been shown to differentially impact cognitive functioning on their own.

Biomarkers/Genetics

Genetic testing for FTD consists of testing for mutations of the *MAPT* gene located on chromosome 17 (Chemali, Withall, & Daffner, 2010; Hutton et al., 1998; van Swieten & Spillantini, 2007). There is a strong familial component with FTD and therefore mutations in the Progranulin (*GRN*) gene are examined due to its association with *TDP-43* positive inclusions (Baker et al., 2006; Cruts et al., 2006). Additional genetic testing includes that of the *VCP* and *CHMP2B* genes (Skibinski et al., 2005; Vance et al., 2006; Watts et al., 2004). With FTD, it is acknowledged that most cases display mutations in the *tau* gene, with familial and sporadic FTD cases showing localization on chromosome 17 (Clark et al., 1998; Dumanchin et al., 1998; Hutton et al., 1998; Poorkaj et al., 1998; Scarmeas & Honig, 2004; Spillantini, Bird, & Ghetti, 1998; Spillantini, Murrell, et al., 1998). Pathologically, FTD is shown to present with neuronal loss and subsequent astrocytic gliosis and spongiosus of the cortical layers of the brain encompassing the frontal and temporal lobes (Foster et al., 1997; Scarmeas & Honig, 2004; Spillantini, Murrell, et al., 1998).

Neuroimaging

Neuroimaging for FTD includes CT and MRI scans in addition to PET scanning to examine metabolic activity in the frontal lobes (Chemali et al., 2010). Additionally, the "knife-edge" atrophy demarcating the frontal and temporal regions from posterior regions of the cortex is considered a key neuroimaging feature (Snowden, Neary, & Mann, 2007).

DEMENTIA WITH LEWY BODIES

Overview

Lewy body disease (LBD) is clinically presented as a cortical dementia referred to as dementia with Lewy bodies (DLB). Symptoms include cognitive impairment, parkinsonism, psychosis (delusions and hallucinations), and remote confusion (Papka, Rubio, & Schiffer, 1998). DLB is the second most prevalent of all neurodegenerative diseases and is often misdiagnosed as AD due to similar diagnostic criteria (McKeith, Fairbairn, Perry, & Thompson, 1994; Perry, Irving, Blessed, Perry, & Fairbairn, 1989). The age of onset is suggested to range from 50 to 83 years with a projected life span ranging from 68 to 92 years of age (Del Ser et al., 2000; Papka et al., 1998). DLB is considered to be an alpha-synuclein metabolism disorder and is characterized by Lewy body inclusions (abnormal cytoplasmic inclusions) throughout the brain (Oda, Yamamoto, & Maeda, 2009). DLB also consists of acetylcholine (ACh) neuronal degeneration, which may account for the cognitive and emotional symptom overlap with AD (Oda et al., 2009). Behavioral symptoms include motor parkinsonism, specifically rigidity and bradykinesia. Additional behavioral symptoms include stooped posture, slow shuffling gait, and hypophonic speech. Clinical symptoms include cognitive impairment with additional psychiatric presentations including delirium and visual hallucination (McKeith et al., 1994).

Diagnosis

Clinical diagnostic criteria outlined by McKeith et al. (1994) state that spontaneous motor features of parkinsonism are required for diagnosis in addition to supportive features such as repeated falls, syncope, and transient loss of consciousness. Furthermore, features required for diagnosis of DLB include neuroleptic sensitivity, systematic delusions, and hallucinations. Two core features are (a) fluctuations in cognitive capacity marked by pronounced variability in attention and alertness and (b) recurrent, well-formed, and detailed visual hallucinations (McKeith et al., 1994).

Neuropsychological Assessment

The neuropsychological symptoms seen with DLB are impairment in remote working memory, executive functioning, language, and visuospatial skills (Byrne, Lennox, Lowe, & Godwin-Austen, 1989; Gibb, Luthert, Janota, & Lantos, 1989). Individuals with DLB also show greater impairment on measures of attention, verbal fluency, and visuospatial skills when compared to those with AD (Hansen et al., 1990). It has also been proposed that DLB patients perform more poorly than AD patients on delayed recognition and paired associate tasks (Sahgal et al., 1992; Zola-Morgan & Squire, 1986).

Differential Diagnosis

It is particularly important to assess the differences that separate DLB from other cortical dementias, such as AD, which include unique pathological components, such as the presence of Lewy body inclusions. Additionally, there is a strong motor component that includes parkinsonism, rigidity, stooped posture, and slow shuffling gait. Furthermore, with DLB, there is often a component of psychosis, which includes both delirium and hallucinations. Those with DLB often experience repeated falls and loss of consciousness and clinically present with deficits in attention and alertness. Neuropsychological assessments should focus specifically on factors such as attention, fluency, and visuospatial abilities due to those factors being commonly shown to differentiate DLB from AD.

Biomarkers/Genetics

Genetic studies have indicated conflicting reports with regard to DLB's association with the E4 (APOEe4) allele, which is a known susceptibility gene for sporadic and late-onset familial AD (Corder et al., 1993; Kalra, Bergeron, & Lang, 1996; Poirier et al., 1993). A complex relationship has been documented between APOE and DLB as reduced Aβ plaque density was shown to occur among DLB cases that are heterozygous for APOEe3, as compared to those with APOEe2 or e4 alleles. Additionally, DLB cases have been shown to have a greater degree of CA2–3 degeneration in cases with the APOEe4 allele than in those with the APOEe3/3 genotype (Kalra et al., 1996). Given that DLB is classified among the synucleinopathies with coexistent AD pathology, the biomarkers receiving the most attention include alpha-synuclein, Aβ, and tau proteins (Johansen, White, Sando, & Aasly, 2010).

Neuroimaging

With DLB, neuronal atrophy is not substantially different from nondemented elders and to date there are no specific structural abnormalities identified that discriminate it from other dementias (Johansen et al., 2010). DLB has been associated with relative preservation of temporal lobe structures, which may aid in differential diagnosis with AD. However, DLB patients seem to have more frontotemporal gray matter atrophy than Parkinson's disease dementia (PDD) patients, which also correlates with cognitive impairment (Johansen et al., 2010; Sanchez-Castaneda et al., 2009). PET scan imaging with N-[^{11}C]-methyl-4-piperidyl acetate has demonstrated extensive cholinergic dysfunction in DLB (Bohnen et al., 2007; Shimada et al., 2009). Recently, dopamine transporter single-photon emission computed tomography (SPECT) has been shown to discriminate DLB from both AD and vascular dementia (McKeith et al., 2007; O'Brien et al., 2009).

PICK'S DISEASE

Overview

Pick bodies have been shown to occur in only 20% of clinically determined FTD cases, suggesting that accurate diagnosis of Pick's disease may only be possible at autopsy (Kertesz & Munoz, 1998). Pick's disease is shown to have localized atrophy of both the frontal lobe and/or the temporal lobe (Dickson, 1998; Snowden et al., 2002). The age of onset ranges from 40 to 80 years and as opposed to AD is more likely to present before the age of 65 years, which is considered to be "presenile" (Dickson, 1998; Heston & Mastri, 1982). Pick's disease is also reported to occur almost equally in both males and females, with some research indicating a possible increased incidence among females. The duration of the disease ranges from 2 to 17 years (Heston, White, & Mastri, 1987). Pick's disease is broken into three different variants depending on the pathological presentation. Type A of the Pick's disease variant is described as having limbic and frontotemporal neurodegeneration, as well as Pick bodies and ballooned neurons (Clark et al., 1986; Dickson, Yen, & Horoupian, 1986; Dickson, Yen, Suzuki et al., 1986; Williams, 1935). Type B presents with frontal atrophy and cortical degeneration with ballooned neurons; however, Pick bodies are not present (Foster et al., 1997; Gibb, Luthert, & Marsden, 1989). Additionally, Type B also manifests with extrapyramidal signs, asymmetrical motor syndromes, and degeneration of the substantia nigra with cortical degeneration (Foster et al., 1997; Gibb et al., 1989). Type C presents with neither Pick bodies nor ballooned neurons; however, circumscribed or diffused cortical atrophy as well as varied involvement of deep gray matter are present (Giannakopoulos, Hof, & Bouras, 1995; Hauw et al., 1996; Knopman, Mastri, Frey, Sung, & Rustan, 1990; Neary & Snowden, 1996).

Neuropsychological Assessment

Features of Pick's disease include impulsivity, hyperorality, and sensory stimulus seeking (Dickson, 1998; Graff-Radford et al., 1990). Presentation of the disease is also likely to include prominent aphasia and paraphasic errors (Graff-Radford et al., 1990; Holland, McBurney, Moossy, & Reinmuth, 1985; Wechsler, Verity, Rosenschein, Fried, & Scheibel, 1982). Other language disturbances include word-finding difficulties, anomia, neologism, phonemic paraphasias, echolalia, and verbal stereotype (Graff-Radford et al., 1990; Holland et al., 1985; Wechsler et al., 1982). Personality changes have also been reported to occur with this disease (Cummings & Duchen, 1981). Additionally, Pick's disease has been shown to have a faster degeneration of functioning with regard to language and global cognitive impairment as compared to those individuals with AD (Binetti, Locascio, Corkin, Vonsattel, & Growdon, 2000).

Differential Diagnosis

In order to differentiate a diagnosis of Pick's disease, it is important to take a multimodal approach utilizing neuroimaging as well as neuropsychological assessment. Pick's disease has an early onset as compared to AD and has been identified as occurring in three different types (Pick's disease Types A, B, and C). Neuroimaging can be useful in differentiating the three different types of Pick's diseases. Type A can be seen as having the presence of Pick bodies and ballooned neurons. While Type B has a similar neurodegeneration pattern as Type A, with frontotemporal and cortical degeneration, however, it is different in that it constitutes the presence of only ballooned neurons but not Pick bodies. Type C of Pick's disease has neither the presence of Pick bodies nor ballooned neurons but cortical atrophy is present. Neuropsychological assessment can further help to differentiate Pick's disease from other cortical dementias such as AD. Particular focus should be placed on utilizing assessments of verbal fluency and global cognitive functioning, which have been shown to decrease at an increased rate when compared to other cortical dementias.

Biomarkers/Genetics

Most cases of Pick's disease that have been documented are considered to be sporadic familial cases (Groen & Endtz, 1982; Heston et al., 1987) and the pattern of inheritance is thought to be autosomal dominant (Dickson, 1998). Due to the rarity of the disease, no gene, to date, has been identified as being associated with Pick's disease (Dickson, 1998).

Neuroimaging

CT and MRI scans are shown to overlap with structural findings of those individuals with AD. Pick's disease, however, is shown to have cerebral atrophy that is more circumscribed (Duara et al., 1992; Wechsler et al., 1982). Additionally, prominent widening of sulcal spaces in both the frontal and temporal lobes can be seen. Furthermore, the lateral ventricles are often shown to be enlarged in the frontal and temporal horns (Groen & Endtz, 1982; Knopman et al., 1989). Moreover, functional imaging using PET or SPECT has shown bifrontal deficits to occur in association with Pick's disease (Kamo et al., 1987; Neary et al., 1987; Salmon & Franck, 1989; Smith, Gallenstein, Layton, Kryscio, & Markesbery, 1993).

PRIMARY PROGRESSIVE APHASIA

Overview

To date, there are no epidemiological studies on the prevalence of PPA; however, the reported prevalence of FTD in clinical settings ranges from 5% to 20% of all dementia cases (Chow et al., 2005). People with this disease do not live any longer than people with other forms of dementia; however, autonomy is maintained until late in the course of the disease unlike other more common dementia syndromes (Le Rhun, Richard, & Pasquier, 2005). PPA is a neurodegenerative disease that produces progressive language disturbance and is present for 2 years prior to the deterioration of other cognitive domains (Mesulam, 1982; Mesulam, Grossman, Hillis, Kertesz, & Weintraub, 2003). Additionally, PPA can present as either fluent or nonfluent, with the nonfluent variant classified as progressive nonfluent aphasia (PNFA; Neary et al., 1998), which is discussed later in this chapter.

Diagnostics

Focal degenerative changes in the frontal and temporal areas are oftentimes associated with PPA, which are areas known to impact neuropsychological domains such as executive functioning (Wicklund, Johnson, & Weintraub, 2004). Further diagnostic criteria for PPA include "an insidious onset and progressive language difficulty presenting for a minimum of two years without present behavioral changes, memory, or visuospatial impairments" (Mesulam, 2001). Additionally, ideomotor apraxia and mild decrements in calculation or copying may be present, although daily functioning of living is not impacted by the symptoms. PPA is characterized by neuropsychological deficits in areas of expressive language, which impact speech production and word retrieval abilities. Furthermore, those with PPA have difficulties with communication tasks requiring them to read or write; however, their ability to understand word meanings is still preserved (Neary et al., 1998). When PPA is suspected, a detailed examination of language abilities is warranted. Tests such as the *Boston Diagnostic Aphasia Examination* (BDAE; Goodglass & Kaplan, 1983) can be useful to assess a wide range of expressive and receptive language skills. A battery containing tests of intellectual abilities (current and premorbid estimates), executive functioning, language, motor skills, and visuospatial abilities (tests described in prior sections) are also necessary for differential diagnostic and longitudinal tracking purposes.

Overview

PNFA presents with alterations in the rhyme and rhythm of speech such that it is telegraphic, halting, or agrammatic (Neary et al., 1998). As with fluent PPA, in PNFA, language difficulties should remain the only feature for at least 2 years before more generalized deficits develop. PNFA is found to reside in multiple brain regions, which can lead to clinical features of dysarthria, ideomotor apraxia, dyscalculia, constructional deficits, and impaired executive functioning as the syndrome spreads (Graff-Radford & Woodruff, 2007). PNFA presents more often in older patients with the age of onset being early 60s and has a survival rate of around 10 years (Hodges, Davies, Xuereb, Kril, & Halliday, 2003; Johnson et al., 2005; Ratnavalli, 2010; Roberson et al., 2005; Snowden et al., 2007).

Diagnostics

According to the diagnostic criteria by Neary et al. (1998), the diagnosis of PNFA can be considered when a patient presents with nonfluent speech that encompasses all or just incorporates one of the following features: agrammatism, phonemic paraphasias, anomia, and/or general dysarthria or apraxia of speech (Neary et al., 1998), and imaging rules out other etiological considerations (e.g., tumor, stroke). Supportive features for the diagnosis of PNFA include language impairments such as stuttering or oral apraxia, perseverations, and alexia with agraphia. Single-word comprehension with PNFA has been shown to remain intact though alternative verbal impairments are seen with regard to syntactic comprehension and phonemic paraphasias on tasks requiring naming of objects (Mesulam, 2001; Turner, Kenyon, Trojanowski, Gonatas, & Grossman, 1996; Weintraub, Rubin, & Mesulam, 1990). Additionally, those in the early stages of PNFA are able to maintain the conservation of word meanings; however, severe difficulties related to speech production have been shown to occur during the later stages of PNFA, which often results in mutism (Gorno-Tempini et al., 2006; Neary et al., 1998). Language impairments associated with PNFA have been indicated to occur in conjunction with preserved cognitive functioning related to memory, visuospatial skills, and orientation (McKinnon et al., 2008; Peelle et al., 2008).

Neuroimaging

In patients with PNFA, asymmetric abnormalities have been seen on neuroimaging (structural or functional), primarily impacting the left dominant hemisphere, similar to the damage observed in those with nonfluent stroke aphasia (Patterson, Graham, Lambon, Ralph, & Hodges, 2006; Reilly, Rodriguez, Lamy, & Neils-Strunjas, 2010).

Differential Diagnosis

A detailed neuropsychological examination covering a range of domains (i.e., intelligence and premorbid intellectual estimates, executive functioning, visuospatial skills, memory, motor abilities, and detailed language evaluation) is necessary to perform a differential diagnosis among PPA, NFPA, and other dementia syndromes, with language tests being among the most important to assess. With the previously mentioned neurocognitive presentation in mind, other important aspects include an informant interview and neuroimaging. Without this additional information, one cannot be certain about the diagnosis as more common neurological events (e.g., stroke) can present with these features.

SEMANTIC DEMENTIA

Overview

SD presents with an age of onset of 55 to 70 years, with equal prevalence seen in men and women (Hodges & Patterson, 2007). With regard to family history, SD is less common when compared to FTD, which has an indicated prevalence rate of only 2% to 10% for early-onset dementia (Hodges et al., 2010). The survival rate has been 50% at 12.8 years (Hodges et al., 2010). Mesulam (2001) proposed two distinct groups of SD patients. One group included those patients who present with fluent aphasia, anomia, and impaired word comprehension, but without agnosia. This group has involvement of the language network in the left posterior temporal–parietal area (Mesulam, 2001). The second group includes those who present with fluent aphasia plus agnosia with involvement of the bilateral inferotemporal-fusiform network in the temporal lobes (Mesulam, 2001), whereas others suggest that patients with fluent aphasia and anomia develop SD and exhibit multimodal object recognition deficits that are indicative of progressive deterioration of an amodal integrative semantic memory system (Adlam et al., 2006; Hodges & Patterson, 2007).

Diagnostics

Diagnostic features include an insidious onset and gradual progression of language disturbance that is characterized by (a) progressive, fluent, empty, spontaneous speech; (b) loss of word meaning, manifest by impaired naming and comprehension; and (c) semantic paraphasias (Garrard & Hodges, 2000; George & Mathuranath, 2005; Neary et al., 1998). Speech is often fluent but circumlocutory (Hodges & Patterson, 2007; Hodges, Patterson, Oxbury, & Funnell, 1992). Associated behavioral changes may include apathy, repetitive behaviors, loss of empathy, and rigidity (Bozeat, Gregory, Ralph, & Hodges, 2000; Rosen et al., 2006; Snowden et al., 2001). Additional supportive features include pressured speech, idiosyncratic word usage, surface dyslexia, and dysgraphia (Neary et al., 1998). Neuroimaging (structural and/or functional) has documented asymmetric abnormalities impacting the language-dominant anterior temporal lobe (Neary et al., 1998).

Differential Diagnosis

As with PPA and NFPA, a comprehensive neuropsychological examination with particular emphasis on language is required for the differential diagnosis. Again, informant report and neuroimaging are necessary to parse out history of presentation as well as rule out other, more common neurological etiologies (i.e., stroke and tumor). It is noteworthy that language disturbances seen in SD can make examination in other cognitive domains challenging, further necessitating the informant report.

CORTICOBASAL GANGLIONIC DEGENERATION

Overview

Corticobasal ganglionic degeneration (CBD) is a form of movement disorder that involves an asymmetric limb in addition to sporadic disturbances in speech and/or gait (Belfor et al., 2006). The most characteristic symptom of CBD is a rigid dystonic jerking hand. Cognitive features of CBD include difficulties with both constructional and visuospatial functions (Tang-Wai et al., 2004), frontal dysfunction, and aphasia, mainly nonfluent (Graham, Bak, & Hodges, 2003; Kertesz, Martinez-Lage, Davidson, & Munoz, 2000).

Neuropsychological Assessment

The most prominent feature of CBD is the limb apraxia, wherein there is a notable inability to execute a skilled movement in the absence of a motor deficit (Belfor et al., 2006). In severe cases, ideomotor and ideational apraxias are present. Further dysfunction with executive functioning and language impairment has been documented in cases with CBD (Belfor et al., 2006). An additional diagnostic criterion includes cortical sensory loss or what is referred to as alien limb, wherein the limb is unidentified by the person as his or her own (Litvan et al., 2003). Left frontal and parietal cortical damage and subcortical white matter and corpus callosum abnormalities have also been identified among cases of CBD (Belfor et al., 2006; Frattali, Grafman, Patronas, Makhlouf, & Litvan, 2000; Graham et al., 2003).

Diagnosis

CBD presents clinically with deficits in motor functioning and is subsequently considered to be a movement disorder. However, individuals with CBD also present with dysfunction in both executive functioning and language. Neuroimaging can be a valuable tool when assessing for a diagnosis of CBD because abnormalities can be detected in both the cortical regions as well as in the corpus callosum. One of the major distinctions of CBD is the occurrence of cortical sensory loss.

PROGRESSIVE SUPRANUCLEAR PALSY
(OR STEELE–RICHARDSON–OLSZEWSKI SYNDROME)

Overview

Progressive supranuclear palsy (PSP) is a neurodegenerative akinetic rigid disorder. Characteristic features of the disorder include axial rigidity, vertical gaze palsy, and recurrent falls. The prevalence of PSP is reported to be 1.39 per 100,000 individuals (Golbe, Davis, Schoenberg, & Duvoisin, 1988). The mean age of occurrence ranges anywhere from 55 to 70 years with a few documented cases commencing prior to 45 years of age (Brusa, Mancardi, & Bugiani, 1980; Litvan et al., 1996). Supportive criteria for PSP include symmetric akinesia or rigidity (proximal rather than distal), abnormal neck posture, absent response of parkinsonism, early dysphagia, and dysarthria (Litvan et al., 1996). Additional supportive criteria include an early onset of cognitive impairment with noted deficits in abstract conceptualization, verbal fluency, and use of imitation behavior or frontal release signs. Behavioral changes are also often noted to occur and include severe apathy (Litvan et al., 1996). Other cognitive features include executive functioning deficits, such as problems in planning and organizing as well as set shifting (Bak, Crawford, Hearn, Mathuranath, & Hodges, 2005; Boeve, Lang, & Litvan, 2003; Grafman, Litvan, & Stark, 1995; Litvan et al., 1996, 2003; Soliveri et al., 1999).

Diagnostics

The National Institute of Neurological Disorders and Stroke (NINDS) held an international workshop to determine criteria for PSP diagnosis. Based on that workshop, it was decided that there were three degrees of diagnoses, which included possible

PSP, probable PSP, and definite PSP (Litvan et al., 1996). Description of each PSP diagnosis based on the NINDS workshop is outlined as follows: (a) Possible PSP requires an insidious onset with gradual progression beginning at or after 40 years of age. Vertical (upward or downward gaze) supranuclear palsy *or* both slowing of vertical saccades and prominent postural instability with falls occurs within the first year of the disease without evidence to suggest other diseases. (b) Probable PSP requires the gradual progression of the disorder with an onset occurring at age 40 years or later. Additionally, there must be evidence of a vertical (upward or downward gaze) supranuclear palsy *and* prominent postural instability with falls occurring within the first year of the disease without evidence suggestive of another disease. (c) Definite PSP is diagnosed at autopsy.

Differential Diagnosis

A differential diagnosis of CBD and FTD would need to be ruled out. PSP presents similarly with regard to being an akinetic rigid disorder with impairment seen in motor movement. Individuals presenting with PSP are shown to experience supranuclear palsy and an increased occurrence of falls. Additionally, neuropsychological assessment of cognitive dysfunction for PSP should focus specifically on signs of severe affective changes, and deficits in verbal fluency and executive functioning. Finally, those with PSP have a difficult time shifting from tasks as well as being able to use higher-order functioning to plan and organize information effectively.

REFERENCES

Adlam, A. L., Patterson, K., Rogers, T. T., Nestor, P. J., Salmond, C. H., Acosta-Cabronero, J., & Hodges, J. R. (2006). Semantic dementia and fluent primary progressive aphasia: Two sides of the same coin? *Brain: A Journal of Neurology, 129*(Pt 11), 3066–3080.

American Psychiatric Association. (2013). *Diagnostic and statistical manual of mental disorders* (5th ed.). Washington, DC: American Psychiatric Association.

Aupperle, R. L., Beatty, W. W., Shelton, F. d. e. N., & Gontkovsky, S. T. (2002). Three screening batteries to detect cognitive impairment in multiple sclerosis. *Multiple Sclerosis, 8*(5), 382–389.

Bak, T. H., Crawford, L. M., Hearn, V. C., Mathuranath, P. S., & Hodges, J. R. (2005). Subcortical dementia revisited: Similarities and differences in cognitive function between progressive supranuclear palsy (PSP), corticobasal degeneration (CBD) and multiple system atrophy (MSA). *Neurocase, 11*(4), 268–273.

Baker, M., Mackenzie, I. R., Pickering-Brown, S. M., Gass, J., Rademakers, R., Lindholm, C.,…Hutton, M. (2006). Mutations in progranulin cause tau-negative frontotemporal dementia linked to chromosome 17. *Nature, 442*(7105), 916–919.

Belfor, N., Amici, S., Boxer, A. L., Kramer, J. H., Gorno-Tempini, M. L., Rosen, H. J., & Miller, B. L. (2006). Clinical and neuropsychological features of corticobasal degeneration. *Mechanisms of Ageing and Development, 127*(2), 203–207.

Binetti, G., Locascio, J. J., Corkin, S., Vonsattel, J. P., & Growdon, J. H. (2000). Differences between Pick disease and Alzheimer disease in clinical appearance and rate of cognitive decline. *Archives of Neurology, 57*(2), 225–232.

Boeve, B. F., Lang, A. E., & Litvan, I. (2003). Corticobasal degeneration and its relationship to progressive supranuclear palsy and frontotemporal dementia. *Annals of Neurology, 54*(Suppl 5), S15–S19.

Bohnen, N. I., Kaufer, D. I., Hendrickson, R., Constantine, G. M., Mathis, C. A., & Moore, R. Y. (2007). Cortical cholinergic denervation is associated with depressive symptoms in Parkinson's disease and parkinsonian dementia. *Journal of Neurology, Neurosurgery, and Psychiatry, 78*(6), 641–643.

Bozeat, S., Gregory, C. A., Ralph, M. A., & Hodges, J. R. (2000). Which neuropsychiatric and behavioural features distinguish frontal and temporal variants of frontotemporal dementia from Alzheimer's disease? *Journal of Neurology, Neurosurgery, and Psychiatry, 69*(2), 178–186.

Brusa, A., Mancardi, G. L., & Bugiani, O. (1980). Progressive supranuclear palsy 1979: An overview. *Italian Journal of Neurological Sciences, 1*(4), 205–222.

Byrne, E. J., Lennox, G., Lowe, J., & Godwin-Austen, R. B. (1989). Diffuse Lewy body disease: Clinical features in 15 cases. *Journal of Neurology, Neurosurgery, and Psychiatry, 52*(6), 709–717.

Callen, D. J., Black, S. E., Gao, F., Caldwell, C. B., & Szalai, J. P. (2001). Beyond the hippocampus: MRI volumetry confirms widespread limbic atrophy in AD. *Neurology, 57*(9), 1669–1674.

Chemali, Z., Withall, A., & Daffner, K. R. (2010). The plight of caring for young patients with frontotemporal dementia. *American Journal of Alzheimer's Disease and Other Dementias, 25*(2), 109–115.

Chow, T. W., Hodges, J. R., Dawson, K. E., Miller, B. L., Smith, V., Mendez, M. F., & Lipton, A. M.; National Alzheimer's Coordinating Center. (2005). Referral patterns for syndromes associated with frontotemporal lobar degeneration. *Alzheimer Disease and Associated Disorders, 19*(1), 17–19.

Clark, A. W., Manz, H. J., White, C. L., Lehmann, J., Miller, D., & Coyle, J. T. (1986). Cortical degeneration with swollen chromatolytic neurons: Its relationship to Pick's disease. *Journal of Neuropathology and Experimental Neurology, 45*(3), 268–284.

Clark, J. H., Hobson, V. L., & O'Bryant, S. E. (2010). Diagnostic accuracy of percent retention scores on RBANS verbal memory subtests for the diagnosis of Alzheimer's disease and mild cognitive impairment. *Archives of Clinical Neuropsychology, 25*(4), 318–326.

Clark, L. N., Poorkaj, P., Wszolek, Z., Geschwind, D. H., Nasreddine, Z. S., Miller, B.,... Wilhelmsen, K. C. (1998). Pathogenic implications of mutations in the tau gene in pallido-ponto-nigral degeneration and related neurodegenerative disorders linked to chromosome 17. *Proceedings of the National Academy of Sciences of the United States of America, 95*(22), 13103–13107.

Corder, E. H., Saunders, A. M., Strittmatter, W. J., Schmechel, D. E., Gaskell, P. C., Small, G. W.,...Pericak-Vance, M. A. (1993). Gene dose of apolipoprotein E type 4 allele and the risk of Alzheimer's disease in late onset families. *Science, 261*(5123), 921–923.

Cruts, M., Gijselinck, I., van der Zee, J., Engelborghs, S., Wils, H., Pirici, D.,...Van Broeckhoven, C. (2006). Null mutations in progranulin cause ubiquitin-positive frontotemporal dementia linked to chromosome 17q21. *Nature, 442*(7105), 920–924.

Cummings, J. L., & Duchen, L. W. (1981). Kluver-Bucy syndrome in Pick disease: Clinical and pathologic correlations. *Neurology, 31*(11), 1415–1422.

De Santi, S., de Leon, M. J., Rusinek, H., Convit, A., Tarshish, C. Y., Roche, A.,...Fowler, J. (2001). Hippocampal formation glucose metabolism and volume losses in MCI and AD. *Neurobiology of Aging, 22*(4), 529–539.

Del Ser, T., McKeith, I., Anand, R., Cicin-Sain, A., Ferrara, R., & Spiegel, R. (2000). Dementia with Lewy bodies: Findings from an international multicentre study. *International Journal of Geriatric Psychiatry, 15*(11), 1034–1045.

Delis, D. C., & Kramer, J. H. (2000). *California verbal learning test: CVLT-II*; Adult Version; Manual. San Antonio, TX: Psychological Corporation.

Dickerson, B. C., Bakkour, A., Salat, D. H., Feczko, E., Pacheco, J., Greve, D. N., . . . Buckner, R. L. (2009). The cortical signature of Alzheimer's disease: Regionally specific cortical thinning relates to symptom severity in very mild to mild AD dementia and is detectable in asymptomatic amyloid-positive individuals. *Cerebral Cortex, 19*(3), 497–510.

Dickson, D. W. (1998). Pick's disease: A modern approach. *Brain Pathology, 8*(2), 339–354.

Dickson, D. W., Yen, S. H., & Horoupian, D. S. (1986). Pick body-like inclusions in the dentate fascia of the hippocampus in Alzheimer's disease. *Acta Neuropathologica, 71*(1–2), 38–45.

Dickson, D. W., Yen, S. H., Suzuki, K. I., Davies, P., Garcia, J. H., & Hirano, A. (1986). Ballooned neurons in select neurodegenerative diseases contain phosphorylated neurofilament epitopes. *Acta Neuropathologica, 71*(3–4), 216–223.

Driscoll, I., Davatzikos, C., An, Y., Wu, X., Shen, D., Kraut, M., & Resnick, S. M. (2009). Longitudinal pattern of regional brain volume change differentiates normal aging from MCI. *Neurology, 72*(22), 1906–1913.

Duara, R., Barker, W. W., Chang, J., Yoshii, F., Loewenstein, D. A., & Pascal, S. (1992). Viability of neocortical function shown in behavioral activation state PET studies in Alzheimer disease. *Journal of Cerebral Blood Flow and Metabolism, 12*(6), 927–934.

Duff, K., Beglinger, L. J., Schoenberg, M. R., Patton, D. E., Mold, J., Scott, J. G., & Adams, R. L. (2005). Test-retest stability and practice effects of the RBANS in a community dwelling elderly sample. *Journal of Clinical and Experimental Neuropsychology, 27*(5), 565–575.

Duff, K., Humphreys Clark, J. D., O'Bryant, S. E., Mold, J. W., Schiffer, R. B., & Sutker, P. B. (2008). Utility of the RBANS in detecting cognitive impairment associated with Alzheimer's disease: Sensitivity, specificity, and positive and negative predictive powers. *Archives of Clinical Neuropsychology, 23*(5), 603–612.

Dumanchin, C., Camuzat, A., Campion, D., Verpillat, P., Hannequin, D., Dubois, B., . . . Brice, A. (1998). Segregation of a missense mutation in the microtubule-associated protein tau gene with familial frontotemporal dementia and parkinsonism. *Human Molecular Genetics, 7*(11), 1825–1829.

Elfgren, C., Passant, U., & Risberg, J. (1993). Neuropsychological findings in frontal lobe dementia. *Dementia, 4*(3–4), 214–219.

Englund, B., Brun, A., Gustafson, L., Passant, U., Mann, D., Neary, D., & Snowden, J. (1994). Clinical and neuropathological criteria for frontotemporal dementia. The Lund and Manchester Groups. *Journal of Neurology, Neurosurgery, and Psychiatry, 57*(4), 416–418.

Folstein, M. F., Folstein, S. E., & McHugh, P. R. (1975). "Mini-Mental State." A practical method for grading the cognitive state of patients for the clinician. *Journal of Psychiatric Research, 12*(3), 189–198.

Foster, N. L., Wilhelmsen, K., Sima, A. A., Jones, M. Z., D'Amato, C. J., & Gilman, S. (1997). Frontotemporal dementia and parkinsonism linked to chromosome 17: A consensus conference. Conference participants. *Annals of Neurology, 41*(6), 706–715.

Fox, N. C., Cousens, S., Scahill, R., Harvey, R. J., & Rossor, M. N. (2000). Using serial registered brain magnetic resonance imaging to measure disease progression in Alzheimer disease: Power calculations and estimates of sample size to detect treatment effects. *Archives of Neurology, 57*(3), 339–344.

Frattali, C. M., Grafman, J., Patronas, N., Makhlouf, F., & Litvan, I. (2000). Language disturbances in corticobasal degeneration. *Neurology, 54*(4), 990–992.

Garrard, P., & Hodges, J. R. (2000). Semantic dementia: Clinical, radiological and pathological perspectives. *Journal of Neurology, 247*(6), 409–422.

George, A., & Mathuranath, P. S. (2005). Primary progressive aphasia: A comparative study of progressive nonfluent aphasia and semantic dementia. *Neurology India, 53*(2), 162–165; discussion 165.

Giannakopoulos, P., Hof, P. R., & Bouras, C. (1995). Dementia lacking distinctive histopathology: Clinicopathological evaluation of 32 cases. *Acta Neuropathologica, 89*(4), 346–355.

Gibb, W. R., Luthert, P. J., Janota, I., & Lantos, P. L. (1989). Cortical Lewy body dementia: Clinical features and classification. *Journal of Neurology, Neurosurgery, and Psychiatry, 52*(2), 185–192.

Gibb, W. R., Luthert, P. J., & Marsden, C. D. (1989). Corticobasal degeneration. *Brain: A Journal of Neurology, 112*(Pt 5), 1171–1192.

Golbe, L. I., Davis, P. H., Schoenberg, B. S., & Duvoisin, R. C. (1988). Prevalence and natural history of progressive supranuclear palsy. *Neurology, 38*(7), 1031–1034.

Goodglass, H., & Kaplan, E. (1983). *Boston diagnostic aphasia examination booklet*. Philadelphia, PA: Lea & Febiger.

Gorno-Tempini, M. L., Ogar, J. M., Brambati, S. M., Wang, P., Jeong, J. H., Rankin, K. P., ... Miller, B. L. (2006). Anatomical correlates of early mutism in progressive nonfluent aphasia. *Neurology, 67*(10), 1849–1851.

Graff-Radford, N. R., Damasio, A. R., Hyman, B. T., Hart, M. N., Tranel, D., Damasio, H., ... Rezai, K. (1990). Progressive aphasia in a patient with Pick's disease: A neuropsychological, radiologic, and anatomic study. *Neurology, 40*(4), 620–626.

Graff-Radford, N. R., & Woodruff, B. K. (2007). Frontotemporal dementia. *Seminars in Neurology, 27*(1), 48–57.

Grafman, J., Litvan, I., & Stark, M. (1995). Neuropsychological features of progressive supranuclear palsy. *Brain and Cognition, 28*(3), 311–320.

Graham, N. L., Bak, T. H., & Hodges, J. R. (2003). Corticobasal degeneration as a cognitive disorder. *Movement Disorders, 18*(11), 1224–1232.

Groen, J. J., & Endtz, L. J. (1982). Hereditary Pick's disease: Second re-examination of the large family and discussion of other hereditary cases, with particular reference to electroencephalography, a computerized tomography. *Brain: A Journal of Neurology, 105*(Pt 3), 443–459.

Hansen, L., Salmon, D., Galasko, D., Masliah, E., Katzman, R., DeTeresa, R., ... Klauber, M. (1990). The Lewy body variant of Alzheimer's disease: A clinical and pathologic entity. *Neurology, 40*(1), 1–8.

Harvan, J. R., & Cotter, V. (2006). An evaluation of dementia screening in the primary care setting. *Journal of the American Academy of Nurse Practitioners, 18*(8), 351–360.

Hauw, J. J., Duyckaerts, C., Seilhean, D., Camilleri, S., Sazdovitch, V., & Rancurel, G. (1996). The neuropathologic diagnostic criteria of frontal lobe dementia revisited. A study of ten consecutive cases. *Journal of Neural Transmission. Supplementum, 47*, 47–59.

Heaton, R. K. (2008). *Wisconsin card sorting test, computer version 4 WVST:CV4*. Odessa, FL: Psychological Assessment Resources.

Heston, L. L., & Mastri, A. R. (1982). Age at onset of Pick's and Alzheimer's dementia: Implications for diagnosis and research. *Journal of Gerontology, 37*(4), 422–424.

Heston, L. L., White, J. A., & Mastri, A. R. (1987). Pick's disease. Clinical genetics and natural history. *Archives of General Psychiatry, 44*(5), 409–411.

Hodges, J. R. (2001). Frontotemporal dementia (Pick's disease): Clinical features and assessment. *Neurology, 56*(11 Suppl 4), S6–10.

Hodges, J. R., Davies, R., Xuereb, J., Kril, J., & Halliday, G. (2003). Survival in frontotemporal dementia. *Neurology, 61*(3), 349–354.

Hodges, J. R., Mitchell, J., Dawson, K., Spillantini, M. G., Xuereb, J. H., McMonagle, P.,...
Patterson, K. (2010). Semantic dementia: Demography, familial factors and survival in a
consecutive series of 100 cases. *Brain: A Journal of Neurology, 133*(Pt 1), 300–306.

Hodges, J. R., & Patterson, K. (2007). Semantic dementia: A unique clinicopathological syndrome. *Lancet Neurology, 6*(11), 1004–1014.

Hodges, J. R., Patterson, K., Oxbury, S., & Funnell, E. (1992). Semantic dementia. Progressive
fluent aphasia with temporal lobe atrophy. *Brain: A Journal of Neurology, 115*(Pt 6),
1783–1806.

Hodges, J. R., Patterson, K., Ward, R., Garrard, P., Bak, T., Perry, R., & Gregory, C. (1999). The
differentiation of semantic dementia and frontal lobe dementia (temporal and frontal
variants of frontotemporal dementia) from early Alzheimer's disease: A comparative
neuropsychological study. *Neuropsychology, 13*(1), 31–40.

Holland, A. L., McBurney, D. H., Moossy, J., & Reinmuth, O. M. (1985). The dissolution of
language in Pick's disease with neurofibrillary tangles: A case study. *Brain and Language,
24*(1), 36–58.

Hutton, M., Lendon, C. L., Rizzu, P., Baker, M., Froelich, S., Houlden, H.,...Heutink, P. (1998).
Association of missense and 5'-splice-site mutations in tau with the inherited dementia
FTDP-17. *Nature, 393*(6686), 702–705.

Jack, C. R., Shiung, M. M., Gunter, J. L., O'Brien, P. C., Weigand, S. D., Knopman, D. S.,...
Petersen, R. C. (2004). Comparison of different MRI brain atrophy rate measures with
clinical disease progression in AD. *Neurology, 62*(4), 591–600.

Jensen, A. R., & Rohwer, W. D. (1966). The Stroop color-word test: A review. *Acta Psychologica,
25*(1), 36–93.

Johansen, K. K., White, L. R., Sando, S. B., & Aasly, J. O. (2010). Biomarkers: Parkinson disease
with dementia and dementia with Lewy bodies. *Parkinsonism & Related Disorders, 16*(5),
307–315.

Johnson, J. K., Diehl, J., Mendez, M. F., Neuhaus, J., Shapira, J. S., Forman, M.,...Miller, B. L.
(2005). Frontotemporal lobar degeneration: Demographic characteristics of 353 patients.
Archives of Neurology, 62(6), 925–930.

Kalra, S., Bergeron, C., & Lang, A. E. (1996). Lewy body disease and dementia. A review.
Archives of Internal Medicine, 156(5), 487–493.

Kamo, H., McGeer, P. L., Harrop, R., McGeer, E. G., Calne, D. B., Martin, W. R., & Pate, B. D.
(1987). Positron emission tomography and histopathology in Pick's disease. *Neurology,
37*(3), 439–445.

Kaplan, E., Goodglass, H., & Weintraub, S. (1983). *Boston naming test*. Philadelphia, PA: Lea &
Febiger.

Kashiwa, Y., Kitabayashi, Y., Narumoto, J., Nakamura, K., Ueda, H., & Fukui, K. (2005).
Anosognosia in Alzheimer's disease: Association with patient characteristics, psychiatric
symptoms and cognitive deficits. *Psychiatry and Clinical Neurosciences, 59*(6), 697–704.

Kertesz, A., Martinez-Lage, P., Davidson, W., & Munoz, D. G. (2000). The corticobasal degeneration syndrome overlaps progressive aphasia and frontotemporal dementia. *Neurology,
55*(9), 1368–1375.

Kertesz, A., & Munoz, D. (1998). Pick's disease, frontotemporal dementia, and Pick complex:
Emerging concepts. *Archives of Neurology, 55*(3), 302–304.

Knight, J. A., & Kaplan, E. (2003). *The handbook of Rey-Osterrieth Complex Figure usage: Clinical
and research applications*. Lutz, FL: Psychological Assessment Resources.

Knopman, D. S., Christensen, K. J., Schut, L. J., Harbaugh, R. E., Reeder, T., Ngo, T., & Frey,
W. (1989). The spectrum of imaging and neuropsychological findings in Pick's disease.
Neurology, 39(3), 362–368.

Knopman, D. S., Mastri, A. R., Frey, W. H., Sung, J. H., & Rustan, T. (1990). Dementia lacking distinctive histologic features: A common non-Alzheimer degenerative dementia. *Neurology, 40*(2), 251–256.

Larson, E., Kirschner, K., Bode, R., Heinemann, A., & Goodman, R. (2005). Construct and predictive validity of the repeatable battery for the assessment of neuropsychological status in the evaluation of stroke patients. *Journal of Clinical and Experimental Neuropsychology, 27*(1), 16–32.

Le Rhun, E., Richard, F., & Pasquier, F. (2005). Natural history of primary progressive aphasia. *Neurology, 65*(6), 887–891.

Lee, A. G., & Martin, C. O. (2004). Neuro-ophthalmic findings in the visual variant of Alzheimer's disease. *Ophthalmology, 111*(2), 376–380; discussion 380.

Lezak, M. D. (2004). *Neuropsychological assessment.* New York, NY: Oxford University Press.

Litvan, I., Agid, Y., Calne, D., Campbell, G., Dubois, B., Duvoisin, R. C.,…Zee, D. S. (1996). Clinical research criteria for the diagnosis of progressive supranuclear palsy (Steele-Richardson-Olszewski syndrome): Report of the NINDS-SPSP international workshop. *Neurology, 47*(1), 1–9.

Litvan, I., Bhatia, K. P., Burn, D. J., Goetz, C. G., Lang, A. E., McKeith, I.,…Wenning, G. K.; Movement Disorders Society Scientific Issues Committee. (2003). Movement Disorders Society Scientific Issues Committee report: SIC Task Force appraisal of clinical diagnostic criteria for Parkinsonian disorders. *Movement Disorders, 18*(5), 467–486.

McKeith, I., O'Brien, J., Walker, Z., Tatsch, K., Booij, J., Darcourt, J.,…Reininger, C.; DLB Study Group. (2007). Sensitivity and specificity of dopamine transporter imaging with 123I-FP-CIT SPECT in dementia with Lewy bodies: A phase III, multicentre study. *Lancet Neurology, 6*(4), 305–313.

McKeith, I. G., Fairbairn, A. F., Perry, R. H., & Thompson, P. (1994). The clinical diagnosis and misdiagnosis of senile dementia of Lewy body type (SDLT). *The British Journal of Psychiatry, 165*(3), 324–332.

McKhann, G. M., Albert, M. S., Grossman, M., Miller, B., Dickson, D., & Trojanowski, J. Q.; Work Group on Frontotemporal Dementia and Pick's Disease. (2001). Clinical and pathological diagnosis of frontotemporal dementia: Report of the Work Group on Frontotemporal Dementia and Pick's Disease. *Archives of Neurology, 58*(11), 1803–1809.

McKhann, G. M., Knopman, D. S., Chertkow, H., Hyman, B. T., Jack, C. R., Kawas, C. H.,… Phelps, C. H. (2011). The diagnosis of dementia due to Alzheimer's disease: Recommendations from the National Institute on Aging-Alzheimer's Association workgroups on diagnostic guidelines for Alzheimer's disease. *Alzheimer's & Dementia, 7*(3), 263–269.

McKinnon, M. C., Nica, E. I., Sengdy, P., Kovacevic, N., Moscovitch, M., Freedman, M.,…Levine, B. (2008). Autobiographical memory and patterns of brain atrophy in frontotemporal lobar degeneration. *Journal of Cognitive Neuroscience, 20*(10), 1839–1853.

Mesulam, M. M. (1982). Slowly progressive aphasia without generalized dementia. *Annals of Neurology, 11*(6), 592–598.

Mesulam, M. M. (2001). Primary progressive aphasia. *Annals of Neurology, 49*(4), 425–432.

Mesulam, M. M., Grossman, M., Hillis, A., Kertesz, A., & Weintraub, S. (2003). The core and halo of primary progressive aphasia and semantic dementia. *Annals of Neurology, 54*(Suppl 5), S11–S14.

Miller, B. L., Cummings, J. L., Villanueva-Meyer, J., Boone, K., Mehringer, C. M., Lesser, I. M., & Mena, I. (1991). Frontal lobe degeneration: Clinical, neuropsychological, and SPECT characteristics. *Neurology, 41*(9), 1374–1382.

Misra, C., Fan, Y., & Davatzikos, C. (2009). Baseline and longitudinal patterns of brain atrophy in MCI patients, and their use in prediction of short-term conversion to AD: Results from ADNI. *NeuroImage, 44*(4), 1415–1422.

Morris, J. C., Edland, S., Clark, C., Galasko, D., Koss, E., Mohs, R., . . . Heyman, A. (1993). The Consortium to Establish a Registry for Alzheimer's Disease (CERAD). Part IV. Rates of cognitive change in the longitudinal assessment of probable Alzheimer's disease. *Neurology, 43*(12), 2457–2465.

Morris, J. C., Heyman, A., Mohns, R. C., Hughes, J. P., van Belle, G., Fillenbaum, G., . . . Clark C. (1989). The Consortium to Establish a Registry for Alzheimer's Disease (CERAD). Part I. Clinical and neuropsychological assessment of Alzheimer's disease. *Neurology, 39*, 1159–1165.

Nasreddine, Z. S., Phillips, N. A., Bédirian, V., Charbonneau, S., Whitehead, V., Collin, I.,… Chertkow, H. (2005). The Montreal Cognitive Assessment, MoCA: A brief screening tool for mild cognitive impairment. *Journal of the American Geriatrics Society, 53*(4), 695–699.

Neary, D., & Snowden, J. (1996). Fronto-temporal dementia: Nosology, neuropsychology, and neuropathology. *Brain and Cognition, 31*(2), 176–187.

Neary, D., Snowden, J. S., Gustafson, L., Passant, U., Stuss, D., Black, S.,… Benson, D. F. (1998). Frontotemporal lobar degeneration: A consensus on clinical diagnostic criteria. *Neurology, 51*(6), 1546–1554.

Neary, D., Snowden, J. S., Northen, B., & Goulding, P. (1988). Dementia of frontal lobe type. *Journal of Neurology, Neurosurgery, and Psychiatry, 51*(3), 353–361.

Neary, D., Snowden, J. S., Shields, R. A., Burjan, A. W., Northen, B., MacDermott, N.,… Testa, H. J. (1987). Single photon emission tomography using 99mTc-HM-PAO in the investigation of dementia. *Journal of Neurology, Neurosurgery, and Psychiatry, 50*(9), 1101–1109.

O'Brien, J. T., McKeith, I. G., Walker, Z., Tatsch, K., Booij, J., Darcourt, J.,… Reininger, C.; DLB Study Group. (2009). Diagnostic accuracy of 123I-FP-CIT SPECT in possible dementia with Lewy bodies. *The British Journal of Psychiatry, 194*(1), 34–39.

O'Bryant, S. E., Lacritz, L. H., Hall, J., Waring, S. C., Chan, W., Khodr, Z. G.,… Cullum, C. M. (2010). Validation of the new interpretive guidelines for the clinical dementia rating scale sum of boxes score in the national Alzheimer's coordinating center database. *Archives of Neurology, 67*(6), 746–749.

O'Bryant, S. E., Waring, S. C., Cullum, C. M., Hall, J., Lacritz, L., Massman, P. J.,… Doody, R.; Texas Alzheimer's Research Consortium. (2008). Staging dementia using Clinical Dementia Rating Scale Sum of Boxes scores: A Texas Alzheimer's research consortium study. *Archives of Neurology, 65*(8), 1091–1095.

Oda, H., Yamamoto, Y., & Maeda, K. (2009). Neuropsychological profile of dementia with Lewy bodies. *Psychogeriatrics, 9*(2), 85–90.

Papka, M., Rubio, A., & Schiffer, R. B. (1998). A review of Lewy body disease, an emerging concept of cortical dementia. *The Journal of Neuropsychiatry and Clinical Neurosciences, 10*(3), 267–279.

Pasquier, F., Lebert, F., Grymonprez, L., & Petit, H. (1995). Verbal fluency in dementia of frontal lobe type and dementia of Alzheimer type. *Journal of Neurology, Neurosurgery, and Psychiatry, 58*(1), 81–84.

Patterson, K., Graham, N. L., Lambon, M. A., Ralph, M., & Hodges, J. R. (2006). Progressive non-fluent aphasia is not a progressive form of non-fluent (post-stroke) aphasia. *Aphasiology, 20*(9), 1018–1034.

Peelle, J. E., Troiani, V., Gee, J., Moore, P., McMillan, C., Vesely, L., & Grossman, M. (2008). Sentence comprehension and voxel-based morphometry in progressive nonfluent aphasia, semantic dementia, and nonaphasic frontotemporal dementia. *Journal of Neurolinguistics,* *21*(5), 418–432.

Perry, R. H., Irving, D., Blessed, G., Perry, E. K., & Fairbairn, A. F. (1989). Senile dementia of Lewy body type and spectrum of Lewy body disease. *Lancet, 1*(8646), 1088.

Perry, R. J., & Hodges, J. R. (2000). Differentiating frontal and temporal variant frontotemporal dementia from Alzheimer's disease. *Neurology, 54*(12), 2277–2284.

Poirier, J., Davignon, J., Bouthillier, D., Kogan, S., Bertrand, P., & Gauthier, S. (1993). Apolipoprotein E polymorphism and Alzheimer's disease. *Lancet, 342*(8873), 697–699.

Poorkaj, P., Bird, T. D., Wijsman, E., Nemens, E., Garruto, R. M., Anderson, L.,...Schellenberg, G. D. (1998). Tau is a candidate gene for chromosome 17 frontotemporal dementia. *Annals of Neurology, 43*(6), 815–825.

Randolph, C. (1998). *Repeatable battery for the assessment of neuropsychological status.* San Antonio, TX: The Psychological Corporation.

Rascovsky, K., Salmon, D. P., Ho, G. J., Galasko, D., Peavy, G. M., Hansen, L. A., & Thal, L. J. (2002). Cognitive profiles differ in autopsy-confirmed frontotemporal dementia and AD. *Neurology, 58*(12), 1801–1808.

Ratnavalli, E. (2010). Progress in the last decade in our understanding of primary progressive aphasia. *Annals of Indian Academy of Neurology, 13*(Suppl 2), S109–S115.

Razani, J., Wong, J. T., Dafaeeboini, N., Edwards-Lee, T., Lu, P., Alessi, C., & Josephson, K. (2009). Predicting everyday functional abilities of dementia patients with the Mini-Mental State Examination. *Journal of Geriatric Psychiatry and Neurology, 22*(1), 62–70.

Reilly, J., Rodriguez, A. D., Lamy, M., & Neils-Strunjas, J. (2010). Cognition, language, and clinical pathological features of non-Alzheimer's dementias: An overview. *Journal of Communication Disorders, 43*(5), 438–452.

Rey, A. (1964). *L'examen clinique en psychologie.* Paris: Presses Universitaires de France.

Roberson, E. D., Hesse, J. H., Rose, K. D., Slama, H., Johnson, J. K., Yaffe, K.,...Miller, B. L. (2005). Frontotemporal dementia progresses to death faster than Alzheimer disease. *Neurology, 65*(5), 719–725.

Robinson, K. M., Adkisson, P., & Weinrich, S. (2001). Problem behaviour, caregiver reactions, and impact among caregivers of persons with Alzheimer's disease. *Journal of Advanced Nursing, 36*(4), 573–582.

Rosen, H. J., Allison, S. C., Ogar, J. M., Amici, S., Rose, K., Dronkers, N.,...Gorno-Tempini, M. L. (2006). Behavioral features in semantic dementia vs other forms of progressive aphasias. *Neurology, 67*(10), 1752–1756.

Rosen, H. J., Hartikainen, K. M., Jagust, W., Kramer, J. H., Reed, B. R., Cummings, J. L.,...Miller, B. L. (2002). Utility of clinical criteria in differentiating frontotemporal lobar degeneration (FTLD) from AD. *Neurology, 58*(11), 1608–1615.

Rosen, W. G., Mohs, R. C., & Davis, K. L. (1984). A new rating scale for Alzheimer's disease. *The American Journal of Psychiatry, 141*(11), 1356–1364.

Roses, A. D., Strittmatter, W. J., Pericak-Vance, M. A., Corder, E. H., Saunders, A. M., & Schmechel, D. E. (1994). Clinical application of apolipoprotein E genotyping to Alzheimer's disease. *Lancet, 343*(8912), 1564–1565.

Royall, D., Mahurin, R. K., & Gray, K. (1992). Bedside assessment of executive cognitive impairment: The Executive Interview (EXIT). *Journal of the American Geriatric Society, 40*(12), 1221–1226.

Royall, D. R., Cordes, J. A., & Polk, M. (1998). CLOX: An executive clock drawing task. *Journal of Neurology, Neurosurgery, and Psychiatry, 64*(5), 588–594.

Sahgal, A., Galloway, P. H., McKeith, I. G., Lloyd, S., Cook, J. H., Ferrier, I. N., & Edwardson, J. A. (1992). Matching-to-sample deficits in patients with senile dementias of the Alzheimer and Lewy body types. *Archives of Neurology, 49*(10), 1043–1046.

Salmon, E., & Franck, G. (1989). Positron emission tomographic study in Alzheimer's disease and Pick's disease. *Archives of Gerontology and Geriatrics. Supplement, 1*, 241–247.

Sanchez-Castaneda, C., Rene, R., Ramirez-Ruiz, B., Campdelacreu, J., Gascon, J., Falcon, C.,... Junque, C. (2009). Correlations between gray matter reductions and cognitive deficits in dementia with Lewy bodies and Parkinson's disease with dementia. *Movement Disorders, 24*(12), 1740–1746.

Scarmeas, N., & Honig, L. S. (2004). Frontotemporal degenerative dementias. *Clinical Neuroscience Research, 3*(6), 449–460.

Schmidt, M. (1996). *Rey Auditory and Verbal Learning Test: A Handbook.* Los Angeles, CA: Western Psychological Services.

Shimada, H., Hirano, S., Shinotoh, H., Aotsuka, A., Sato, K., Tanaka, N.,...Irie, T. (2009). Mapping of brain acetylcholinesterase alterations in Lewy body disease by PET. *Neurology, 73*(4), 273–278.

Silverman, J. M., Schnaider-Beeri, M., Grossman, H. T., Schmeidler, J., Wang, J. Y., & Lally, R. C. (2008). A phenotype for genetic studies of successful cognitive aging. *American Journal of Medical Genetics. Part B, Neuropsychiatric Genetics, 147B*(2), 167–173.

Skibinski, G., Parkinson, N. J., Brown, J. M., Chakrabarti, L., Lloyd, S. L., Hummerich, H.,...Collinge, J. (2005). Mutations in the endosomal ESCRTIII-complex subunit CHMP2B in frontotemporal dementia. *Nature Genetics, 37*(8), 806–808.

Smith, C. D., Gallenstein, L. G., Layton, W. J., Kryscio, R. J., & Markesbery, W. R. (1993). 31P magnetic resonance spectroscopy in Alzheimer's and Pick's disease. *Neurobiology of Aging, 14*(1), 85–92.

Snowden, J. S., Bathgate, D., Varma, A., Blackshaw, A., Gibbons, Z. C., & Neary, D. (2001). Distinct behavioural profiles in frontotemporal dementia and semantic dementia. *Journal of Neurology, Neurosurgery, and Psychiatry, 70*(3), 323–332.

Snowden, J. S., Neary, D., & Mann, D. M. (2002). Frontotemporal dementia. *The British Journal of Psychiatry, 180*, 140–143.

Snowden, J., Neary, D., & Mann, D. (2007). Frontotemporal lobar degeneration: Clinical and pathological relationships. *Acta Neuropathologica, 114*(1), 31–38.

Soininen, H. S., Partanen, K., Pitkänen, A., Vainio, P., Hänninen, T., Hallikainen, M.,...Riekkinen, P. J. (1994). Volumetric MRI analysis of the amygdala and the hippocampus in subjects with age-associated memory impairment: Correlation to visual and verbal memory. *Neurology, 44*(9), 1660–1668.

Soliveri, P., Monza, D., Paridi, D., Radice, D., Grisoli, M., Testa, D.,...Girotti, F. (1999). Cognitive and magnetic resonance imaging aspects of corticobasal degeneration and progressive supranuclear palsy. *Neurology, 53*(3), 502–507.

Spering, C. C., Hobson, V., Lucas, J. A., Menon, C. V., Hall, J. R., & O'Bryant, S. E. (2012). Diagnostic accuracy of the MMSE in detecting probable and possible Alzheimer's disease in ethnically diverse highly educated individuals: An analysis of the NACC database. *The Journals of Gerontology. Series A, Biological Sciences and Medical Sciences, 67*(8), 890–896.

Spillantini, M. G., Bird, T. D., & Ghetti, B. (1998). Frontotemporal dementia and Parkinsonism linked to chromosome 17: A new group of tauopathies. *Brain Pathology, 8*(2), 387–402.

Spillantini, M. G., Murrell, J. R., Goedert, M., Farlow, M. R., Klug, A., & Ghetti, B. (1998). Mutation in the tau gene in familial multiple system tauopathy with presenile dementia. *Proceedings of the National Academy of Sciences of the United States of America, 95*(13), 7737–7741.

Starkstein, S. E., Mizrahi, R., & Power, B. D. (2008). Depression in Alzheimer's disease: Phenomenology, clinical correlates and treatment. *International Review of Psychiatry, 20*(4), 382–388.

Strauss, E., Sherman, E. M. S., & Spreen, O. (2006). *A compendium of neuropsychological tests: Administration, norms, and commentary* (3rd ed.). Oxford: Oxford University Press.

Stroop, J. R. (1935). Studies of interference in serial verbal reactions. *Journal of Experimental Psychology, 18*(6), 643–662.

Tang-Wai, D. F., Graff-Radford, N. R., Boeve, B. F., Dickson, D. W., Parisi, J. E., Crook, R.,... Petersen, R. C. (2004). Clinical, genetic, and neuropathologic characteristics of posterior cortical atrophy. *Neurology, 63*(7), 1168–1174.

Tariq, S. H., Tumosa, N., Chibnall, J. T., Perry, M. H., & Morley, J. E. (2006). Comparison of the Saint Louis University mental status examination and the Mini-Mental State Examination for detecting dementia and mild neurocognitive disorder—a pilot study. *The American Journal of Geriatric Psychiatry, 14*(11), 900–910.

Thambisetty, M., Wan, J., Carass, A., An, Y., Prince, J. L., & Resnick, S. M. (2010). Longitudinal changes in cortical thickness associated with normal aging. *NeuroImage, 52*(4), 1215–1223.

Thies, W., & Bleiler, L. (2011). 2011 Alzheimer's disease facts and figures. *Alzheimer's & Dementia, 7*(2), 208–244.

Turner, R. S., Kenyon, L. C., Trojanowski, J. Q., Gonatas, N., & Grossman, M. (1996). Clinical, neuroimaging, and pathologic features of progressive nonfluent aphasia. *Annals of Neurology, 39*(2), 166–173.

van Swieten, J., & Spillantini, M. G. (2007). Hereditary frontotemporal dementia caused by Tau gene mutations. *Brain Pathology, 17*(1), 63–73.

Vance, C., Al-Chalabi, A., Ruddy, D., Smith, B. N., Hu, X., Sreedharan, J.,...Shaw, C. E. (2006). Familial amyotrophic lateral sclerosis with frontotemporal dementia is linked to a locus on chromosome 9p13.2–21.3. *Brain: A Journal of Neurology, 129*(Pt 4), 868–876.

Watts, G. D., Wymer, J., Kovach, M. J., Mehta, S. G., Mumm, S., Darvish, D.,...Kimonis, V. E. (2004). Inclusion body myopathy associated with Paget disease of bone and frontotemporal dementia is caused by mutant valosin-containing protein. *Nature Genetics, 36*(4), 377–381.

Wechsler, A. F., Verity, M. A., Rosenschein, S., Fried, I., & Scheibel, A. B. (1982). Pick's disease. A clinical, computed tomographic, and histologic study with golgi impregnation observations. *Archives of Neurology, 39*(5), 287–290.

Wechsler, D. (2009). *Wechsler Memory Scale (WMS-IV)*. San Antonio, TX: Psychological Corporation.

Weintraub, S., Rubin, N. P., & Mesulam, M. M. (1990). Primary progressive aphasia. Longitudinal course, neuropsychological profile, and language features. *Archives of Neurology, 47*(12), 1329–1335.

Wicklund, A. H., Johnson, N., & Weintraub, S. (2004). Preservation of reasoning in primary progressive aphasia: Further differentiation from Alzheimer's disease and the behavioral presentation of frontotemporal dementia. *Journal of Clinical and Experimental Neuropsychology, 26*(3), 347–355.

Williams, H. W. (1935). The peculiar cells of Pick's disease: Their pathogenesis and distribution in disease. *Archives of Neurology & Psychiatry, 34*(3), 508–519.

Yamauchi, H., Fukuyama, H., Nagahama, Y., Katsumi, Y., Hayashi, T., Oyanagi, C.,...Shio, H. (2000). Comparison of the pattern of atrophy of the corpus callosum in frontotemporal dementia, progressive supranuclear palsy, and Alzheimer's disease. *Journal of Neurology, Neurosurgery, and Psychiatry, 69*(5), 623–629.

Zola-Morgan, S., & Squire, L. R. (1986). Memory impairment in monkeys following lesions limited to the hippocampus. *Behavioral Neuroscience, 100*(2), 155–160.

Types of Cortical Dementias and Related Presentations

CHAPTER 4

Alzheimer's Disease

Steven W. Anderson and Martin D. Cassell

In 1906, German psychiatrist and neuropathologist Alois Alzheimer described abnormal extracellular accumulations of protein (neuritic plaques) and tangled bundles of intracellular protein fibers (neurofibrillary tangles [NFTs]) on postmortem examination of the brain of a patient who had developed progressive memory, language, and behavioral problems. His discovery attracted limited attention from the medical or neuroscience community at the time, in part because his patient had developed dementia at a relatively young age (50 years), suggesting that this pathology was responsible only for a rare condition. Alzheimer went on to confirm the finding of plaques and tangles as the pathological substrate of dementia in a second patient a few years later, and his influential colleague, Emil Kraepelin, introduced the term *Alzheimer's disease* (AD) in the next edition of his textbook. For many years, this disorder was rarely reported, while "senility" was considered to be an expected, if not inevitable, consequence of brain aging or age-related cerebrovascular disease. With further study, however, it became increasingly clear that Alzheimer's findings applied not just to early-onset dementia, but also to the much more common dementia associated with old age.

The causes of age-related dementia are myriad, but the most common neuropathological finding, either in isolation or in combination with other pathologies, is a gradual accumulation of the plaques and tangles first linked to dementia by Alzheimer. When the concentration of plaques and tangles, along with the related neuronal loss, neurotransmitter depletion, and vascular damage of AD, become sufficient to disrupt the neural circuitry underlying cognition, dementia ensues. The typical behavioral profile associated with AD involves an insidious onset after the age of 70 years, initially expressed as mildly increased difficulty remembering recent events or recently presented information, losing one's train of thought, and word-finding problems. These cognitive difficulties gradually worsen over a period of months or years until they begin to interfere with the performance of normal daily activities. Worsening memory impairment usually remains prominent, but impairments also become apparent in nearly all aspects of cognition, accompanied by changes in emotion and personality. Further disease progression leads to impaired perception, skilled movement, and communication. Eventually, assistance is required for even basic daily activities, and the individual becomes bedridden. Death typically occurs within 5 to 7 years after diagnosis. With good reason, AD is among the most feared diseases in developed countries.

Increased age is the greatest risk factor for AD; hence, as the life expectancy of the population has increased, so too has the prevalence of AD. It is estimated that more than 35 million people worldwide have AD, including 5.4 million Americans. Almost 50% of U.S. citizens older than 85 years are affected by AD (Hebert, Scherr, Bienias, Bennett, & Evans, 2003), and this number will rise as the average age of the population continues to increase. Although estimates vary across studies due to different cohorts, criteria, and methodologies, autopsy studies indicate that AD accounts for 40% to 56% of cases of dementia, with an additional 15% to 40% accounted for by AD combined with other pathologies (e.g., Jellinger & Attems, 2010a). It is estimated that AD and related disorders cost more than $183 billion in the United States annually (Alzheimer's Association, 2011). AD occurs in men and women across racial and ethnic groups, geographic areas, and all levels of socioeconomic status and education. The high prevalence of AD has resulted in nearly all adults having personal familiarity with the disease in family or friends, and everyone fortunate enough to live into old age faces the risk of losing his or her mental capacities to AD.

NEUROPATHOLOGY

The neuropathological hallmarks of AD are senile plaques (SP), NFTs, and cell and synapse loss in multiple brain areas. Recent studies have included inflammation, marked by the presence of microglia, as a consistent finding in AD, and the presence of cerebral amyloid angiopathy (CAA) and granulovacuolar degeneration (GVD). The first three characteristic pathological features of AD were identified in the earliest descriptions of the disease. Alois Alzheimer's first report of his findings in the brain of patient Auguste Deter on November 3, 1906, mentioned fibrils in otherwise normal neurons and neuritic plaques (described as "miliary foci"). These were identified in sections from the cerebral cortex of the patient using a silver stain (Bielschowsky's). A later description of AD in the eighth edition of Emil Kraeplin's *Psychiatrie* additionally referred to significant cell loss in the cortex.

The pathological features of AD cause the physical and behavioral signs presented in AD because they disrupt, and eventually destroy, the neural networks in the central nervous system (CNS) that analyze incoming sensory information, disseminate information in a modified form to other brain areas, store information, and generate behavioral strategies that are transmitted to the motor and autonomic nervous systems (Savioz, Leuba, Vallet, & Walzer, 2009). In addition, changes in brain circuitry that are made to compensate for the effects of AD pathology may in fact contribute to some of the signs seen in AD. The presence of NFTs and SPs in the brain is not in itself lethal and AD patients do not die of AD per se but of the consequences of loss of motor and autonomic control. Most AD patients die of bronchopneumonia, septicaemia following infected bed sores (the cause of death in Alzheimer's patient Auguste Deter), or cardiovascular disease.

Although early work focused on the presence of SPs and NFTs in the cerebral cortex as a characteristic feature of AD, subsequent work has identified the presence of SPs, NFTs, and cell loss in the amygdala, basal forebrain (particularly acetylcholine-containing neurons), thalamic nuclei associated with the limbic system, hypothalamus, and brain stem (including the colliculi, acetylcholine, and monoamine-containing neurons; Figure 4.1). Only the basal ganglia and cerebellum appear relatively spared, although NFTs, diffuse amyloid deposits (though not SPs), and shrinkage of the putamen in AD are well documented (Braak & Braak, 1991),

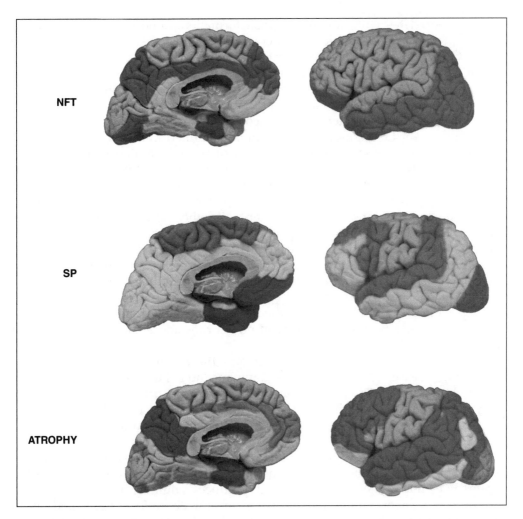

FIGURE 4.1 (*See color insert.*) Representation of the progression of the spread of NFTs, SPs, and atrophy through the early (red), middle (green), and late (purple) stages of Alzheimer's disease. Based on Braak and Braak (1991) and other sources cited in the text.

NFTs, neurofibrillary tangles; SPs, senile plaques.

and SPs (though not NFTs), cell loss, and inflammatory changes have been identified in the cerebellum in AD (Larner, 1997). In the substantia nigra, which is severely affected in Parkinson's disease, NFTs and cell loss have been found in AD, and are associated with extrapyramidal motor signs (e.g., rigidity, tremor, and parkinsonian gait) in the later stages of AD (Burns, Galvin, Roe, Morris, & McKeel, 2005).

Amyloid (Senile or Neuritic) Plaques

Many researchers believe that brain amyloidosis is the first pathological event leading to all aspects of subsequent AD pathology, even though the exact link to these aspects is unclear (Hardy & Allsop, 1991). Amyloidosis can occur in any organ as a consequence of inflammation and genetic factors; in the brain, amyloid deposits are usually associated with increased numbers of glial cells (microglia and astrocytes) that mediate inflammatory responses. Experimental studies indicate that microglia activation correlates with amyloid deposit formation, although there is evidence that the numbers of resting microglia increase prior to plaque formation (Rodríguez, Witton, Olabarria, Noristani, & Verkhratsky, 2010).

SPs are extracellular deposits of amyloid, an insoluble fibrillar protein, though the term *amyloid*—"starch-like"—refers to the early belief that the deposits were composed of carbohydrates. Plaques are generally spheroid structures, between 50 µm and 0.3 mm in diameter, and some contain fragments of axons and dendrites, the so-called neuritic plaques. Plaques can be identified in histological sections of postmortem brain tissue by using a number of special staining methods. Simple dyes like thioflavin S and Congo Red stain amyloid fibrils, while silver stains additionally reveal the fragments of neurites contained within plaques. However, antibodies to components of the amyloid-beta (Aβ) protein (see below) reveal a much greater number of plaques than those seen with other staining methods. This has led to the idea of "staging" of plaque development; the first stage is a deposit of amyloid, detectable by immunocytochemistry using antibodies to Aβ protein but not by silver stains, thioflavin S, or Congo Red; the next plaque form is additionally stainable by silver methods and thioflavin S, but no neurites are identifiable ("primitive"); the third stage is the neuritic plaque with staining of neurites by silver methods ("mature"); the final, or "burned out" stage, now stainable by Congo Red, consists of a dense core of amyloid with no neurites and a substantial number of nearby glia.

The principal amyloid protein found in the SP of AD is Aβ, whereas in Parkinson's disease, alpha-synuclein is dominant and in Huntington's disease, huntingtin. Alpha-synuclein is the principal amyloid protein found in Lewy bodies. Lewy bodies are found in the brains of approximately 60% of patients with early-onset and sporadic AD, with a particularly heavy concentration in the amygdala (Hamilton, 2000).

Aβ is formed from amyloid precursor protein (APP), a glycoprotein found in cell membranes, by a sequence of enzymes, the β- and γ-secretases. The critical action appears to be that of the γ-secretase, which produces a number of different Aβs that vary in their number of amino acids. $A\beta_{42}$ is most likely to form fibrils and insoluble deposits and is the form associated with SPs. SPs are fairly evenly distributed throughout the cortex with the fewest numbers being found in the hippocampal and parahippocampal regions of the temporal lobe where NFTs are found early in AD (see the following text). The greatest numbers of SPs are to be found in the lateral temporal and occipital lobes (Arnold, Hyman, Flory, Damasio, & Van Hoesen, 1991). As described in the following text, advances in PET imaging have now made it possible to estimate brain amyloidosis (Aβ load) in vivo.

Neurofibrillary Tangles

NFTs are intracellular accumulations of a hyperphosphorylated microtubule-associated protein, tau, which self-aggregates as paired helical filaments (King, Ahuja, Binder, & Kuret, 1999). The exact mechanism behind the formation of NFTs and their relationship to AD has not been firmly established. NFTs have been found in the brains of very old individuals with no or mild cognitive impairment, and may be part of normal aging (Jellinger & Attems, 2010a). One school of thought suggests that they are a protective response to other pathological events rather than a cause of neuron death (Lee et al., 2005). The correlation between cell loss and the presence of NFTs is weak and NFTs may only contribute to about 10% of cell loss in AD (Kril, Patel, Harding, & Halliday, 2002).

The pattern and time course of NFT formation differs from that of SP (Arnold et al., 1991). In early and mid-stage AD, NFTs are confined to the cortex surrounding the rhinal sulcus and the anterior part of the collateral sulcus (the transentorhinal region) and the hippocampus. In these regions, NFTs predominate in layers II and IV. In later stages, NFTs may be found in the neocortex, but the distribution is uneven. In late-stage AD, proisocortical areas (e.g., insular and cingulate cortices) have the most NFTs, followed by association areas in the frontal (e.g., prelimbic [Brodmann area 32]) and temporal lobes (e.g., Wernicke's area). The fewest NFTs are found in sensory association areas (e.g., Brodmann areas 18 and 19 in the occipital lobe, and areas 20 and 21 in the temporal lobe), motor and premotor regions (including Broca's area), and the primary sensory cortex (e.g., areas 17 [visual] and 1, 2, and 3 [somatosensory]). NFTs in the cortex are mostly located in layers III and V.

Cell Loss

Progressive and regional atrophy of brain structures constitutes the most obvious pathological change in AD (Figure 4.2). While there is a slight decline in overall brain volume with normal aging—and is largely attributable to a decline in white matter (e.g., Double et al., 1996)—overall brain volume decreases by between 15% and 25% in AD patients. Most of this volume reduction appears to arise from atrophy of the

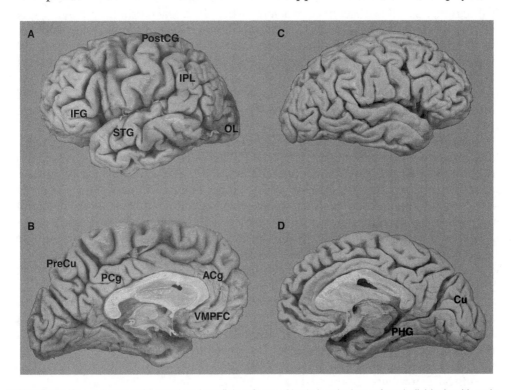

FIGURE 4.2 (*See color insert.*) Lateral and medial surfaces of brain hemispheres from individuals with early-stage Alzheimer's disease (left hemisphere, A, B) and late-stage Alzheimer's disease (right hemisphere, C, D) showing the extent of atrophy. The presence of NFTs and SPs was histologically confirmed in the opposite hemisphere.

ACg, anterior cingulate gyrus; Cu, cuneus of occipital lobe; IFG, inferior frontal gyrus; IPL, inferior parietal lobule; NFT, neurofibrillary tangles; OL, occipital lobe; PCg, posterior cingulate gyrus; PHG, parahippocampal gyrus; PostCG, postcentral gyrus; PreCu, precuneus of parietal lobe; SP, senile plaques; STG, superior temporal gyrus; VMPFC, ventromedial prefrontal cortex.

gray matter of the cerebral cortex. Moreover, atrophy is greatest in the hippocampal formation (dentate gyrus, hippocampus, and subiculum) and the cortex of the medial temporal lobe. In fact, a 20% to 25% reduction in the volume of the hippocampus and entorhinal cortex has been demonstrated in presymptomatic patients and those with mild cognitive impairment (e.g., Bobinski et al., 2000; Jack et al., 1997; Scahill, Schott, Stevens, Rossor, & Fox, 2002). However, atrophy, even at early stages of AD, is not confined to the medial temporal lobe. Reduction in the volume of the precuneus region of the medial parietal lobe and adjacent posterior cingulate cortex has been observed in patients with early-stage AD (e.g., Scahill et al., 2002). Patients with middle- and late-stage AD show additional atrophy in the inferior and superior temporal gyri, the insula, and orbitofrontal and dorsolateral frontal cortices. The pattern and progression of atrophy in AD is consistent enough for sophisticated pattern recognition algorithms to be able to discriminate AD from other forms of dementia (e.g., Davatzikos, Xu, An, Fan, & Resnick, 2009; Fan, Batmanghelich, Clark, & Davatzikos; Alzheimer's Disease Neuroimaging Initiative, 2008).

Although white matter thinning (leukoaraiosis) has been associated with AD, the bulk of the brain atrophy seen in AD is attributable to loss of neurons and loss of neuropil (dendrites, dendritic spines, and axons) in both cortical and subcortical regions. Loss of neurons and associated neuropil will both disrupt local neuronal network function, that is, the functioning within a particular neuronal nucleus or cortical region, as well as disconnect nuclei/cortical from each other, destroying global network function. Neuronal/neuropil loss can affect systems processing and relaying activity with high information content as well as those affecting signal-to-noise ratios or general arousal. For example, disconnection of the hippocampus from the parahippocampal gyrus due to neuronal/neuropil loss in AD leads to loss of episodic memory (high information content); the loss of substantial numbers of hypocretin/orexin neurons in the hypothalamus in AD is thought to be behind the frequent sleep disturbances found in AD patients (Fronczek et al., 2012).

Surprisingly, the *overall* number of cortical neurons declines only marginally in AD (Regeur, Jensen, Pakkenberg, Evans, & Pakkenberg, 1994), reflecting two features of AD-associated cell loss: The cell loss is heaviest in specific cortical regions, and particular cortical cell types are especially vulnerable to AD pathology. Cell loss in AD appears to be greatest in the temporal cortices followed by the parietal, frontal, and posterior cingulate cortices (e.g., Coleman & Flood, 1987; Terry, Peck, DeTeresa, Schechter, & Horoupian, 1981). In the neocortex, a subpopulation of large pyramidal neurons (identifiable by antibodies to a neurofilament-associated protein, SMI32) located in layers III and V suffer the greatest loss in AD (e.g., Hof, Cox, & Morrison, 1990). These particular pyramidal neurons give rise to associative and commissural cortico-cortical connections, and their loss disrupts large-scale network function. Additionally, these neurons are also components of "mini-columns," vertically organized functional units found in most cortical areas; thus *local* intrinsic networks are also disrupted by pyramidal cell loss. The presence of abundant NFTs in layers III and V provides a strong link between NFTs and cell loss, although cell loss greatly exceeds NFT numbers (Gómez-Isla et al., 1997).

Heavy cell loss also occurs in limbic system structures, but again, specific regions are more vulnerable. In the entorhinal cortex region of the parahippocampal gyrus, major cell loss is evident even in patients with mild clinical signs of AD, and more advanced stages of the disease are associated with almost total loss of layer II neurons (e.g., Hyman, Van Hoesen, Kromer, & Damasio, 1986). This layer-specific loss is of particular importance as layer II cells of the entorhinal cortex are the origin of most of the perforant path, the largest input to the hippocampus. Loss of these cells effectively disconnects the hippocampus from the network activity of the neocortex. Additional heavy cell loss in the CA1 and subicular regions of the hippocampus also destroys the output link from the hippocampus itself to entorhinal and neocortical areas (e.g., West, Coleman, Flood, & Troncoso, 1994).

Atrophy has been reported in the amygdala in early stages of AD with magnitudes of volume changes comparable to those found for the hippocampus (Poulin et al., 2011). In addition to the presence of NFTs and SPs (e.g., Herzog & Kemper, 1980), significant cell loss has also been reported in the amygdala of AD patients (Scott, DeKosky, Sparks, Knox, & Scheff, 1992), although it appears to be confined to those components included in the amygdala that have a cortical-like structure (e.g., the cortical and basomedial nuclei [the periamygdaloid cortex] and basal nucleus).

NFTs and SPs are found in the basal telencephalon, the diencephalon, midbrain, and pons and medulla in AD, but cell loss has been only well documented in two subcortical nuclei: the nucleus basalis of Meynert (NBM) in the basal telencephalon and the locus ceruleus in the pons.

The NBM is a scattered group of cholinergic (acetylcholine-containing) and GABAergic (γ-amino butyric acid-containing) neurons located lateral to the anterior hypothalamus and ventral to the globus pallidus. Both types of neurons innervate the cerebral cortex and the NBM is the source of more than 80% of cortical acetylcholine. Cortical acetylcholine is required for consolidation of memories and general neural activity. Progressive loss of neurons occurs in the NBM in late-stage AD (e.g., Whitehouse, Price, Clark, Coyle, & DeLong, 1981), and the degree of loss correlates with the degree of dementia (e.g., Lehéricy et al., 1993) although little change in NBM cell numbers is seen in mild cognitive impairment and early AD (Gilmor et al., 1999). This loss of cholinergic NBM neurons leads to a dramatic decline in cortical acetylcholine levels (less than 10% of normal age-matched peers). Loss of cholinergic fibers is greatest in the entorhinal and superior temporal gyrus and lowest in primary sensory areas (with the exception of the primary auditory cortex), motor and premotor cortices, and the anterior cingulate cortex (Geula & Mesulam, 1996). The numbers of both nicotinic and muscarinic acetylcholine receptors (e.g., Shimohama, Taniguchi, Fujiwara, & Kameyama, 1986; Whitehouse et al., 1986) decline in AD and the changes in AD in the α7 class of nicotinic receptor may relate to the binding of Aβ to the receptor (e.g., Wang et al., 2010).

Loss of the pigmented, noradrenaline-containing neurons of the locus ceruleus occurs during normal aging (e.g., Chan-Palay & Asan, 1989); however, greater loss occurs in AD, particularly among the subpopulation of locus ceruleus neurons innervating the cerebral cortex and limbic system (Marcyniuk, Mann, & Yates, 1989).

Neuropil and Synapse Loss

The pathological event that correlates most with cognitive decline in AD is loss of synapses, nerve terminals, and dendritic spines in the cortex and hippocampus. Ultrastructural analyses of biopsy and postmortem tissue from the frontal cortex of AD patients have revealed more than 50% decline in volumetric synaptic density with the loss showing a strong positive correlation (r = circa 0.8) with scores on the Mini-Mental State Examination (MMSE; e.g., DeKosky & Scheff, 1990; Terry et al., 1991). Losses in synaptic volume density from 25% to 33% have been found in superior temporal and posterior cingulate cortices (e.g., Scheff & Price, 2003). In the outer molecular layer of the dentate gyrus of the hippocampus, the area targeted by inputs from layer II of the entorhinal cortex, synapse number is positively correlated with scores on the MMSE and delayed word list recall and recognition (Scheff, Price,

Schmitt, & Mufson, 2006), as well as the packing density of NFTs in the entorhinal cortex. In addition, synapse density in the outer molecular layer has been reported to be an average of 13% lower in patients with mild cognitive impairment compared to controls and an average of 44% lower in patients with early AD (Scheff et al., 2006), indicating that the synapse number has declined significantly prior to diagnosis.

In addition to actual physical loss of synapses and associated pre- and postsynaptic elements, numerous studies have reported declines in neurotransmitter levels and the density and ratios of proteins required for assembly and maintenance of synaptic contact in AD brains (e.g., Reddy et al., 2005). While some synaptic loss may be attributable to the loss of the cells of origin of the synapse (e.g., as in the case of the entorhinal input to the dentate gyrus), most modern researchers postulate that synapse loss is due directly to the toxic effects of the soluble forms of Aβ. There is a wealth of evidence for Aβ negatively affecting synapse formation, neurotransmitter release, and long-term potentiation (e.g., Koffie et al., 2009), although the exact mechanism(s) are controversial. Aβ may have its major influence on the protein kinase C (PKC) group of enzymes, particularly the PKCα and PKCε isoforms, which are found abundantly in synaptic terminals. Recent studies on an animal model of AD have shown that administration of two drugs, bryostatin-1 and the linoleic acid derivative (DCP-LA), which specifically activate the PKCα and PKCε isoforms, prevents synaptic loss, formation of SPs, and a decline in spatial memory (Hongpaisan, Sun, & Alkon, 2011).

Cerebral Amyloid Angiopathy

In addition to forming SPs in nervous tissue, Aβ can be deposited within the walls of small cerebral arteries and arterioles. Initially, Aβ deposits cause progressive narrowing of the internal lumen of the vessels, but eventually the whole of the vessel wall is compromised and the vessel ruptures, resulting in disruption of the blood–brain barrier and microhemorrhages (Attems, Jellinger, Thal, & Van Nostrand, 2011). The most heavily affected vessels are small arteries and arterioles in the cortex, with vessels in the occipital lobe being the most affected and those in the parahippocampal and hippocampal regions the least (or latest) to be affected. The precise relationship of CAA to AD is not clear. In one study, 57% of demented patients presented CAA at autopsy compared to only 24% of nondemented patients (Matthews et al., 2009). CAA is a common finding in elderly patients with or without AD although, nonetheless, it is a strong predictor of cognitive decline (Jellinger & Attems, 2010b).

Granulovacuolar Degeneration

GVD has long been recognized to be present in the brains of AD patients, although the relationship to the other pathological features of AD is unclear, in part because GVD occurs in other late-onset dementias, for example, frontotemporal dementia and Pick's disease, as well as normal aging. GVD is characterized by the presence of small vacuoles, roughly 3 to 5 μm in diameter, in the cytoplasm of neurons. These vacuoles also contain a single, small basophilic granule. Immunostaining indicates that the granules contain the tau protein, suggesting that the vacuoles in GVD may be related to the sequestering of abnormal protein complexes that contribute to the formation of NFTs. Indeed, the anatomical progression of GVD follows closely that of NFTs and to a lesser extent SPs (Thal et al., 2011). GVD is found first in the CA1 subfield of the hippocampus and the subiculum, followed by the entorhinal (area 28) and perirhinal (area 35) areas of the medial temporal lobe. Subsequent areas affected include the NBM, the amygdala, and diencephalon (hypothalamus and thalamus).

Outside of the medial temporal and cingulate cortices, GVD is only found occasionally in frontal, parietal, and occipital areas. While the presence of GVD correlates with the presence of NFTs and SPs, the link between them is not known. Recent studies (e.g., Thal et al., 2011) have pointed out that GVD occurs in brain regions innervated by the locus ceruleus, a collection of monoaminergic neurons in the pons and midbrain that exhibits NFTs at very early stages of AD. The locus ceruleus is important in maintaining wakefulness and is strongly activated during stress.

Eosinophilic Rod-Like Inclusions (Hirano Bodies)

Hirano bodies are crystalline, rod-like intraneuronal inclusions that consist of actin and actin-related proteins (including APP) and, like the vacuoles found in GVD, they are found in the brains of patients with AD and other degenerative diseases, including Creutzfeldt–Jakob disease, as well as normal aging. Actin is the most important element of the cytoskeleton and its rapid conversion from a globular to filamentous form and back is key to many intracellular processes. This conversion is regulated by a number of factors, the most important being cofilin. Phosphorylation of cofilin enhances the formation of filamentous actin. Hirano bodies are cofilin-actin-enriched inclusions and are found in most neurodegenerative diseases. Cofilin-actin rods are formed in many cell types in response to cellular stressors such as excessive glutamate and peroxide, and increased sodium, but the clearance of the rods appears to be particularly difficult in neurons. Of relevance is the fact that the presence of Aβ induces cofilin-actin rod formation in hippocampal neurons in culture. Hirano bodies are found in neurons at normal levels in the case of normal aging but increased numbers are found in AD, particularly in neurons of the hippocampus. As previously noted, synaptic loss is a hallmark of AD; experimental studies have shown that increased levels of cofilin affect synaptic transmission and number as well as the functioning of the critically important postsynaptic structure, the dendritic spine. It has been suggested that dysregulation of cofilin and subsequent alterations in actin dynamics may be the major cause of synaptic loss in AD (Bamburg & Bloom, 2009).

RISK FACTORS

The evidence to date suggests that AD develops as a result of multiple risk factors rather than from one cause. Advanced age carries the greatest risk, but even when age is considered together with known genetic risk factors, there is considerable variability in susceptibility to AD that remains unexplained. Except in the relatively rare cases of familial early-onset AD and in persons with Down syndrome (DS), no single risk factor is strongly predictive of developing AD. However, several factors influence the probability of developing AD. Consideration of these factors is important both for understanding the causal mechanisms of the disorder, and because scientific and societal attention to risk factors that are potentially modifiable (e.g., mental and physical activity, depression, diabetes) could substantially reduce the prevalence of AD in future generations.

Age

Age is the single greatest risk factor for developing AD, with approximately 1 in 8 people (13%) older than 65 years with probable AD, but nearly half (43%) of those aged 85 years or older afflicted by the disease (Alzheimer's Association, 2011). It is possible that altered regulation of the mechanisms of brain aging may contribute to the pathogenesis of AD, but the relationships between the development of AD pathology and brain aging are not fully understood. Disentangling the linkages between aging and the development of AD is complicated because of the widespread effects of aging on other factors that directly or indirectly influence brain health and expression of functional deficits (e.g., sensory loss, cerebrovascular disease, social isolation). Normal aging is accompanied by structural and physiological changes in the brain and variable cognitive decline, with several features of healthy brain aging resembling milder versions of the more drastic changes found in AD. The pathological hallmarks of AD, including NFT, neuritic plaques, and loss of synapses, are found to varying degrees in aged persons without dementia (e.g., Aizenstein et al., 2008; Braak & Braak, 1991; Katzman et al., 1989). Normal aging also is associated with shrinkage and decreased resting-state metabolism in the hippocampal formation, although the pattern of involvement of hippocampal subregions varies between AD and healthy aging. The impact of AD is seen particularly in the entorhinal cortex, where greater than 50% loss of layer II neurons has been found in mild AD (Gómez-Isla et al., 1996), whereas healthy aging is associated with involvement of the dentate gyrus and CA3, with relatively little change in the entorhinal cortex (Mueller et al., 2010; Mueller & Weiner, 2009).

Although increased age is the strongest predictor of developing AD, and despite the neurophysiological similarities between AD and aging, AD is not an inevitable consequence of aging. Dissociations between advanced age and AD take various forms (e.g., Nelson et al., 2011). First are the instances of early-onset AD, where dementia due to AD pathology can occur in persons as early as in their 30s. Second are those persons who survive into their 10th decade without developing dementia or significant AD neuropathology. Clearly, aging as a risk factor for AD must be considered in the context of genetic predispositions and lifestyle and environmental factors.

Genetic Factors

The heritability of the common late-onset form of AD may be as high as 70%, based on twin studies (Gatz et al., 2006; Meyer & Breitner, 1998). Individuals with a parent or sibling with AD are at increased risk of developing the disease, and those with more than one first-degree relative with AD are at even greater risk (Green et al., 2002; Mayeux, Sano, Chen, Tatemichi, & Stern, 1991). However, the disease is genetically heterogeneous, with no simple mode of transmission. The first genetic risk factor established for late-onset AD is the gene that encodes apolipoprotein E (ApoE). ApoE guides development of a protein that carries cholesterol in the bloodstream, and may contribute to B-amyloid deposition and plaque formation (Blennow, de Leon, & Zetterberg, 2006). The ApoE gene comes in three common forms (e2, e3, and e4), and all persons have two copies, one inherited from each of his or her parents. Individuals with one copy of the ApoE-e4 form of the gene are at two- to threefold increased risk of developing late-onset AD, and those who inherit two ApoE-e4 genes are at even higher risk (five- to tenfold). ApoE-e4 is associated with decreased age of onset of dementia in a gene dosage-dependent manner (Reitz & Mayeux, 2009). Although ApoE status may account for as much as 20% to 50% of late-onset dementia risk and can serve as a stratification factor for clinical trials and other research, it is not sufficiently predictive to be useful in most clinical situations. AD can develop in persons with no ApoE-e4 gene, and persons with one or two copies of this gene may not develop AD. More than 500 other genes have been evaluated as potential risk factors for developing AD, and although meta-analyses point to several genes with marginally significant associations with disease risk, none has been proven to consistently affect disease risk or onset age (Bertram & Tanzi, 2008). However, two recent large genome-wide association studies have identified three new potential genetic risk factors for late-onset AD, which are possibly involved in clearance of amyloid from the brain (Harold et al., 2009; Lambert et al., 2009). Overall, the evidence to date suggests that the neuropathology of common late-onset AD arises through the effects of multiple genes with small effects each, in interaction with environmental factors.

Genetic factors play a more direct role in the development of AD in two special populations, persons with DS and the rare families in which early-onset (or "presenile") AD is transmitted in an autosomal-dominant fashion. DS is caused by trisomy of chromosome 21. Dementia is common in DS, often with onset in the 50s, and plaques and tangles are found in the brains of most elderly persons with DS. Chromosome 21 has been found to include the *APP* gene involved in production of the Aβ peptide.

Three genes have been found to affect the small number of families with autosomal-dominant early-onset AD (1%–2% of the total AD population). Although these genes do not seem to be directly relevant to the vast majority of people who develop AD later in life, they do provide clues as to the mechanisms of the disease. Early- and late-onset AD are generally considered to be the same disease, as it is not possible to differentiate early-onset AD from late-onset AD on the basis of neuropathological findings. The three genes that have been linked to early-onset forms of the disease (the *APP* gene—APP, and two presenilin genes—*PSEN1* and *PSEN2*) all alter production of the Aβ peptide, which is the principal component of SP. Although the majority of AD patients show no mutations in the genes coding for either APP or presenilins, these findings still provide critical support for the amyloid cascade hypothesis, which posits that an accumulation of Aβ triggers AD, as well as the subsequent formation of tangles and neural degeneration (Hardy & Selkoe, 2002).

Race and Gender

In the United States, African Americans and Hispanics are proportionately more likely to develop dementia than older Whites, but poor health conditions, lower education, and other socioeconomic risk factors likely account for these differences (Dilworth-Anderson et al., 2008; Gurland et al., 1999; Plassman et al., 2007). Likewise, gender does not appear to substantially influence the risk of AD, despite the fact that women tend to live longer than men. Almost two thirds of Americans with AD are women, reflecting the greater longevity of women, but the incidence of AD at any given age does not differ between men and women (e.g., Barnes et al., 2003; Hebert, Scherr, McCann, Beckett, & Evans, 2001).

Potentially Modifiable Factors

In addition to the risks of advanced age and genetic factors, several potentially modifiable risk factors have been reported to show an association with AD. The strength of these associations is low, and the overall scientific quality of the evidence remains limited (Daviglus et al., 2011; National Institutes of Health [NIH], 2010). Furthermore, it is not clear that the factors associated with AD contribute causally to the disease, or are related for other reasons. For example, it has become increasingly clear that brain physiology and function in aging are closely linked to overall health of the heart and blood vessels. Thus, although factors such as diabetes, obesity, elevated blood cholesterol, high blood pressure, and physical inactivity have been linked to increased risk of dementia, these factors are likely to exert their effects primarily through increased cerebrovascular disease, which commonly co-occurs with AD. An autopsy study of 80 people with clinically diagnosed probable AD found that more than half of the tissue samples showed evidence of AD together with other brain disease, primarily infarcts and Lewy body disease (Schneider, Arvanitakis, Bang, & Bennett, 2007). However, it would be wrong to think of AD and vascular disease as simply two co-occurring and additive sources of brain damage in old age. Rather, there is an interaction and synergy of pathologies not yet fully understood. As described earlier, most patients with AD have vascular damage in the form of CAA, and resultant disruption of the blood–brain barrier and cerebral blood flow are important features of AD (Zlokovic, 2011).

The probability of developing AD is elevated in persons with a history of depression, but the nature of the link between depression and AD is not well understood (e.g., Devanand et al., 1996; Saczynski et al., 2010). Depression may reflect the behavioral expression of an early stage of AD, or an emotional response to increasing cognitive impairment, rather than a causal factor. Traumatic brain injury (TBI), particularly repeated blows to the head such as those experienced by boxers, hockey players, and football players, can lead to a condition of dementia and chronic traumatic encephalopathy, including tau tangles (e.g., Guskiewicz et al., 2005; Roberts, Allsop, & Bruton, 1990). A history of a single moderate TBI also may increase the risk of developing AD twofold, and severe TBI increases the risk even more. ApoE-e4 carriers with a history of TBI may be at greater risk of developing AD than ApoE-e4 carriers with no history of TBI (Lye & Shores, 2000; Plassman et al., 2000). Exposure to environmental toxins, such as commonly used pesticides, also may increase the risk of AD (e.g., Hayden et al., 2010), but no environmental factor has yet shown a strong association with AD.

Consistent with the growing literature on neural and cognitive plasticity, there is increasing evidence that cognitive and physical activity throughout one's life and into old age can have a positive influence on brain health in aging. For example, level of participation in exercise has been found to be inversely correlated with the onset of cognitive impairment (Jedrziewski, Ewbank, Wang, & Trojanowski, 2010). Engaging in cognitively stimulating leisure activities may help preserve memory abilities in individuals with early dementia (Hall et al., 2009). Even if the mechanisms linking modifiable risk factors to AD and dementia are not fully understood, reducing these risk factors in the population could have a significant effect on the prevalence of AD-related dementia (e.g., Barnes & Yaffe, 2011).

Cognitive Reserve

Reduced risk of developing dementia due to AD has been linked to higher education, intelligence quotient (IQ), and occupational attainment (e.g., Stern, 2006). These observations, together with the repeated finding that many older individuals with high levels of plaques and tangles at autopsy, or with high levels of Aβ on labeled PET imaging, do not show signs of dementia (e.g., Aizenstein et al., 2008; Katzman et al., 1989; Knopman et al., 2003; Price & Morris, 1999), have been used to support the notion that there are individual differences in "reserve" against the effects of AD pathology. This reserve might be based on anatomical differences (e.g., brain size or synapse count), whereby a certain threshold of extent of damage must be reached before there are clinically observable consequences. It might also be the case that there are individual differences in cognitive processing approaches that are more or less effective in recruiting alternate brain areas or otherwise coping with brain damage, even in the absence of significant anatomical differences.

FUNCTIONAL IMPACT

All patients with AD will encounter difficulties in their daily real-world behavioral repertoire, and it is inevitable that these difficulties will worsen as the disease progresses. Although AD pathology is not limited to the cortex, the predominantly cortical distribution leads to the prototypical "cortical dementional syndrome." The early and prominent deficits occur specifically in the realm of cognition and behavior, with other aspects of the neurologic examination remaining normal until much later in the progression. However, AD is associated with an increased risk of seizures that may occur at any stage of the disease, particularly in cases with early onset (Palop & Mucke, 2009). There is variability across individuals in the behavioral expression of AD, but the most common presentation begins with gradually worsening difficulty in anterograde memory. These initial symptoms appear after a lengthy presymptomatic phase of neurodegeneration that may span 20 years or more. By the time patients are diagnosed with mild AD, they may have undergone more than 50% loss of neurons in layer II of the entorhinal cortex (Gómez-Isla et al., 1996). This damage deprives the hippocampal formation of cortical input and weakens the ability to distinguish between recently presented stimuli and retain new information over brief delays.

Initially indistinguishable from the occasional lapses in recall or attention that characterize normal cognition, the memory problems of AD worsen to a point where they attract the attention of others or begin to disrupt normal daily activities. Common early signs of the memory impairment include losing personal items, not returning to an ongoing activity or line of thought following an interruption, forgetting about upcoming appointments or responsibilities, and failure to recall recent conversations and activities.

Onset and Early AD

The detection of AD in its earliest stages is a research and clinical priority, based on general agreement that any disease-modifying intervention is likely to be most effective if introduced earlier in the course of the disease. It has become apparent that subtle impairments in memory or other cognitive abilities may be detectable before a person with AD meets the criteria for dementia, that is, before there is significant impairment in daily functional abilities. For example, a person may notice that tasks are more difficult or take more time, but are still achievable, or that they have become more reliant on notes, schedules, and other people in order to accomplish familiar tasks. These earliest signs of cognitive decline often reflect a transition stage from normal mentation to dementia, termed *mild cognitive impairment* (MCI). MCI is discussed in detail in Chapter 14.

Although all persons who develop dementia due to AD must pass through a stage of MCI, this stage may go undetected. Compensatory behaviors may hide cognitive changes from friends and relatives, and clinical evaluation is unlikely to be pursued. Even if the individual is presented with one of the commonly used screening evaluations, such as the MMSE, there is a good chance that subtle and isolated memory problems will not be detected.

When MCI reflects an early stage of AD, memory worsens and impairments gradually begin to appear and worsen in other domains of cognition, including language, problem solving, perception, and behavior initiation. As cognition worsens during the early stages of AD, patients and care providers are presented with numerous decisions that can have major implications for autonomy, safety, and quality of life. One key decision faced by most U.S. citizens with AD is when to stop driving an automobile. Decisions regarding driving after a diagnosis of AD present particular challenges, due to the importance of driving for independence in modern society balanced against the public safety risk posed by the growing number of impaired older drivers. Previously experienced drivers are able to continue performing most aspects of operating a vehicle even after developing severe hippocampal damage and dense amnesia, likely due to the dependence of driving on preserved procedural memory (Anderson et al., 2007). Thus, drivers with AD often are capable of starting a car, backing it down the driveway, and pulling into traffic long after their dementia has progressed beyond a point of safe driving. Drivers with AD show considerable variability in driving performance, but on average they make more safety errors (e.g., lane crossings) than do elderly drivers without AD; they also have greater difficulty with vehicle control when multitasking (e.g., route following) and show poorer responses in common high-risk situations such as intersections and rear-end collision avoidance (e.g., Rizzo, McGehee, Dawson, & Anderson, 2001; Uc, Rizzo, Anderson, Shi, & Dawson, 2004; Uc, Rizzo, Anderson, Shi, & Dawson, 2006). The extent of driving safety risk in drivers with early AD is correlated with the degree of cognitive impairment on standardized testing (Anderson et al., 2012; Dawson, Anderson, Uc, Dastrup, & Rizzo, 2009), providing a means for neuropsychologists to provide patients and families with guidance on this complex issue. Curtailment of driving is just one example of functional challenges and decisions that must be considered over the course of AD. These issues are discussed in detail in Chapter 20.

Course of Dementia

The time course of progressive dementia in AD varies considerably, with death occurring from 4 to 20 years after diagnosis. As AD progresses beyond the early phase, worsening amnesia is accompanied by changes in virtually all aspects of cognition. Language impairments can substantially interfere with communication and complicate caregiving. Word-finding problems gradually worsen, and speech becomes increasingly vague, sparse, and repetitive. However, speech prosody and articulation tend to be relatively preserved in early stages of the disease, and conversational skills (e.g., turn-taking, eye contact) and other social graces may be preserved, often allowing the disease to go undetected by others in casual social interactions. Aural comprehension declines, as does the ability to detect humor or sarcasm. Although reading comprehension may not be affected early in the course of the disease, it becomes difficult for patients to remember recently read information. Reading comprehension eventually declines, although the ability to read words and passages aloud often persists even when there is little or no comprehension of what is being read. Writing tends to follow a parallel course of decline, typically marked by gradually worsening perseveration, micrographia, agrammatism, and spelling errors. Production becomes slowed and sparse.

Perceptual impairments typically appear later than memory and language problems, but gradual decline in multiple aspects of perception often introduce problems in several aspects of daily function. Difficulties with contrast sensitivity, spatial perception, and allocation of visual attention can lead to falls and contribute to misperception of environmental stimuli, confusion, and hallucinations (Rizzo, Anderson, Dawson, Myers, & Ball, 2000a; Rizzo, Anderson, Dawson, & Nawrot, 2000b). Visual agnosia leads to confusion in the use of household objects, and can be dangerous (e.g., if cleaning substances are mistaken for food). Prosopagnosia often extends to even the patient's closest relatives. Auditory agnosia also is a common source of confusion. The higher-order perceptual impairments caused by AD often are worsened by age-related peripheral hearing and vision problems. Apraxia typically appears in a subtle form in early AD, where it may be detected by clinical testing (e.g., demonstrating how to use tools and utensils not actually present), yet does not interfere with normal activities. Eventually, apraxia progresses to a point of interfering with daily activities such as getting dressed, toileting, and feeding.

Over time, social withdrawal, apathy, and other changes in mood and personality are common. Many of these behavioral changes resemble those seen in depressed persons, although mood may or may not be sad in AD. Agitation, irritability, anxiety, and disinhibition also may occur at any stage of the disease (e.g., Lyketsos et al., 2011). Wandering is common, and can be dangerous when combined with poor awareness of environmental conditions (e.g., bad weather, dangerous traffic). Sleep disturbances (e.g., night-time wake ups, daytime drowsiness, excess daytime sleeping) may occur in a quarter of patients with mild-to-moderate AD, likely due in large part to hypothalamic cell loss, and often are associated with other behavioral problems (Moran et al., 2005; Tractenberg, Singer, & Kaye, 2006). There is considerable variability in AD patients' awareness of their condition. Self-awareness of progressing cognitive deficits varies across individuals with AD, and within individuals over time, and may be influenced on a moment-to-moment basis by the demands of the current activity and how awareness is assessed (Anderson & Tranel, 1989; Kotler-Cope & Camp, 1995).

In late-stage AD, patients become immobile, unable to feed or clean themselves, and unable to respond to the environment or communicate their needs. Reflexes become abnormal, and muscles become rigid. Swallowing becomes impaired. Advanced-stage AD patients are at significantly increased risk of death, which commonly occurs within 4 to 8 years after diagnosis (Larson et al., 2004). AD has been reported as the fifth leading cause of death for those 65 years and older (Heron, Hoyert, Xu, Scott, & Tejada-Vera, 2008), and the percent of death certificates recording AD as the underlying cause continues to increase. This likely reflects both the increased prevalence of AD and changes in death certificate recording practices. The presence of AD pathology in the brain is not in itself lethal, but the loss of motor and autonomic control can lead to death through complications such as immobility, swallowing disorders, and malnutrition, which in turn increase the risk of bronchopneumonia, other infections, or cardiovascular disease.

Atypical Profiles

Although the most common presentation of AD involves an initial gradual onset of memory problems as previously described, AD can vary in initial signs and course. Focal cortical symptoms other than amnesia may remain relatively pure or isolated for years (Alladi et al., 2007). Atypical presentations occur in both early-onset and late-onset AD, but may be particularly common in early-onset AD, where one third of cases may have atypical symptoms (Balasa et al., 2011). The most common variant involves early problems with language that precede and outweigh memory difficulties, known as primary progressive aphasia (PPA). PPA is discussed in detail in Chapter 11. Infrequently, AD presents initially with visual perceptual problems (visual variant AD) that may include agnosia, simultanagnosia, alexia, and impaired ability to guide hand movements. These perceptual impairments may gradually worsen over a period of 2 to 3 years before memory problems become evident. AD also may present with early prominent changes in personality, mood, or social behavior, and some patients with clinical diagnoses of frontotemporal dementia have been found to have AD pathology at autopsy (Snowden et al., 2011). The initial presentation and course of AD also may vary as a function of comorbid neurodegenerative conditions (mixed dementia), premorbid personality, psychiatric conditions, and other health factors, resulting in as much variability in presentation of AD as there is in the behavior of the general public.

CLINICAL PRACTICES

Diagnosis and Assessment

Because there is no definitive diagnostic biomarker for AD, diagnosis of definite AD can be made only with histopathological evidence obtained from a brain autopsy. As previously described, the key histological changes described by Alzheimer himself, the accumulation of NFT and Aβ plaques in the cortex, remain the diagnostic hallmarks of the disease. The formal criteria for diagnosing probable AD in living persons were proposed in 1984 by the National Institute of Neurological and Communicative Disorders and Stroke—Alzheimer's Disease and Related Disorders Association (NINCDS-ADRDA). Scientific advances, a growing emphasis on earlier diagnosis, and evolving clinical practices have spurred efforts to revise these criteria. Diagnosis of probable AD using the NINCDS-ADRDA criteria begins with determination of the presence of dementia, defined as impairment of memory and at least one other cognitive domain, with the impairments being of sufficient severity to disrupt normal social or occupational function (*Diagnostic and Statistical Manual of Mental Disorders—Fourth Edition—Text Revised* [*DSM-IV-TR*] criteria; American Psychiatric Association, 2000). A dementia diagnostic evaluation involves a medical history, neuropsychological evaluation, physical evaluation, CT and/or MRI of the brain, and laboratory tests. Following determination of dementia, the second step in diagnosis of AD is application of criteria based on the clinical features of the AD phenotype. These criteria (McKhann et al., 1984) require an insidious onset, progressively worsening dementia, and other brain diseases or systemic disorders that could account for the deficits to be ruled out. In most persons diagnosed with dementia, the underlying cause is AD, either alone or in combination with other neuropathological processes. However, there are several other conditions that can cause or simulate dementia and which must be considered in the differential diagnosis. Although most instances of dementia not due to AD are caused by other neurodegenerative conditions currently lacking effective treatment, it is particularly important to consider potentially treatable conditions that may cause or exacerbate dementia, such as adverse drug reactions, metabolic or systemic disorders, depression, hydrocephalus, or intracranial neoplasm.

Although the NINCDS-ADRDA diagnostic guidelines have been proven to be useful since their development more than 25 years ago, there is broad agreement that scientific advances since then necessitate revisions (Dubois et al., 2007). First, as described in other chapters in this volume, the operational definitions, characterization, and diagnostic criteria for non-AD dementias have improved since publication of the NINCDS-ADRDA criteria (e.g., the concept of Lewy body dementia did not exist). Second, the growing emphasis on early diagnosis as an important step toward eventual effective treatment, together with our growing understanding of MCI (see Chapter 14), argues against waiting until dementia has developed before making a diagnosis. Lastly, several biomarkers for AD are being investigated and are beginning to impact on clinical practice.

To illustrate one of the difficulties with the current diagnostic criteria, consider the case of an otherwise healthy 70-year-old man who presents with complaints of recent gradual onset and worsening of memory problems and who demonstrates a mild but significant memory impairment on neuropsychological testing. All other neuropsychological test performances are normal, and he is still able to function with his normal activities. Even if all other aspects of this case pointed to the early stages of AD, he would meet criteria for MCI but not AD. If, in fact, he has AD, a binary diagnostic decision must be made at some point during a continuous process of gradual dementia. By current criteria, this would not occur until impairment could be measured in another cognitive domain in addition to memory, and when he began to have functional problems in his normal activities. Identifying a second domain of cognitive impairment likely would require a follow-up neuropsychological evaluation after a wait of at least 6 months, and determination of when daily functioning is impaired is an imprecise process that may be influenced by several factors. There is considerable variability across persons in the cognitive demands of daily life; for example, between an active business person and a retired and relatively sedentary individual engaged only in familiar routines. Determination of functional impairment also may be influenced by how carefully this is assessed, by a patient's insight and memory, or by access to an involved family member.

Proposed revisions to the diagnostic criteria applied to this case would take into account the prototypical gradual onset and progression of episodic memory problems, together with the fact that memory problems in AD often are isolated in the early stages. By not waiting for "full blown" dementia to develop, a diagnosis of probable AD could likely be made at least a year or more earlier if current criteria were applied. In addition, supportive evidence for the diagnosis of AD could take into account MRI evidence of medial temporal lobe atrophy, specific patterns of reduced glucose metabolism in bilateral temporoparietal regions on PET, and other biomarkers suggestive of AD (de Jager, Honey, Birks, & Wilcock, 2010; Dubois et al., 2007).

Neuroimaging and Other Biomarkers

Neuroimaging plays an increasingly important role in the diagnosis of AD, based on advances in structural MRI (e.g., volumetric methods of quantifying atrophy in the hippocampal formation and cortex), imaging of reduced cerebral metabolism (PET) and perfusion (single-photon emission computed tomography [SPECT]), and molecular imaging. Recent advances in imaging technology now allow in vivo estimation of brain amyloidosis (Aβ load). Using intravenous injections of a radionuclide-tagged compound, Pittsburgh Compound B (PiB), which binds to Aβ, PET can be used to estimate the amount of amyloid present in the brain. In early studies (e.g., Mintun et al., 2006), the great majority of individuals with AD had elevated PiB binding, notably in the cortex, though elevated PiB binding was found in a small proportion of non-AD controls. A recent study (Jack et al., 2010) showed that approximately 50% of a patient sample with MCI and who had amyloid deposits in the brain progressed to dementia within 2 years, whereas only 19% of patients with MCI and no brain amyloid deposits did so. However, the degree of amyloid load was not a good predictor of the extent of underlying disease and thus not a good predictor of the time taken to progress to dementia. Neuroimaging is discussed further in Chapter 2.

In addition to new neuroimaging approaches to diagnosing AD, the identification of practical and reliable chemical biomarkers is a research priority. Biomarkers are parameters derived from tissue or fluid such as blood or cerebrospinal fluid (CSF) that can be measured in vivo and reflect specific features of the pathological processes.

Because AD pathology precedes clinical symptomatology by several years, biomarkers may be able to serve as early diagnostic indicators. For AD, the focus has been on biomarkers linked to the primary neuropathological features of the disease; the buildup of Aβ in plaques and tau deposition in NFT. CSF markers of amyloid and tau have been found to discriminate between AD and controls and to predict disease progression, with a combination of CSF markers and neuroimaging further improving reliability of diagnosis (e.g., Mormino et al., 2009). Elevations in amyloid appear to be more specific to AD than are tau markers, and also appear more likely to mark the early stages of the disease (McKhann et al., 2011). At this time, biomarkers for AD are proposed as research criteria with potential to impact on clinical practice in the near future. Considerable work remains to be done before chemical biomarkers become part of the standard AD diagnostic evaluation, given that alterations in both Aβ and tau may be seen in other neurological disorders, and that all biomarkers exist on a continuum, requiring establishment and validation of cutoffs. Furthermore, because lumbar puncture is not always well tolerated, efforts are underway to identify less-invasive blood-based biomarkers.

Neuropsychological Assessment

Because there are no sensory, motor, or other neurological deficits in the early stages of AD, careful examination of cognitive status is essential to diagnosis and monitoring of disease progression. Serial evaluations with standardized neuropsychological tests provide a noninvasive means of characterizing the profile of cognitive deficits and measuring change in disease status over time. As previously described, episodic memory impairment is typically the earliest and most pronounced deficit in AD, characterized by rapid forgetting of recently presented information with limited benefit from recognition testing relative to free recall (e.g., Delis et al., 1991). The finding that impairment of delayed recall is the hallmark of AD is consistent with the early and strong impact of the disease on the entorhinal cortex, which has been linked by various approaches to activation during brief retention intervals (e.g., Gallagher & Koh, 2011; Small, Schobel, Buxton, Witter, & Barnes, 2011). In addition to the anterograde memory deficit, patients with AD show a temporally graded retrograde amnesia (e.g., Hodges, Salmon, & Butters, 1993; Sagar, Sullivan, Gabrieli, Corkin, & Growdon, 1988), which may be caused by interruption of a long-term consolidation process dependent on the hippocampal system, together with relatively poor learning of information during the decade or so of preclinical memory impairment prior to diagnosis. Procedural memory, for example, as assessed by rotor pursuit or mirror-tracing tests, often is preserved in the face of amnesia in AD, and this can have important implications for maintaining activities of daily life, exercise, and stress management (e.g., Suhr et al., 1999).

Beyond the emphasis on assessment of memory systems, the neuropsychological evaluation of patients with suspected AD is generally similar to the evaluation of other dementias. Because of the variability in the presentation of AD, and the tendency of AD dementia to gradually progress to encompass multiple cognitive domains, it is important that all key domains of cognition as well as mood and personality characteristics be evaluated. Neuropsychological assessment is discussed in detail in Chapter 3.

One population that warrants special consideration with regard to neuropsychological assessment of AD is persons with DS. As described earlier in this chapter, persons with DS are substantially more likely than the general population to develop AD. Diagnosis of dementia in DS presents special challenges. First, there is considerable intraindividual variability in baseline cognitive abilities, often with little reliable documentation. Establishment of a neuropsychological baseline at age 35 years can be valuable in this regard. A second issue is that the behavioral expression of AD may be more variable in DS, with memory deficits not as consistently being the prominent feature. Behavioral changes such as uncooperativeness, apathy, or diminished function in daily activities may appear before obvious memory deficits. Interviews with family, caretakers, and employers are essential for determining the baseline level of function and assessing possible changes in adaptive behavior. Because of low baseline abilities, floor effects limit the utility of many standardized tests normally used for dementia evaluation. Tests with simple early items (e.g., Benton Visual Retention Test [BVRT], Digit Span) and cued production tests (e.g., Animal Fluency, writing to dictation), as well as tests designed specifically for persons with DS or other developmental disabilities (e.g., Cambridge Cognitive Examination-Revised [CAMCOG-R]; Revised Cambridge Examination for Mental Disorders [CAMDEX-R]; Dementia Scale for DS; see Nieuwenhuis-Mark, 2009, for review), can be informative.

Intervention

No therapy has yet been found to stop or substantially slow the deterioration of neurons and subsequent dementia of AD, and as such, AD is the only leading cause of death for which no disease-modifying treatment is available. There currently are five Food and Drug Administration (FDA)-approved medications for AD that may temporarily improve cognitive and behavioral function in some patients, including cholinesterase inhibitors and memantine (an N-methyl-D-aspartic acid [NMDA] receptor antagonist), but their benefits are limited. The cholinesterase inhibitors block the activity of acetylcholinesterase, the main enzyme that breaks down acetylcholine. This increases the availability of this key neurotransmitter that is depleted in AD, but does nothing to stop the steady loss of cholinergic neurons. Donepezil (Aricept), a reversible acetylcholinesterase inhibitor, has been extensively used to treat AD and is currently the world's best-selling treatment for AD. Memantine is the only approved AD medication that influences a different pathway, likely by protecting against excess glutamate by blocking NMDA receptors, and currently is approved only for patients with moderate to severe (not mild) AD.

Several new drugs for AD are in various stages of development and testing, with an emphasis on drugs that may prevent the buildup of Aβ. To date, drugs designed to either inhibit secretase activity (e.g., Tarenflurbil and Semagacestat) or Aβ aggregation (e.g., Galantamine) have not been proved to be successful in controlling AD progression in clinical trials. Other new approaches are based on the fact that NBM cholinergic neurons require neurotrophic support from the nerve growth factor (NGF). In animal experiments, intracerebral application of NGF promotes survival of damaged cholinergic neurons, and reverses age-related atrophy in the NBM. Clinical trials of NGF cell-mediated gene therapy have demonstrated attenuation of the rate of decline on the MMSE as well as increased general cortical activity (Tuszynski et al., 2005). Studies of virus-mediated transfer of *NGF* genes are ongoing. More recently, several laboratories have successfully converted human stem cells into functional cholinergic neurons (e.g., Bissonnette et al., 2011), potentially paving the way for stem cell transplants into the NBM.

At present, pharmacological intervention in AD often is directed at management of specific problem behaviors, relying on medications that have been developed for management of psychiatric conditions. These issues are discussed in Chapter 16. In addition to pharmacological interventions, behavioral and environmental interventions can substantially improve quality of life and help optimize remaining cognitive abilities in AD patients. Finally, when considering care of AD patients, it is important to attend to the growing segment of the population being placed in the role of care providers (nearly 15 million unpaid providers). Education, support, and continued research can help lessen the enormous burden of caring for individuals with AD.

SUMMARY

AD presents one of the most urgent health care issues of our time. Despite substantial research progress, AD remains untreatable and incompletely understood. The pathological correlates of the cognitive decline of AD have been well defined, but the causal chain of events in the initiation and progression of the disease remains a mystery. AD is a disease of the brain and mind, and as such, neuropsychology has an essential and evolving role to play in addressing this growing public health concern. Measurement of key cognitive functions, such as delayed recall of recently presented information, is crucial in the diagnosis and monitoring of the disease. Progress in the development of biomarkers is likely to provide additional diagnostic information in the coming years, but this will not change the fact that the functional expression of AD is in the realm of cognition. The trend toward earlier diagnosis presents additional challenges for neuropsychology, particularly in the need to develop evidence-based predictions of real-world competencies (e.g., driving) for those in early stages of cognitive decline. In addition to the importance of advancing scientifically informed disease-specific measurement of cognition, neuropsychology has a growing role to play in the design and implementation of nonpharmacological interventions for AD. Drawing upon principles of behavioral change, known influences on neuroplasticity, and the unique neuropsychology of AD (e.g., the preservation of procedural memory), practical and inexpensive behavioral and environmental interventions are available, but remain underused. In the absence of a cure on the near horizon, it is essential that effort and resources be directed at reducing the burden of AD by improving diagnostic techniques and outcome monitoring, as well as development of neuropsychologically informed approaches to modifying risk factors and optimizing function and quality of life in the face of dementia.

REFERENCES

Aizenstein, H. J., Nebes, R. D., Saxton, J. A., Price, J. C., Mathis, C. A., Tsopelas, N. D.,... Klunk, W. E. (2008). Frequent amyloid deposition without significant cognitive impairment among the elderly. *Archives of Neurology, 65*(11), 1509–1517.

Alladi, S., Xuereb, J., Bak, T., Nestor, P., Knibb, J., Patterson, K., & Hodges, J. R. (2007). Focal cortical presentations of Alzheimer's disease. *Brain: A Journal of Neurology, 130*(Pt 10), 2636–2645.

Alzheimer's Association. (2011). 2011 Alzheimer's disease facts and figures. *Alzheimers & Dementia, 7*, 1–63.

American Psychiatric Association. (2000). *Diagnostic and Statistical Manual of Mental Disorders, 4th Edition –Text Revised (IV-TR)*. Washington, DC: American Psychiatric Press.

Anderson, S. W., Aksan, N., Dawson, J. D., Uc, E. Y., Johnson, A. M., & Rizzo, M. (2012). Neuropsychological assessment of driving safety risk in older adults with and without neurologic disease. *Journal of Clinical and Experimental Neuropsychology, 34*(9), 895–905.

Anderson, S. W., Rizzo, M., Skaar, N., Stierman, L., Cavaco, S., Dawson, J., & Damasio, H. (2007). Amnesia and driving. *Journal of Clinical and Experimental Neuropsychology, 29*(1), 1–12.

Anderson, S. W., & Tranel, D. (1989). Awareness of disease states following cerebral infarction, dementia, and head trauma: Standardized assessment. *The Clinical Neuropsychologist, 3,* 327–339.

Arnold, S. E., Hyman, B. T., Flory, J., Damasio, A. R., & Van Hoesen, G. W. (1991). The topographical and neuroanatomical distribution of neurofibrillary tangles and neuritic plaques in the cerebral cortex of patients with Alzheimer's disease. *Cerebral Cortex, 1*(1), 103–116.

Attems, J., Jellinger, K., Thal, D. R., & Van Nostrand, W. (2011). Review: Sporadic cerebral amyloid angiopathy. *Neuropathology and Applied Neurobiology, 37*(1), 75–93.

Balasa, M., Gelpi, E., Antonell, A., Rey, M. J., Sánchez-Valle, R., Molinuevo, J. L., & Lladó, A.; Neurological Tissue Bank/University of Barcelona/Hospital Clínic NTB/UB/HC Collaborative Group. (2011). Clinical features and ApoE genotype of pathologically proven early-onset Alzheimer disease. *Neurology, 76*(20), 1720–1725.

Bamburg, J. R., & Bloom, G. S. (2009). Cytoskeletal pathologies of Alzheimer disease. *Cell Motility and the Cytoskeleton, 66*(8), 635–649.

Barnes, D. E., & Yaffe, K. (2011). The projected effect of risk factor reduction on Alzheimer's disease prevalence. *Lancet Neurology, 10*(9), 819–828.

Barnes, L. L., Wilson, R. S., Schneider, J. A., Bienias, J. L., Evans, D. A., & Bennett, D. A. (2003). Gender, cognitive decline, and risk of AD in older persons. *Neurology, 60*(11), 1777–1781.

Bertram, L., & Tanzi, R. E. (2008). Thirty years of Alzheimer's disease genetics: The implications of systematic meta-analyses. *Nature Reviews. Neuroscience, 9*(10), 768–778.

Bissonnette, C. J., Lyass, L., Bhattacharyya, B. J., Belmadani, A., Miller, R. J., & Kessler, J. A. (2011). The controlled generation of functional basal forebrain cholinergic neurons from human embryonic stem cells. *Stem Cells, 29*(5), 802–811.

Blennow, K., de Leon, M., & Zetterberg, H. (2006). Alzheimer's disease. *Lancet, 368,* 387–403.

Bobinski, M., de Leon, M. J., Wegiel, J., Desanti, S., Convit, A., Saint Louis, L. A., ... Wisniewski, H. M. (2000). The histological validation of post mortem magnetic resonance imaging-determined hippocampal volume in Alzheimer's disease. *Neuroscience, 95*(3), 721–725.

Braak, H., & Braak, E. (1991). Neuropathological stageing of Alzheimer-related changes. *Acta Neuropathologica, 82*(4), 239–259.

Burns, J. M., Galvin, J. E., Roe, C. M., Morris, J. C., & McKeel, D. W. (2005). The pathology of the substantia nigra in Alzheimer disease with extrapyramidal signs. *Neurology, 64*(8), 1397–1403.

Chan-Palay, V., & Asan, E. (1989). Alterations in catecholamine neurons of the locus coeruleus in senile dementia of the Alzheimer type and in Parkinson's disease with and without dementia and depression. *The Journal of Comparative Neurology, 287*(3), 373–392.

Coleman, P. D., & Flood, D. G. (1987). Neuron numbers and dendritic extent in normal aging and Alzheimer's disease. *Neurobiology of Aging, 8*(6), 521–545.

Davatzikos, C., Xu, F., An, Y., Fan, Y., & Resnick, S. M. (2009). Longitudinal progression of Alzheimer's-like patterns of atrophy in normal older adults: The SPARE-AD index. *Brain: A Journal of Neurology, 132*(Pt 8), 2026–2035.

Daviglus, M. L., Plassman, B. L., Pirzada, A., Bell, C. C., Bowen, P. E., Burke, J. R., ... Williams, J. W. (2011). Risk factors and preventive interventions for Alzheimer disease: State of the science. *Archives of Neurology, 68*(9), 1185–1190.

Dawson, J. D., Anderson, S. W., Uc, E. Y., Dastrup, E., & Rizzo, M. (2009). Predictors of driving safety in early Alzheimer disease. *Neurology, 72*(6), 521–527.

de Jager, C. A., Honey, T. E., Birks, J., & Wilcock, G. K. (2010). Retrospective evaluation of revised criteria for the diagnosis of Alzheimer's disease using a cohort with post-mortem diagnosis. *International Journal of Geriatric Psychiatry, 25*(10), 988–997.

DeKosky, S. T., & Scheff, S. W. (1990). Synapse loss in frontal cortex biopsies in Alzheimer's disease: Correlation with cognitive severity. *Annals of Neurology, 27*(5), 457–464.

Delis, D. C., Massman, P. J., Butters, N., Salmon, D. P., Cermak, L. S. & Kramer, J. H. (1991). Profiles of demented and amnesic patients on the California verbal learning test: Implications for the assessment of memory disorders. *Psychological Assessment, 3,* 19–26.

Devanand, D. P., Sano, M., Tang, M. X., Taylor, S., Gurland, B. J., Wilder, D., . . . Mayeux, R. (1996). Depressed mood and the incidence of Alzheimer's disease in the elderly living in the community. *Archives of General Psychiatry, 53*(2), 175–182.

Dilworth-Anderson, P., Hendrie, H. C., Manly, J. J., Khachaturian, A. S., & Fazio, S.; Social, Behavioral and Diversity Research Workgroup of the Alzheimer's Association. (2008). Diagnosis and assessment of Alzheimer's disease in diverse populations. *Alzheimer's & Dementia: The Journal of the Alzheimer's Association, 4*(4), 305–309.

Double, K. L., Halliday, G. M., Kril, J. J., Harasty, J. A., Cullen, K., Brooks, W. S., . . . , & Broe, G. A. (1996). Topography of brain atrophy during normal aging and Alzheimer's disease. *Neurobiology of Aging, 17*(4), 513–521.

Dubois, B., Feldman, H. H., Jacova, C., Dekosky, S. T., Barberger-Gateau, P., Cummings, J., . . . Scheltens, P. (2007). Research criteria for the diagnosis of Alzheimer's disease: Revising the NINCDS-ADRDA criteria. *Lancet Neurology, 6*(8), 734–746.

Fan, Y., Batmanghelich, N., Clark, C. M., & Davatzikos, C.; Alzheimer's Disease Neuroimaging Initiative. (2008). Spatial patterns of brain atrophy in MCI patients, identified via high-dimensional pattern classification, predict subsequent cognitive decline. *NeuroImage, 39*(4), 1731–1743.

Fronczek, R., van Geest, S., Frölich, M., Overeem, S., Roelandse, F. W., Lammers, G. J., & Swaab, D. F. (2012). Hypocretin (orexin) loss in Alzheimer's disease. *Neurobiology of Aging, 33*(8), 1642–1650.

Gallagher, M., & Koh, M. T. (2011). Episodic memory on the path to Alzheimer's disease. *Current Opinion in Neurobiology, 21*(6), 929–934.

Gatz, M., Reynolds, C. A., Fratiglioni, L., Johansson, B., Mortimer, J. A., Berg, S., . . . Pedersen, N. L. (2006). Role of genes and environments for explaining Alzheimer disease. *Archives of General Psychiatry, 63*(2), 168–174.

Geula, C., & Mesulam, M. M. (1996). Systematic regional variations in the loss of cortical cholinergic fibers in Alzheimer's disease. *Cerebral Cortex, 6*(2), 165–177.

Gilmor, M. L., Erickson, J. D., Varoqui, H., Hersh, L. B., Bennett, D. A., Cochran, E. J., . . . Levey, A. I. (1999). Preservation of nucleus basalis neurons containing choline acetyltransferase and the vesicular acetylcholine transporter in the elderly with mild cognitive impairment and early Alzheimer's disease. *The Journal of Comparative Neurology, 411*(4), 693–704.

Gómez-Isla, T., Price, J. L., McKeel, D. W., Morris, J. C., Growdon, J. H., & Hyman, B. T. (1996). Profound loss of layer II entorhinal cortex neurons occurs in very mild Alzheimer's disease. *The Journal of Neuroscience: The Official Journal of the Society for Neuroscience, 16*(14), 4491–4500.

Gómez-Isla, T., Hollister, R., West, H., Mui, S., Growdon, J. H., Petersen, R. C., . . . Hyman, B. T. (1997). Neuronal loss correlates with but exceeds neurofibrillary tangles in Alzheimer's disease. *Annals of Neurology, 41*(1), 17–24.

Green, R. C., Cupples, L. A., Go, R., Benke, K. S., Edeki, T., Griffith, P. A., . . . Farrer, L. A.; MIRAGE Study Group. (2002). Risk of dementia among white and African American relatives of patients with Alzheimer disease. *The Journal of the American Medical Association, 287*(3), 329–336.

Gurland, B. J., Wilder, D. E., Lantigua, R., Stern, Y., Chen, J., Killeffer, E. H., & Mayeux, R. (1999). Rates of dementia in three ethnoracial groups. *International Journal of Geriatric Psychiatry, 14*(6), 481–493.

Guskiewicz, K. M., Marshall, S. W., Bailes, J., McCrea, M., Cantu, R. C., Randolph, C., & Jordan, B. D. (2005). Association between recurrent concussion and late-life cognitive impairment in retired professional football players. *Neurosurgery, 57*(4), 719–726; discussion 719.

Hall, C. B., Lipton, R. B., Sliwinski, M., Katz, M. J., Derby, C. A., & Verghese, J. (2009). Cognitive activities delay onset of memory decline in persons who develop dementia. *Neurology, 73*(5), 356–361.

Hamilton, R. L. (2000). Lewy bodies in Alzheimer's disease: A neuropathological review of 145 cases using alpha-synuclein immunohistochemistry. *Brain Pathology, 10*(3), 378–384.

Hardy, J., & Allsop, D. (1991). Amyloid deposition as the central event in the aetiology of Alzheimer's disease. *Trends in Pharmacological Sciences, 12*(10), 383–388.

Hardy, J., & Selkoe, D. J. (2002). The amyloid hypothesis of Alzheimer's disease: Progress and problems on the road to therapeutics. *Science, 297*(5580), 353–356.

Harold, D., Abraham, R., Hollingworth, P., Sims, R., Gerrish, A., Hamshere, M. L.,…Williams, J. (2009). Genome-wide association study identifies variants at CLU and PICALM associated with Alzheimer's disease. *Nature Genetics, 41*(10), 1088–1093.

Hayden, K. M., Norton, M. C., Darcey, D., Ostbye, T., Zandi, P. P., Breitner, J. C., & Welsh-Bohmer, K. A.; Cache County Study Investigators. (2010). Occupational exposure to pesticides increases the risk of incident AD: The Cache County study. *Neurology, 74*(19), 1524–1530.

Hebert, L. E., Scherr, P. A., Bienias, J. L., Bennett, D. A., & Evans, D. A. (2003). Alzheimer disease in the US population: Prevalence estimates using the 2000 census. *Archives of Neurology, 60*(8), 1119–1122.

Hebert, L. E., Scherr, P. A., McCann, J. J., Beckett, L. A., & Evans, D. A. (2001). Is the risk of developing Alzheimer's disease greater for women than for men? *American Journal of Epidemiology, 153*(2), 132–136.

Heron, M. P., Hoyert, D. L., Xu, J., Scott, C., & Tejada-Vera, B. (2008). Deaths: Preliminary data for 2006. *National Vital Statistics Reports*, Vol. 56, No. 16. Hyattsville, MD: National Center for Health Statistics.

Herzog, A. G., & Kemper, T. L. (1980). Amygdaloid changes in aging and dementia. *Archives of Neurology, 37*(10), 625–629.

Hodges, J. R., Salmon, D. P., & Butters, N. (1993). Recognition and naming of famous faces in Alzheimer's disease: A cognitive analysis. *Neuropsychologia, 31*(8), 775–788.

Hof, P. R., Cox, K., & Morrison, J. H. (1990). Quantitative analysis of a vulnerable subset of pyramidal neurons in Alzheimer's disease: I. Superior frontal and inferior temporal cortex. *The Journal of Comparative Neurology, 301*(1), 44–54.

Hongpaisan, J., Sun, M. K., & Alkon, D. L. (2011). PKC e activation prevents synaptic loss, Aß elevation, and cognitive deficits in Alzheimer's disease transgenic mice. *The Journal of Neuroscience: The Official Journal of the Society for Neuroscience, 31*(2), 630–643.

Hyman, B. T., Van Hoesen, G. W., Kromer, L. J., & Damasio, A. R. (1986). Perforant pathway changes and the memory impairment of Alzheimer's disease. *Annals of Neurology, 20*(4), 472–481.

Jack, C. R., Petersen, R. C., Xu, Y. C., Waring, S. C., O'Brien, P. C., Tangalos, E. G.,…Kokmen, E. (1997). Medial temporal atrophy on MRI in normal aging and very mild Alzheimer's disease. *Neurology, 49*(3), 786–794.

Jack, C. R., Wiste, H. J., Vemuri, P., Weigand, S. D., Senjem, M. L., Zeng, G., …Knopman, D. S.; Alzheimer's Disease Neuroimaging Initiative. (2010). Brain beta-amyloid measures and magnetic resonance imaging atrophy both predict time-to-progression from mild cognitive impairment to Alzheimer's disease. *Brain: A Journal of Neurology, 133*(11), 3336–3348.

Jedrziewski, M. K., Ewbank, D. C., Wang, H., & Trojanowski, J. Q. (2010). Exercise and cognition: Results from the National Long Term Care Survey. *Alzheimer's & Dementia: The Journal of the Alzheimer's Association, 6*(6), 448–455.

Jellinger, K. A., & Attems, J. (2010a). Prevalence of dementia disorders in the oldest-old: An autopsy study. *Acta Neuropathologica, 119*(4), 421–433.

Jellinger, K. A., & Attems, J. (2010b). Is there pure vascular dementia in old age? *Journal of the Neurological Sciences, 299*(1–2), 150–154.

Katzman, R., Aronson, M., Fuld, P., Kawas, C., Brown, T., Morgenstern, H., …Ooi, W. L. (1989). Development of dementing illnesses in an 80-year-old volunteer cohort. *Annals of Neurology, 25*(4), 317–324.

King, M. E., Ahuja, V., Binder, L. I., & Kuret, J. (1999). Ligand-dependent tau filament formation: Implications for Alzheimer's disease progression. *Biochemistry, 38*(45), 14851–14859.

Knopman, D. S., Parisi, J. E., Salviati, A., Floriach-Robert, M., Boeve, B. F., Ivnik, R. J., …Petersen, R. C. (2003). Neuropathology of cognitively normal elderly. *Journal of Neuropathology and Experimental Neurology, 62*(11), 1087–1095.

Koffie, R. M., Meyer-Luehmann, M., Hashimoto, T., Adams, K. W., Mielke, M. L., Garcia-Alloza, M., …Spires-Jones, T. L. (2009). Oligomeric amyloid beta associates with postsynaptic densities and correlates with excitatory synapse loss near senile plaques. *Proceedings of the National Academy of Sciences of the United States of America, 106*(10), 4012–4017.

Kotler-Cope, S., & Camp, C. J. (1995). Anosognosia in Alzheimer disease. *Alzheimer Disease and Associated Disorders, 9*(1), 52–56.

Kril, J. J., Patel, S., Harding, A. J., & Halliday, G. M. (2002). Neuron loss from the hippocampus of Alzheimer's disease exceeds extracellular neurofibrillary tangle formation. *Acta Neuropathologica, 103*(4), 370–376.

Lambert, J. C., Heath, S., Even, G., Campion, D., Sleegers, K., Hiltunen, M., …Amouyel, P.; European Alzheimer's Disease Initiative Investigators. (2009). Genome-wide association study identifies variants at CLU and CR1 associated with Alzheimer's disease. *Nature Genetics, 41*(10), 1094–1099.

Larner, A. J. (1997). The cerebellum in Alzheimer's disease. *Dementia and Geriatric Cognitive Disorders, 8*(4), 203–209.

Larson, E. B., Shadlen, M. F., Wang, L., McCormick, W. C., Bowen, J. D., Teri, L., & Kukull, W. A. (2004). Survival after initial diagnosis of Alzheimer disease. *Annals of Internal Medicine, 140*(7), 501–509.

Lee, H. G., Perry, G., Moreira, P. I., Garrett, M. R., Liu, Q., Zhu, X., …Smith, M. A. (2005). Tau phosphorylation in Alzheimer's disease: Pathogen or protector? *Trends in Molecular Medicine, 11*(4), 164–169.

Lehéricy, S., Hirsch, E. C., Cervera-Piérot, P., Hersh, L. B., Bakchine, S., Piette, F., …Agid, Y. (1993). Heterogeneity and selectivity of the degeneration of cholinergic neurons in the basal forebrain of patients with Alzheimer's disease. *The Journal of Comparative Neurology, 330*(1), 15–31.

Lye, T. C., & Shores, E. A. (2000). Traumatic brain injury as a risk factor for Alzheimer's disease: A review. *Neuropsychology Review, 10*(2), 115–129.

Lyketsos, C. G., Carrillo, M. C., Ryan, J. M., Khachaturian, A. S., Trzepacz, P., Amatniek, J., …Miller, D. S. (2011). Neuropsychiatric symptoms in Alzheimer's disease. *Alzheimer's & Dementia: The Journal of the Alzheimer's Association, 7*(5), 532–539.

Marcyniuk, B., Mann, D. M., & Yates, P. O. (1989). The topography of nerve cell loss from the locus caeruleus in elderly persons. *Neurobiology of Aging, 10*(1), 5–9.

Matthews, F. E., Brayne, C., Lowe, J., McKeith, I., Wharton, S. B., & Ince, P. (2009). Epidemiological pathology of dementia: Attributable-risks at death in the Medical Research Council Cognitive Function and Ageing Study. *PLoS Medicine, 6*(11), e1000180.

Mayeux, R., Sano, M., Chen, J., Tatemichi, T., & Stern, Y. (1991). Risk of dementia in first-degree relatives of patients with Alzheimer's disease and related disorders. *Archives of Neurology, 48*(3), 269–273.

McKhann, G., Drachman, D., Folstein, M., Katzman, R., Price, D., & Stadlan, E. M. (1984). Clinical diagnosis of Alzheimer's disease: Report of the NINCDS-ADRDA Work Group under the auspices of Department of Health and Human Services Task Force on Alzheimer's Disease. *Neurology, 34*(7), 939–944.

McKhann, G. M., Knopman, D. S., Chertkow, H., Hyman, B. T., Jack, C. R. Jr., Kawas, C. H.,…Phelps, C. H. (2011). The diagnosis of dementia due to Alzheimer's disease: Recommendations from the National Institute on Aging and the Alzheimer's Association workgroups on diagnostic guidelines for Alzheimer's disease. *Alzheimer's and Dementia, 7*(3), 263–269.

Meyer, J. M., & Breitner, J. C. (1998). Multiple threshold model for the onset of Alzheimer's disease in the NAS-NRC twin panel. *American Journal of Medical Genetics, 81*(1), 92–97.

Mintun, M. A., Larossa, G. N., Sheline, Y. I., Dence, C. S., Lee, S. Y., Mach, R. H.,…Morris, J. C. (2006). [^{11}C]PIB in a nondemented population: Potential antecedent marker of Alzheimer disease. *Neurology, 67*(3), 446–452.

Moran, M., Lynch, C. A., Walsh, C., Coen, R., Coakley, D., & Lawlor, B. A. (2005). Sleep disturbance in mild to moderate Alzheimer's disease. *Sleep Medicine, 6*(4), 347–352.

Mormino, E. C., Kluth, J. T., Madison, C. M., Rabinovici, G. D., Baker, S. L., Miller, B. L.,…Jagust, W. J.; Alzheimer's Disease Neuroimaging Initiative. (2009). Episodic memory loss is related to hippocampal-mediated beta-amyloid deposition in elderly subjects. *Brain: A Journal of Neurology, 132*(Pt 5), 1310–1323.

Mueller, S. G., Schuff, N., Yaffe, K., Madison, C., Miller, B., & Weiner, M. W. (2010). Hippocampal atrophy patterns in mild cognitive impairment and Alzheimer's disease. *Human Brain Mapping, 31*(9), 1339–1347.

Mueller, S. G., & Weiner, M. W. (2009). Selective effect of age, Apo e4, and Alzheimer's disease on hippocampal subfields. *Hippocampus, 19*(6), 558–564.

National Institutes of Health (NIH). (2010). *State-of-the-Science Conference: Preventing Alzheimer's disease and cognitive decline.* National Institutes of Health, April 28, 2010.

Nelson, P. T., Head, E., Schmitt, F. A., Davis, P. R., Neltner, J. H., Jicha, G. A.,…Scheff, S. W. (2011). Alzheimer's disease is not "brain aging": neuropathological, genetic, and epidemiological human studies. *Acta Neuropathologica, 121*(5), 571–587.

Nieuwenhuis-Mark, R. E. (2009). Diagnosing Alzheimer's dementia in Down syndrome: Problems and possible solutions. *Research in Developmental Disabilities, 30*(5), 827–838.

Palop, J. J., & Mucke, L. (2009). Epilepsy and cognitive impairments in Alzheimer disease. *Archives of Neurology, 66*(4), 435–440.

Plassman, B. L., Havlik, R. J., Steffens, D. C., Helms, M. J., Newman, T. N., Drosdick, D.,…Breitner, J. C. (2000). Documented head injury in early adulthood and risk of Alzheimer's disease and other dementias. *Neurology, 55*(8), 1158–1166.

Plassman, B. L., Langa, K. M., Fisher, G. G., Heeringa, S. G., Weir, D. R., Ofstedal, M. B.,…Wallace, R. B. (2007). Prevalence of dementia in the United States: The aging, demographics, and memory study. *Neuroepidemiology, 29*(1–2), 125–132.

Poulin, S. P., Dautoff, R., Morris, J. C., Barrett, L. F., & Dickerson, B. C.; Alzheimer's Disease Neuroimaging Initiative. (2011). Amygdala atrophy is prominent in early Alzheimer's disease and relates to symptom severity. *Psychiatry Research, 194*(1), 7–13.

Price, J. L., & Morris, J. C. (1999). Tangles and plaques in nondemented aging and "preclinical" Alzheimer's disease. *Annals of Neurology, 45*(3), 358–368.

Reddy, P. H., Mani, G., Park, B. S., Jacques, J., Murdoch, G., Whetsell, W., . . . Manczak, M. (2005). Differential loss of synaptic proteins in Alzheimer's disease: Implications for synaptic dysfunction. *Journal of Alzheimer's Disease, 7*(2), 103–117; discussion 173.

Regeur, L., Jensen, G. B., Pakkenberg, H., Evans, S. M., & Pakkenberg, B. (1994). No global neocortical nerve cell loss in brains from patients with senile dementia of Alzheimer's type. *Neurobiology of Aging, 15*(3), 347–352.

Reitz, C., & Mayeux, R. (2009). Use of genetic variation as biomarkers for Alzheimer's disease. *Annals of the New York Academy of Sciences, 1180*, 75–96.

Rizzo, M., Anderson, S. W., Dawson, J., Myers, R., & Ball, K. (2000a). Visual attention impairments in Alzheimer's disease. *Neurology, 54*(10), 1954–1959.

Rizzo, M., Anderson, S. W., Dawson, J., & Nawrot, M. (2000b). Vision and cognition in Alzheimer's disease. *Neuropsychologia, 38*(8), 1157–1169.

Rizzo, M., McGehee, D. V., Dawson, J. D., & Anderson, S. N. (2001). Simulated car crashes at intersections in drivers with Alzheimer disease. *Alzheimer Disease and Associated Disorders, 15*(1), 10–20.

Roberts, G. W., Allsop, D., & Bruton, C. (1990). The occult aftermath of boxing. *Journal of Neurology, Neurosurgery, and Psychiatry, 53*(5), 373–378.

Rodríguez, J. J., Witton, J., Olabarria, M., Noristani, H. N., & Verkhratsky, A. (2010). Increase in the density of resting microglia precedes neuritic plaque formation and microglial activation in a transgenic model of Alzheimer's disease. *Cell Death & Disease, 1*, e1.

Saczynski, J. S., Beiser, A., Seshadri, S., Auerbach, S., Wolf, P. A., & Au, R. (2010). Depressive symptoms and risk of dementia: The Framingham Heart Study. *Neurology, 75*(1), 35–41.

Sagar, H. J., Sullivan, E. V., Gabrieli, J. D., Corkin, S., & Growdon, J. H. (1988). Temporal ordering and short-term memory deficits in Parkinson's disease. *Brain: A Journal of Neurology, 111*(Pt 3), 525–539.

Savioz, A., Leuba, G., Vallet, P. G., & Walzer, C. (2009). Contribution of neural networks to Alzheimer disease's progression. *Brain Research Bulletin, 80*(4–5), 309–314.

Scahill, R. I., Schott, J. M., Stevens, J. M., Rossor, M. N., & Fox, N. C. (2002). Mapping the evolution of regional atrophy in Alzheimer's disease: Unbiased analysis of fluid-registered serial MRI. *Proceedings of the National Academy of Sciences of the United States of America, 99*(7), 4703–4707.

Scheff, S. W., & Price, D. A. (2003). Synaptic pathology in Alzheimer's disease: A review of ultrastructural studies. *Neurobiology of Aging, 24*(8), 1029–1046.

Scheff, S. W., Price, D. A., Schmitt, F. A., & Mufson, E. J. (2006). Hippocampal synaptic loss in early Alzheimer's disease and mild cognitive impairment. *Neurobiology of Aging, 27*(10), 1372–1384.

Schneider, J. A., Arvanitakis, Z., Bang, W., & Bennett, D. A. (2007). Mixed brain pathologies account for most dementia cases in community-dwelling older persons. *Neurology, 69*(24), 2197–2204.

Scott, S. A., DeKosky, S. T., Sparks, D. L., Knox, C. A., & Scheff, S. W. (1992). Amygdala cell loss and atrophy in Alzheimer's disease. *Annals of Neurology, 32*(4), 555–563.

Shimohama, S., Taniguchi, T., Fujiwara, M., & Kameyama, M. (1986). Changes in nicotinic and muscarinic cholinergic receptors in Alzheimer-type dementia. *Journal of Neurochemistry, 46*(1), 288–293.

Small, S. A., Schobel, S. A., Buxton, R. B., Witter, M. P., & Barnes, C. A. (2011). A pathophysi-ological framework of hippocampal dysfunction in ageing and disease. *Nature Reviews. Neuroscience, 12*(10), 585–601.

Snowden, J. S., Thompson, J. C., Stopford, C. L., Richardson, A. M., Gerhard, A., Neary, D., & Mann, D. M. (2011). The clinical diagnosis of early-onset dementias: Diagnostic accu-racy and clinicopathological relationships. *Brain: A Journal of Neurology, 134*(Pt 9), 2478–2492.

Stern, Y. (2006). Cognitive reserve and Alzheimer disease. *Alzheimer Disease and Associated Disorders, 20*(2), 112–117.

Suhr, J. A., Anderson, S. W., & Tranel, D. (1999). Progressive muscle relaxation in the manage-ment of behavioral disturbance in Alzheimer's disease. *Neuropsychological Rehabilitation, 9,* 31–44.

Terry, R. D., Peck, A., DeTeresa, R., Schechter, R., & Horoupian, D. S. (1981). Some morpho-metric aspects of the brain in senile dementia of the Alzheimer type. *Annals of Neurology, 10*(2), 184–192.

Terry, R. D., Masliah, E., Salmon, D. P., Butters, N., DeTeresa, R., Hill, R., … Katzman, R. (1991). Physical basis of cognitive alterations in Alzheimer's disease: Synapse loss is the major correlate of cognitive impairment. *Annals of Neurology, 30*(4), 572–580.

Thal, D. R., Del Tredici, K., Ludolph, A. C., Hoozemans, J. J., Rozemuller, A. J., Braak, H., & Knippschild, U. (2011). Stages of granulovacuolar degeneration: Their relation to Alzheimer's disease and chronic stress response. *Acta Neuropathologica, 122*(5), 577–589.

Tractenberg, R. E., Singer, C. M., & Kaye, J. A. (2006). Characterizing sleep problems in persons with Alzheimer's disease and normal elderly. *Journal of Sleep Research, 15*(1), 97–103.

Tuszynski, M. H., Thal, L., Pay, M., Salmon, D. P., U, H. S., Bakay, R., … Conner, J. (2005). A phase 1 clinical trial of nerve growth factor gene therapy for Alzheimer disease. *Nature Medicine, 11*(5), 551–555.

Uc, E. Y., Rizzo, M., Anderson, S. W., Shi, Q., & Dawson, J. D. (2004). Driver route-following and safety errors in early Alzheimer disease. *Neurology, 63*(5), 832–837.

Uc, E. Y., Rizzo, M., Anderson, S. W., Shi, Q., & Dawson, J. D. (2006). Unsafe rear-end col-lision avoidance in Alzheimer's disease. *Journal of the Neurological Sciences, 251*(1–2), 35–43.

Wang, H. Y., Bakshi, K., Shen, C., Frankfurt, M., Trocmé-Thibierge, C., & Morain, P. (2010). S 24795 limits beta-amyloid-alpha7 nicotinic receptor interaction and reduces Alzheimer's disease-like pathologies. *Biological Psychiatry, 67*(6), 522–530.

West, M. J., Coleman, P. D., Flood, D. G., & Troncoso, J. C. (1994). Differences in the pattern of hippocampal neuronal loss in normal ageing and Alzheimer's disease. *Lancet, 344*(8925), 769–772.

Whitehouse, P. J., Price, D. L., Clark, A. W., Coyle, J. T., & DeLong, M. R. (1981). Alzheimer disease: Evidence for selective loss of cholinergic neurons in the nucleus basalis. *Annals of Neurology, 10*(2), 122–126.

Whitehouse, P. J., Martino, A. M., Antuono, P. G., Lowenstein, P. R., Coyle, J. T., Price, D. L., & Kellar, K. J. (1986). Nicotinic acetylcholine binding sites in Alzheimer's disease. *Brain Research, 371*(1), 146–151.

Zlokovic, B. V. (2011). Neurovascular pathways to neurodegeneration in Alzheimer's disease and other disorders. *Nature Reviews. Neuroscience, 12*(12), 723–738.

CHAPTER 5

Vascular-Based Cognitive Disorders: Vascular Dementias, CADASIL, and Moyamoya

Chad A. Noggle, Lokesh Shahani, and Mark T. Barisa

Vascular dementia (VaD) is an umbrella term representing a clinical grouping with inherent heterogeneity in its clinical manifestations reflecting a variability in its underlying etiology. No diagnostic neuropsychological pattern has been identified for VaD (Looi & Sachdev, 1999). As noted by Knopman and Selnes (2003), the dementia due to a series of large cortical infarctions will present significantly different clinically from dementia due to lacunar infarctions in the striatum and thalamus. The commonality of these presentations that may fall under this umbrella of VaD is that their pathology involves the cerebrovascular system in some way, shape, or form.

Dementia related to vascular disorders was first described as *arteriosclerotic dementia* (McMenemey, 1961). This term was later replaced by *multi-infarct dementia* (MID; Hachinski, Lassen, & Marshall, 1974) and then "VaD" (Garcia & Brown, 1992). More recently, the term *vascular cognitive impairment* (VCI) has been proposed (Rincon & Wright, 2013).

In this chapter, we discuss specific presentations that *can* fall under the VaD heading. This will include discussion of MID and dementia associated with lacunar states (LSs), as well as Binswanger's disease (BD), which remains embroiled in controversy. For comparison, we also discuss cerebral autosomal dominant arteriopathy with subcortical infarcts and leukoencephalopathy (CADASIL) and moyomoya disease due to their clinical overlap.

VASCULAR DEMENTIA

Research has consistently demonstrated that stroke is a risk factor for cognitive deterioration and dementia. Cognitive impairment occurs after stroke in 6% to 41% of patients, but can also arise from covert cerebrovascular disease (CVD; Pendlebury & Rothwell, 2009). While it is more common within the clinical setting to observe a mixed dementia presentation, in which vascular disease is intermixed with the neuropathological changes associated with Alzheimer's disease (AD), dementia with a pure vascular pathology is possible, although far less common (Holmes,

Cairns, Lantos, & Mann, 1999). VaD is the second most common form of dementia, behind AD, accounting for approximately 15% to 20% of dementia cases (Román et al., 1993). As implied by the name, the common causal factor in VaD is the CVD lesion resulting from vascular and circulatory pathology (Román, 2002). The primary lesions are hemorrhage (due to hypertension, cerebral amyloid angiopathy or hematological causes, subarachnoid hemorrhage, posthemorrhagic obstructive hydrocephalus, subdural hematoma), ischemia (complete ischemia resulting from arterial occlusion leading to necrosis, liquefaction, and cavitation, or incomplete ischemia resulting from hypoperfusion secondary to medullary arteriolar stenosis and cardiac or circulatory disorders), and combinations of ischemia and hemorrhage (such as that in cortical vein and sinus thromboses; Román, 2003). Thus, VaD encompasses different clinical and pathological subtypes. Subtypes are classified based on their neuropathological correlates. A rather straightforward dichotomy involves the classification of multifocal/diffuse disease versus focal disease. In this chapter, we primarily focus on multifocal/diffuse disease. Beyond this, multifocal disease can be further separated into large-vessel disease and small-vessel disease. Hypoxic–ischemic dementia, venous infarct dementia, and hemorrhagic dementia have also been discussed to a lesser extent.

Within the large-vessel subtype, poststroke dementia is the most common form of acute-onset VaD, and the term MID is used when the dementia develops after multiple large-vessel, cortico-subcortical thrombotic or embolic strokes (Román, 2002). Previously, primary focus was placed on the cumulative effects of multiple infarctions; however, single, strategically located infarctions may also cause acute-onset, poststroke dementia. This usually stems from a cortico-subcortical stroke affecting a large-vessel arterial territory (usually right posterior cerebral artery, anterior cerebral artery, or left gyrus angularis). In small-vessel subtypes of VaD, more often the dementia has a slow, subacute-onset, although an abrupt course may be seen following single strategic lacunes, for example, when they involve the capsular genu, intralaminary nuclei of the thalamus, or head of the caudate nucleus. BD and the LS both have a slow, subacute onset and fall into this small-vessel subtype, as they are both characterized by multiple lacunes and ischemic periventricular leukoencephalopathy that typically spares the arcuate subcortical U fibers (Román, Erkinjuntti, Wallin, Pantoni, & Chui, 2002). Due to differences in the underlying pathology of VaDs, clinical characteristics may vary. Nevertheless, VaD has been most consistently associated with psychomotor slowing, visuoconstructional abnormalities, executive dysfunction, and less prominent involvement of functions such as language and calculations (Desmond, 1996). Executive dysfunction in relationship to VaD has often been emphasized as the deficits often exceed those experienced by AD (Looi & Scahdev, 1999). Lamar, Price, Giovannetti, Swenson, and Libon (2014) address executive dysfunction in association with VaD in greater depth in Chapter 6 of this book. Deficits in new learning in VaD are similar to those in AD, at times even extending to similar deficits in free delayed recall, although VaD is associated with significantly better outcomes in delayed recognition (Cummings, 1994).

A prominent issue in the discussion of VaD stems from a lack of consensus in the classification of VaD. While some classification systems such as the one proposed by the National Institutes of Neurological Disease and Stroke stipulates an onset of dementia within 3 months following a recognized stroke; abrupt deterioration in cognitive functioning; and a stepwise decline in cognitive functioning, in combination with confirmed CVD on neuroimaging, the Tenth Revision of the International Classification of Diseases merely stipulates that cognitive or memory symptoms have been present for at least 6 months with no requirement of neuroimaging findings.

The diagnostic criteria for VaD as defined in the *Diagnostic and Statistical Manual of Mental Disorders, Fourth Edition—Text Revision* (*DSM-IV-TR*) include memory impairment and aphasia, apraxia, agnosia, and/or executive functioning deficits, which result in social or occupational impairment as well as focal neurological signs and symptoms or laboratory findings of CVD, the cause of dementia (American Psychiatric Association [APA], 2000).

MULTIFOCAL/DIFFUSE DISEASE

Large-Vessel Dementia

The most commonly discussed form of large-vessel VaD is MID. The term *multi-infarct dementia* was coined by Hachinski et al. (1974) when they described the relationship between artherosclerosis and mental deterioration. Based on their observations they suggested that atherosclerosis may lead to recurring small infarcts that can cause mental deterioration. The term incorrectly implies that multiple cerebrovascular events are needed for cognitive deterioration. As discussed previously, dementia may stem from singular infarcts and even the cumulative effects of lacunar events. In the *DSM-IV* (APA, 1994), the term *multi-infarct dementia* was replaced with *vascular dementia,* to be inclusive of other etiologies and not suggest that only multiple events can lead to dementia.

Estimates of poststroke dementia have varied. Research has demonstrated that the prevalence of poststroke dementia depends on the age and characteristics of the study population, the time between stroke and assessment, and the diagnostic criteria used. Regarding the latter, one large study from Canada identified a poststroke dementia prevalence of 29% according to *DSM-III* criteria, compared with 17% using *DSM-III-R* criteria and 14% using *DSM-IV* criteria (Erkinjuntti, Ostbye, Steenhuis, & Hachinski, 1997). Similar results were found elsewhere (e.g., Pendlebury & Rothwell, 2009; Pohjasvaara, Erkinjuntti, Vataja, & Kaste, 1997). While there is disparity across different studies, the general finding is that there is clear evidence that suffering a stroke increases a person's risk of subsequent dementia.

Neuropathology and Pathophysiology of MID

The etiology of MID is in many ways the same as the etiology of CVD in general and even late-life dementia. Hypertension (Knopman & Roberts, 2010; Wiseman et al., 2004), hypercholesterolemia (Kivipelto et al., 2005), diabetes (Götz, Ittner, & Lim, 2009; Verdelho et al., 2010), and obesity (Kivipelto et al., 2005) have all been associated with changes in brain volume and increased risks of dementia. Genetics may also serve as a risk factor, or mediator of the impact these other risk factors have on individuals. In particular, the apolipoprotein-e4 allele (ApoE-e4), which is commonly discussed in relation to the risk of AD, has been found to increase the risk of vascular disease, including the progression of chronic ischemic white matter lesion load and even the potential for poststroke cognitive decline (Godin et al., 2009; Wagle et al., 2010).

The term MID itself is used to describe a disorder characterized by a stepwise deterioration of cognitive functioning associated with strokes or accumulated transient ischemic attacks (TIAs). Thus, the underlying neuroanatomical abnormalities largely suggest the diagnosis of MID. As described by Hachinski et al. (1974), MID stems from the "occurrence of multiple small or large cerebral infarcts." There is no stipulation placed on the site of infarcts. Rather, the term is linked with a history and imaging confirmation of multiple large-vessel strokes in the gray matter of the cortex and subcortical regions associated with a stepwise progression of cognitive deficits. While it has long been suggested that functional impairments vary based on the site, size, and number of lesions, this has not always held up in the research (e.g., Sachdev, Brodaty, Valenzuela, Lorentz, & Koschera, 2004; Sachdev et al., 2009). In a large stroke study done in Australia, cognitive impairment was associated with deep white matter hyperintensities (WMH) but not with volume or number of infarctions. Additional trends have been noted within this patient population. For example, Neshige, Barrett, and Shibasaki (1988) found that MID and result- ing decreases in cognitive functioning were associated with longer P300 latencies of event-related potentials. Decreases in cerebral blood flow (CBF) and lower cere- bral oxygen metabolism have been noted in the cerebral cortex, basal ganglia, and thalamus in general and are not necessarily dependent on infarction sites (De Reuck et al., 1998). Reductions in the genu of the corpus callosum have been noted on MRI (Lyoo, Satlin, Lee, & Renshaw, 1997).

Hippocampal atrophy is also commonly observed. Laakso et al. (1996) found that hippocampal atrophy was not specific to AD as it was observed in a series of nine patients with VaD. In this sample, four patients had bilateral hippocampal atro- phy, three had unilateral hippocampal atrophy, and only two had no hippocampal atrophy. However, this is not to suggest that the hippocampal atrophy is observed at the same level of severity as that seen in AD. For example, Fein et al. (2000) observed significant atrophy of both the hippocampal formation and cortical gray matter in a sample of patients with subcortical ischemic vascular disease that presented with lacunes and dementia. These authors noted that the hippocampal atrophy was less than that observed in a group of patients with probable AD. While these findings have been reported, they do not always correspond to cognitive decline. While Fein et al. found a correlation between cortical gray matter atrophy and hippocampal atrophy in patients with subcortical ischemic vascular disease, Mungas et al. (2002) found no evidence that hippocampal atrophy or even white matter signal hyperintensities predicted cognitive decline in cases with lacunes. These authors did, however, report that cortical gray matter atrophy predicted cognitive decline regardless of whether lacunes were present.

Comorbidity of MID

Another issue stems from the fact that stroke and CVD are not only associated with dementia (as broadly defined) but also with dementia of the Alzheimer's type. The Rochester study demonstrated that risk of dementia was doubled in the stroke cohort over the 25-year follow-up while the risk of AD was also doubled over this period, indicating that the association between stroke and dementia could not be accounted for by VCI alone (Kokmen, Whisnant, O'Fallon, Chu, & Beard, 1996). The well-known Nun Study indicated that the presence of CVD may determine the expression and severity of clinical dementia symptoms in AD. Among the 61 par- ticipants who met neuropathological criteria for AD, those with brain infarcts had poorer cognitive function and a higher prevalence of dementia than those with- out infarcts (Snowdon et al., 1997). Lacunar infarcts in the basal ganglia, thala- mus, or deep white matter demonstrated the greatest link with poorer cognition. When considering individual contributions, Schneider, Wilson, Bienias, Evans, and Bennett (2004) found that each unit of AD pathology increased dementia risk more than fourfold and the presence of one or more infarctions independently increased dementia risk by two- to eightfold, but there was no interaction between them to increase dementia risk.

Clinical Features of MID

There is no pure functional profile of MID. The hallmark of MID is a stepwise progression, corresponding to additional functional decline in conjunction with new cerebrovascular events. Cognitive, psychological, and motor impairment may all occur. Symptoms of MID include confusion, seizures, focal neurological signs, memory deficits, motor impairment, hemiparesis, sleep disturbances, gait abnormalities, pseudobulbar palsy, extensor plantar responses, exaggerated deep tendon reflexes, speech impairment, somatic complaints, and psychological symptoms, including depression and anxiety as well as psychosis (Barker, Musso, & Gouvier, 2011).

Within the cognitive realm, variability is observed across patients. However, reductions in information processing speed, attention, learning efficiency, delayed recall, and executive functioning are among the most common features (Selnes & Vinters, 2006) being attributed to the propensity of CVD burden toward frontal-subcortical circuits (Chui, 2007; Jokinen et al., 2009). Studies have further demonstrated neuroanatomical correlates to these cognitive issues including associations between the severity of WMH in fronto-striato-thalamic circuits (Burton et al., 2003) and associations with the severity of volumetric reductions in gray matter, particularly in the thalamus and cingulated gyrus (Stebbins et al. 2008). Gold et al. (2005) found that lacunar infarcts in the thalamus and basal ganglia had a larger impact on cognition than infarcts in the deep white matter (Gold et al., 2005). In the Rotterdam Scan Study, periventricular but not subcortical white matter lesions were associated with both cognitive function (de Groot et al., 2000) and cognitive decline during follow-up (de Groot et al., 2002), although it should be noted that this finding remains controversial (Delano-Wood et al., 2008). In this same study cohort, thalamic infarcts were associated with a decline in memory performance, whereas nonthalamic infarcts were linked with a decline in psychomotor speed (Vermeer et al., 2003).

Diagnosing MID

Diagnostic criteria for MID was originally included in the third edition of the *DSM* (APA, 1987). Criteria included a stepwise pattern of progression associated with CVD and infarctions. Focal neurological signs and differential deficits in various cognitive domains corresponding to dementia represented the clinical features. However, when the *DSM* moved into its fourth edition (APA, 2000), the term MID was set aside in favor of *vascular dementia,* as research and numerous case studies demonstrated that dementia could stem from CVD without multiple infarctions, as well as from multiple infarctions exclusively. As noted previously, the diagnostic criteria for VaD as defined in the *DSM-IV-TR* include memory impairment and aphasia, apraxia, agnosia, and/or executive functioning deficits, which result in social or occupational impairment as well as focal neurological signs and symptoms or laboratory findings of CVD, the cause of dementia (APA, 2000). To make a diagnosis of VaD, such as MID, three elements are necessary: cognitive loss, presence of cerebrovascular lesions as shown by brain imaging (or as inferred from a history of stroke and presence of focal neurological signs), and onset of dementia within 3 months of a symptomatic stroke (this criterion is waived in patients with subacute VaD; Román, 2003).

Differentiation of MID from other forms of dementia, such as AD, can oftentimes be difficult. MID and AD may present in relatively similar ways clinically. Further complicating the matter is the fact that the two presentations are not mutually exclusive as the two disorders may present comorbidly. Nevertheless, VaD (including MID) and AD are two conditions that can be distinguished in the clinic due to their differences in onset and progression. In VaD, the onset can be sudden or gradual and the progression is slow and stepwise, often increasing in severity with each ischemic event (Román, 2003).

Unlike the typical early and severe memory deficits of AD, memory may be only mildly affected or remain intact in VaD, including MID (Geldmacher & Whitehouse, 1996). A comparison of neuropsychological performance between individuals with AD and individuals with MID found that while individuals in both groups showed broad impairment, those with AD obtained significantly lower overall mean scores on the neuropsychological battery. The largest differences between the groups were observed on measures of memory and learning, including orientation, paragraph recall, picture recognition memory, and face-name learning, on which individuals with AD performed more poorly. In fact, because memory may be minimally affected in VaD, it is usually recommended that two other areas of cognition be impaired for an appropriate diagnosis (Román, 2003).

Psychomotor deficits, however, may be more pronounced in individuals with MID (Taylor, Gilleard, & McGuire, 1996). Individuals with MID may also demonstrate poorer performance on measures of executive function and speech mechanics than individuals with AD, while speech and calculation abilities are involved earlier in AD (Looi & Sachdev, 1999; Powell, Cummings, Hill, & Benson, 1988; Román & Royall, 1999). While individuals with AD show poverty of content of speech, individuals with MID produce shorter utterances with less grammatical complexity. Research also reveals that individuals with MID display more severe behavioral retardation, expressive verbal impairment, and greater levels of psychopathology than individuals with AD. Psychopathology is not correlated with cognitive impairment in individuals with MID, but this correlation has been demonstrated in individuals with AD (Sultzer, Levin, Mahler, High, & Cummings, 1993).

Small-Vessel Dementia

Subcortical ischemic VaD (SVD), also commonly referred to as small-vessel dementia, stems from small-artery vascular disease and hypoperfusion and is one of the major causes of cognitive impairment and dementia (Erkinjuntti, 2007; Román et al., 2002). Research has demonstrated SVD accounts for the presence of silent ischemia in neuroimaging studies in 20% of the elderly (Vermeer et al., 2003) and 25% of symptomatic ischemic strokes (Petty et al., 1999).

There are two primary SVD pathological subtypes, the LS and BD, which will be the focus of this section. Both presentations share risk factors and present with typical radiological correlates (Boiten, Lodder, & Kessels, 1993). While significant overlap is seen between these two presentations, they are differentiated based on the amount of white matter ischemic disease. That is, BD is associated with greater cognitive burden due to the additional burden of white matter ischemic disease; thus, individuals may present with dementia, whereas the cognitive impairment associated with the LS does not reach the degree of dementia.

The LS concept may well be traced back to the 1800s; however, Fisher's work in the 1960s brought the issue into the clinical light. The definition of a "lacunar" infarct is a lesion that is less than 15 mm in diameter in the perfusion territory of a small penetrating artery (Fisher, 1982). LSs can result in damage to cortical, subcortical, or both regions, but are due to ischemia or chronic hypoperfusion of the microvasculature (Haaland & Swanda, 2008). Clinical features are generally dependent on the severity of the pathological impact. Unless the damage is in strategically important areas, the condition may not produce obvious deficits that are reported by patients, and the clinical significance of the damaged areas is often less certain (Haaland & Swanda, 2008).

BD is a controversial disorder that is considered by some a VaD subtype. The disorder was first described by Otto Binswanger in 1894 who described a subset of eight patients that included one patient in particular who demonstrated significant atrophy of the white matter while the cortex and basal ganglia remained relatively spared. Binswanger posited that the result of sporadic stroke-like events stemmed from an insufficiency of blood supply to the subcortical white matter (Blass, Hoyer, & Nitsch, 1991). He termed the disorder *encephalitis subcorticalis chronica progressiva*. Based on his observations, Binswanger proposed that ischemic damage to the white matter alone could result in mental impairment (Filley, 2001).

Alois Alzheimer in 1902 described another series of patients with progressive dementias stemming from arteriosclerotic subcortical white matter changes (Alzheimer, 1902). Alzheimer named the disorder after Binswanger in recognition of his seminal work (Román, 1987). Olszewski (1962) expanded on the work of both Binswanger and Alzheimer when he presented two additional cases. In his writings, Olszewski (1962) spoke of the role of lacunar infarctions in the disease and suggested the term *subcortical arteriosclerotic encephalopathy* as a more appropriate label, although BD remains the most commonly cited name under which diagnostic criteria have also been proposed (Bennett, Wilson, Gilley, & Fox, 1990).

The controversy surrounding BD stems from professionals in the field arguing that cases are actually undiagnosed AD (Haaland & Swanda, 2008). Others have questioned whether BD actually represents a distinct subtype of VaD and whether differentiation of dementias associated with white matter disease is even necessary (Caplan, 1995; Hurley, Tomimoto, Akiguchi, Fisher, & Taber, 2000). Nevertheless, BD continues to be regarded as a form of VaD characterized by prominent involvement of the white matter (Filley, 2001).

Neuropathology of SVDs

LSs and BD are similar in that they both correspond to small-artery vascular disease and hypoperfusion. LSs result in multiple small areas of infarction, white matter demyelination, and axonal loss (Haaland & Swanda, 2008) that most commonly affect the corticostriatal circuits and deep white matter connections (Haaland & Swanda, 2008; Moody, Santamore, & Bell, 1991).

BD constitutes a disorder of the cerebral white matter of an unknown etiology (Caplan, 1995; Hurley et al., 2000). More specifically, BD is characterized pathologically by a combination of diffuse white matter disease lesions and lacunar infarcts in the basal ganglia and white matter. The fact that a unique etiology has not been described has been a primary source of the controversy surrounding BD as there is no clear distinction between the disease and other subtypes of VaD. Filley (2001) noted that while white matter changes on neuroimaging for a diagnosis of BD is necessary, such findings are not mutually exclusive findings as they are not uncommon for a multitude of other diseases and even normal aging. The vast majority of clinical neuroscience professionals working within the adult and geriatric setting, including these authors, could likely attest to the fact that findings of small-vessel ischemic changes involving the white matter on neuroimaging can be relatively common. The reality is that the incidence of findings of WMH on MRI increases with age in nondemented patients (de Groot et al., 2000; Ylikoski et al., 1995). Therefore, a "diagnostic" feature of BD is something that many older adults may demonstrate. As a result of this lack of diagnostic uncertainty, prevalence rates of BD are unknown. Santamaria Ortiz and Knight (1994) reported that on autopsy, as many as 4% of the general population and 35% of dementia patients present with pathological markers of BD.

As noted, the etiology of BD remains unknown. Hypertension is seen as a primary risk factor along with other vascular risk factors (e.g., high cholesterol, diabetes, etc.). One proposal for the etiology of BD has been a reduction in the functionality of the long-penetrating arterioles of the deep cerebral white matter (Hurley et al., 2000). The arterioles are affected by hyalinization of the vessel walls that leads to a narrowing of the lumen, but not complete occlusion (Babikian & Ropper, 1987). As a result, there is subtle reduction of the blood supply to the deep white matter, possibly leading to individuals experiencing repeated hypoxic–ischemic events (Caplan, 1995). Over time, this leads to reductions in the density of nerve fibers along with axonal damage within the lesions. In early-stage disease, pathological changes may only be noted in the myelin pallor, but as the disease progresses, widespread loss of myelin, particularly within periventricular regions, axons, and oligodendrocytes, is commonly observed along with atrocytic gliosis and cavitation of the white matter (Babikian & Ropper, 1987; Caplan, 1995; Hurley et al., 2000). Truly, research has demonstrated the vulnerability of white matter to ischemia (Pantoni, Garcia, & Gutierrez, 1996). While in Binswanger's original description the white matter lesions predominately involved the occipital and temporal lobes (Binswanger, 1894), additional studies have noted significant white matter lesions at varying degrees throughout all the lobes (Bogousslavsky, 1992; Goto, Ishii, & Fukasawa, 1981; Kitani, Tomonaga, Yoshimura, Mori, & Yamanouchi, 1986; Olszewski, 1962; Révész, Hawkins, du Boulay, Barnard, & McDonald, 1989; Yamanouchi & Nagura, 1997). The ischemic process in BD may also involve the brain stem to a lesser extent (Pullicino, Ostrow, Miller, Snyder, & Munschauer, 1995).

On autopsy, the white matter often is firm, rubbery, puckered, granular, wrinkled, and discolored in severe cases (Caplan, 1995). The external surface of the brain may remain normal in appearance, although diffuse atrophy and enlargement of the ventricles have been noted (Caplan, 1995). Lacunar infarcts involving the basal ganglia, thalamus, pons, and internal capsule are commonly found (Caplan, 1995). While some previous research has found an association between cognitive deficits and even dementia and the extent of pathological markers including subcortical white matter degeneration, cerebral hypoperfusion, and cerebral atrophy (Shyu et al., 1996), others have failed to find a strong association between the two (Hurley et al., 2000). Still, others have suggested a threshold in relation to the association between white matter pathology and cognitive impairment. For example, Román et al. (1993) suggested that once 25% or more of the white matter is involved, dementia is observed.

The white matter lesions in BD have been associated with compromised axonal transport, blood–brain barrier function, regressive changes in the astroglia, the frequent infiltration of T-lymphocytes, and activated microglia (Akiguchi, Tomimoto, Suenaga, Wakita, & Budka, 1997, 1998; Akiguchi et al., 1999).

Clinical Features of SVDs

Clinically, SVD translates into subcortical ischemic disease, which is the most common and most homogeneous form of VCI (Rockwood et al., 2000). While a stepwise decline of functioning is considered synonymous with MID and is often described in BD, a pattern of progressive decline has been described in certain cases (Caplan, 1995). Neurological features include the subacute onset of focal pyramidal or extrapyramidal signs, acute lacunar syndromes, gait disorder, pseudobulbar signs, and sometimes seizures (Filley, 2001). Deficits in cognitive, motor, and behavioral functioning all become increasingly apparent over time. Symptoms may include slowed cognitive processing, memory deficits reflecting reduced new learning and retrieval-based memory impairment, executive dysfunction, disturbances in mood, inertia, abulia, apathy, and poor judgment and insight (Filley, 2001; Hurley et al., 2000). Román (1987) classified BD as a subcortical dementia, which has been supported by others (e.g., Stuss & Cummings, 1990) due to the fact that aphasia, apraxia, and agnosia are rarely seen aside from severe cases. Stuss and Cummings (1990) have spoken of this being the primary difference between BD and MID as the latter more commonly involves these cortical signs.

The clinical features of BD overlap with many other presentations, particularly those that impede frontal system functioning. While impairment in memory, language, and visuospatial processing is commonly noted in relation to BD, it is much less severe than that seen in AD (Caplan, 1995). Motor symptoms are parkinsonian in nature, including slowed walking, unsteadiness, taking small steps, flexion posture, rigidity, and pseudobulbar palsy (Caplan, 1995). Behaviorally and emotionally, individuals with BD often manifest depression (Bennett, Gilley, Lee, & Cochran, 1994). Individuals become disinterested in previously enjoyed activities and interests, have decreased spontaneity in action and conversation, and are generally apathetic (Caplan, 1995; Santamaria Ortiz & Knight, 1994). Based on these clinical features and neuroradiological findings, BD is best conceptualized as a disease primarily affecting frontal-subcortical circuitry.

Executive functioning is one area in which, functionally, BD and LS oftentimes differ. This corresponds to the greater burden on the white matter in BD compared to LS, particularly in the dorsolateral prefrontal cortex, and its connections with basal ganglia (Charlton, Morris, Nitkunan, & Markus, 2006; Grau-Olivares, Arboix, Bartrés-Faz, & Junqué, 2007; O'Sullivan, Morris, & Markus, 2005; Sachdev et al., 2006). Consequently, Ramos-Estebanez et al. (2011) found that BD was associated with greater deficits in executive functioning than LS.

Diagnosing SVD

Diagnostic criteria for LS and BD remain largely dependent on neuroradiological findings supplemented by clinical data regarding an individual's health history, including risk factors and observation of cognitive, behavioral, and motor symptoms. The criteria for a diagnosis of BD include evidence of a subcortical dementia based on neurocognitive testing, bilateral abnormalities (e.g., lesions, infarcts) on imaging (CT or MRI), and two or more of the following: (a) vascular risk factors or vascular disease (e.g., hypertension); (b) focal CVD (e.g., evidence of stroke); and/or (c) subcortical cerebral deficits (e.g., gait abnormalities; Thakur, Verma, Mokta, Aggarwal, & Sharma, 2007). Regarding findings on neuroimaging, MRI is considered supportive of a diagnosis of BD if it reveals variable combinations of white matter ischemia and infarcts on T2-weighted scans (Filley, 2001).

Treatment of VaD

In many ways, regardless of the pathological basis, VaD subtypes are treated similarly. Focus is placed on the reduction of disease progression and symptom relief. It has been established that vascular risk factors (e.g., diabetes, hypertension, obesity, etc.) increase the potential of stroke and CVD. Up to 75% of the risk of cardiovascular disease can be prevented by management of these risk factors (Hachinski, 2002; Yusuf, 2002). Specifically, research has demonstrated that interventions directed at reducing these vascular risk factors correspond to reductions in VaD. For example, calcium-channel blockers have demonstrated neuroprotective effects in VaD although this protection has been found to go beyond blood pressure control (Morich et al. 1996; Pantoni et al., 2000).

Heparin-induced extracorporeal low-density lipoprotein (LDL)/fibrinogen precipitation (HELP) has been found to ameliorate the pathological hemorheologic state associated with MID (Walzl, 2000). In one study, the odds of incident cognitive impairment were reduced by roughly 38% in relation to antihypertensive treatment (Murray et al., 2002). Antihypertensive therapy has also been associated with a 28% reduction in the risk of recurrent stroke and a 38% to 55% reduction in the risk of dementia (PROGRESS Collaborative Group, 2001). Finally, discontinuing smoking not only reduces vascular risk, but it may improve cognition. Smokers show worse cognitive performances than nonsmokers, including reduced psychomotor speed and reduced cognitive flexibility (Kalmijn, van Boxtel, Verschuren, Jolles, & Launer, 2002). This effect is observed in subjects as young as 45 years.

Beyond a reduction of vascular risk factors, interventions to improve cognitive functioning have also been assessed. In general, VaD, regardless of the pathological subtype, is chronic and irreversible. Nevertheless, several drug classes have been used for the symptomatic treatment of VaD including vasodilators, calcium-channel blockers, nootropic agents, pentoxifylline, antiplatelet agents, and cholinesterase inhibitors (Román, 2000). As a result of research demonstrating that VaD is oftentimes associated with cholinergic deficits, likely due to disruption of cholinergic pathways because of cerebrovascular lesions, cholinesterase inhibitors have grown in popularity as the first-line pharmacological agents used to stabilize VaD (Román, 2003) including memantine, donepezil, galantamine, and rivastigmine.

Memantine has shown some efficacy in patients with mild to moderate VaD. In a randomized, placebo-controlled clinical trial, memantine was associated with a significant improvement on both the Alzheimer's Disease Assessment Scale—cognitive subscale (ADAS-COG) and Mini-Mental State Examination (MMSE) in patients with mild to moderate VaD, whereas further deterioration was seen in relation to the placebo (Orgogozo, Rigaud, Stöffler, Möbius, & Forette, 2002). In addition, patients receiving memantine demonstrated stable global functioning scores on the Clinician's Interview-Based Impression of Change-plus version (CIBIC-plus) and their frequency of disturbed behavior as measured on The Nurses' Observation Scale for Geriatric Patients ratings went down.

Donepezil has likely received the most attention in research, having also proven its effectiveness in treating VaD. In a large clinical trial, patients diagnosed with VaD were treated over the course of 24 weeks (Pratt & Perdomo, 2002). Only patients with possible or probable VaD were included while patients with preexisting AD were excluded, as were patients with AD plus CVD. Patients were randomized into one of three groups: placebo, 5 mg/d of donepezil, or 10 mg/d of donepezil. The latter group started out at 5 mg/d for 4 weeks prior to being titrated up to 10 mg/d. When compared to placebo, both groups receiving donepezil, regardless of dosage, showed statistically significant improvement in cognitive functioning measured with the ADAS-COG. The MMSE also showed statistically significant improvement versus placebo. Significant improvements were noted in global function on the CIBIC-plus and on the Sum of the Boxes of the Clinical Dementia Rating.

Galantamine is a reversible cholinesterase inhibitor and a modulator of nicotinic acetylcholine receptors in the brain that has also demonstrated effectiveness in treating VaD (Santos et al., 2002). In a large clinical trial, patients with VaD were randomly assigned to either placebo or galantamine (Erkinjuntti et al., 2002). Overall, 294 subjects in the galantamine group and 163 in the placebo group completed the study. The treatment group received 4 mg/d of galantamine for 1 week, titrated up to 24 mg/d by week 6. By the end of the study, the galantamine group had shown a statistically significant improvement in overall cognitive functioning on the ADAS-COG compared to the placebo group. Galantamine was also associated with a significant improvement in behavioral symptoms.

Finally, rivastigmine, which is a dual inhibitor of acetylcholinesterase (AChE) and butyryl-cholinesterase, has also demonstrated efficacy in the treatment of VaD. An open-label study demonstrated sustained cognitive improvement 22 months post-initiation of treatment with rivastigmine compared to aspirin in patients with subcortical VaD (Moretti, Torre, Antonello, & Cazzato, 2001; Moretti, Torre, Antonello, Cazzato, & Bava, 2002). These improvements were noted even in executive functioning and behavioral symptoms. Baseline scores of global response, cognition, word fluency, and activities of daily living (ADL) were maintained in patients receiving rivastigmine, and there was no increase in benzodiazepine or neuroleptic intake. Rivastigmine has also been shown to be more effective than nimodipine in improving behavioral symptoms associated with MID, including hallucinations, aberrant behavior, sleep disturbances, and anxiety disorders (Moretti, Torre, Antonello, Cazzato, & Pizzolato, 2008). Individuals with MID who are treated with rivastigmine also show a reduced reliance on other medications, including neuroleptics and benzodiazepines (Moretti et al., 2008).

SIMILAR NEUROLOGICAL PRESENTATIONS

Cerebral Autosomal Dominant Arteriopathy With Subcortical Infarcts and Leukoencephalopathy

CADASIL is an inherited small-vessel disease of the brain due to mutations in the *Notch3* gene on chromosome 19p13. The prevalence of CADASIL is estimated to be about 2 to 4 individuals in 100,000 (Chabriat, Joutel, Dichgans, Tournier-Lasserve, & Bousser, 2009; Razvi, Davidson, Bone, & Muir, 2005). CADASIL is quite similar to BD clinically but is differentiated based on the fact that it stems from a genetic mutation rather than cerebral arteriosclerosis (Filley, 2001). Andreadou, Papadimas, and Sfagos (2008) note that CADASIL is a common, yet underdiagnosed, cause of inherited stroke in young patients lacking other established cardiovascular risk factors. The disorder was first described by van Bogaert (1955), who wrote on his observations of two sisters, both of whom presented with disease processes similar to BD. Research has since linked the presentation with a hereditary mutation of the *Notch3* gene on chromosome 19. The *Notch3* gene is responsible for encoding a transmembrane receptor that is predominantly expressed in arterial smooth muscle cells and is essential for vascular development. The mutation leads to a progressive degeneration of arteriole smooth muscles within the cerebrum, as well as the skin. Fibrosis occurs over time, leading to a narrowing of the vessel walls, thus reducing blood flow to the deep white matter and eventually leading to repeated ischemic events (Rein Gustavsen, Reinholt, & Schlosser, 2006).

CADASIL's clinical spectrum includes recurrent subcortical ischemic stroke, TIAs, migraine with or without aura, psychiatric disturbances, stroke, and dementia, with an age of onset in mid-to-late adulthood (Chabriat, Bousser, & Pappata, 1995; Liem et al., 2007). Other disturbances, including epilepsy, acute reversible encephalopathy, and myopathy, have also been reported.

Mood disruptions are commonly observed in relation to CADASIL. They have even been found to precede neurological symptoms and cognitive decline and dementia in some cases, although not often (Filley et al., 1999; Liem et al., 2007).

As white matter pathology increases, individuals commonly manifest symptoms consistent with frontal-subcortical involvement. Abulia, deficits in sustained attention, impaired memory retrieval, and perseveration develop (Filley et al., 1999). Dementia is often diagnosed at the end stage of the disorder, and is associated with motor dysfunction, pseudobulbar palsy, and incontinence. The mean age of death is around 60 to 65 years.

The disease manifestation most often occurs between the third and sixth decades. Pathologically, MRI reveals diffuse areas of hyperintensities of the white matter predominantly located subcortically. Lacunar infarcts, microbleeds, and subcortical lacunar lesions are also observed (van den Boom, Oberstein, Ferrari, Haan, & van Buchem, 2003). Temporal pole hyperintensities and involvement of the external capsule may help to distinguish patients with CADASIL from subcortical arteriosclerotic encephalopathy (O'Sullivan et al., 2001), although diagnosis is made by way of genetic testing. Of interest, regarding radiological findings, is the fact that abnormalities can oftentimes be observed prior to the emergence of clinical symptoms (Coulthard, Blank, Bushby, Kalaria, & Burn, 2000).

Neuropathology of CADASIL

CADASIL represents a genetic, non-arteriosclerotic, non-amyloid arteriopathy, a disorder that primarily affects small cerebral arteries and arterioles. The disorder was first discussed by van Bogaert (1955) following his observation of two sisters presenting with similar disease courses. Both demonstrated involvement of the white matter that was not linked to cerebral arteriosclerosis. Van Bogaert suggested a possible genetic root. In time, CADASIL was mapped to chromosome 19q12 across groups from around the world (Tournier-Lasserve et al., 1993). More specifically, CADASIL is caused by mutations in the *Notch3* gene on chromosome 19 (Tournier-Lasserve et al., 1993), which encodes for the Notch3 protein, a member of a highly conserved transmembrane receptor family (Notch signaling; Joutel et al., 1996). The *Notch3* gene is responsible for encoding a transmembrane receptor that is predominantly expressed in arterial smooth muscle cells and essential for vascular development (Andreadou et al., 2008; Tournier-Lasserve et al., 1993). In a British CADASIL study carried out on 83 potential cases (in 48 families) with symptoms characteristic of the disease, 15 different point mutations were identified: 73% in exon 4, 8% in exon 3, and 6% in each of exons 5 and 6 (Markus et al., 2002). In another study, genetic testing was done on the same exons on patients with simple cerebral infarcts. In this case, a single mutation on exon 4 was found in the 218 consecutive cases studied (Dong et al., 2003).

The mutations lead to the development of an odd number of cysteine residues within the *Notch3* extracellular domain that are believed to be related to abnormalities in protein folding and disulfide bridging, resulting in a disruption of ligand binding and, consequently, receptor activation and signal transduction (Federico, Bianchi, & Dotti, 2005). Over time this leads to a degeneration of smooth muscles within the deep penetrating arterioles of the cerebrum and skin. Fibrosis occurs in response to this degeneration and, in doing so, the vessels grow more narrow, thereby reducing blood flow to the brain, particularly to the deep white matter (Rein Gustavsen et al., 2006). As noted by Filley (2001), in some cases, these ultrastructural changes consisting of granular osmiophilic inclusions of the vascular smooth muscle can be seen using electron microscopy (EM) of the skin obtained by biopsy, although these changes are not always seen. Cases have been reported that involve a mixture of subcortical white matter and gray matter disease, although there are reported cases of pure white matter pathology (Hedera & Friedland, 1997). Neuropathological changes associated with CADASIL most typically include a combination of WMH, lacunar lesions, and cerebral microhemorrhages (Federico et al., 2005; Jouvent et al., 2007). Viswanathan, Gray, Bousser, Baudrimont, and Chabriat (2006) found widespread neuronal apoptosis in the cerebral cortex of CADASIL brains, demonstrating that the degree of neuronal apoptosis is related to the underlying subcortical white matter damage. The typical lesion of CADASIL is the presence of granular osmiophilic material (GOM) in white matter and leptomeningeal arteries (Guidetti, Casali, Mazzei, & Dotti, 2006). GOMs are located close to vascular smooth muscles, nerves, and skin cells. The white matter infarcts may cause cortical cholinergic denervation. Primary disease burden involves frontal lobes, anterior temporal lobes, and the periventricular caps. MRI in symptomatic patients is always abnormal and, oftentimes, even in presymptomatic patients. T2-weighted images often show punctuated and nodular hypersignals with a symmetrical distribution. They predominate in periventricular areas and in centrum semiovale, but they also are present in the basal ganglia, brain stem, and corpus callosum. Ischemic leukoaraiosis is common in advanced cases and increases remarkably with age (Iannucci et al., 2001). Temporal lobe hyperintensity is a radiological marker of CADASIL, with a sensitivity of 89% for CADASIL diagnosis in the British study (Guidetti et al., 2006). Another pathological hallmark, present only in about 45% of cases (Iannucci et al., 2001), is a dense, darkly stained GOM in the arterial walls, identified by EM. *Notch3* immunohistochemistry is considered an alternative to EM in skin biopsies (Liebetrau, Herzog, Kloss, Hamann, & Dichgans, 2002).

Clinical Features of CADASIL

As noted previously, CADASIL is clinically marked by recurrent subcortical ischemic stroke, TIAs, cognitive decline, and migraine with aura, with an age of onset in mid-to-late adulthood (Chabriat et al., 1995; Liem et al., 2007). Migraines, TIAs, and strokes are often cited as the most frequent symptoms. The aura experienced in conjunction with migraines is commonly visual, but often it is atypical, long lasting, or exceptionally severe (Guidetti et al., 2006). Interestingly, in the majority of patients with migraine plus stroke, headache either ceased at the time of the first stroke or migraine attacks became markedly less frequent (Guidetti et al., 2006). However, different types of migraine have been reported. While migraine with typical aura accounts for the majority of cases, migraine without aura, migraine aura without headache, basilar migraine, hemiplegic migraine, acute-onset aura without headache, migraine with acute-onset aura, migraine with prolonged aura, and retinal migraine have all been reported (Chabriat et al., 1995; Desmond et al., 1999; Dichgans et al., 1998; Vahedi et al., 2004; Valko, Siccoli, Schiller, Wieser, & Jung, 2007).

The main feature of CADASIL remains the occurrence of recurrent episodes of stroke that early on present as TIAs. In about 70% of patients, the disease began with TIAs or strokes. Often strokes are lacunar and almost invariably subcortical, located in white matter or basal ganglia. They also may affect the brain stem in 45% of symptomatic cases (Chabriat et al., 1999). Recurrent infarctions are linked with pseudobulbar paresis, difficulties in locomotion, dysarthria, dysphagia, spasticity, gait ataxia, emotional lability, and spasmodic laughing or crying (Guidetti et al., 2006).

One feature of the presentation that distinguishes CADASIL from cortical dementias is the relative age of onset. Individuals with CADASIL typically demonstrate cognitive deficits by the age of 35 years, and in more than 80% of cases, there is a progressive decline in cognitive functions before 60 years of age (Liem et al., 2007). However, mood disruptions may occur even earlier, prior to the development of neurological symptoms or cognitive decline and dementia (Filley et al., 1999; Liem et al., 2007). Changes in executive function and working memory have been found among mutation carriers even in the prestroke phase. As white matter pathology increases, individuals commonly manifest symptoms consistent with frontal-subcortical dysfunction including abulia, deficits in sustained attention, impaired memory retrieval, and perseveration development (Filley et al., 1999). Individuals also commonly demonstrate impaired executive and organizing abilities, slowing of mental abilities, poor concentration, or slowing of motor functions (Tournier-Lasserve et al., 1993). Language remains relatively spared (Filley et al., 1999) likely aside from issues with verbal fluency, which may correspond to additional deficits in executive functioning. Over time, CADASIL leads to a subcortical-type dementia (Trojano, Ragno, Manca, & Caruso, 1998). In 10% to 15% of patients, dementia develops without acute episodes of clinical stroke (Davous & Bequet, 1995).

Dichgans et al. (1999) demonstrated that a correlation exists between cognitive decline and white matter lesion burden in CADASIL. Rein Gustavsen et al. (2006) noted that lacunar infarct lesion load, rather than WMH or microbleeds, is the most important MRI finding associated with the severity of cognitive dysfunction in individuals with CADASIL. They reported that the number of infarcts observed is significantly associated with neuropsychological test results of global cognitive functioning, including language, praxis, memory, and executive functions. Furthermore, individuals who have had multiple strokes demonstrate declines in perceptual speed, visuospatial skills, and working memory (Rein Gustavsen et al., 2006). In a similar fashion, Reyes et al. (2009) demonstrated that apathy is not only commonly present in CADASIL, but the degree of apathy along with other neuropsychiatric symptoms (e.g., depression, agitation, irritability, and aggression) is related to the volume of subcortical lesions present and the overall clinical severity of subsequent cognitive and motor disability. Dementia is often diagnosed at the end stage of the disorder, and is associated with motor dysfunction, pseudobulbar palsy, and incontinence. The mean age of death is around 60 to 65 years.

In their study, Buffon et al. (2006) noted three specific findings: (a) The cognitive profile in CADASIL patients is heterogeneous and involves only a few cognitive domains at the onset of the disease, while it is homogeneous after the age of 60 years with significant deficits in all cognitive domains; (b) patients with dementia have additional impairment in skills such as reasoning compared to subjects without dementia; and (c) memory impairment even at the late stage of the disorder does not involve the encoding process (retrieval significantly improved with cues), which is relatively preserved compared to that reported in other types of dementia with degeneration of the hippocampus.

While the clinical expression of CADASIL is mostly neurological, psychiatric disturbances are also commonly observed. One review showed that the reported frequency of psychiatric disturbances in CADASIL ranges between 20% and 41% (Valenti, Poggesi, Pescini, Inzitari, & Pantoni, 2008). While these disturbances predominantly involve affective and adjustment disorders, agoraphobia, substance abuse and addiction, and psychotic disturbances have also been decribed in the literature (Dichgans et al., 1998; Joutel et al., 1997; Razvi et al., 2005; Reyes et al., 2009). Some studies have noted that depressive episodes can oftentimes represent the initial clinical manifestation of CADASIL on retrospective analysis (Rufa et al., 2004). Apathy has been commonly observed as a major symptom in CADASIL (Reyes et al., 2009). Psychiatric manifestations are not necessarily surprising given the involvement of frontal systems.

Diagnosing CADASIL

Although CADASIL has been recognized as the most common cause of hereditary stroke, it remains underdiagnosed (Dichgans, 2002, 2007). A diagnosis of CADASIL is suggested through MRI findings and neuropsychological testing, but definitive diagnosis is confirmed by the presence of GOMs in smooth muscle cells of the skin and muscle vessels (Jung et al., 1995; Ruchoux, Chabriat, Bousser, Baudrimont, & Tournier-Lasserve, 1994) or molecular genetic analysis allowing identification of the pathogenic mutation in the *Notch3* gene (Ruchoux et al., 1994). Numerous mutations have been reported, mostly located within the 23 exons that encode the 34 epidermal growth factor-like (EGF-like) repeats (Joutel et al., 1997). The sensitivity of this mutational screening is so high that cases of CADASIL may be confirmed even at presymptomatic stages (Peters et al., 2005). Skin biopsy, examined by EM, can also detect the degeneration and loss of smooth muscle cells as well as deposits of GOM in the external basal lamina in the extracellular matrix of arterioles and small arteries (Rein Gustavsen et al., 2006).

MRI of CADASIL presents with symmetrical and extensive WMH in T2-weighted images and well-defined hypointense lesions in T1 images (Jouvent et al., 2007). Specific findings consistent with CADASIL involve white matter changes in the anterior temporal lobe and hyperintensities in the external capsule along with an absence of spinal cord involvement and no oligoclonal bands in the cerebrospinal fluid (Andreadou et al., 2008; Markus et al., 2002; Rein Gustavsen et al., 2006). The latter two (i.e., no spinal cord involvement and no oligoclonal bands) allow for differentiation from multiple sclerosis. When the aforementioned MRI findings are noted in the absence of vascular risk factors and a family history consistent with autosomal dominant inheritance, the possibility of the pathological findings being related to CADASIL increases (Andreadou et al., 2008). Single-photon emission computed tomography (SPECT) and PET scans have also shown some promise as studies have demonstrated hypoperfusion and decreased vasoreactivity in relation to CADASIL corresponding to the increasing impairment of adaptive vasodilation, especially of the small brain arteries, due to the progressive degeneration of the smooth muscle cells in blood vessels (Chabriat et al., 1995; Mellies et al., 1998; Pfefferkorn et al., 2001). Proton magnetic resonance spectroscopy studies often demonstrate metabolic abnormalities that suggest axonal injury, enlarged extracellular spaces, myelin loss, and gliosis due to microinfarctions and stroke episodes (Auer et al., 2001; Kemp, 2000; Macrì et al., 2006; Oliveri et al., 2001).

Treatment of CADASIL

Treatment of CADASIL is focused on symptom relief as there exists no evidence-based treatment for the disorder itself. Antidepressants have shown some efficiency in reducing the mood disturbances that often coincide with CADASIL. Migraines have also demonstrated responsiveness to medicinal intervention.

Akhvlediani et al. (2010) reported on a case study of a patient in which migrainosus status and the persistent aura without infarction resolved after intravenous treatment with lorazepam and mannitol. Phenytoin, an antiepileptic agent, has also shown some benefit in resolving prolonged attacks of migraine in a small series of patients (Chabriat et al., 1995).

The possible benefit of AChE inhibitors has been suggested. As noted previously, the white matter infarcts occurring in association with CADASIL may cause cortical cholinergic denervation, thus suggesting the possible utility of AChE inhibitors such as donepezil (Keverne et al., 2007). However, studies have failed to identify a significant benefit of donepezil in treating patients with CADASIL (Dichgans et al., 2008).

MOYAMOYA

Moyamoya is an uncommon chronic unremitting cerebrovasculopathy, which is characterized by progressive occlusion of the supraclinoid internal carotid artery and its main branches within the circle of Willis. Reduced blood flow to the anterior regions of the brain results in the compensatory development of the collateral arterial network. This develops near the apex of the carotid, on the cortical surface, leptomeninges, and the branches of the external carotid artery (ECA) supplying the dura and the base of the skull.

Takeuchi and Shimizu (1957) first described in 1957 a case of "hypoplasia of the bilateral internal carotid arteries." Later in 1968, Kudo described a similar presentation, which he described as "spontaneous occlusion of the circle of Willis" (Kudo, 1968). Finally in 1969, Suzuki and Takaku used the term *moyamoya*, a Japanese term expressing "something hazy, like a puff of cigarette smoke" (Suzuki & Takaku, 1969). This best described the characteristic appearance of the associated network of abnormally dilated collateral vessels on angiography. Although "spontaneous occlusion of the circle of Willis" has recently been suggested as an alternative to the more evocative name *moyamoya*, the International Classification of Diseases recognizes *moyamoya* as the specific name for this condition (Fukui, 1997a, 1997b).

In 1997, the Research Committee on Spontaneous Occlusion of the Circle of Willis (Moyamoya Disease) published guidelines for the diagnosis of moyamoya disease in English (Fukui, 1997a, 1997b). According to these guidelines, moyamoya disease is characterized by stenosis or occlusion at the terminal portions of the internal carotid artery (ICA) or the proximal areas of the anterior or the middle cerebral arteries and abnormal vascular networks in the arterial territories near the occlusive or stenotic lesions, as shown by cerebral angiography. Definite cases of moyamoya disease are diagnosed in patients with bilateral lesions, whereas patients with unilateral lesions are diagnosed as probable cases. Because the etiology of moyamoya disease is unknown, so-called quasi-moyamoya diseases or moyamoya syndromes need to be eliminated (Kuroda & Houkin, 2008).

Although initial descriptions and studies initially centered on the Asian population, moyamoya is currently observed throughout the world in people of various ethnic backgrounds (Caldarelli, Di Rocco, & Gaglini, 2001; Suzuki & Kodama, 1983). Japan presents the highest rate of moyamoya disease, with an annual prevalence and incidence estimated at 3.16 to 10.5 per 100,000 and 0.35 to 0.94 per 100,000, respectively (Baba, Houkin, & Kuroda, 2008; Wakai et al., 1997). It is the most common pediatric CVD in that country. Results from a 2005 American review suggest an incidence of 0.086 case per 100,000 persons. Reported incidence-rate ratios are 4.6 for Asian Americans, 2.2 for Blacks, and 0.5 for Hispanics, as compared with Whites (Uchino, Johnston, Becker, & Tirschwell, 2005). Moyamoya has bimodal age of onset: children who are approximately 5 years of age and adults in their mid-40s (Baba et al., 2008; Han, Nam, & Oh, 1997; Han et al., 2000; Wakai et al., 1997). There are nearly twice as many female patients as male patients (Baba et al., 2008; Scott et al., 2004; Wakai et al., 1997).

Neuropathology of Moyamoya

Pathophysiology

The stenosis associated with moyamoya arises in the supraclinoid part of the internal carotid artery and later progresses distally to bifurcation and in later stages to the proximal branches of the anterior and middle cerebral arteries. Stenosis of the proximal portions of the posterior cerebral arteries and basilar artery has been observed in rare cases (Miyamoto et al., 1986).

Histologically, the vascular changes described include endothelial hyperplasia, fibrocellular thickening of the intima, and tortuosity and duplication of the internal elastic lamina (Fukui, Kono, Sueishi, & Ikezaki, 2000; Ikeda, 1991; Scott & Smith, 2009; Smith, 2009). Occlusion due to progressive vascular stenosis is a result of smooth muscle hyperplasia and formation of intraluminal hyperplasia (Ikeda, 1991; Scott & Smith, 2009), rather than from any inflammatory infiltrate of atheromatous plaque (Fukui et al., 2000). The media are often attenuated with irregular elastic laminae, and capase-dependant apoptosis has been associated with the degradation of the arterial wall (Takagi, Kikuta, Nozaki, & Hashimoto, 2007; Takagi, Kikuta, Sadamasa, Nozaki, & Hashimoto, 2006). The collateral vessels in moyamoya constitute a compensatory mechanism acting in response to the cerebral ischemia secondary to the vascular stenosis. They originate from the various perforating vessels including the medial and lateral lenticulostriate, anterior and posterior choroidal, thalamoperforating, and thalamogenic arteries (Miyamoto et al., 1986; Takahashi, 1980). In the latter stages of moyamoya, transdural collaterals derived from the ECAs, including the middle meningeal, superficial temporal, occipital, and internal maxillary arteries, and from the ophthalmic arteries, including the anterior and posterior ethmoid, recurrent meningeal, and anterior falx arteries, are noted (Takahashi, 1980). The collateral vessels are also categorized as follows (Matsushima & Inaba, 1986): (a) intracerebral anastomoses, which arise from basal and convexity perforating arteries that penetrate brain parenchyma and anastomose at the external angle of the lateral ventricles; (b) dilated basal collateral networks, which develop directly from circle of Willis vessels and perforating carotid artery–basilar artery anastomoses; (c) cortical-leptomeningeal end-to-end anastomoses, which form over the surface of the brain at watershed areas of the major cerebral artery territories; (d) dural networks, which arise from dural vessels and perfuse ischemic brain through anastomoses with the cortical leptomeningeal system; and (e) extracranial networks, which arise from transdural vessels and connect scalp arteries to the cortical leptomeningeal system.

Moyamoya-associated collateral vessels are generally dilated perforating vessels, which are believed to be a combination of preexisting and newly developed vessels (Kono, Oka, & Sueishi, 1990; Lim, Cheshier, & Steinberg, 2006).

A postmortem study of collateral vessel specimens reveals overall thinned walls; atrophy of the media secondary to damaged smooth muscle cells; increased matrix deposition with cellular debris; and tortuosity, fragmentation, and thinning of the internal elastic lamina (Takebayashi, Matsuo, & Kaneko, 1984). Microaneurysm formation within the weakened moyamoya vessels is a potential source of intracranial hemorrhage, and has been found on both the anterior and posterior choroidal arteries (Smith, 2009).

Etiology

Although the pathogenesis and etiology of moyamoya remain unknown, genetic and acquired or environmental factors are implicated in the development of this rare disease. The previously noted characteristic pathological change seen in the vasculature suggests an altered expression of certain mitogen, adhesion molecules, and angiogenic factors. Alteration in cellular response to growth factor and cytokines in the vascular cells has also been implicated in the development of the moyamoya pathology (Smith, 2009). Levels of many growth factors, enzymes, and other peptides such as basic fibroblast growth factor (bFGF), transforming growth factor-β1 (TGF-β1), hepatocyte growth factor, matrix, metalloproteinases, intracellualar adhesion molecules, and hypoxia-inducing factor 1α have been shown to be altered (Scott & Smith, 2009). Mutation in the region affects the tissue inhibitor of matrix metalloproteinase type 2 (TIMP-2), which is a regulator of matrix metalloproteinases of particular interest, given the important role of extracellular-matrix remodeling and angiogenesis in both the primary arteriopathy and subsequent response of the ischemic brain (Kang et al., 2006; Lim et al., 2006). Due to the collateral formation in moyamoya, angiogenic factors are currently being examined for their potential role in the disease (Burke et al., 2009). Vascular endothelial growth factor (VEGF) has been shown to lead to cerebral angiogenesis during ischemia; however, its role in moyamoya has been inconclusive (Sakamoto et al., 2008; Takekawa, Umezawa, Ueno, Sawada, & Kobayashi, 2004). bFGF has been found to be elevated in patients with moyamoya and has been postulated to be specific to the particular disease (Yoshimoto, Houkin, Takahashi, & Abe, 1996). bFGF has been associated with migration and activation of smooth muscle cells, which result in intimal thickening and neovascularization (Hoshimaru, Takahashi, Kikuchi, Nagata, & Hatanaka, 1991). TGF-β has been shown to be elevated in the cerebrospinal fluid (CSF) and in expression in superior temporal artery (STA) in moyamoya. It has been shown to increase the elastin synthesis and could lead to intimal thickening (Hojo et al., 1998; Yamamoto et al., 1997). Furthermore, hypoxia inducible factor-1α (HIF-1α) and endoglin have been found to be significantly higher in patients with myotonic muscular dystrophy (MMD). Endoglin modulates cellular response to TGF-β and is involved in vascular morphogenesis. HIF-1α regulates TGF-β transcription. In addition, HIF-1α in the presence of bFGF or hepatocyte growth factor, both of which are elevated in the CSF, promotes thickening of the intima and the proliferation of smooth muscle cells (Takagi et al., 2007). Additionally, intercellular adhesion molecule-1 (ICAM-1) and vascular cell adhesion molecule-1 (VCAM-1) have been shown to be increased in the CSF of patients with moyamoya disease (Soriano, Cowan, Proctor, & Scott, 2002). Protein S deficiency, lupus anticoagulant, and anticardiolipin antibodies found in other cases suggest a possible autoimmune mechanism in MMD as the antibodies could contribute to thrombus formation in strokes (Bonduel, Hepner, Sciuccati, Torres, & Tenembaum, 2001; Kuroda & Houkin, 2008).

Genetic factors appear to play a major role in the development of moyamoya disease. The proportion of patients who have affected first-degree relatives is 10% in Japan, and a rate of 6% was reported in a U.S. series (Fukui et al., 2000; Scott et al., 2004). Most familial cases appear to be polygenic or inherited in an autosomal dominant fashion with incomplete penetrance. A 2008 study reported a major gene locus for autosomal dominant moyamoya disease on chromosome 17q25 (Mineharu et al., 2008). Associations with loci on chromosomes 3, 6, 8, and 17, as well as specific HLA haplotypes, have been described (Scott & Smith, 2009). A number of genome-wide linkage studies have been carried out in Japanese families with diagnoses of familial moyamoya that suggest linkage to at least five different chromosomal regions: 3p24.2-p26, 6q25, 8q23, 12p12, and 17q25 (Achrol et al., 2009). The differences in loci identified by these linkage studies may represent locus heterogeneity. Chromosome linkage analyses provide further support for genetic factors in the etiology of moyamoya disease. Linkage study using markers on chromosome 6, where the HLA gene resides, have identified an allele that appears to be linked with moyamoya disease (Kelly, Bell-Stephens, Marks, Do, & Steinberg, 2006). Clinical observation of the association of moyamoya disease and sometimes neurofibromatosis type 1, whose causative gene (i.e., *NF1*) has been assigned to 17q11.2, led to microsatellite linkage analyses to ascertain whether a gene related to moyamoya disease is also located on chromosome 17 (Yamauchi et al., 2000). Such analyses detected a gene for familial moyamoya disease on 17q. Microsatellite linkage analyses have also shown linkages between moyamoya disease and markers located on 3p, 6q, and 8q (Smith, 2009). Interestingly, a locus for Marfan syndrome and von Hippel Lindau disease tumor suppressor gene maps to 3p (Collod et al., 1994; Latif et al., 1993). The gene product of the moyamoya gene mapping to 3p is postulated to be fundamental to the formation and maintenance of vascular wall homeostasis (Smith, 2009). Mutation in genes *neurofibromatosis type-1* (*NF1*) and *ACTA2* predispose the affected individuals to various vascular diseases. They promote increased smooth muscle cell proliferation and could lead to hyperplastic vasculopathy. Association between the *NF1* gene and *ACTA2* gene, and predisposition to develop moyamoya, has been postulated (Friedman et al., 2002; Guo et al., 2009). The loss of BRCC3 deubiquitinating enzyme has been postulated to cause abnormal angiogenesis and to be associated with moyamoya angiopathy (Miskinyte et al., 2011).

Associated Conditions

Moyamoya syndrome is a term used when radiographic features similar to those of idiopathic moyamoya disease coexist with other medical conditions that can explain the vasculopathy. Catheter angiograms performed after a stroke in children with sickle cell disease reported a moyamoya pattern; the risk is estimated to be around 20% to 35% (Moritani et al., 2004). Red blood cells containing deoxygenated hemoglobin become abnormally adherent to the walls of blood vessels in sickle cell disease. Subsequent vascular stasis produces platelet aggregation and fibrin deposition, resulting in ischemia and infarction. Continued damage to the blood vessels results in fibrosis and narrowing of the cerebral vasculature, further exacerbating the stenoses, and leading to an eventual progression to occlusion. Collateral vessels are likely to develop at the points of greatest metabolic demand (Meyers, Halbach, & Barkovich, 2000). Down syndrome and Turner syndrome, because of higher incidence of vascular dysplasia, have been associated with moyamoya syndrome (Mito & Becker, 1992; Spengos et al., 2006). Infectious causes such as tuberculous meningitis and other causes of viral vasculitis result in inflammatory exudative fluid and reduced caliber of the vessels (Barkovich, 2000; Sharfstein, Ahmed, Islam, Najjar, & Ratushny, 2007).

Radiation-induced vasculopathy has been a well-recognized late complication of radiation therapy. Intimal thickening and medial necrosis are the hallmark histological changes seen in radiation-induced damage to the large vessels (Aoki et al., 2002). Higher incidence of radiation-induced moyamoya has been seen in younger patients, probably due to the vascular immaturity (Maruyama et al., 2000; Rudoltz et al., 1998). Correlation between the treatment volume and the latent period and their effects on development of radiation-induced moyamoya syndrome has not been documented (Desai, Paulino, Mai, & Teh, 2006). Chemotherapy combined with radiation increases vascular inflammation and may induce local vasculopathy (Mitchell et al., 1991).

Posterior fossa malformations–hemangiomas–arterial anomalies–cardiac defects–eye abnormalities–sternal cleft and supraumbilical raphe syndrome (PHACES) is a neurocutaneous disorder characterized by large cervicofacial infantile hemangiomas and associated anomalies of the brain, cerebrovasculature, aorta, heart, and eyes; it has been associated with moyamoya-like vasculopathy and consequent ischemic strokes (Heyer, Millar, Ghatan, & Garzon, 2006). Mitochondrial disorders are usually multisystem diseases, and the central nervous system (CNS) is the most commonly affected organ (Finsterer, Jarius, & Eichberger, 2001). Various case reports have described moyamoya disease in patients with mitochondrial disease (Finsterer, 2009).

Several studies have shown the relationship between Graves' disease and stenosis/occlusion of the intracranial arteries; however, the underlying mechanism is not elucidated (Ohba, Nakagawa, & Murakami, 2011). Thyroid hormones might augment vascular sensitivity to the sympathetic nervous system and induce pathological changes in the arterial walls (Liu, Juo, Chen, Chang, & Chen, 1994) such as increased stiffness of the internal carotid artery (Czarkowski, Hilgertner, Powalowski, & Radomski, 2002; Inaba et al., 2002). Another hypothesis is that an immune-mediated mechanism may play a role in the pathogenesis of the disease (Ni, Gao, Cui, & Li, 2006; Panegyres, Morris, O'Neill, & Balleine, 1993). A common pathogenic link involving T-cell dysregulation resulting in cellular proliferation and vascular dysregulation in moyamoya disease and immunologic stimulation of the thyroid in Graves' disease has been suggested (Tendler et al., 1997). Elevated thyroid autoantibodies are frequently observed in patients with MMD and suggest the role of immune abnormalities associated with or underlying thyroid autoimmunity, which play a role in developing moyamoya (Kim et al., 2010). The other hypothesis is that atherosclerosis may be a key link between these disorders (Sasaki, Nogawa, & Amano, 2006). The positive correlation between the levels of free thyroxine and both homocysteine and methylmalonic acid suggests that thyrotoxicosis may induce hyperhomocysteinemia (Colleran, Ratliff, & Burge, 2003). Because homocysteinemia has been implicated in patients with ischemic stroke and lacunar infarction (Iso et al., 2004), this would be another key factor in the pathophysiology of moyamoya syndrome. Cerebrovascular hemodynamic changes induced by thyrotoxicosis were considered to be responsible for infarctions.

In the thyrotoxic state, excessive production of thyroid hormones is believed to increase cerebral metabolism and oxygen consumption, resulting in impairment of cerebral perfusion. Because the cerebrovascular perfusion reserve capacity is reduced in moyamoya disease, impairment of cerebral perfusion is considered to occur more frequently in such cases (Im, Oh, Kwon, Kim, & Han, 2005). In addition, hypercoagulability, which is reported to be induced during thyrotoxicosis, may influence ischemic events (Siegert, Smelt, & de Bruin, 1995).

Clinical Features of Moyamoya

Presentation

Moyamoya disease usually presents with symptoms and signs secondary to the changes in blood flow in the internal carotid artery. Fukui defined four types of MMD with the following presentation percentages—ischemic: 63.4%; hemorrhagic: 21.6%; epileptic: 7.6%; and "other": 7.4% (Fukui, 1997a). In the United States, most adults and children present with ischemic symptoms, although the rate of hemorrhage is approximately seven times greater in adults (20% vs. 2.8%; Fukui, 1997a; Kelly et al., 2006). Some degree of geographic variability exists; reports from Asian populations indicate that adults have much higher rates of hemorrhage as a presenting symptom (42%) compared with U.S. populations (20%; Scott & Smith, 2009).

In contrast, it is extremely rare for children to present with hemorrhage (2.8%); they predominantly present with TIAs or ischemic strokes (68%; Fukui, 1997a; Scott & Smith, 2009). Cerebrovascular homeostasis is maintained by the process of autoregulation through the interplay among CBF, cerebral perfusion pressure (CPP), and vascular resistance. Extreme fall in CPP results in reduced CBF despite compensatory mechanisms and can cause ischemic symptoms (Currie, Raghavan, Batty, Connolly, & Griffiths, 2011). Moyamoya disease usually causes some cerebral ischemia in the territory of the ICA, particularly in the frontal lobe. Therefore, most patients with moyamoya disease present with focal neurological signs, such as dysarthria, aphasia, or hemiparesis (Kuroda & Houkin, 2008). However, moyamoya disease might also cause other atypical symptoms such as syncope, paraparesis, visual symptoms, or involuntary movements, particularly in children (Karasawa, Touho, Ohnishi, Miyamoto, & Kikuchi, 1993; Miyamoto et al., 1986; Zheng et al., 2006). Some pediatric patients develop intellectual impairment owing to frontal lobe ischemia, infarct, or both (Bowen, Marks, & Steinberg, 1998; Kuroda et al., 2004). In rare cases, adult patients can develop cognitive dysfunction, such as short-term memory disturbance, irritability, or agitation; patients who present with these symptoms are commonly misdiagnosed with psychiatric disorders, such as schizophrenia, depression, or personality disorder (Kuroda & Houkin, 2008; Lubman, Pantelis, Desmond, Proffitt, & Velakoulis, 2003; Nagata et al., 2007). In pediatric patients, ischemic attacks are characteristically induced by hyperventilation, for example, when crying or playing a wind instrument. The reduced partial pressure of carbon dioxide results in reduced CBF because of vasoconstriction. The fall in CBF compromises the already reduced cerebral perfusion and causes ischemic symptoms (Currie et al., 2011). Following a TIA, children have a much higher rate of completed infarcts when compared to their adult counterparts. This tendency is likely due to immature verbal skills in younger children, making it difficult to communicate symptoms associated with TIAs, delaying the diagnosis of moyamoya, and increasing the likelihood of completed stroke on presentation (Jea, Smith, Robertson, & Scott, 2005). Stenosis in the posterior circulation has been associated with visual symptoms such as temporary and permanent blindness, visual field deficits, homonymous hemianopsia, quadrantanopsia, scintillating scotomata, blurred vision, and amaurosis fugax. Disturbances in the visual pathway are more likely to occur in children as opposed to adults (Miyamoto et al., 1986). About half of the adult patients with moyamoya disease develop intracranial bleeding (Miyamoto et al., 1986). There are two main causes of intracranial bleeding in moyamoya disease: rupture of dilated, fragile moyamoya vessels or rupture of saccular aneurysms in the circle of Willis. In the first case, the rupture is due to persistent hemodynamic stress of the moyamoya vessels and occurs in the basal ganglia, thalamus, or periventricular region (Irikura et al., 1996; Iwama et al., 1997). In the second case, rupture of saccular aneurysms located around the circle of Willis occurs most commonly at the basilar artery bifurcation or the junction of the basilar artery and the superior cerebellar artery (Kawaguchi, Sakaki, Morimoto, Kakizaki, & Kamada, 1996). There is increasing evidence that moyamoya disease in adults might induce subarachnoid hemorrhage over the cerebral cortex despite the absence of an intracranial aneurysm (Dietrichs et al., 1992; Marushima, Yanaka, Matsuki, Kojima, & Nose, 2006; Osanai et al., 2008). A third cause of intracranial bleeding in adult patients with moyamoya disease is therefore rupture of the dilated collateral arteries on the brain surface, although this is rare (Kuroda & Houkin, 2008).

Headache is a frequent symptom presenting in patients with moyamoya. Dilatation of the meningeal and leptomeningeal collateral vessels, which stimulates the dural nociceptors, has been suggested as the most likely mechanism (Seol et al., 2005). Hypoperfusion-induced activation of pain-sensitive structures also gives rise to headaches (Seol et al., 2005). The headache is most likely migraine-like in quality and has variable response to surgery for moyamoya (Scott & Smith, 2009). Movement disorders as the presenting feature probably arise from ischemia or changes in the excitatory and inhibitory circuits interconnecting the basal ganglia and cerebral cortex (Pandey, Bell-Stephens, & Steinberg, 2010). Choreiform movements secondary to dilatation of the collateral vessels in the basal ganglia are seen in children (Parmar, Bavdekar, Muranjan, & Limaye, 2000; Scott et al., 2004; Scott & Smith, 2009). "Morning glory disc," an opthalmologic finding of enlarged optic disc and concomitant retinovascular anomalies, is occasionally seen with moyamoya (Massaro et al., 1998). Seizures, both focal and generalized, have been associated with moyamoya and are likely related to hypoperfusion.

Neuropsychological Changes

Cognitive dysfunction and loss of intellectual capacity are commonly described in children with moyamoya (Imaizumi, Imaizumi, Osawa, Fukuyama, & Takeshita, 1999; Matsushima, Aoyagi, Masaoka, Suzuki, & Ohno, 1990). Experience in children shows that cognitive deficits improve after surgery, and revascularization has been associated with the improvement (Matsushima et al., 1990). A recent review of the literature suggested significant loss of intellectual capacity at the time of diagnosis (Karzmark et al., 2008). Long-term intellectual deficits have been shown in children who have been managed conservatively without surgery (Imaizumi et al., 1999; Matsushima et al., 1990). Lesions in the left cerebral hemisphere have been shown to result in diminished verbal abilities, whereas lesions on the right side have been shown to impair visual-spatial function, resulting in a lower performance intelligent quotient (PIQ) score (Bornstein, 1983; Iverson, Mendrek, & Adams, 2004). Surgery has been shown to be beneficial in patients with moyamoya. Improvements in visual memory and visual-motor coordination with surgery also have been demonstrated (Lee et al., 2011). The presence of infarction has been related to poorer intellectual functioning (Matsushima et al., 1990). Patients with infarction have been shown to have the worst postoperative cognitive functions; however, further deterioration of the remaining cognitive ability could be prevented through surgery (Kuroda et al., 2004; Lee et al., 2011).

Cognitive dysfunction in adults is less well described, with much of the information coming by way of case studies (e.g., Bornstein, McLean, & Ho, 1985; Hoare & Keogh, 1974; Jefferson, Glosser, Detre, Sinson, & Liebeskind, 2006; Komiyama et al., 2001; Lubman et al., 2003; Ogasawara et al., 2005). The highest rate of cognitive impairment has been described for executive functions, processing speed, verbal memory, and verbal fluency, and lowest rate of cognitive impairment for memory and perception measures (Bornstein et al., 1985; Festa et al., 2010; Hoare & Keogh, 1974; Jefferson et al., 2006; Karzmark et al., 2008; Komiyama et al., 2001; Lubman et al., 2003; Ogasawara et al., 2005). This pattern of deficits is more typical for diffuse small-vessel disease, which may be caused by small-vessel disease, and is similar to deficits found in VCI. General impairment in intelligence has also been noted in one case (Lubman et al., 2003) but was not found in a larger series of adults (Karzmark et al., 2008). Problems with executive functioning are mostly reported, and use of Trail Making tests may be a useful tool to screen for the deficits (Calviere et al., 2010; Karzmark et al., 2008). Memory impairment and severe amnestic states have been reported in patients with intraventricular hemorrhage (Darby, Donnan, Saling, Walsh, & Bladin, 1988); however, in presurgical, nonhemorrhagic patients, relatively intact memory functioning has been reported (Komiyama et al., 2001; Lubman et al., 2003; Ogasawara et al., 2005). Frontal lobe pathology as a cause of impairment in short-term, free-recall memory for temporal order and source memory has been postulated (Shimamura, Janosky, & Squire, 1991). Cognitive impairment in such patients is often expressed as mood disorder, irritability, or agitation, and is misdiagnosed as being psychiatric in nature (Kuroda & Houkin, 2008).

Disease Progression

Asymptomatic moyamoya has been described, and the most important clinical implication in this case includes treatment to prevent future cerebrovascular events such as TIAs, ischemic stroke, and hemorrhages. Asymptomatic moyamoya is not considered a silent disorder but a potentially progressive disease that could lead to serious cerebrovacular events as described in the Japanese literature (Kuroda et al., 2007). Progression of disease is more common in children than in adults (Kuroda et al., 2007; Suzuki & Kodama, 1983). Similarly, progression from unilateral to bilateral disease has been shown to be common, and the average time of progression has been estimated to be between 1.5 and 2.2 years (Kelly et al., 2006; Kuroda et al., 2007; Smith & Scott, 2008).

Diagnosing Moyamoya

Diagnosis

Conventional angiography remains the gold standard for both the diagnosis and surgical planning for patients with suspected moyamoya disease. A five- or six-vessel study should be performed, including imaging of the bilateral ECA, ICA, and one or two vertebral injections. Angiographic imaging of the bilateral ECAs is of utmost importance for preoperative planning to prevent disruption of these collaterals during the surgical revascularization. Classical findings on angiogram include stenosis of the supraclinoid ICA, proximal anterior cerebral artery (ACA), and middle cerebral artery (MCA), associated with basal ICA, leptomeningeal, and transdural collaterals, giving rise to the classic "puff of smoke" appearance (Suzuki & Takaku, 1969). Angiographic appearance of moyamoya disease progresses through one of six stages as originally defined by Suzuki and Takaku in 1969: (a) carotid stenosis in the absence of moyamoya collaterals; (b) initial appearance of basal collateral vessels; (c) progressive stenosis of the distal ICA, with increasing prominence of the basal collaterals; (d) severe stenosis or occlusion of the anterior circulation with the formation of ECA collaterals; (e) prominence of the ECA collaterals, reduction, and stenosis of the basal moyamoya collaterals; and (f) complete occlusion of the ICA, disappearance of the basal moyamoya collaterals, with cortical blood supply solely provided through ECA collaterals.

Workup of a patient with moyamoya disease typically begins with a head CT. CT in a patient with moyamoya disease may show small areas of hypodensity suggestive of hemorrhage or of a stroke in the cortical watershed zones, basal ganglia, deep white matter, or periventricular regions (Scott et al., 2004). However, the CT scan can be normal, particularly in patients presenting solely with TIAs.

MRI has become a reliable diagnostic modality in moyamoya disease. Acute cerebral infarctions are easily recognized on diffusion-weighted imaging, with chronic infarcts delineated by both T1- and T2-weighted imaging (Chabbert et al., 1998). T2-weighted MRI is also useful to identify occlusive lesions around the circle of Willis and dilated moyamoya vessels as well as asymptomatic microbleeds (Harada et al., 2001; Ishikawa et al., 2005; Kikuta et al., 2005; Yamada, Suzuki, & Matsushima, 1995a). T1-weighted MRI can be used to identify dilated moyamoya vessels in the basal ganglia and thalamus (Kuroda & Houkin, 2008). Fluid-attenuated inversion recovery MRI, which demonstrates linear high-signal intensity following a sulcal pattern (ivy sign), has been used to infer cortical ischemia and is felt to represent slow flow in the poorly perfused cortical circulation in children with moyamoya (Fujiwara, Momoshima, & Kuribayashi, 2005; Scott & Smith, 2009). Leptomeningeal enhancement or ivy sign as previously described is a characteristic sign for moyamoya. MRA has been used to accurately characterize both the stenosis and basal collateral formation associated with moyamoya disease (Yamada, Suzuki, & Matsushima, 1995b). The MRA findings most suggestive of moyamoya disease remain diminished-flow voids in the ICA, ACA, and MCA bilaterally, with concurrent large-flow voids in the basal ganglia and thalamus representing collateral moyamoya vessel formation (Yamada, Matsushima, & Suzuki, 1992; Yamada et al., 1995b). Recently, MRI/MRA has been suggested as a reliable alternative to conventional angiography for diagnosis of moyamoya, based on the ease and fewer procedure-associated risks (Ibrahimi, Tamargo, & Ahn, 2010).

Blood oxygen level–dependent MRI can be used to map cerebrovascular reactivity in cases with arterial steno-occlusive disease. Blood oxygen level–dependent MRI is based on the decrease in T2 signal changes that occurs with an increased concentration of intravoxel deoxyhemoglobin, which is related to either reduced perfusion or increased metabolic activity (Shimizu, Shirane, Fujiwara, Takahashi, & Yoshimoto, 1997). Arterial spin labeling is an alternative noncontrast perfusion technique utilizing an inversion pulse to magnetically label intravascular water protons upstream to the region of interest and has been extensively studied due to its noninvasive nature (Kodama, Aoki, Hiraga, Wada, & Suzuki, 1979). In accordance with the guidelines of the Research Committee on Spontaneous Occlusion of the Circle of Willis (Moyamoya Disease), cerebral angiography is not mandatory if MRI and MRA show all of the following findings: stenosis or occlusion at the end of the ICA or at the proximal part of the ACAs and MCAs on MRA, and an abnormal vascular network seen in the basal ganglia with MRA; an abnormal vascular network that is evident from ipsilateral flow voids seen in the basal ganglia with MRI; and bilateral presentation of the above two findings (Fukui, 1997b). However, the quality of MRA largely depends on the strength of the static magnetic field. The new criteria of the Research Committee for Diagnosis of Moyamoya Disease recommend MRA with a 1.5 T machine; MRA scans with 0.5 T or 1.0 T machines are not recommended (Kuroda & Houkin, 2008). Data from several studies have shown specific patterns of cerebral hemodynamics and metabolism in patients with moyamoya disease such as lower CBF after ischemic stroke, and the distribution of CBF typically shows posterior dominance (Kuroda et al., 1993; Ogawa, Yoshimoto, Suzuki, & Sakurai, 1990). The cerebrovascular reactivity to acetazolamide or carbon dioxide is widely impaired in the territory of the ICA, which suggests reduced CPP (Kuroda & Houkin, 2008; Kuroda, Houkin, Kamiyama, Abe, & Mitsumori, 1995; Kuwabara et al. 1997; Matheja et al., 2002; Ogawa, Yoshimoto, et al., 1990; Ogawa, Nakamura, Yoshimoto, & Suzuki, 1990). SPECT is a long-established, whole-brain radioisotope axial perfusion study that provides relative perfusion compared with the opposite side. Use of SPECT in patients with moyamoya disease shows low perfusion in the upper and lower frontal, parietal, and temporal regions, especially in cases at Stages 2 and 3. SPECT helps to measure CBF, especially in vessels that cannot be visualized angiographically (Burke et al., 2009; Shimizu et al., 1997).

EEG is a diagnostic tool used in the evaluation of moyamoya, as specific alterations are found in children affected with this condition. Characteristic findings include posterior and/or centrotemporal slowing, and a re-build-up phenomenon after the end of hyperventilation (Kodama et al., 1979). In all children, hyperventilation induces a diffuse pattern of high voltage, monophasic slow waves, referred to as build up, which terminate after hyperventilation has ceased. In 50% of children with moyamoya, there is a return of the high-voltage, monophasic slow waves following the end of hyperventilation, termed re-build-up, which is thought to represent a diminished cerebral perfusion reserve. Essentially, hyperventilation induces cerebral vasoconstriction and, on its cessation, cerebrovascular dilation (build-up). In children with moyamoya, re-build-up occurs as a steal phenomenon as blood is diverted from the dilated cortical vessels to the moyamoya-associated collaterals, creating a cortical ischemic state, represented as the reappearance of the high-voltage, monophasic slow waves on the EEG. Over time, re-build-up resolves and the EEG returns to baseline (Ibrahimi et al., 2010; Kodama et al., 1979; Scott & Smith, 2009; Smith, 2009).

Screening

There are no data to support indiscriminate screening for moyamoya, and there is little evidence to warrant the screening of first-degree relatives of patients with moyamoya when only a single family member is affected. However, data concerning patients with unilateral moyamoya showed a decreased stroke burden and better clinical outcome when this specific population underwent imaging at specific intervals, providing evidence in support of selective screening (Scott & Smith, 2009; Smith & Scott, 2008). There are Class III data that support the premise of prospective noninvasive screening for moyamoya syndrome in patients with neurofibromatosis 1, Down syndrome, and sickle cell disease because of the association with moyamoya (Jea et al., 2005; Kirkham & DeBaun, 2004; Roach, 2000; Rosser, Vezina, & Packer, 2005).

There is compelling Class I data to support the use of transcranial Doppler ultrasonography (TCD) as an initial screening study for stroke in the sickle cell population. In a recent randomized trial (Adams et al., 2004), the stroke prevention trial in sickle cell anemia (STOP) evaluated more than 2,000 children with sickle cell disease and validated the use of TCD as a screening study for stroke in this patient group. Use of the information resulted in a more than 90% decreased risk of strokes through the use of transfusions (Gebreyohanns & Adams, 2004). The American Heart Association recognizes the need for more frequent monitoring of young children (aged 2–10 years) and those with relatively high velocities on transcranial Doppler imaging. Recommendations include annual surveillance of patients with normal transcranial Doppler imaging (time-averaged mean velocity less than 170 cm/sec) and monthly follow-up for children with abnormal transcranial Doppler imaging results (greater than 200 cm/sec). For children with results between these two velocities, transcranial Doppler imaging should be repeated at 3 months (transcranial Doppler imaging: 185–199 cm/sec) and 6 months (transcranial Doppler imaging: 170–184 cm/sec; Adams et al., 2004; Roach et al., 2008). There is less compelling evidence to suggest some usefulness in screening first-degree relatives of patients with moyamoya (Smith & Scott, 2010).

Treatment for Moyamoya

Medical Therapies

Currently, there is no definitive medical treatment to reverse or stabilize the course of moyamoya disease (Ibrahimi et al., 2010). Medical therapy has been used in patients with moyamoya, particularly when surgery has been considered to present a high risk or the patient has had relatively mild disease, but there are few data showing either its short-term or long-term efficacy. A recent review revealed that 38% of 651 patients with moyamoya who were initially treated medically ultimately underwent surgery because of progressive symptoms (Ikezaki, 2000). There are two classes of medications that play an adjuvant role in the treatment of moyamoya; antiplatelet agents and calcium-channel blockers (Ohaegbulam, Magge, & Scott, 2001; Scott, 2000, 2001). A proportion of the ischemic symptoms associated with moyamoya disease has been attributed to microthrombus formation due to emboli arising from sites of arterial stenosis. Daily, lifelong aspirin use is prescribed to prevent the ischemia associated with this embolic phenomenon. The second class of medications used in moyamoya disease is calcium-channel blockers, and evidence exists to support their use in the treatment of persistent postoperative TIAs and intractable headaches. The mechanism of action remains unknown, but calcium-channel blockers are shown to reduce the frequency and severity of refractory TIAs as well as to ameliorate intractable headaches (Scott & Smith, 2009; Smith, 2009; Smith & Scott, 2008). Although currently there is no evidence that medical management alters the clinical course or outcome of individuals with moyamoya disease, future treatment will likely include the use of medical therapy.

Surgical Interventions

Surgical interventions have been devised with goals of promoting neoangiogenesis, inducing collateral vessel formation and restoring perfusion to oxygen-deprived areas of the brain. Furthermore, relieving the hemodynamic stress on the moyamoya vessel at the base of the brain may reduce the risk of future hemorrhage from these abnormal vessels. The arteriopathy of moyamoya affects the internal carotid artery while sparing the ECA. Surgical treatment of patients with moyamoya typically uses the ECA as a source of new blood to the ischemic hemispheres.

Two general methods of revascularization are used: direct and indirect. In direct revascularization, a branch of the ECA (usually the superficial temporal artery) is directly anastomosed to a cortical artery. Indirect techniques involve the placement of vascularized tissue supplied by the ECA (e.g., dura, temporalis muscle, or the superficial temporal artery itself) in direct contact with the brain, leading to an ingrowth of new blood vessels to the underlying cerebral cortex (Scott & Smith, 2009). In direct revascularization, a branch of the ECA (usually the STA) is directly anastomosed to a cortical artery. The direct bypass techniques that have been proposed include STA to the MCA, occipital artery to the MCA, and the middle meningeal artery to the MCA anastomoses. Direct vascularization has been shown to drastically improve CBF and thus prevent brain infarctions. Although the direct revascularization procedure has a distinct advantage over indirect revascularization procedures by providing immediate high-flow revascularization to ischemic brain regions, there are limitations to its widespread use in children (Smith, 2009). First, the small diameters of the STA and MCA in children make it technically very challenging to accomplish a successful anastomosis that supplies meaningful blood flow to the operated hemisphere. Second, the risk of intraoperative stroke is increased, which is related to the temporary MCA occlusion required for anastomosis and also to the potential damage that can occur to existing transdural anastomoses between the distal STA and cortical arteries. Third, unless the proximal MCA circulation is relatively intact, the amount of blood flow to the entire MCA territory that can be achieved by STA–MCA bypass is severely limited.

Indirect procedures were developed as an alternative to bypass due to the difficulties encountered in the pediatric population with direct STA–MCA anastomosis.

Indirect procedures tend to be less invasive; are technically easier, resulting in a shorter operative time; do not restrict treatment to solely the MCA distribution; and most importantly, do not involve clamping of recipient vessels (Smith, 2009). However, collateral formation and angiogenesis take longer to develop after indirect revascularization. Various techniques of indirect revascularization have been described in the literature (Patel, Mangano, & Klimo, 2010). Some commonly practiced procedures are described below.

The Encephalo-Duro-Arterio-Syangiosis Procedure. The indirect (nonanastomotic) revascularization technique that is most commonly used to treat moyamoya disease in children is the encephalo-duro-arterio-syangiosis (EDAS) procedure (Matsushima et al., 1981, 1998). In this technique, the intact STA (usually parietal STA branch or other scalp donor artery such as the OA or the anterior STA branch) is sutured by its adventitia into a linear opening in the dura subjacent to a small elliptical craniotomy. Recent studies have criticized the EDAS technique because of insufficient collateral flow on postoperative angiograms and persistence of ischemic symptoms (Smith, 2009).

Pial Syangiosis. Another widely used indirect revascularization procedure is pial synangiosis. This technique, which represents a modification of the EDAS procedure, can be used to treat moyamoya disease in children and adults. Pial synangiosis allows for greater induction of extradural collateral vessels by placing the donor scalp artery in direct contact with the pial vasculature stripped of its meningeal coverings (Smith, 2009). A retrospective case study showed that patients treated with pial synangiosis stop having strokes and TIAs and have an excellent long-term prognosis (Scott et al., 2004).

Omental Transplantation. Another indirect revascularization technique occasionally used in the treatment of moyamoya disease is intracranial transplantation of the omentum. This involves tunneling an intact omental flap from the abdomen and placing it on the surface of the brain or anastomosing a free flap of omentum via the gastroepiploic artery and vein end to end with the superficial temporal artery and vein, respectively. Omental transplantation is typically reserved for treatment of moyamoya disease after a direct or other indirect revascularization procedure has failed to alleviate ischemic symptoms or for revascularization of the frontal pole or medial cortical surface. Omental transplants also provide good collateralization and resolution of ischemic symptoms (Scott et al., 2004).

Multiple Burr Holes. The multiple cranial burr hole technique is an additional indirect technique that can be used to treat moyamoya disease. Until recently, this technique has been used in combination with other techniques, such as the STA–MCA bypass, EMS, EDAS, or pial synangiosis, to provide supplemental collateralization, especially to the frontal and occipital lobes, which typically are not well vascularized by these other techniques.

Encephalomyosynangiosis. Encephalomyosynangiosis (EMS) was first used in the treatment of moyamoya disease in the late 1970s, and involves a frontotemporal craniotomy, dural opening, followed by the removal of the arachnoid over the region to be treated. The temporalis muscle is placed over the exposed pia and the dura approximated over the muscle. Angiogenesis occurs over several weeks to months due to the rich blood supply of the temporalis muscle by the deep temporal artery. Even though EMS is a less-invasive procedure, there are distinct disadvantages, including the necessity of a larger craniotomy and dural opening, cosmetic deformation, and, more importantly, postoperative complications such as seizure, brain edema, and symptomatic mass effect associated with the large space-occupying muscle (Ibrahimi et al., 2010).

Surgical Outcomes

Long-term follow-up studies have shown a good safety profile for patients' postsurgical treatment. The risk of stroke is highest in the first month postsurgery; however, it decreases considerably over time; in fact, 96% of the patients remain stroke free over the next 5 years (Scott et al., 2004; Yamada et al., 1995b). A 2005 meta-analysis demonstrated that 87% of the patients benefited from surgical revascularization, and all revascularization techniques demonstrated equal effectiveness (Fung, Thompson, & Ganesan, 2005). Reduction in hemorrhagic events postsurgery has not been as well studied in comparison to ischemic events. It has been hypothesized that the bypass procedure may reduce the stress on the perforating vessel and in turn reduce the risk of hemorrhage (Burke et al., 2009). Neuroimaging studies have demonstrated an increase in the caliber of the deep temporal and middle meningeal arteries with reciprocal regression of moyamoya vessel postsurgery (Houkin, Nakayama, Kuroda, Ishikawa, & Nonaka, 2004). Similarly, postsurgical reduction in the "ivy sign," a characteristic radiological sign of moyamoya, has been demonstrated and indicated to improve cerebral hemodynamic status postsurgery (Komiyama et al., 2001).

SUMMARY

Stroke and CVD, whether affecting large or small vessels, can correspond to an array of functional impairment. There is truly no pure profile, and the features can demonstrate significant overlap with other neurological presentations. Within this grouping, controversy abounds whether it be related to the consideration of BD as a distinct neurological entity, or a more specific debate regarding the link between white matter lesions and cognitive functioning. The best advice for practicing neuropsychologists is to not lose sight of the power of assessment in identifying the strengths and weaknesses of patients in order to either aid in diagnosis or treatment planning. VaDs are heterogeneous in nature; thus, a one-size-fits-all approach will likely fall woefully short of the necessary mark.

REFERENCES

Achrol, A. S., Guzman, R., Varga, M., Adler, J. R., Steinberg, G. K., & Chang, S. D. (2009). Pathogenesis and radiobiology of brain arteriovenous malformations: Implications for risk stratification in natural history and posttreatment course. *Neurosurgical Focus, 26*(5), E9.

Adams, R. J., Brambilla, D. J., Granger, S., Gallagher, D., Vichinsky, E., Abboud, M. R., . . . Roach, E. S.; STOP Study. (2004). Stroke and conversion to high risk in children screened with transcranial Doppler ultrasound during the STOP study. *Blood, 103*(10), 3689–3694.

Akhvlediani, T., Henning, A., Sándor, P. S., Boesiger, P., & Jung, H. H. (2010). Adaptive metabolic changes in CADASIL white matter. *Journal of Neurology, 257*(2), 171–177.

Akiguchi, I., Tomimoto, H., Suenaga, T., Wakita, H., & Budka, H. (1997). Alterations in glia and axons in the brains of Binswanger's disease patients. *Stroke, 28*(7), 1423–1429.

Akiguchi, I., Tomimoto, H., Suenaga, T., Wakita, H., & Budka, H. (1998). Blood-brain barrier dysfunction in Binswanger's disease; an immunohistochemical study. *Acta Neuropathologica, 95*(1), 78–84.

Akiguchi, I., Tomimoto, H., Wakita, H., Yamamoto, Y., Suenaga, T., Ueno, M., & Budka, H. (1999). Cytopathological alterations and therapeutic approaches in Binswanger's disease. *Neuropathology, 19*(1), 119–128.

Alzheimer, A. (1902). Mental disturbances of arteriosclerotic origin (Forstl, H., Howard, R., Levy, R., tr.), *Neuropsychiatry, Neuropsychology, and Behavioral Neurology, 5*, 1–6.

American Psychiatric Association (APA). (1987). *Diagnostic and statistical manual of mental disorders* (3rd ed.). Washington, DC: Author.

American Psychiatric Association (APA). (1994). *Diagnostic and statistical manual of mental disorders* (4th ed.). Washington, DC: Author.

American Psychiatric Association (APA). (2000). *Diagnostic and statistical manual of mental disorders* (4th ed., text rev.). Washington, DC: Author.

Andreadou, E., Papadimas, G., & Sfagos, C. (2008). A novel heterozygous mutation in the Notch3 gene causing CADASIL. *Swiss Medical Weekly, 138*(41–42), 614–617.

Aoki, S., Hayashi, N., Abe, O., Shirouzu, I., Ishigame, K., Okubo, T.,…Araki, T. (2002). Radiation-induced arteritis: Thickened wall with prominent enhancement on cranial MR images report of five cases and comparison with 18 cases of Moyamoya disease. *Radiology, 223*(3), 683–688.

Auer, D. P., Schirmer, T., Heidenreich, J. O., Herzog, J., Pütz, B., & Dichgans, M. (2001). Altered white and gray matter metabolism in CADASIL: A proton MR spectroscopy and 1H-MRSI study. *Neurology, 56*(5), 635–642.

Baba, T., Houkin, K., & Kuroda, S. (2008). Novel epidemiological features of moyamoya disease. *Journal of Neurology, Neurosurgery, and Psychiatry, 79*(8), 900–904.

Babikian, V., & Ropper, A. H. (1987). Binswanger's disease: A review. *Stroke, 18*(1), 2–12.

Barker, A., Musso, M., & Gouvier, W. D. (2011). Multi-infarct dementia. In C. A. Noggle, R. S. Dean, & A. M. Horton Jr. (Eds.), *The encyclopedia of neuropsychological disorders* (pp. 485–487). New York, NY: Springer Publishing Company.

Barkovich, A. (2000). Infection of the nervous system. In A. Barkovich (ed.), *Pedaitric neuroimaging* (3rd ed., p. 735). Philadelphia, PA: Lippincott Williams and Wilkins.

Bennett, D. A., Gilley, D. W., Lee, S., & Cochran, E. J. (1994). White matter changes: Neurobehavioral manifestations of Binswanger's disease and clinical correlates in Alzheimer's disease. *Dementia, 5*(3–4), 148–152.

Bennett, D. A., Wilson, R. S., Gilley, D. W., & Fox, J. H. (1990). Clinical diagnosis of Binswanger's disease. *Journal of Neurology, Neurosurgery, and Psychiatry, 53*(11), 961–965.

Binswanger, O. (1894). Die Abgrenzung der allgemeinen progressive Paralyse. *Berl Klin Wochenschr, 31*, 1103–1105, 1137–1139, 1180–1186.

Blass, J. P., Hoyer, S., & Nitsch, R. (1991). A translation of Otto Binswanger's article, "The delineation of the generalized progressive paralyses" 1894. *Archives of Neurology, 48*(9), 961–972.

Bogousslavsky, J. (1992). Binswanger's disease. In H. J. M. Barnett, J. P. Mohr, & B. M. Stein (Eds.), *Stroke: Pathophysiology, diagnosis, and management* (2nd ed., pp. 805–819). New York: Churchill Livingstone.

Boiten, J., Lodder, J., & Kessels, F. (1993). Two clinically distinct lacunar infarct entities? A hypothesis. *Stroke, 24*(5), 652–656.

Bonduel, M., Hepner, M., Sciuccati, G., Torres, A. F., & Tenembaum, S. (2001). Prothrombotic disorders in children with moyamoya syndrome. *Stroke, 32*(8), 1786–1792.

Bornstein, R. A. (1983). Verbal IQ-performance IQ discrepancies on the Wechsler Adult Intelligence Scale-Revised in patients with unilateral or bilateral cerebral dysfunction. *Journal of Consulting and Clinical Psychology, 51*(5), 779–780.

Bornstein, R. A., McLean, D. R., & Ho, K. (1985). Neuropsychological and electrophysiological examination of a patient with Wilson's disease. *The International Journal of Neuroscience, 26*(3–4), 239–247.

Bowen, M., Marks, M. P., & Steinberg, G. K. (1998). Neuropsychological recovery from childhood moyamoya disease. *Brain & Development, 20*(2), 119–123.

Buffon, F., Porcher, R., Hernandez, K., Kurtz, A., Pointeau, S., Vahedi, K., . . . Chabriat, H. (2006). Cognitive profile in CADASIL. *Journal of Neurology, Neurosurgery, and Psychiatry, 77*(2), 175–180.

Burke, G. M., Burke, A. M., Sherma, A. K., Hurley, M. C., Batjer, H. H., & Bendok, B. R. (2009). Moyamoya disease: A summary. *Neurosurgical Focus, 26*(4), E11.

Burton, E., Ballard, C., Stephens, S., Kenny, R. A., Kalaria, R., Barber, R., & O'Brien, J. (2003). Hyperintensities and fronto-subcortical atrophy on MRI are substrates of mild cognitive deficits after stroke. *Dementia and Geriatric Cognitive Disorders, 16*(2), 113–118.

Caldarelli, M., Di Rocco, C., & Gaglini, P. (2001). Surgical treatment of moyamoya disease in pediatric age. *Journal of Neurosurgical Sciences, 45*(2), 83–91.

Calviere, L., Catalaa, I., Marlats, F., Viguier, A., Bonneville, F., Cognard, C., & Larrue, V. (2010). Correlation between cognitive impairment and cerebral hemodynamic disturbances on perfusion magnetic resonance imaging in European adults with moyamoya disease. Clinical article. *Journal of Neurosurgery, 113*(4), 753–759.

Caplan, L. R. (1995). Binswanger's disease—revisited. *Neurology, 45*(4), 626–633.

Chabbert, V., Ranjeva, J. P., Sevely, A., Boetto, S., Berry, I., & Manelfe, C. (1998). Diffusion- and magnetisation transfer-weighted MRI in childhood moya-moya. *Neuroradiology, 40*(4), 267–271.

Chabriat, H., Bousser, M. G., & Pappata, S. (1995). Cerebral autosomal dominant arteriopathy with subcortical infarcts and leukoencephalopathy: A positron emission tomography study in two affected family members. *Stroke, 26*(9), 1729–1730.

Chabriat, H., Joutel, A., Dichgans, M., Tournier-Lasserve, E., & Bousser, M. G. (2009). Cadasil. *Lancet Neurology, 8*(7), 643–653.

Chabriat, H., Mrissa, R., Levy, C., Vahedi, K., Taillia, H., Iba-Zizen, M. T., . . . Bousser, M. G. (1999). Brain stem MRI signal abnormalities in CADASIL. *Stroke, 30*(2), 457–459.

Chabriat, H., Vahedi, K., Iba-Zizen, M. T., Joutel, A., Nibbio, A., Nagy, T. G., . . . Ducrocq, X. (1995). Clinical spectrum of CADASIL: A study of 7 families. Cerebral autosomal dominant arteriopathy with subcortical infarcts and leukoencephalopathy. *Lancet, 346*(8980), 934–939.

Charlton, R. A., Morris, R. G., Nitkunan, A., & Markus, H. S. (2006). The cognitive profiles of CADASIL and sporadic small vessel disease. *Neurology, 66*(10), 1523–1526.

Chui, H. C. (2007). Subcortical ischemic vascular dementia. *Neurologic Clinics, 25*(3), 717–740, vi.

Colleran, K. M., Ratliff, D. M., & Burge, M. R. (2003). Potential association of thyrotoxicosis with vitamin B and folate deficiencies, resulting in risk for hyperhomocysteinemia and subsequent thromboembolic events. *Endocrine Practice, 9*(4), 290–295.

Collod, G., Babron, M. C., Jondeau, G., Coulon, M., Weissenbach, J., Dubourg, O., . . . Boileau, C. (1994). A second locus for Marfan syndrome maps to chromosome 3p24.2-p25. *Nature Genetics, 8*(3), 264–268.

Coulthard, A., Blank, S. C., Bushby, K., Kalaria, R. N., & Burn, D. J. (2000). Distribution of cranial MRI abnormalities in patients with symptomatic and subclinical CADASIL. *The British Journal of Radiology, 73*(867), 256–265.

Cummings, J. L. (1994). Vascular subcortical dementias: Clinical aspects. *Dementia, 5*(3–4), 177–180.

Currie, S., Raghavan, A., Batty, R., Connolly, D. J., & Griffiths, P. D. (2011). Childhood moyamoya disease and moyamoya syndrome: A pictorial review. *Pediatric Neurology, 44*(6), 401–413.

Czarkowski, M., Hilgertner, L., Powalowski, T., & Radomski, D. (2002). The stiffness of the common carotid artery in patients with Graves' disease. *International Angiology: A Journal of the International Union of Angiology, 21*(2), 152–157.

Darby, D. G., Donnan, G. A., Saling, M. A., Walsh, K. W., & Bladin, P. F. (1988). Primary intraventricular hemorrhage: Clinical and neuropsychological findings in a prospective stroke series. *Neurology, 38*(1), 68–75.

Davous, P., & Bequet, D. (1995). [CADASIL—a new model for subcortical dementia]. *Revue Neurologique, 151*(11), 634–639.

de Groot, J. C., de Leeuw, F. E., Oudkerk, M., Van Gijn, J., Hofman, A., Jolles, J., & Breteler, M. M. (2002). Periventricular cerebral white matter lesions predict rate of cognitive decline. *Annals of Neurology, 52*(3), 335–341.

de Groot, J. C., de Leeuw, F. E., Oudkerk, M., van Gijn, J., Hofman, A., Jolles, J., & Breteler, M. M. (2000). Cerebral white matter lesions and cognitive function: The Rotterdam Scan Study. *Annals of Neurology, 47*(2), 145–151.

De Reuck, J., Decoo, D., Marchau, M., Santens, P., Lemahieu, I., & Strijckmans, K. (1998). Positron emission tomography in vascular dementia. *Journal of the Neurological Sciences, 154*(1), 55–61.

Delano-Wood, L., Abeles, N., Sacco, J. M., Wierenga, C. E., Horne, N. R., & Bozoki, A. (2008). Regional white matter pathology in mild cognitive impairment: Differential influence of lesion type on neuropsychological functioning. *Stroke, 39*(3), 794–799.

Desai, S. S., Paulino, A. C., Mai, W. Y., & Teh, B. S. (2006). Radiation-induced moyamoya syndrome. *International Journal of Radiation Oncology, Biology, Physics, 65*(4), 1222–1227.

Desmond, D. W. (1996). Vascular dementia: A construct in evolution. *Cerebrovascular and Brain Metabolism Reviews, 8*(4), 296–325.

Desmond, D. W., Moroney, J. T., Lynch, T., Chan, S., Chin, S. S., & Mohr, J. P. (1999). The natural history of CADASIL: A pooled analysis of previously published cases. *Stroke, 30*(6), 1230–1233.

Dichgans, M. (2002). Cerebral autosomal dominant arteriopathy with subcortical infarcts and leukoencephalopathy: Phenotypic and mutational spectrum. *Journal of the Neurological Sciences, 203–204*, 77–80.

Dichgans, M. (2007). Genetics of ischaemic stroke. *Lancet Neurology, 6*(2), 149–161.

Dichgans, M., Filippi, M., Bruning, R., Iannucci, G., Berchtenbreiter, C., Minicucci, L., . . . Yousry, T. A. (1999). Quantitative MRI in CADASIL: Correlation with disability and cognitive performance. *Neurology, 52*, 1361–1367.

Dichgans, M., Markus, H. S., Salloway, S., Verkkoniemi, A., Moline, M., Wang, Q., . . . Chabriat, H. S. (2008). Donepezil in patients with subcortical vascular cognitive impairment: A randomised double-blind trial in CADASIL. *Lancet Neurology, 7*(4), 310–318.

Dichgans, M., Mayer, M., Uttner, I., Brüning, R., Müller-Höcker, J., Rungger, G., . . . Gasser, T. (1998). The phenotypic spectrum of CADASIL: Clinical findings in 102 cases. *Annals of Neurology, 44*(5), 731–739.

Dietrichs, E., Dahl, A., Nyberg-Hansen, R., Russell, D., Rootwelt, K., & Veger, T. (1992). Cerebral blood flow findings in moyamoya disease in adults. *Acta Neurologica Scandinavica, 85*(5), 318–322.

Dong, Y., Hassan, A., Zhang, Z., Huber, D., Dalageorgou, C., & Markus, H. S. (2003). Yield of screening for CADASIL mutations in lacunar stroke and leukoaraiosis. *Stroke, 34*(1), 203–205.

Erkinjuntti, T. (2007). Vascular cognitive deterioration and stroke. *Cerebrovascular Diseases, 24*(Suppl 1), 189–194.

Erkinjuntti, T., Kurz, A., Gauthier, S., Bullock, R., Lilienfeld, S., & Damaraju, C. V. (2002). Efficacy of galantamine in probable vascular dementia and Alzheimer's disease combined with cerebrovascular disease: A randomised trial. *Lancet, 359*(9314), 1283–1290.

Erkinjuntti, T., Ostbye, T., Steenhuis, R., & Hachinski, V. (1997). The effect of different diagnostic criteria on the prevalence of dementia. *The New England Journal of Medicine, 337*(23), 1667–1674.

Federico, A., Bianchi, S., & Dotti, M. T. (2005). The spectrum of mutations for CADASIL diagnosis. *Neurological Sciences, 26*(2), 117–124.

Fein, G., Di Sclafani, V., Tanabe, J., Cardenas, V., Weiner, M. W., Jagust, W. J.,...Chui, H. (2000). Hippocampal and cortical atrophy predict dementia in subcortical ischemic vascular disease. *Neurology, 55*(11), 1626–1635.

Festa, J. R., Schwarz, L. R., Pliskin, N., Cullum, C. M., Lacritz, L., Charbel, F. T.,...Lazar, R. M. (2010). Neurocognitive dysfunction in adult moyamoya disease. *Journal of Neurology, 257*(5), 806–815.

Filley, C. M. (2001). *The behavioral neurology of white matter.* New York, NY: Oxford University Press.

Filley, C. M., Thompson, L. L., Sze, C. I., Simon, J. A., Paskavitz, J. F., & Kleinschmidt-DeMasters, B. K. (1999). White matter dementia in CADASIL. *Journal of the Neurological Sciences, 163*(2), 163–167.

Finsterer, J. (2009). Central nervous system imaging in mitochondrial disorders. *The Canadian Journal of Neurological Sciences, 36*(2), 143–153.

Finsterer, J., Jarius, C., & Eichberger, H. (2001). Phenotype variability in 130 adult patients with respiratory chain disorders. *Journal of Inherited Metabolic Disease, 24*(5), 560–576.

Fisher, C. M. (1982). Hydrocephalus as a cause of disturbances of gait in the elderly. *Neurology, 32*(12), 1358–1363.

Friedman, J. M., Arbiser, J., Epstein, J. A., Gutmann, D. H., Huot, S. J., Lin, A. E.,...Korf, B. R. (2002). Cardiovascular disease in neurofibromatosis 1: Report of the NF1 Cardiovascular Task Force. *Genetics in Medicine, 4*(3), 105–111.

Fujiwara, H., Momoshima, S., & Kuribayashi, S. (2005). Leptomeningeal high signal intensity (ivy sign) on fluid-attenuated inversion-recovery (FLAIR) MR images in moyamoya disease. *European Journal of Radiology, 55*(2), 224–230.

Fukui, M., Kono, S., Sueishi, K., & Ikezaki, K. (2000). Moyamoya disease. *Neuropathology, 20*(Suppl), S61–S64.

Fukui, M. (1997a). Guidelines for the diagnosis and treatment of spontaneous occlusion of the circle of Willis ("moyamoya" disease). Research Committee on Spontaneous Occlusion of the Circle of Willis (Moyamoya Disease) of the Ministry of Health and Welfare, Japan. *Clinical Neurology and Neurosurgery, 99*(Suppl 2), S238–S240.

Fukui, M. (1997b). Current state of study on moyamoya disease in Japan. *Surgical Neurology, 47*(2), 138–143.

Fung, L. W., Thompson, D., & Ganesan, V. (2005). Revascularisation surgery for paediatric moyamoya: A review of the literature. *Child's Nervous System, 21*(5), 358–364.

Furuta, A., Ishii, N., Nishihara, Y., & Horie, A. (1991). Medullary arteries in aging and dementia. *Stroke, 22*(4), 442–446.

Garcia, J. H., & Brown, G. G. (1992). Vascular dementia: Neuropathologic alterations and metabolic brain changes. *Journal of the Neurological Sciences, 109*(2), 121–131.

Gebreyohanns, M., & Adams, R. J. (2004). Sickle cell disease: Primary stroke prevention. *CNS Spectrums, 9*(6), 445–449.

Geldmacher, D. S., & Whitehouse, P. J. (1996). Evaluation of dementia. *New England Journal of Medicine, 335,* 330–336.

Godin, O., Tzourio, C., Maillard, P., Alpérovitch, A., Mazoyer, B., & Dufouil, C. (2009). Apolipoprotein E genotype is related to progression of white matter lesion load. *Stroke, 40*(10), 3186–3190.

Gold, G., Kövari, E., Herrmann, F. R., Canuto, A., Hof, P. R., Michel, J. P.,...Giannakopoulos, P. (2005). Cognitive consequences of thalamic, basal ganglia, and deep white matter lacunes in brain aging and dementia. *Stroke, 36*(6), 1184–1188.

Goto, K., Ishii, N., & Fukasawa, H. (1981). Diffuse white-matter disease in the geriatric population. A clinical, neuropathological, and CT study. *Radiology, 141*(3), 687–695.

Götz, J., Ittner, L. M., & Lim, Y. A. (2009). Common features between diabetes mellitus and Alzheimer's disease. *Cellular and Molecular Life Sciences: CMLS, 66*(8), 1321–1325.

Grau-Olivares, M., Arboix, A., Bartrés-Faz, D., & Junqué, C. (2007). Neuropsychological abnormalities associated with lacunar infarction. *Journal of the Neurological Sciences, 257*(1–2), 160–165.

Guidetti, D., Casali, B., Mazzei, R. L., & Dotti, M. T. (2006). Cerebral autosomal dominant arteriopathy with subcortical infarcts and leukoencephalopathy. *Clinical and Experimental Hypertension, 28*(3–4), 271–277.

Guo, D. C., Papke, C. L., Tran-Fadulu, V., Regalado, E. S., Avidan, N., Johnson, R. J.,...Milewicz, D. M. (2009). Mutations in smooth muscle alpha-actin (ACTA2) cause coronary artery disease, stroke, and Moyamoya disease, along with thoracic aortic disease. *American Journal of Human Genetics, 84*(5), 617–627.

Haaland, K. Y. & Swanda, R. M. (2008). Vascular dementia. In J. E. Morgan & J. H. Ricker, *Textbook of clinical neuropsychology*. New York, NY: Taylor & Francis.

Hachinski, V. (2002). Stroke: The next 30 years. *Stroke, 33*(1), 1–4.

Hachinski, V. C., Lassen, N. A., & Marshall, J. (1974). Multi-infarct dementia. A cause of mental deterioration in the elderly. *Lancet, 2*(7874), 207–210.

Han, D. H., Kwon, O. K., Byun, B. J., Choi, B. Y., Choi, C. W., Choi, J. U.,...Yim, M. B.; Korean Society for Cerebrovascular Disease. (2000). A co-operative study: Clinical characteristics of 334 Korean patients with moyamoya disease treated at neurosurgical institutes (1976–1994). The Korean Society for Cerebrovascular Disease. *Acta Neurochirurgica, 142*(11), 1263–1273; discussion 1273.

Han, D. H., Nam, D. H., & Oh, C. W. (1997). Moyamoya disease in adults: Characteristics of clinical presentation and outcome after encephalo-duro-arterio-synangiosis. *Clinical Neurology and Neurosurgery, 99*(Suppl 2), S151–S155.

Harada, A., Fujii, Y., Yoneoka, Y., Takeuchi, S., Tanaka, R., & Nakada, T. (2001). High-field magnetic resonance imaging in patients with moyamoya disease. *Journal of Neurosurgery, 94*(2), 233–237.

Hedera, P., & Friedland, R. P. (1997). Cerebral autosomal dominant arteriopathy with subcortical infarcts and leukoencephalopathy: Study of two American families with predominant dementia. *Journal of the Neurological Sciences, 146*(1), 27–33.

Heyer, G. L., Millar, W. S., Ghatan, S., & Garzon, M. C. (2006). The neurologic aspects of PHACE: Case report and review of the literature. *Pediatric Neurology, 35*(6), 419–424.

Hoare, A. M., & Keogh, A. J. (1974). Cerebrovascular moyamoya disease. *British Medical Journal, 1*(5905), 430–432.

Hojo, M., Hoshimaru, M., Miyamoto, S., Taki, W., Nagata, I., Asahi, M.,...Hashimoto, N. (1998). Role of transforming growth factor-beta1 in the pathogenesis of moyamoya disease. *Journal of Neurosurgery, 89*(4), 623–629.

Holmes, C., Cairns, N., Lantos, P., & Mann, A. (1999). Validity of current clinical criteria for Alzheimer's disease, vascular dementia and dementia with Lewy bodies. *The British Journal of Psychiatry, 174*, 45–50.

Hoshimaru, M., Takahashi, J. A., Kikuchi, H., Nagata, I., & Hatanaka, M. (1991). Possible roles of basic fibroblast growth factor in the pathogenesis of moyamoya disease: An immunohistochemical study. *Journal of Neurosurgery, 75*(2), 267–270.

Houkin, K., Nakayama, N., Kuroda, S., Ishikawa, T., & Nonaka, T. (2004). How does angiogenesis develop in pediatric moyamoya disease after surgery? A prospective study with MR angiography. *Child's Nervous System, 20*(10), 734–741.

Hurley, R. A., Tomimoto, H., Akiguchi, I., Fisher, R. E., & Taber, K. H. (2000). Binswanger's disease: An ongoing controversy. *The Journal of Neuropsychiatry and Clinical Neurosciences, 12*(3), 301–304.

Iannucci, G., Dichgans, M., Rovaris, M., Brüning, R., Gasser, T., Giacomotti, L.,...Filippi, M. (2001). Correlations between clinical findings and magnetization transfer imaging metrics of tissue damage in individuals with cerebral autosomal dominant arteriopathy with subcortical infarcts and leukoencephalopathy. *Stroke, 32*(3), 643–648.

Ibrahimi, D. M., Tamargo, R. J., & Ahn, E. S. (2010). Moyamoya disease in children. *Child's Nervous System, 26*(10), 1297–1308.

Ikeda, E. (1991). Systemic vascular changes in spontaneous occlusion of the circle of Willis. *Stroke, 22*(11), 1358–1362.

Ikezaki, K. (2000). Rational approach to treatment of moyamoya disease in childhood. *Journal of Child Neurology, 15*(5), 350–356.

Im, S. H., Oh, C. W., Kwon, O. K., Kim, J. E., & Han, D. H. (2005). Moyamoya disease associated with Graves disease: Special considerations regarding clinical significance and management. *Journal of Neurosurgery, 102*(6), 1013–1017.

Imaizumi, C., Imaizumi, T., Osawa, M., Fukuyama, Y., & Takeshita, M. (1999). Serial intelligence test scores in pediatric moyamoya disease. *Neuropediatrics, 30*(6), 294–299.

Inaba, M., Henmi, Y., Kumeda, Y., Ueda, M., Nagata, M., Emoto, M.,...Nishizawa, Y. (2002). Increased stiffness in common carotid artery in hyperthyroid Graves' disease patients. *Biomedicine & Pharmacotherapy, 56*(5), 241–246.

Irikura, K., Miyasaka, Y., Kurata, A., Tanaka, R., Fujii, K., Yada, K., & Kan, S. (1996). A source of haemorrhage in adult patients with moyamoya disease: The significance of tributaries from the choroidal artery. *Acta Neurochirurgica, 138*(11), 1282–1286.

Ishikawa, T., Kuroda, S., Nakayama, N., Terae, S., Kudou, K., & Iwasaki, Y. (2005). Prevalence of asymptomatic microbleeds in patients with moyamoya disease. *Neurologia Medico-Chirurgica, 45*(10), 495–500; discussion 500.

Iso, H., Moriyama, Y., Sato, S., Kitamura, A., Tanigawa, T., Yamagishi, K.,...Shimamoto, T. (2004). Serum total homocysteine concentrations and risk of stroke and its subtypes in Japanese. *Circulation, 109*(22), 2766–2772.

Iverson, G. L., Mendrek, A., & Adams, R. L. (2004). The persistent belief that VIQ-PIQ splits suggest lateralized brain damage. *Applied Neuropsychology, 11*(2), 85–90.

Iwama, T., Morimoto, M., Hashimoto, N., Goto, Y., Todaka, T., & Sawada, M. (1997). Mechanism of intracranial rebleeding in moyamoya disease. *Clinical Neurology and Neurosurgery, 99*(Suppl 2), S187–S190.

Jea, A., Smith, E. R., Robertson, R., & Scott, R. M. (2005). Moyamoya syndrome associated with Down syndrome: Outcome after surgical revascularization. *Pediatrics, 116*(5), e694–e701.

Jefferson, A. L., Glosser, G., Detre, J. A., Sinson, G., & Liebeskind, D. S. (2006). Neuropsychological and perfusion MR imaging correlates of revascularization in a case of moyamoya syndrome. *AJNR, 27*(1), 98–100.

Jokinen, H., Kalska, H., Ylikoski, R., Madureira, S., Verdelho, A., van der Flier, W. M.,...Erkinjuntti, T.; LADIS group. (2009). Longitudinal cognitive decline in subcortical ischemic vascular disease—the LADIS Study. *Cerebrovascular Diseases, 27*(4), 384–391.

Joutel, A., Corpechot, C., Ducros, A., Vahedi, K., Chabriat, H., Mouton, P., … Tournier-Lasserve, E. (1996). Notch3 mutations in CADASIL, a hereditary adult-onset condition causing stroke and dementia. *Nature, 383*(6602), 707–710.

Joutel, A., Corpechot, C., Ducros, A., Vahedi, K., Chabriat, H., Mouton, P., … Tournier-Lasserve, E. (1997). Notch3 mutations in cerebral autosomal dominant arteriopathy with subcortical infarcts and leukoencephalopathy (CADASIL), a mendelian condition causing stroke and vascular dementia. *Annals of the New York Academy of Sciences, 826*, 213–217.

Jouvent, E., Viswanathan, A., Mangin, J. F., O'Sullivan, M., Guichard, J. P., Gschwendtner, A., … Chabriat, H. (2007). Brain atrophy is related to lacunar lesions and tissue microstructural changes in CADASIL. *Stroke, 38*(6), 1786–1790.

Jung, H. H., Bassetti, C., Tournier-Lasserve, E., Vahedi, K., Arnaboldi, M., Arifi, V. B., & Burgunder, J. M. (1995). Cerebral autosomal dominant arteriopathy with subcortical infarcts and leukoencephalopathy: A clinicopathological and genetic study of a Swiss family. *Journal of Neurology, Neurosurgery, and Psychiatry, 59*(2), 138–143.

Kalmijn, S., van Boxtel, M. P., Verschuren, M. W., Jolles, J., & Launer, L. J. (2002). Cigarette smoking and alcohol consumption in relation to cognitive performance in middle age. *American Journal of Epidemiology, 156*(10), 936–944.

Kang, H. S., Kim, S. K., Cho, B. K., Kim, Y. Y., Hwang, Y. S., & Wang, K. C. (2006). Single nucleotide polymorphisms of tissue inhibitor of metalloproteinase genes in familial moyamoya disease. *Neurosurgery, 58*(6), 1074–1080; discussion 1074.

Karasawa, J., Touho, H., Ohnishi, H., Miyamoto, S., & Kikuchi, H. (1993). Cerebral revascularization using omental transplantation for childhood moyamoya disease. *Journal of Neurosurgery, 79*(2), 192–196.

Karzmark, P., Zeifert, P. D., Tan, S., Dorfman, L. J., Bell-Stephens, T. E., & Steinberg, G. K. (2008). Effect of moyamoya disease on neuropsychological functioning in adults. *Neurosurgery, 62*(5), 1048–1051; discussion 1051.

Kawaguchi, S., Sakaki, T., Morimoto, T., Kakizaki, T., & Kamada, K. (1996). Characteristics of intracranial aneurysms associated with moyamoya disease. A review of 111 cases. *Acta Neurochirurgica, 138*(11), 1287–1294.

Kelly, M. E., Bell-Stephens, T. E., Marks, M. P., Do, H. M., & Steinberg, G. K. (2006). Progression of unilateral moyamoya disease: A clinical series. *Cerebrovascular Diseases, 22*(2–3), 109–115.

Kemp, G. J. (2000). Non-invasive methods for studying brain energy metabolism: What they show and what it means. *Developmental Neuroscience, 22*(5–6), 418–428.

Keverne, J. S., Low, W. C., Ziabreva, I., Court, J. A., Oakley, A. E., & Kalaria, R. N. (2007). Cholinergic neuronal deficits in CADASIL. *Stroke, 38*(1), 188–191.

Kikuta, K., Takagi, Y., Nozaki, K., Hanakawa, T., Okada, T., Mikuni, N., … Hashimoto, N. (2005). Asymptomatic microbleeds in moyamoya disease: T2*-weighted gradient-echo magnetic resonance imaging study. *Journal of Neurosurgery, 102*(3), 470–475.

Kim, S. J., Heo, K. G., Shin, H. Y., Bang, O. Y., Kim, G. M., Chung, C. S., … Lee, K. H. (2010). Association of thyroid autoantibodies with moyamoya-type cerebrovascular disease: A prospective study. *Stroke, 41*(1), 173–176.

Kirkham, F. J., & DeBaun, M. R. (2004). Stroke in children with sickle cell disease. *Current Treatment Options in Neurology, 6*(5), 357–375.

Kitani, M., Tomonaga, M., Yoshimura, M., Mori, H., & Yamanouchi, H. (1986). [A clinicopathological study of progressive subcortical vascular encephalopathy (Binswanger type) observed in elderly persons—classification of PSVE based on white-matter degeneration]. *Japanese Journal of Geriatrics, 23*(2), 155–162.

Kivipelto, M., Ngandu, T., Fratiglioni, L., Viitanen, M., Kåreholt, I., Winblad, B.,...Nissinen, A. (2005). Obesity and vascular risk factors at midlife and the risk of dementia and Alzheimer disease. *Archives of Neurology, 62*(10), 1556–1560.

Knopman, D., & Selnes, O. (2003). Neuropsychology of dementia. In K. M. Heilman & E. Valenstein (Eds.), *Clinical neuropsychology* (4th ed., pp. 574–616). New York, NY: Oxford University Press.

Knopman, D. S., & Roberts, R. (2010). Vascular risk factors: Imaging and neuropathologic correlates. *Journal of Alzheimer's Disease, 20*(3), 699–709.

Kodama, N., Aoki, Y., Hiraga, H., Wada, T., & Suzuki, J. (1979). Electroencephalographic findings in children with moyamoya disease. *Archives of Neurology, 36*(1), 16–19.

Kokmen, E., Whisnant, J. P., O'Fallon, W. M., Chu, C. P., & Beard, C. M. (1996). Dementia after ischemic stroke: A population-based study in Rochester, Minnesota (1960–1984). *Neurology, 46*(1), 154–159.

Komiyama, M., Nakajima, H., Nishikawa, M., Yasui, T., Kitano, S., & Sakamoto, H. (2001). Leptomeningeal contrast enhancement in moyamoya: Its potential role in postoperative assessment of circulation through the bypass. *Neuroradiology, 43*(1), 17–23.

Kono, S., Oka, K., & Sueishi, K. (1990). Histopathologic and morphometric studies of leptomeningeal vessels in moyamoya disease. *Stroke, 21*(7), 1044–1050.

Kudo, T. (1968). Spontaneous occlusion of the circle of Willis. A disease apparently confined to Japanese. *Neurology, 18*(5), 485–496.

Kuroda, S., Hashimoto, N., Yoshimoto, T., & Iwasaki, Y.; Research Committee on Moyamoya Disease in Japan. (2007). Radiological findings, clinical course, and outcome in asymptomatic moyamoya disease: Results of multicenter survey in Japan. *Stroke, 38*(5), 1430–1435.

Kuroda, S., & Houkin, K. (2008). Moyamoya disease: Current concepts and future perspectives. *Lancet Neurology, 7*(11), 1056–1066.

Kuroda, S., Houkin, K., Ishikawa, T., Nakayama, N., Ikeda, J., Ishii, N.,...Iwasaki, Y. (2004). Determinants of intellectual outcome after surgical revascularization in pediatric moyamoya disease: A multivariate analysis. *Child's Nervous System, 20*(5), 302–308.

Kuroda, S., Houkin, K., Kamiyama, H., Abe, H., & Mitsumori, K. (1995). Regional cerebral hemodynamics in childhood moyamoya disease. *Child's Nervous System, 11*(10), 584–590.

Kuroda, S., Kamiyama, H., Abe, H., Yamauchi, T., Kohama, Y., Houkin, K., & Mitsumori, K. (1993). Cerebral blood flow in children with spontaneous occlusion of the circle of Willis (moyamoya disease): Comparison with healthy children and evaluation of annual changes. *Neurologia Medico-Chirurgica, 33*(7), 434–438.

Kuwabara, Y., Ichiya, Y., Sasaki, M., Yoshida, T., Masuda, K., Ikezaki, K.,...Fukui, M. (1997). Cerebral hemodynamics and metabolism in moyamoya disease—a positron emission tomography study. *Clinical Neurology and Neurosurgery, 99*(Suppl 2), S74–S78.

Laakso, M. P., Partanen, K., Riekkinen, P., Lehtovirta, M., Helkala, E. L., Hallikainen, M.,...Soininen, H. (1996). Hippocampal volumes in Alzheimer's disease, Parkinson's disease with and without dementia, and in vascular dementia: An MRI study. *Neurology, 46*(3), 678–681.

Lamar, M., Price, C. G., Giovannetti, T., Swenson, R., & Liboin, D. J. (2014). Dysexecutive impairment associated with vascular dementia. In C. A. Noggle & R. S. Dean with S. Bush & S. Anderson (Eds.), *The neuropsychology of cortical dementias*. New York, NY: Springer Publishing Company.

Latif, F., Tory, K., Gnarra, J., Yao, M., Duh, F. M., Orcutt, M. L.,...Geil, L. (1993). Identification of the von Hippel-Lindau disease tumor suppressor gene. *Science, 260*(5112), 1317–1320.

Lee, J. Y., Phi, J. H., Wang, K. C., Cho, B. K., Shin, M. S., & Kim, S. K. (2011). Neurocognitive profiles of children with moyamoya disease before and after surgical intervention. *Cerebrovascular Diseases, 31*(3), 230–237.

Liebetrau, M., Herzog, J., Kloss, C. U., Hamann, G. F., & Dichgans, M. (2002). Prolonged cerebral transit time in CADASIL: A transcranial ultrasound study. *Stroke, 33,* 509–512.

Liem, M. K., van der Grond, J., Haan, J., van den Boom, R., Ferrari, M. D., Knaap, Y. M., ... Lesnik Oberstein, S. A. (2007). Lacunar infarcts are the main correlate with cognitive dysfunction in CADASIL. *Stroke, 38*(3), 923–928.

Lim, M., Cheshier, S., & Steinberg, G. K. (2006). New vessel formation in the central nervous system during tumor growth, vascular malformations, and moyamoya. *Current Neurovascular Research, 3*(3), 237–245.

Liu, J. S., Juo, S. H., Chen, W. H., Chang, Y. Y., & Chen, S. S. (1994). A case of Graves' diseases associated with intracranial moyamoya vessels and tubular stenosis of extracranial internal carotid arteries. *Journal of the Formosan Medical Association, 93*(9), 806–809.

Looi, J. C., & Sachdev, P. S. (1999). Differentiation of vascular dementia from AD on neuropsychological tests. *Neurology, 53*(4), 670–678.

Lubman, D. I., Pantelis, C., Desmond, P., Proffitt, T. M., & Velakoulis, D. (2003). Moyamoya disease in a patient with schizophrenia. *Journal of the International Neuropsychological Society, 9*(5), 806–810.

Lyoo, I. K., Satlin, A., Lee, C. K., & Renshaw, P. F. (1997). Regional atrophy of the corpus callosum in subjects with Alzheimer's disease and multi-infarct dementia. *Psychiatry Research, 74*(2), 63–72.

Macrì, M. A., Colonnese, C., Garreffa, G., Fattapposta, F., Restuccia, R., Bianco, F., ... Maraviglia, B. (2006). A chemical shift imaging study on regional metabolite distribution in a CADASIL family. *Magnetic Resonance Imaging, 24*(4), 443–447.

Markus, H. S., Martin, R. J., Simpson, M. A., Dong, Y. B., Ali, N., Crosby, A. H., & Powell, J. F. (2002). Diagnostic strategies in CADASIL. *Neurology, 59*(8), 1134–1138.

Marushima, A., Yanaka, K., Matsuki, T., Kojima, H., & Nose, T. (2006). Subarachnoid hemorrhage not due to ruptured aneurysm in moyamoya disease. *Journal of Clinical Neuroscience, 13*(1), 146–149.

Maruyama, K., Mishima, K., Saito, N., Fujimaki, T., Sasaki, T., & Kirino, T. (2000). Radiation-induced aneurysm and moyamoya vessels presenting with subarachnoid haemorrhage. *Acta Neurochirurgica, 142*(2), 139–143.

Massaro, M., Thorarensen, O., Liu, G. T., Maguire, A. M., Zimmerman, R. A., & Brodsky, M. C. (1998). Morning glory disc anomaly and moyamoya vessels. *Archives of Ophthalmology, 116*(2), 253–254.

Matheja, P., Weckesser, M., Debus, O., Franzius, C. H., Löttgen, J., Schober, O., & Kurlemann, G. (2002). Moyamoya syndrome: Impaired hemodynamics on ECD SPECT after EEG controlled hyperventilation. *Nuklearmedizin. Nuclear Medicine, 41*(1), 42–46.

Matsushima, T., Inoue, T., Ikezaki, K., Matsukado, K., Natori, Y., Inamura, T., & Fukui, M. (1998). Multiple combined indirect procedure for the surgical treatment of children with moyamoya disease. A comparison with single indirect anastomosis and direct anastomosis. *Neurosurgical Focus, 5*(5), e4.

Matsushima, Y., Fukai, N., Tanaka, K., Tsuruoka, S., Inaba, Y., Aoyagi, M., & Ohno, K. (1981). A new surgical treatment of moyamoya disease in children: A preliminary report. *Surgical Neurology, 15*(4), 313–320.

Matsushima, Y., & Inaba, Y. (1986). The specificity of the collaterals to the brain through the study and surgical treatment of moyamoya disease. *Stroke, 17*(1), 117–122.

McMenemey, W. H. (1961). The dementias and progressive diseases of the basal ganglia. In J. G. Greenfield (Ed.), *Neuropathology* (3rd ed., pp. 475–521). London: Arnold.

Mellies, J. K., Bäumer, T., Müller, J. A., Tournier-Lasserve, E., Chabriat, H., Knobloch, O.,...Haller, P. (1998). SPECT study of a German CADASIL family: A phenotype with migraine and progressive dementia only. *Neurology, 50*(6), 1715–1721.

Meyers, P., Halbach, V., & Barkovich, A. (2000). Anomalies of cerebral vasculature: Diagnostic and endovascular considerations. In A. Barkovich (ed.), *Pediatric neuroimaging* (3rd ed., p. 806). Philadelphia, PA: Lippincott Williams & Wilkins.

Mineharu, Y., Liu, W., Inoue, K., Matsuura, N., Inoue, S., Takenaka, K.,...Koizumi, A. (2008). Autosomal dominant moyamoya disease maps to chromosome 17q25.3. *Neurology, 70*(24 Pt 2), 2357–2363.

Miskinyte, S., Butler, M. G., Hervé, D., Sarret, C., Nicolino, M., Petralia, J. D.,...Tournier-Lasserve, E. (2011). Loss of BRCC3 deubiquitinating enzyme leads to abnormal angiogenesis and is associated with syndromic moyamoya. *American Journal of Human Genetics, 88*(6), 718–728.

Mitchell, W. G., Fishman, L. S., Miller, J. H., Nelson, M., Zeltzer, P. M., Soni, D., & Siegel, S. M. (1991). Stroke as a late sequela of cranial irradiation for childhood brain tumors. *Journal of Child Neurology, 6*(2), 128–133.

Mito, T., & Becker, L. E. (1992). Vascular dysplasia in Down syndrome: A possible relationship to moyamoya disease. *Brain & Development, 14*(4), 248–251.

Miyamoto, S., Kikuchi, H., Karasawa, J., Nagata, I., Ihara, I., & Yamagata, S. (1986). Study of the posterior circulation in moyamoya disease. Part 2: Visual disturbances and surgical treatment. *Journal of Neurosurgery, 65*(4), 454–460.

Moody, D. M., Santamore, W. P., & Bell, M. A. (1991). Does tortuosity in cerebral arterioles impair down-autoregulation in hypertensives and elderly normotensives? A hypothesis and computer model. *Clinical Neurosurgery, 37*, 372–387.

Moretti, R., Torre, P., Antonello, R. M., & Cazzato, G. (2001). Rivastigmine in subcortical vascular dementia: A comparison trial on efficacy and tolerability for 12 months follow-up. *European Journal of Neurology, 8*(4), 361–362.

Moretti, R., Torre, P., Antonello, R. M., Cazzato, G., & Bava, A. (2002). Rivastigmine in subcortical vascular dementia: An open 22-month study. *Journal of the Neurological Sciences, 203–204*, 141–146.

Moretti, R., Torre, P., Antonello, R. M., Cazzato, G., & Pizzolato, G. (2008). Different responses to rivastigmine in subcortical vascular dementia and multi-infarct dementia. *American Journal of Alzheimer's Disease and Other Dementias, 23*(2), 167–176.

Morich, F. J., Bieber, F., Lewis, J. M., Kaiser, L., Cutler, N. R., Escobar, J. I.,...Reisberg, B. (1996). Nimodipine in the treatment of probable Alzheimer's disease: Results of two multi-centre trials. *Clinical Drug Investigation, 11*, 185–195.

Moritani, T., Numaguchi, Y., Lemer, N. B., Rozans, M. K., Robinson, A. E., Hiwatashi, A., & Westesson, P. L. (2004). Sickle cell cerebrovascular disease: Usual and unusual findings on MR imaging and MR angiography. *Clinical Imaging, 28*(3), 173–186.

Mungas, D., Reed, B. R., Jagust, W. J., DeCarli, C., Mack, W. J., Kramer, J. H.,...Chui, H. C. (2002). Volumetric MRI predicts rate of cognitive decline related to AD and cerebrovascular disease. *Neurology, 59*(6), 867–873.

Murray, M. D., Lane, K. A., Gao, S., Evans, R. M., Unverzagt, F. W., Hall, K. S., & Hendrie, H. (2002). Preservation of cognitive function with antihypertensive medications: A longitudinal analysis of a community-based sample of African Americans. *Archives of Internal Medicine, 162*(18), 2090–2096.

Nagata, T., Harada, D., Aoki, K., Kada, H., Miyata, H., Kasahara, H., & Nakayama, K. (2007). Effectiveness of carbamazepine for benzodiazepine-resistant impulsive aggression in a patient with frontal infarctions. *Psychiatry and Clinical Neurosciences*, *61*(6), 695–697.

Neshige, R., Barrett, G., & Shibasaki, H. (1988). Auditory long latency event-related potentials in Alzheimer's disease and multi-infarct dementia. *Journal of Neurology, Neurosurgery, and Psychiatry*, *51*(9), 1120–1125.

Ni, J., Gao, S., Cui, L. Y., & Li, S. W. (2006). Intracranial arterial occlusive lesion in patients with Graves' disease. *Chinese Medical Sciences Journal*, *21*(3), 140–144.

O'Sullivan, M., Jarosz, J. M., Martin, R. J., Deasy, N., Powell, J. F., & Markus, H. S. (2001). MRI hyperintensities of the temporal lobe and external capsule in patients with CADASIL. *Neurology*, *56*(5), 628–634.

O'Sullivan, M., Morris, R. G., & Markus, H. S. (2005). Brief cognitive assessment for patients with cerebral small vessel disease. *Journal of Neurology, Neurosurgery, and Psychiatry*, *76*(8), 1140–1145.

Ogasawara, K., Komoribayashi, N., Kobayashi, M., Fukuda, T., Inoue, T., Yamadate, K., & Ogawa, A. (2005). Neural damage caused by cerebral hyperperfusion after arterial bypass surgery in a patient with moyamoya disease: Case report. *Neurosurgery*, *56*(6), E1380; discussion E1380.

Ogawa, A., Nakamura, N., Yoshimoto, T., & Suzuki, J. (1990). Cerebral blood flow in moyamoya disease. Part 2: Autoregulation and CO2 response. *Acta Neurochirurgica*, *105*(3–4), 107–111.

Ogawa, A., Yoshimoto, T., Suzuki, J., & Sakurai, Y. (1990). Cerebral blood flow in moyamoya disease. Part 1: Correlation with age and regional distribution. *Acta Neurochirurgica*, *105*(1–2), 30–34.

Ohaegbulam, C., Magge, S., & Scott, R. M. (2001). Moyamoya syndrome. In D. G. McLone (ed.), *Pediatric neurosurgery. Surgery of the developing nervous system* (4th ed., pp. 1077–1092). Philadelphia, PA: WB Saunders.

Ohba, S., Nakagawa, T., & Murakami, H. (2011). Concurrent Graves' disease and intracranial arterial stenosis/occlusion: Special considerations regarding the state of thyroid function, etiology, and treatment. *Neurosurgical Review*, *34*(3), 297–304; discussion 304.

Oliveri, R. L., Muglia, M., De Stefano, N., Mazzei, R., Labate, A., Conforti, F. L., . . . Quattrone, A. (2001). A novel mutation in the Notch3 gene in an Italian family with cerebral autosomal dominant arteriopathy with subcortical infarcts and leukoencephalopathy: Genetic and magnetic resonance spectroscopic findings. *Archives of Neurology*, *58*(9), 1418–1422.

Olszewski, J. (1962). Subcortical arteriosclerotic encephalopathy. Review of the literature on the so-called Binswanger's disease and presentation of two cases. *World Neurology*, *3*, 359–375.

Orgogozo, J. M., Rigaud, A. S., Stöffler, A., Möbius, H. J., & Forette, F. (2002). Efficacy and safety of memantine in patients with mild to moderate vascular dementia: A randomized, placebo-controlled trial (MMM 300). *Stroke*, *33*(7), 1834–1839.

Osanai, T., Kuroda, S., Nakayama, N., Yamauchi, T., Houkin, K., & Iwasaki, Y. (2008). Moyamoya disease presenting with subarachnoid hemorrhage localized over the frontal cortex: Case report. *Surgical Neurology*, *69*(2), 197–200.

Pandey, P., Bell-Stephens, T., & Steinberg, G. K. (2010). Patients with moyamoya disease presenting with movement disorder. *Journal of Neurosurgery. Pediatrics*, *6*(6), 559–566.

Panegyres, P. K., Morris, J. G., O'Neill, P. J., & Balleine, R. (1993). Moyamoya-like disease with inflammation. *European Neurology*, *33*(3), 260–263.

Pantoni, L., Garcia, J. H., & Gutierrez, J. A. (1996). Cerebral white matter is highly vulnerable to ischemia. *Stroke*, *27*(9), 1641–1646; discussion 1647.

Pantoni, L., Rossi, R., Inzitari, D., Bianchi, C., Beneke, M., Erkinjuntti, T., & Wallin, A. (2000). Efficacy and safety of nimodipine in subcortical vascular dementia: A subgroup analysis of the Scandinavian Multi-Infarct Dementia Trial. *Journal of the Neurological Sciences, 175*(2), 124–134.

Parmar, R. C., Bavdekar, S. B., Muranjan, M. N., & Limaye, U. (2000). Chorea: An unusual presenting feature in pediatric moyamoya disease. *Indian Pediatrics, 37*(9), 1005–1009.

Patel, N. N., Mangano, F. T., & Klimo, P. (2010). Indirect revascularization techniques for treating moyamoya disease. *Neurosurgery Clinics of North America, 21*(3), 553–563.

Pendlebury, S. T., & Rothwell, P. M. (2009). Prevalence, incidence, and factors associated with pre-stroke and post-stroke dementia: A systematic review and meta-analysis. *Lancet Neurology, 8*(11), 1006–1018.

Peters, N., Opherk, C., Danek, A., Ballard, C., Herzog, J., & Dichgans, M. (2005). The pattern of cognitive performance in CADASIL: A monogenic condition leading to subcortical ischemic vascular dementia. *The American Journal of Psychiatry, 162*(11), 2078–2085.

Petty, G. W., Brown, R. D., Whisnant, J. P., Sicks, J. D., O'Fallon, W. M., & Wiebers, D. O. (1999). Ischemic stroke subtypes: A population-based study of incidence and risk factors. *Stroke, 30*(12), 2513–2516.

Pfefferkorn, T., von Stuckrad-Barre, S., Herzog, J., Gasser, T., Hamann, G. F., & Dichgans, M. (2001). Reduced cerebrovascular CO(2) reactivity in CADASIL: A transcranial Doppler sonography study. *Stroke, 32*(1), 17–21.

Pohjasvaara, T., Erkinjuntti, T., Vataja, R., & Kaste, M. (1997). Dementia three months after stroke: Baseline frequency and effect of different definitions for dementia in the Helsinki Stroke Aging Memory Study (SAM) stroke cohort. *Stroke, 28*, 785–792.

Powell, A. L., Cummings, J. L., Hill, M. A., & Benson, D. F. (1988). Speech and language alterations in multi-infarct dementia. *Neurology, 38*(5), 717–719.

Pratt, R. D., & Perdomo, C. A. (2002). Results of clinical studies with donepezil in vascular dementia. *The American Journal of Geriatric Psychiatry, 10*(Suppl 1), 88–89.

PROGRESS Collaborative Group. (2001). Randomised trial of perindopril-based blood-pressure lowering regimen among 6105 individuals with prior stroke or transient ischaemic attack. *Lancet, 358*, 1033–1041.

Pullicino, P., Ostrow, P., Miller, L., Snyder, W., & Munschauer, F. (1995). Pontine ischemic rarefaction. *Annals of Neurology, 37*(4), 460–466.

Ramos-Estebanez, C., Moral-Arce, I., Gonzalez-Mandly, A., Dhagubatti, V., Gonzalez-Macias, J., Munoz, R., & Hernadez-Hernandez, J. L. (2011). Vascular cognitive impairment in small vessel disease: Clinical and neuropsychological features of lacunar state and Binswanger's disease. *Age and Ageing, 40*(2), 175–180.

Razvi, S. S., Davidson, R., Bone, I., & Muir, K. W. (2005). The prevalence of cerebral autosomal dominant arteriopathy with subcortical infarcts and leucoencephalopathy (CADASIL) in the west of Scotland. *Journal of Neurology, Neurosurgery, and Psychiatry, 76*(5), 739–741.

Rein Gustavsen, W., Reinholt, F. P., & Schlosser, A. (2006). Skin biopsy findings and results of neuropsychological testing in the first confirmed cases of CADASIL in Norway. *European Journal of Neurology, 13*(4), 359–362.

Révész, T., Hawkins, C. P., du Boulay, E. P., Barnard, R. O., & McDonald, W. I. (1989). Pathological findings correlated with magnetic resonance imaging in subcortical arteriosclerotic encephalopathy (Binswanger's disease). *Journal of Neurology, Neurosurgery, and Psychiatry, 52*(12), 1337–1344.

Reyes, S., Viswanathan, A., Godin, O., Dufouil, C., Benisty, S., Hernandez, K.,…Chabriat, H. (2009). Apathy: A major symptom in CADASIL. *Neurology, 72*(10), 905–910.

Rincon, F., & Wright, C. B. (2013). Vascular cognitive impairment. *Current Opinion in Neurology*, *26*(1), 29–36.

Roach, E. S. (2000). Etiology of stroke in children. *Seminars in Pediatric Neurology*, *7*(4), 244–260.

Roach, E. S., Golomb, M. R., Adams, R., Biller, J., Daniels, S., Deveber, G.,...Smith, E. R.; American Heart Association Stroke Council; Council on Cardiovascular Disease in the Young. (2008). Management of stroke in infants and children: A scientific statement from a Special Writing Group of the American Heart Association Stroke Council and the Council on Cardiovascular Disease in the Young. *Stroke*, *39*(9), 2644–2691.

Rockwood, K., Wentzel, C., Hachinski, V., Hogan, D. B., MacKnight, C., & McDowell, I. (2000). Prevalence and outcomes of vascular cognitive impairment. Vascular Cognitive Impairment Investigators of the Canadian Study of Health and Aging. *Neurology*, *54*(2), 447–451.

Román, G. C. (1987). Senile dementia of the Binswanger type. A vascular form of dementia in the elderly. *The Journal of American Medical Association*, *258*(13), 1782–1788.

Román, G. (2000). Perspectives in the treatment of vascular dementia. *Drugs of Today*, *36*(9), 641–653.

Román, G. C. (2002). Vascular dementia revisited: Diagnosis, pathogenesis, treatment, and prevention. *The Medical Clinics of North America*, *86*(3), 477–499.

Román, G. C. (2003). Vascular dementia: Distinguishing characteristics, treatment, and prevention. *Journal of the American Geriatrics Society*, *51*(5 Suppl Dementia), S296–S304.

Román, G. C., Erkinjuntti, T., Wallin, A., Pantoni, L., & Chui, H. C. (2002). Subcortical ischaemic vascular dementia. *Lancet Neurology*, *1*(7), 426–436.

Román, G. C., & Royall, D. R. (1999). Executive control function: A rational basis for the diagnosis of vascular dementia. *Alzheimer Disease and Associated Disorders*, *13*(Suppl 3), S69–S80.

Román, G. C., Tatemichi, T. K., Erkinjuntti, T., Cummings, J. L., Masdeu, J. C., Garcia, J. H.,...Hofman, A. (1993). Vascular dementia: Diagnostic criteria for research studies. Report of the NINDS-AIREN International Workshop. *Neurology*, *43*(2), 250–260.

Rosser, T. L., Vezina, G., & Packer, R. J. (2005). Cerebrovascular abnormalities in a population of children with neurofibromatosis type 1. *Neurology*, *64*(3), 553–555.

Ruchoux, M. M., Chabriat, H., Bousser, M. G., Baudrimont, M., & Tournier-Lasserve, E. (1994). Presence of ultrastructural arterial lesions in muscle and skin vessels of patients with CADASIL. *Stroke*, *25*(11), 2291–2292.

Rudoltz, M. S., Regine, W. F., Langston, J. W., Sanford, R. A., Kovnar, E. H., & Kun, L. E. (1998). Multiple causes of cerebrovascular events in children with tumors of the parasellar region. *Journal of Neuro-Oncology*, *37*(3), 251–261.

Rufa, A., De Stefano, N., Dotti, M. T., Bianchi, S., Sicurelli, F., Stromillo, . . . Federico, A. (2004). Acute unilateral visual loss as the first symptom of cerebral autosomal dominant arteriopathy with subcortical infarcts and leukoencephalopathy. *Archives of Neurology*, *61*, 577–580.

Sachdev, P. S., Brodaty, H., Valenzuela, M. J., Lorentz, L., Looi, J. C., Berman, K.,...Zagami, A. S. (2006). Clinical determinants of dementia and mild cognitive impairment following ischaemic stroke: The Sydney Stroke Study. *Dementia and Geriatric Cognitive Disorders*, *21*(5–6), 275–283.

Sachdev, P. S., Brodaty, H., Valenzuela, M. J., Lorentz, L. M., & Koschera, A. (2004). Progression of cognitive impairment in stroke patients. *Neurology*, *63*(9), 1618–1623.

Sachdev, P. S., Chen, X., Brodaty, H., Thompson, C., Altendorf, A., & Wen, W. (2009). The determinants and longitudinal course of post-stroke mild cognitive impairment. *Journal of the International Neuropsychological Society*, *15*(6), 915–923.

Sakamoto, S., Kiura, Y., Yamasaki, F., Shibukawa, M., Ohba, S., Shrestha, P.,...Kurisu, K. (2008). Expression of vascular endothelial growth factor in dura mater of patients with moyamoya disease. *Neurosurgical Review, 31*(1), 77–81; discussion 81.

Santamaria Ortiz, J., & Knight, P. V. (1994). Review: Binswanger's disease, leukoaraiosis and dementia. *Age and Ageing, 23*(1), 75–81.

Santos, M. D., Alkondon, M., Pereira, E. F., Aracava, Y., Eisenberg, H. M., Maelicke, A., & Albuquerque, E. X. (2002). The nicotinic allosteric potentiating ligand galantamine facilitates synaptic transmission in the mammalian central nervous system. *Molecular Pharmacology, 61*(5), 1222–1234.

Sasaki, T., Nogawa, S., & Amano, T. (2006). Co-morbidity of moyamoya disease with Graves' disease. Report of three cases and a review of the literature. *Internal Medicine, 45*(9), 649–653.

Schneider, J. A., Wilson, R. S., Bienias, J. L., Evans, D. A., & Bennett, D. A. (2004). Cerebral infarctions and the likelihood of dementia from Alzheimer disease pathology. *Neurology, 62*(7), 1148–1155.

Scott, R. M. (2000). Moyamoya syndrome: A surgically treatable cause of stroke in the pediatric patient. *Clinical Neurosurgery, 47*, 378–384.

Scott, R. M. (2001). Surgery for moyamoya syndrome? Yes. *Archives of Neurology, 58*(1), 128–129.

Scott, R. M., & Smith, E. R. (2009). Moyamoya disease and moyamoya syndrome. *The New England Journal of Medicine, 360*(12), 1226–1237.

Scott, R. M., Smith, J. L., Robertson, R. L., Madsen, J. R., Soriano, S. G., & Rockoff, M. A. (2004). Long-term outcome in children with moyamoya syndrome after cranial revascularization by pial synangiosis. *Journal of Neurosurgery, 100*(2 Suppl. Pediatrics), 142–149.

Selnes, O. A., & Vinters, H. V. (2006). Vascular cognitive impairment. *Nature Clinical Practice. Neurology, 2*(10), 538–547.

Seol, H. J., Wang, K. C., Kim, S. K., Hwang, Y. S., Kim, K. J., & Cho, B. K. (2005). Headache in pediatric moyamoya disease: Review of 204 consecutive cases. *Journal of Neurosurgery, 103*(5 Suppl), 439–442.

Sharfstein, S. R., Ahmed, S., Islam, M. Q., Najjar, M. I., & Ratushny, V. (2007). Case of moyamoya disease in a patient with advanced acquired immunodeficiency syndrome. *Journal of Stroke and Cerebrovascular Diseases, 16*(6), 268–272.

Shimamura, A. P., Janosky, J. S., & Squire, L. R. (1991). What is the role of frontal lobe damage in amnesic disorders? In H. S. Levin, H. M. Eisenberg, & A. L. Benton (Eds.), *Frontal lobe functioning and dysfunction*. Oxford, UK: Oxford University Press.

Shimizu, H., Nakasato, N., Mizoi, K., & Yoshimoto, T. (1997). Localizing the central sulcus by functional magnetic resonance imaging and magnetoencephalography. *Clinical Neurology and Neurosurgery, 99*(4), 235–238.

Shimizu, H., Shirane, R., Fujiwara, S., Takahashi, A., & Yoshimoto, T. (1997). Proton magnetic resonance spectroscopy in children with Moyamoya disease. *Clinical Neurology and Neurosurgery, 99*(Suppl. 2), S64–S67.

Shyu, W. C., Lin, J. C., Shen, C. C., Hsu, Y. D., Lee, C. C., Shiah, I. S., & Tsao, W. L. (1996). Vascular dementia of Binswanger's type: Clinical, neuroradiological and 99mTc-HMPAO SPET study. *European Journal of Nuclear Medicine, 23*(10), 1338–1344.

Siegert, C. E., Smelt, A. H., & de Bruin, T. W. (1995). Superior sagittal sinus thrombosis and thyrotoxicosis. Possible association in two cases. *Stroke, 26*(3), 496–497.

Smith, E. R., & Scott, R. M. (2010). Moyamoya: Epidemiology, presentation, and diagnosis. *Neurosurgery Clinics of North America, 21*(3), 543–551.

Smith, E. R., & Scott, R. M. (2008). Progression of disease in unilateral moyamoya syndrome. *Neurosurgical Focus, 24*(2), E17.

Smith, J. L. (2009). Understanding and treating moyamoya disease in children. *Neurosurgical Focus, 26*(4), E4.

Snowdon, D. A., Greiner, L. H., Mortimer, J. A., Riley, K. P., Greiner, P. A., & Markesbery, W. R. (1997). Brain infarction and the clinical expression of Alzheimer disease. The Nun Study. *The Journal of the American Medical Association, 277*(10), 813–817.

Soriano, S. G., Cowan, D. B., Proctor, M. R., & Scott, R. M. (2002). Levels of soluble adhesion molecules are elevated in the cerebrospinal fluid of children with moyamoya syndrome. *Neurosurgery, 50*(3), 544–549.

Spengos, K., Kosmaidou-Aravidou, Z., Tsivgoulis, G., Vassilopoulou, S., Grigori-Kostaraki, P., & Zis, V. (2006). Moyamoya syndrome in a Caucasian woman with Turner's syndrome. *European Journal of Neurology, 13*(10), e7–e8.

Stebbins, G. T., Nyenhuis, D. L., Wang, C., Cox, J. L., Freels, S., Bangen, K.,...Gorelick, P. B. (2008). Gray matter atrophy in patients with ischemic stroke with cognitive impairment. *Stroke, 39*(3), 785–793.

Stuss, D., & Cummings, J. (1990). Subcortical vascular dementias. In J. L. Cummings (Ed.), *Subcortical dementia* (pp. 145–163). New York, NY: Oxford University Press

Sultzer, D. L., Levin, H. S., Mahler, M. E., High, W. M., & Cummings, J. L. (1993). A comparison of psychiatric symptoms in vascular dementia and Alzheimer's disease. *The American Journal of Psychiatry, 150*(12), 1806–1812.

Suzuki, J., & Kodama, N. (1983). Moyamoya disease—a review. *Stroke, 14*(1), 104–109.

Suzuki, J., & Takaku, A. (1969). Cerebrovascular "moyamoya" disease. Disease showing abnormal net-like vessels in base of brain. *Archives of Neurology, 20*(3), 288–299.

Takagi, Y., Kikuta, K., Nozaki, K., & Hashimoto, N. (2007). Histological features of middle cerebral arteries from patients treated for moyamoya disease. *Neurologia Medico-Chirurgica, 47*(1), 1–4.

Takagi, Y., Kikuta, K., Sadamasa, N., Nozaki, K., & Hashimoto, N. (2006). Proliferative activity through extracellular signal-regulated kinase of smooth muscle cells in vascular walls of cerebral arteriovenous malformations. *Neurosurgery, 58*(4), 740–748; discussion 740.

Takahashi, M. (1980). Magnification angiography in moyamoya disease: New observations on collateral vessels. *Radiology, 36*, 379–386.

Takebayashi, S., Matsuo, K., & Kaneko, M. (1984). Ultrastructural studies of cerebral arteries and collateral vessels in moyamoya disease. *Stroke, 15*(4), 728–732.

Takekawa, Y., Umezawa, T., Ueno, Y., Sawada, T., & Kobayashi, M. (2004). Pathological and immunohistochemical findings of an autopsy case of adult moyamoya disease. *Neuropathology, 24*(3), 236–242.

Takeuchi, K., & Shimizu, K. (1957). Hypoplasia of the bilateral internal carotid arteries. *Brain Nerve, 9*, 37–43.

Taylor, R., Gilleard, C. J., & McGuire, R. J. (1996). Patterns of neuropsychological impairment in dementia of the Alzheimer type and multi-infarct dementia. *Archives of Gerontology and Geriatrics, 23*(1), 13–26.

Tendler, B. E., Shoukri, K., Malchoff, C., MacGillivray, D., Duckrow, R., Talmadge, T., & Ramsby, G. R. (1997). Concurrence of Graves' disease and dysplastic cerebral blood vessels of the moyamoya variety. *Thyroid, 7*(4), 625–629.

Thakur, S., Verma, B., Mokta, J., Aggarwal, P., & Sharma, A. (2007). Binswanger's disease. *The Journal of the Association of Physicians of India, 55*, 285.

Tournier-Lasserve, E., Joutel, A., Melki, J., Weissenbach, J., Lathrop, G. M., Chabriat, H.,...Maciazek, J. (1993). Cerebral autosomal dominant arteriopathy with subcortical infarcts and leukoencephalopathy maps to chromosome 19q12. *Nature Genetics, 3*(3), 256–259.

Trojano, L., Ragno, M., Manca, A., & Caruso, G. (1998). A kindred affected by cerebral autosomal dominant arteriopathy with subcortical infarcts and leukoencephalopathy (CADASIL). A 2-year neuropsychological follow-up. *Journal of Neurology, 245*(4), 217–222.

Uchino, K., Johnston, S. C., Becker, K. J., & Tirschwell, D. L. (2005). Moyamoya disease in Washington State and California. *Neurology, 65*(6), 956–958.

Vahedi, K., Chabriat, H., Levy, C., Joutel, A., Tournier-Lasserve, E., & Bousser, M. G. (2004). Migraine with aura and brain magnetic resonance imaging abnormalities in patients with CADASIL. *Archives of Neurology, 61*(8), 1237–1240.

Valenti, R., Poggesi, A., Pescini, F., Inzitari, D., & Pantoni, L. (2008). Psychiatric disturbances in CADASIL: A brief review. *Acta Neurologica Scandinavica, 118*(5), 291–295.

Valko, P. O., Siccoli, M. M., Schiller, A., Wieser, H. G., & Jung, H. H. (2007). Non-convulsive status epilepticus causing focal neurological deficits in CADASIL. *Journal of Neurology, Neurosurgery, and Psychiatry, 78*(11), 1287–1289.

van Bogaert, L. (1955). Encephalopathie sous corticale progressive (Binswanger) a evolution rapide chez des soeurs. *Med Hellen, 24*, 961–972.

van den Boom, R., Oberstein, S. A., Ferrari, M. D., Haan, J., & van Buchem, M. A. (2003). Cerebral autosomal dominant arteriopathy with subcortical infarcts and leukoencephalopathy: MR imaging findings at different ages—3rd-6th decades. *Radiology, 229*(3), 683–690.

Verdelho, A., Madureira, S., Moleiro, C., Ferro, J. M., Santos, C. O., Erkinjuntti, T., … Inzitari, D.; LADIS Study. (2010). White matter changes and diabetes predict cognitive decline in the elderly: The LADIS study. *Neurology, 75*(2), 160–167.

Vermeer, S. E., Prins, N. D., den Heijer, T., Hofman, A., Koudstaal, P. J., & Breteler, M. M. (2003). Silent brain infarcts and the risk of dementia and cognitive decline. *The New England Journal of Medicine, 348*(13), 1215–1222.

Viswanathan, A., Gray, F., Bousser, M. G., Baudrimont, M., & Chabriat, H. (2006). Cortical neuronal apoptosis in CADASIL. *Stroke, 37*(11), 2690–2695.

Wagle, J., Farner, L., Flekkøy, K., Wyller, T. B., Sandvik, L., Eiklid, K. L., … Engedal, K. (2010). Cognitive impairment and the role of the ApoE epsilon4-allele after stroke—a 13 months follow-up study. *International Journal of Geriatric Psychiatry, 25*(8), 833–842.

Wakai, K., Tamakoshi, A., Ikezaki, K., Fukui, M., Kawamura, T., Aoki, R., … Ohno, Y. (1997). Epidemiological features of moyamoya disease in Japan: Findings from a nationwide survey. *Clinical Neurology and Neurosurgery, 99*(Suppl 2), S1–S5.

Walzl, M. (2000). A promising approach to the treatment of multi-infarct dementia. *Neurobiology of Aging, 21*(2), 283–287.

Wiseman, R. M., Saxby, B. K., Burton, E. J., Barber, R., Ford, G. A., & O'Brien, J. T. (2004). Hippocampal atrophy, whole brain volume, and white matter lesions in older hypertensive subjects. *Neurology, 63*(10), 1892–1897.

Yamada, I., Matsushima, Y., & Suzuki, S. (1992). Moyamoya disease: Diagnosis with three-dimensional time-of-flight MR angiography. *Radiology, 184*(3), 773–778.

Yamada, I., Suzuki, S., & Matsushima, Y. (1995a). Moyamoya disease: Comparison of assessment with MR angiography and MR imaging versus conventional angiography. *Radiology, 196*(1), 211–218.

Yamada, I., Suzuki, S., & Matsushima, Y. (1995b). Moyamoya disease: Diagnostic accuracy of MRI. *Neuroradiology, 37*(5), 356–361.

Yamamoto, M., Aoyagi, M., Tajima, S., Wachi, H., Fukai, N., Matsushima, Y., & Yamamoto, K. (1997). Increase in elastin gene expression and protein synthesis in arterial smooth muscle cells derived from patients with moyamoya disease. *Stroke, 28*(9), 1733–1738.

Yamanouchi, H., & Nagura, H. (1997). Neurological signs and frontal white matter lesions in vascular parkinsonism. A clinicopathologic study. *Stroke, 28*(5), 965–969.

Yamauchi, T., Tada, M., Houkin, K., Tanaka, T., Nakamura, Y., Kuroda, S.,... Fukui, M. (2000). Linkage of familial moyamoya disease (spontaneous occlusion of the circle of Willis) to chromosome 17q25. *Stroke, 31*(4), 930–935.

Ylikoski, A., Erkinjuntti, T., Raininko, R., Sarna, S., Sulkava, R., & Tilvis, R. (1995). White matter hyperintensities on MRI in the neurologically nondiseased elderly. Analysis of cohorts of consecutive subjects aged 55 to 85 years living at home. *Stroke, 26*(7), 1171–1177.

Yoshimoto, T., Houkin, K., Takahashi, A., & Abe, H. (1996). Angiogenic factors in moyamoya disease. *Stroke, 27*(12), 2160–2165.

Yusuf, S. (2002). Two decades of progress in preventing vascular disease. *Lancet, 360*(9326), 2–3.

Zheng, W., Wanibuchi, M., Onda, T., Liu, H., Koyanagi, I., Fujimori, K., & Houkin, K. (2006). A case of moyamoya disease presenting with chorea. *Child's Nervous System, 22*(3), 274–278.

CHAPTER 6

Dysexecutive Impairment Associated With Vascular Dementia

Melissa Lamar, Catherine C. Price, Tania Giovannetti,
Rod Swenson, and David J. Libon

HISTORY OF VASCULAR DEMENTIA

Interest in the neuropsychological and behavioral alterations associated with cerebrovascular pathology is usually traced to the work of Otto Binswanger (1894; translated by Blass, Hoyer, & Nitsch, 1991). Binswanger suggested the notion that white matter atrophy, associated with vascular insufficiency, could cause cognitive impairment and described a series of patients who presented with slowly deteriorating cognitive decline along with focal neurological signs, enlarged ventricles, and significant white matter loss (see Blass et al., 1991). Unfortunately, a detailed pathological description of these series of cases was never published. Nonetheless, Alzheimer essentially corroborated Binswanger's work (Román et al., 1993), labeling the disorder as *Binswanger's disease*. During the late 19th and early 20th centuries, cerebrovascular dementia was a well-established clinical syndrome. Alzheimer wrote at least five papers on vascular dementia (VaD) and described clinical aspects of VaD that continue to be debated today (Libon, Price, Heilman, & Grossman, 2006).

The modern history of VaD dates from the seminal work of Hachinski (Hachinski, Lassen, & Marshall, 1974), who described what is now understood as multi-infarct dementia (MID; Hachinski, Lassen, N. A., & Marshall, 1974, Hachinski et al., 1975). Unfortunately, MID generally became associated with all types of vascular syndromes. Newer diagnostic criteria for VaD, including those from the Alzheimer's Disease Diagnostic and Treatment Centers (ADDTC; Chui et al., 1992) and the National Institute of Neurological Communicative Disorders and Stroke— Association Internationale pour la Recherché et l'Enseignement en Neurosciences (NINDS -AIREN criteria; Román et al., 1993), have reshaped our thinking about the role of cerebrovascular disease as related to dementia and normal aging.

Despite these advances, large-scale autopsy studies suggest that not all structural brain alterations related to cerebrovascular disease fit within a single diagnostic entity. Recent research suggests the presence of considerable overlap between the neuropathology underlying Alzheimer's disease (AD) and VaD (Cosentino, Jefferson, Chute, Kaplan, & Libon, 2004; Jellinger, 2002a; Pantoni & Garcia, 1997). This research indicates that subcortical white matter neuropathology can influence the symptoms and presentation of a dementia irrespective of dementia subtype (Jellinger, 2002a, 2002b; Libon et al., 2008; Luchsinger et al., 2005; Price, Jefferson, Merino, Heilman, & Libon, 2005).

DYSEXECUTIVE IMPAIRMENT ASSOCIATED WITH VAD

The Production of Perseverations

Consistent with theoretical models put forth by many other researchers (i.e., Dias, Robbins, & Roberts, 1997; Rogers, Andrews, Grasby, Brooks, & Robbins, 2000), the ability to establish and maintain a mental set can be operationally defined within the context of the the patient's ability to understand the nature of a task and to respond within the parameters of a task until the task is completed. When this cognitive function is disrupted, perseverations often emerge (Sandson & Albert, 1984). Prior research suggests that patients with VaD generate more perseverations than seen in patients with AD. Moreover, perseverations produced by patients with VaD are very different compared to the perseverations generated by patients with AD (Lamar et al., 1997). This is illustrated by observing the perseverations produced by VaD and AD when assessed with the Graphical Sequence Test (GST; Goldberg, 1986; Lamar et al., 1997). The GST is based on research originally carried out by Luria (1980; see Figure 6.1).

Individuals With VaD Consistently Produced *Hyperkinetic/Interminable* Perseverations

Patients diagnosed with VaD tend to produce *hyperkinetic/interminable* perseverations, suggesting an inability to appropriately terminate a motor response. On the other hand, patients with AD tend to produce "higher-order" or conceptual perseverations related to derailed or disrupted semantic access. For example, when presented with commands such as "draw a circle, draw a circle, draw a circle…" patients with VaD often continue to produce circles and fail to terminate their activity as requested (Figure 6.1, left panel). In VaD, these types of perseverations have been

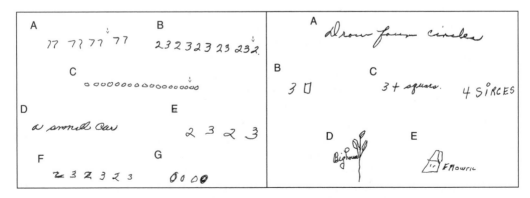

FIGURE 6.1 Left panel displays various hyperkinetic perseverations (A–G) made by individuals with vascular dementia (VaD) associated with white matter alterations. Right panel displays various semantic perseverations (A–E) made by individuals with Alzheimer's disease (AD) with little to no white matter alterations.

shown to correlate with impaired performance on tests of executive and motor functioning. Patients with AD produce very different perseverative errors. Thus, when asked to *write* the sentence "three squares and two circles," AD patients might *draw* three squares and two circles; or when asked to *draw* a house to the right of a flower, AD patients may write the word "house" next to the picture of a flower or vice versa (Figure 6.1, right panel). In AD, such perseverative errors have been shown to correlate with impaired performance on tests of naming and semantic knowledge. These contrasting patterns of dysexecutive impairment suggest that VaD is characterized by severe impairment involving the conscious termination of motor acts, whereas AD is characterized by the production of conceptual errors.

Higher-Order Verbal Concept Formation

This distinction between impairment in higher-order conceptual impairment versus lower-level pervasive impairment in appreciating mental set has also been observed on tests of verbal concept formation such as the Wechsler Adult Intelligence Scale-Revised (WAIS-R) Similarities subtest (Wechsler, 1997). When Giovannetti et al. (2001) recoded zero-point responses from the Similarities subtest to measure the ability to reflect proper mental set, patients with VaD generated proportionally more *out of* set errors that were clearly incorrect (i.e., *dog–lion—one barks and the other growls*). This is in contrast to patients with AD who generated errors that were vague, that is, *in-set*, but nonetheless superficially related to the given word pair (i.e., *dog–lion—they're alive*). The in-set errors produced by patients with AD were associated with poor performance on measures of language and semantic knowledge (Giovannetti et al., 2001). In sum, both studies indicate that patients with VaD present with a dysexecutive syndrome characterized by a pervasive impairment in the ability to engage and/ or terminate behavior as required by task demands.

Maintaining Mental Set and Inhibitory Control

Other aspects of the dysexecutive syndrome associated with VaD revolve around constructs related to interference inhibition, flexibility of response selection, and sustained attention. The differential impairment of these constructs related to executive control in VaD were observed in studying tests that assess mental control as measured with the Boston Revision of the Wechsler Memory Scale (WMS) Mental Control subtest (Wechsler, 1945). Research has demonstrated that VaD patients make more total errors than AD patients. Also, VaD patients tend to make more errors of commission than patients with AD (Lamar, Price, Davis, Kaplan, & Libon, 2002). The pattern of impairment in VaD was most evident at the beginning and end of each mental control task, whereas errors in AD were equally distributed across time points of the task (Lamar et al., 2002), suggesting that vascular disease derails the ability to select target stimuli and reject or inhibit erroneous responses.

This pattern of behavior has also been observed on tests of letter fluency ("FAS") where output was analyzed across the four 15-second test epochs. When controlled for total output, patients with VaD generated their larger percentage of words in the first 15 seconds of the test as compared to AD patients and healthy controls (Lamar et al., 2002; Figure 6.2). After the first 15 seconds, epoch patients with VaD demonstrated a precipitous drop in output. In contrast, AD patients were no different from healthy controls regarding their percentage of output for the rest of the test (Figure 6.2).

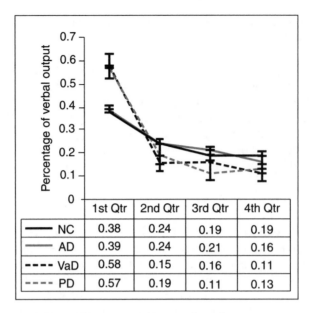

	1st Qtr	2nd Qtr	3rd Qtr	4th Qtr
NC	0.38	0.24	0.19	0.19
AD	0.39	0.24	0.21	0.16
VaD	0.58	0.15	0.16	0.11
PD	0.57	0.19	0.11	0.13

FIGURE 6.2 The proportion of letter "S" output per 15-second epoch.
VaD, vascular dementia; PD, Parkinson's disease; NC, normal controls.

Thus, in VaD, such behavior suggests an inability to actively engage inhibitory mechanisms as well as a more overarching difficulty initiating and maintaining cognitive control for the duration of performance. As with their performance on the Mental Control test described previously, the majority of errors made by VaD patients were errors of commission, suggesting differential impairment in inhibitory control.

Working Memory and Temporal Reordering

The model of working memory put forth by Baddeley, Logie, Bressi, Della Sala, and Spinnler (1986) suggests that the brain has multiple, sensory-specific, lower-level buffer systems involved in the storage and rehearsal of information and a higher-level central executive mechanism responsible for overseeing these buffer systems and the mental manipulation of information (Baddeley & Hitch, 1994). In prior research, we have found that these cognitive processes are particularly impaired in VaD compared to AD, suggesting significant problems with disengagement and temporal reordering (Lamar, Swenson, Kaplan, & Libon, 2004). Recently, we have developed and administered a new Backward Digit Task (BDT) to patients with VaD and AD to disambiguate specific components of Baddeley's model of working memory. This new BDT (Lamar et al., 2007) asked patients to repeat 3, 4, and 5 numbers in reverse order. However, responses were specifically scored to distinguish lower-level short-term storage and rehearsal deficits versus higher-level disengagement and temporal reordering deficits. It is interesting to note that when VaD and AD patients were compared, there were no differences in indices designed to measure lower-level short-term storage and rehearsal. In contrast, VaD patients displayed significant deficits in higher-level disengagement and temporal reordering compared to AD patients (Lamar et al., 2007). This pattern of deficits appears to be due to an inability to disengage from or inhibit overlearned and automatic memories (Lamar et al., 1997; Stuss, Shallice, Alexander, & Picton, 1995).

THEORETICAL AND NEUROANATOMICAL CONSIDERATIONS

When viewed as a whole, the clinical presentations outlined on the previous pages suggest that the dysexecutive syndrome associated with VaD is rather pervasive, involving a variety of important theoretical constructs such as pathological inertia, mental bradyphrenia and disengagement, and temporal reordering deficits. In contrast, dysexecutive syndrome associated with AD appears to be restricted, context specific, and related to lexical/semantic operations. As suggested by Luria (1980) and others (Goldberg, 1986; Goldberg & Bilder, 1987), our data support the idea that some aspects of executive functioning are related to specific, higher-level disorders of cognition while other aspects of executive control are more rudimentary and pervasive. From the view point of diagnosis, the neuropathology of VaD often differentially impacts the frontal lobes, whereas the neuropathology associated with AD revolves more around circumscribed temporal lobe involvement. This model suggests that disruption of these prefrontal–basal ganglia–thalamic pathways (Alexander, DeLong, & Strick, 1986) explains the pervasive dysexecutive syndrome associated with VaD. It should be noted that comorbid vascular diseases can be present in patients with AD.

SUMMARY

In sum, the research reviewed in this chapter suggests that the dysexecutive syndrome associated with VaD is caused by impairment in separate but related cognitive concepts; that is, pathological inertia, mental bradyphrenia, disengagement, and temporal reordering. Data from our laboratory suggest that the dysexecutive syndrome seen in VaD tends to be pervasive regardless of the task at hand or the modality used. In VaD, underlying disease processes prohibit adequate engagement in task demands and, when engaged, impair the preservation of relevant behavior and disrupt the inhibition of irrelevant responses.

REFERENCES

Alexander, G. E., DeLong, M. R., & Strick, P. L. (1986). Parallel organization of functionally segregated circuits linking basal ganglia and cortex. *Annual Review` of Neuroscience, 9,* 357–381.

Baddeley, A., & Hitch, G. J. (1994). Developments in the concept of working memory. *Neuropsychology, 8,* 485–493.

Baddeley, A., Logie, R., Bressi, S., Della Sala, S., & Spinnler, H. (1986). Dementia and working memory. *The Quarterly Journal of Experimental Psychology, 38*(4), 603–618.

Blass, J. P., Hoyer, S., & Nitsch, R. (1991). A translation of Otto Binswanger's article, "The delineation of the generalized progressive paralyses" 1894. *Archives of Neurology, 48*(9), 961–972.

Chui, H. C., Victoroff, J. I., Margolin, D., Jagust, W., Shankle, R., & Katzman, R. (1992). Criteria for the diagnosis of ischemic vascular dementia proposed by the State of California Alzheimer's Disease Diagnostic and Treatment Centers. *Neurology, 42*(3 Pt 1), 473–480.

Cosentino, S., Jefferson, A., Chute, D. L., Kaplan, E., & Libon, D. J. (2004). Clock drawing errors in dementia: Neuropsychological and neuroanatomical considerations. *Cognitive and Behavioral Neurology, 17*(2), 74–84.

Dias, R., Robbins, T. W., & Roberts, A. C. (1997). Dissociable forms of inhibitory control within prefrontal cortex with an analog of the Wisconsin Card Sort Test: restriction to novel situations and independence from "on-line" processing. *The Journal of Neuroscience, 17*(23), 9285–9297.

Giovannetti, T., Lamar, M., Cloud, B. S., Swenson, R., Fein, D., Kaplan, E., & Libon, D. J. (2001). Different underlying mechanisms for deficits in concept formation in dementia. *Archives of Clinical Neuropsychology, 16*(6), 547–560.

Goldberg, E. (1986). Varieties of perseveration: A comparison of two taxonomies. *Journal of Clinical and Experimental Neuropsychology, 8*(6), 710–726.

Goldberg, E., & Bilder, R. (1987). The frontal lobes and hierarchical organization of cognitive control. In E. Perecman (Ed.), *The frontal lobes revised* (pp. 159–187). New York, NY: IRBN Press.

Hachinski, V. C., Iliff, L. D., Zilhka, E., Du Boulay, G. H., McAllister, V. L., Marshall, J., . . . Symon, L. (1975). Cerebral blood flow in dementia. *Archives of Neurology, 32*(9), 632–637.

Hachinski, V. C., Lassen, N. A., & Marshall, J. (1974). Multi-infarct dementia. A cause of mental deterioration in the elderly. *Lancet, 2*(7874), 207–210.

Jellinger, K. A. (2002a). Alzheimer disease and cerebrovascular pathology: An update. *Journal of Neural Transmission, 109*(5–6), 813–836.

Jellinger, K. A. (2002b). The pathology of ischemic-vascular dementia: An update. *Journal of the Neurological Sciences, 203–204*, 153–157.

Lamar, M., Podell, K., Carew, T. G., Cloud, B. S., Resh, R., Kennedy, C., . . . Libon, D. J. (1997). Perseverative behavior in Alzheimer's disease and subcortical ischemic vascular dementia. *Neuropsychology, 11*(4), 523–534.

Lamar, M., Price, C. C., Davis, K. L., Kaplan, E., & Libon, D. J. (2002). Capacity to maintain mental set in dementia. *Neuropsychologia, 40*(4), 435–445.

Lamar, M., Price, C. C., Libon, D. J., Penney, D. L., Kaplan, E., Grossman, M., & Heilman, K. M. (2007). Alterations in working memory as a function of leukoaraiosis in dementia. *Neuropsychologia, 45*(2), 245–254.

Lamar, M., Swenson, R., Kaplan, E., & Libon, D. J. (2004). Characterizing alterations in executive functioning across distinct subtypes of cortical and subcortical dementia. *The Clinical Neuropsychologist, 18*(1), 22–31.

Libon, D. J., Price, C. C., Giovannetti, T., Swenson, R., Bettcher, B. M., Heilman, K. M., & Pennisi, A. (2008). Linking MRI hyperintensities with patterns of neuropsychological impairment: Evidence for a threshold effect. *Stroke, 39*(3), 806–813.

Libon, D. J., Price, C. C., Heilman, K. M., & Grossman, M. (2006). Alzheimer's "other dementia." *Cognitive and Behavioral Neurology, 19*(2), 112–116.

Luchsinger, J. A., Reitz, C., Honig, L. S., Tang, M. X., Shea, S., & Mayeux, R. (2005). Aggregation of vascular risk factors and risk of incident Alzheimer disease. *Neurology, 65*(4), 545–551.

Luria, A. R. (1980). *Higher cortical functions* (pp. 246–360). New York, NY: Basic Books.

Pantoni, L., & Garcia, J. H. (1997). Pathogenesis of leukoaraiosis: A review. *Stroke, 28*(3), 652–659.

Price, C. C., Jefferson, A. L., Merino, J. G., Heilman, K. M., & Libon, D. J. (2005). Subcortical vascular dementia: Integrating neuropsychological and neuroradiologic data. *Neurology, 65*(3), 376–382.

Rogers, R. D., Andrews, T. C., Grasby, P. M., Brooks, D. J., & Robbins, T. W. (2000). Contrasting cortical and subcortical activations produced by attentional-set shifting and reversal learning in humans. *Journal of Cognitive Neuroscience, 12*(1), 142–162.

Román, G. C., Tatemichi, T. K., Erkinjuntti, T., Cummings, J. L., Masdeu, J. C., Garcia, J. H.,...Hofman, A. (1993). Vascular dementia: Diagnostic criteria for research studies. Report of the NINDS-AIREN International Workshop. *Neurology, 43*(2), 250–260.

Sandson, J., & Albert, M. L. (1984). Varieties of perseveration. *Neuropsychologia, 22*(6), 715–732.

Stuss, D. T., Shallice, T., Alexander, M. P., & Picton, T. W. (1995). A multidisciplinary approach to anterior attentional functions. *Annals of the New York Academy of Sciences, 769*, 191–211.

Wechsler, D. A. (1945). A standardized memory scale for clinical use. *Journal of Psychology, 19*, 87–95.

Wechsler, D. A. (1997). *The Wechsler Adult Intelligence Scale-III*. San Antonio, TX: Psychology Corporation.

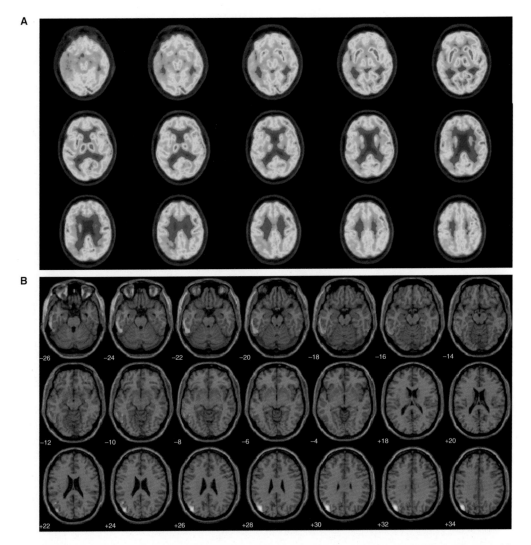

FIGURE 2.2 ^{18}FDG-PET imaging (A) and the relative SPM analysis at *p* < .001 threshold (B) of a 58-year-old man affected by amnestic MCI. The images show hypometabolism of the left medial and inferior temporal cortex and inferior parietal lobule. The patient clinically converted to AD after 18 months, as seen from PET acquisition.

AD, Alzheimer's disease; FDG, fluorodeoxyglucose; MCI, mild cognitive impairment.

Images courtesy of Prof. D. Perani, Nuclear Medicine, Vita-Salute University and San Raffaele Scientific Institute, Milan, Italy.

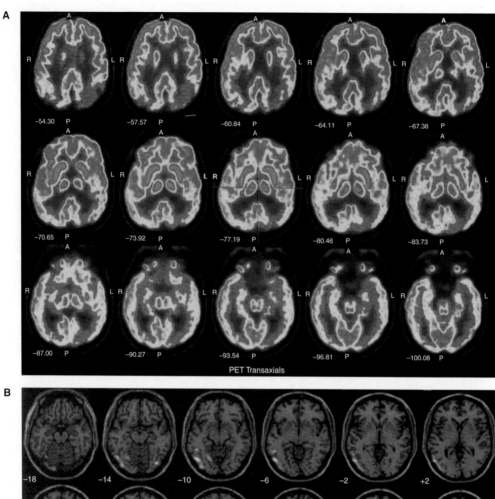

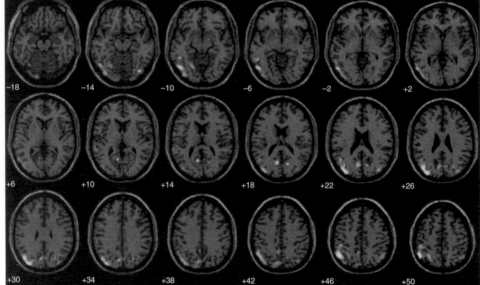

FIGURE 2.3 ¹⁸FDG-PET imaging (A) and the relative SPM analysis at $p < .001$ threshold (B) of a 67-year-old man affected by PCA. The image shows prominent hypometabolism of the posterior brain regions bilaterally, involving the temporoparietal and occipital cortex bilaterally, mostly on the left side.

FDG, fluorodeoxyglucose; PCA, posterior cortical atrophy; SPM, statistical parametric mapping.

Images courtesy of Prof. D. Perani, Nuclear Medicine, Vita-Salute University and San Raffaele Scientific Institute, Milan, Italy.

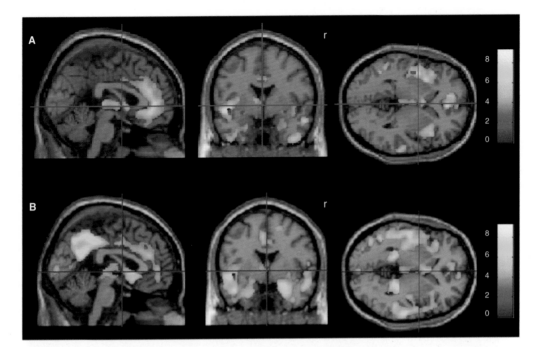

FIGURE 2.5 VBM analysis on bvFTD (A) and AD (B) samples, compared to healthy matched subjects, showing different patterns of gray matter density loss. (A) bvFTD: anterior cingulated cortex, medial and orbitobasal frontal cortex, temporal poles, and amygdala and insula bilaterally; (B) AD: hippocampus, para-hippocampal regions, amygdala bilaterally, and parietal and lateral posterior superior temporal regions. All images are displayed at $p < .005$ corrected threshold.

AD, Alzheimer's disease; bvFTD, behavioral variant of frontotemporal dementia; r, right; VBM, voxel-based morphometry.

Images courtesy of Dr. A. Canessa, Vita-Salute University, Milan, Italy.

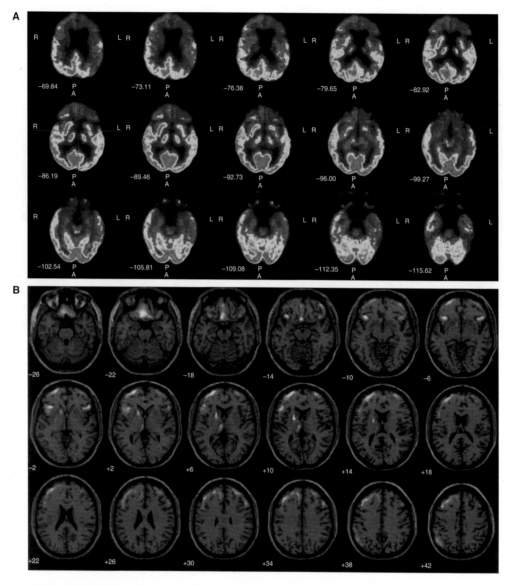

FIGURE 2.6 [18]FDG-PET imaging (A) and the relative SPM analysis at $p < .001$ threshold (B) of a 53-year-old woman affected by bvFTD. The image shows bilateral cortico-subcortical hypometabolism, more pronounced on the left side and mostly involving the orbitobasal, dorsolateral, medial frontal, and inferior parietal cortices.

bvFTD, behavioral variant of frontotemporal dementia; FDG, fluorodeoxyglucose; SPM, statistical parametric mapping.

Images courtesy of Prof. D. Perani, Nuclear Medicine, Vita-Salute University and San Raffaele Scientific Institute, Milan, Italy.

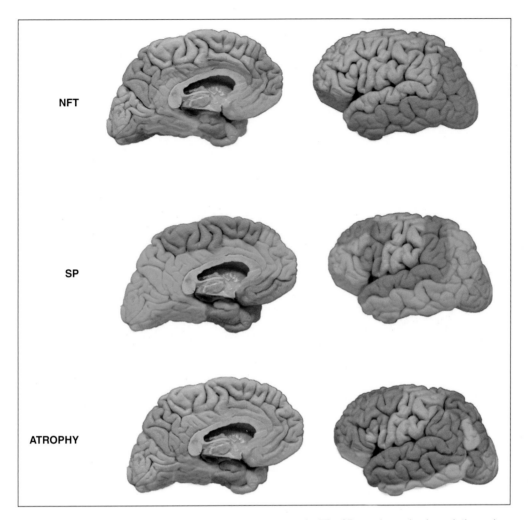

FIGURE 4.1 Representation of the progression of the spread of NFTs, SPs, and atrophy through the early (red), middle (green), and late (purple) stages of Alzheimer's disease. Based on Braak and Braak (1991) and other sources cited in the text.

NFTs, neurofibrillary tangles; SPs, senile plaques.

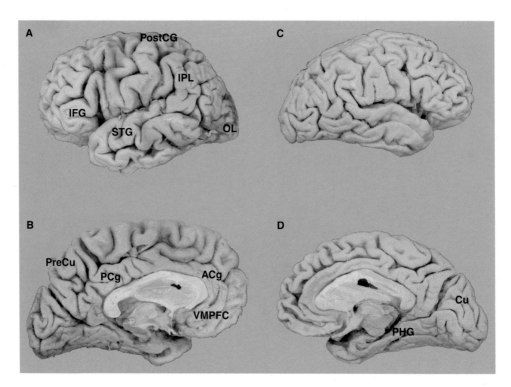

FIGURE 4.2 Lateral and medial surfaces of brain hemispheres from individuals with early-stage Alzheimer's disease (left hemisphere, A, B) and late-stage Alzheimer's disease (right hemisphere, C, D) showing the extent of atrophy. The presence of NFTs and SPs was histologically confirmed in the opposite hemisphere.

ACg, anterior cingulate gyrus; Cu, cuneus of occipital lobe; IFG, inferior frontal gyrus; IPL, inferior parietal lobule; NFT, neurofibrillary tangles; OL, occipital lobe; PCg, posterior cingulate gyrus; PHG, parahippocampal gyrus; PostCG, postcentral gyrus; PreCu, precuneus of parietal lobe; SP, senile plaques; STG, superior temporal gyrus; VMPFC, ventromedial prefrontal cortex.

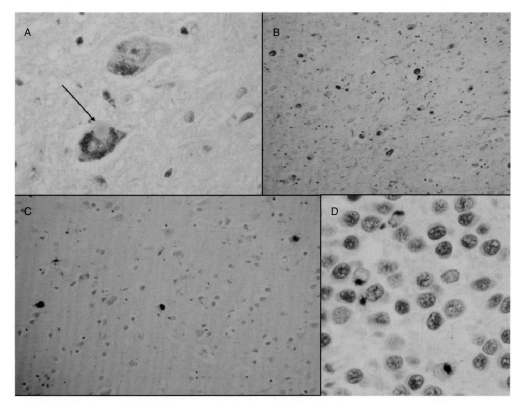

FIGURE 7.1 Neuropathology of an 88-year-old female with dementia with Lewy bodies. (A) Hematoxylin and eosin histological staining showing a classical Lewy body (arrow) in the substantia nigra; (B) alpha-synuclein immunostaining in the amygdala showing cortical Lewy bodies and Lewy neurites; (C) alpha-synuclein immunostaining in the frontal cortex showing cortical Lewy bodies; (D) TDP-43-positive inclusions in the dentate gyrus. The neuropathological study in this patient also showed amyloid plaques in the neocortex and neuritic plaques and neurofibrillary tangles in the hippocampus.

Courtesy of Dr. R. L. Hamilton, Department of Pathology (Neuropathology Division), University of Pittsburgh Medical Center, Pittsburgh, PA.

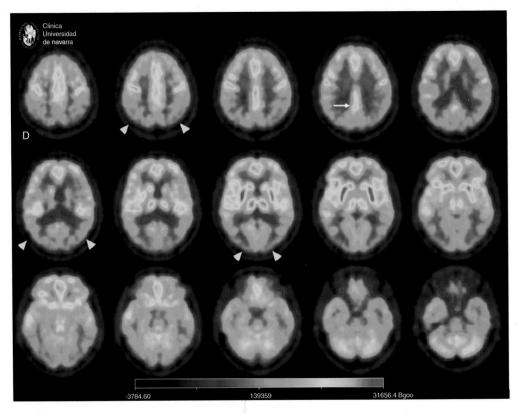

FIGURE 7.2 ^{18}F-FDG PET scan showing parietotemporal and occipital cortices, hypometabolism in a patient with DLB (white head arrows). The white arrow points to the posterior cingulated cortex, demonstrating the cingulate island sign.

DLB, dementia with Lewy bodies.

Courtesy of Dr. Javier Arbizu, Department of Nuclear Medicine, Clínica Universidad de Navarra, Pamplona, Spain.

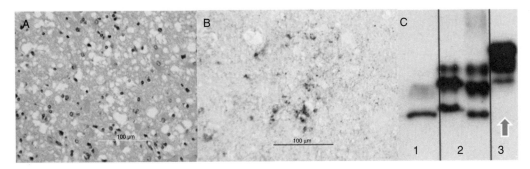

FIGURE 12.2 Definite diagnosis of prion disease requires neuropathological examination. (A) Hematoxylin and eosin stain of the temporal lobe of a patient with prion disease. (B) Immunohistochemistry using 3F4 antibody of the hippocampus of a patient with prion disease. (C) Western blot of a brain homogenate subjected to proteinase K; lanes 1 and 2 display a PrP$^{27-30}$ band seen in prion disease compared to lane 3 from a normal control (arrow).

CHAPTER 7

Dementia With Lewy Bodies

Mario Riverol and Oscar L. López

Dementia with Lewy bodies (DLB) is a clinical syndrome characterized by progressive dementia, cognitive fluctuations, visual hallucinations (VH), and parkinsonism. Other associated features are auditory and olfactory hallucinations; delusions; hypersomnia; frequent falls; syncope, transient loss of consciousness; neuroleptic sensitivity (McKeith et al., 1996); major depression (Klatka, Louis, & Schiffer, 1996); rapid eye movement (REM); sleep behavior disorder (Ferman et al., 1999); an abnormal EEG (Briel et al., 1999); and urinary incontinence (Del-Ser, Munoz, & Hachinski, 1996). Although neuropathological series suggested that DLB is the second most common type of neurodegenerative dementia in older people after Alzheimer's disease (AD; McKeith et al., 1996), there are few population-based studies assessing its prevalence and incidence. The estimated prevalence of DLB was in a range from 0% to 5% with regard to the general population, and from 0% to 30.5% of all dementia cases, while incidence was estimated in 100 to 112 cases per 100,000 person-years (Perez, Helmer, Dartigues, Auriacombe, & Tison, 2010; Zaccai, McCracken, & Brayne, 2005). DLB incidence increases with age and is higher in men (Perez et al., 2010).

The first reports of DLB cases took place during the 1960s and 1970s in Japan. In 1961, Okazaki, Lipkin, and Aronson reported two patients with dementia and parkinsonism with cortical neuronal inclusions similar to the brain-stem Lewy bodies (LB) seen in Parkinson's disease (PD). Kosaka, Oyanagi, Matsushita, and Hori (1976) and Kosaka (1978) later described three patients with dementia and parkinsonism who presented LB-like inclusions in the brain cortex as well as AD pathology at autopsy. In 1984, Kosaka, Yoshimura, Ikeda, and Budka (1984) and Kosaka (1990) proposed the term *diffuse Lewy body disease* for this neuropathological entity characterized clinically by a dementia–parkinsonism syndrome. However, nowadays the term DLB (McKeith et al., 1996) is preferred from a series of diagnostic names given to this entity that included *cortical LB dementia* (Gibb, Luthert, Janota, & Lantos, 1989), *dementia associated with cortical LB* (Byrne, Lennox, & Goodwin-Austen, 1991), *senile dementia of LB type* (Perry, Irving, Blessed, Fairbairn, & Perry, 1990), and *diffuse LB disease* (Kosaka, 1990). The term *Lewy variant of AD* has been used to describe cases where the LB coexist with AD pathology (Hansen et al., 1990), and LB disease has been used to describe all the disorders that are characterized by the presence of LB in the nervous system such as PD (with and without dementia), DLB, pure autonomic failure, and LB dysphagia (Kövari, Horvath, & Bouras, 2009).

NEUROPATHOLOGY

Neuropathological Features

DLB is characterized by the presence of LB pathology (brain stem and cortical LBs, and also Lewy neurites) throughout the brain (Table 7.1 and Figure 7.1). LBs are intra-cytoplasmic neuronal inclusions containing α-synuclein and ubiquitin. Brain stem or classic LBs are large, spherical, eosinophilic inclusions surrounded by a clear halo located in the locus coeruleus, the dopaminergic neurons of the substantia nigra, and other subcortical nuclei (McKeith et al., 1996). Cortical LBs are less eosinophilic and less well-defined inclusions predominantly situated in the hypothalamus, basal fore-brain, amygdala, and temporal cortex, with smaller involvement of frontal and pos-terior cortices (Braak et al., 2003; Kosaka et al., 1984; Kosaka, 1990). Cortical LBs are not easy to identify with classic histological staining and are best detected by inmu-nohistochemistry with anti-ubiquitin and anti-α-synuclein antibodies. Interestingly, cortical LBs can also be detected in up to 60% of AD cases, mainly in the amygdala (Hamilton, 2000). Lewy neurites are α-synuclein inclusions detected by inmunohis-tochemistry and situated in neural processes, mainly in limbic and temporal lobe structures but also in the striatum (Dickson et al., 1991; Kövari et al., 2009; Tsuboi, Uchikado, & Dickson, 2007).

There are other associated pathological features in DLB such as spongiform change (or microvacuolation), neuronal loss, and AD pathology (amyloid plaques and neurofibrillary tangles [NFTs]). Microvacuolization, as seen in prion diseases, is observed in the amygdala and basal forebrain (Dickson et al., 1987) and neural loss is especially important in the substantia nigra, locus coeruleus, and nucleus basalis of Meynert (McKeith et al., 1996). AD pathology is seen in most, but not all, DLB cases (pure diffuse LB pathology forms vs. diffuse LB pathology and concomitant AD pathology forms). Amyloid plaques in DLB differ from AD by a near lack of neuritic changes and when detected, they are circumscribed to limbic areas accompanying

TABLE 7.1 Major Pathological Features of Lewy Body Disease

PATHOLOGICAL FINDINGS	PD	PDD	DLB	AD
Substantia nigra cell loss	Prominent (mainly in the medioventral part)	Prominent (mainly in the medioventral part)	Milder (mainly in the dorsolateral part)	Minimal or none
Lewy bodies	Brain stem	Diffuse neocortical and transitional	Diffuse neocortical and transitional	Amygdala (in up to 60% of cases)
Amyloid plaques	None	Variable (less frequent than in DLB); mostly diffuse plaques	Variable; mostly diffuse plaques	Many neuritic plaques
NFT (Braak stage)	0–III	0–IV	0–IV	V–VI
Striatal LB pathology	Minimal	Extensive	Extensive	None

AD, Alzheimer's disease; DLB, dementia with Lewy bodies; LB, Lewy body; NFT, neurofibrillary tangle; PD, Parkinson's disease; PDD, Parkinson's disease dementia.

Source: Data from Kövari et al. (2009) and Tsuboi et al. (2007).

NFTs (Dickson et al., 1989). NFTs are less frequent in DLB than in AD, and they are usually confined to limbic regions (Hansen et al., 1990). Interestingly, those DLB patients with AD pathology have a higher prevalence of the apolipoprotein E (ApoE) ε4 allele (Singleton et al., 2002). The relative importance of concomitant AD pathology in DLB remains unclear, but some authors suggest that AD and PD represent the end points of a spectrum with intermediate stages (Hansen et al., 1990). More intriguing is the presence of transactive response (TAR)-DNA-binding protein-43 (TDP-43) inclusions in a subgroup of patients with DLB and AD pathology (Figure 7.1D), suggesting that all these abnormal proteins can synergistically promote the aggregation and deposition of each other (Nakashima-Yasuda et al., 2007).

Neuropathological Classification

There are two classification systems to assess LB pathology distribution in LB disorders. In 2003, Braak et al. proposed a staging for the LB pathology of idiopathic PD. Stages 1 and 2 specify involvement of the olfactory regions and lower brain stem. In Stages 3 and 4, α-synuclein aggregations spread to the midbrain, affecting first

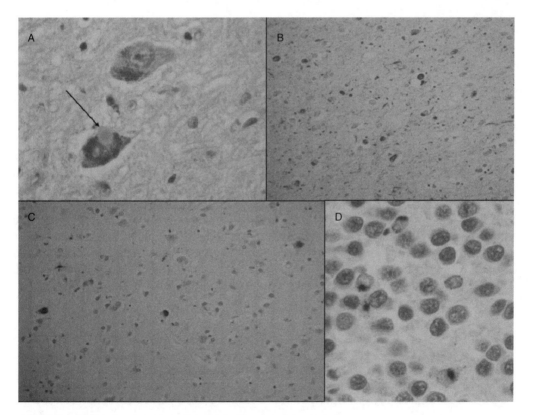

FIGURE 7.1 *(See color insert.)* Neuropathology of an 88-year-old female with dementia with Lewy bodies. (A) Hematoxylin and eosin histological staining showing a classical Lewy body (arrow) in the substantia nigra; (B) alpha-synuclein immunostaining in the amygdala showing cortical Lewy bodies and Lewy neurites; (C) alpha-synuclein immunostaining in the frontal cortex showing cortical Lewy bodies; (D) TDP-43-positive inclusions in the dentate gyrus. The neuropathological study in this patient also showed amyloid plaques in the neocortex and neuritic plaques and neurofibrillary tangles in the hippocampus.

Courtesy of Dr. R. L. Hamilton, Department of Pathology (Neuropathology Division), University of Pittsburgh Medical Center, Pittsburgh, PA.

the substantia nigra and the basal forebrain, and then the transenthorhinal cortex and CA2 region of the hippocampus. Finally, Stages 5 and 6 indicate a progressive spread of LB pathology into the neocortex. These authors suggested that LB pathology follows a caudo-rostral pattern, which is correlated with symptoms and clinical progression, giving a unitary concept of the pathogenesis of LB disease. However, only young-onset PD cases follow the Braak staging scheme, while those patients with PD who develop an early dementia syndrome present severe diffuse neocortical α-synuclein pathology (Halliday, Hely, Reid, & Morris, 2008).

The revised consensus pathological guidelines for DLB diagnosis proposed a semiquantitative assessment of LB density based on α-synuclein immunohistochemistry and took into account the extent of AD pathology (Table 7.2). LB pathology staging distinguishes three different patterns: brain stem predominant, limbic/transitional, and diffuse neocortical. This classification system indicates the likelihood that the neuropathological findings explain the clinical syndrome of DLB; this is directly related to the severity of LB pathology, and inversely related to AD pathology (McKeith et al., 2005). Nevertheless, this classification fails to categorize a large number of dementia subjects with LB pathology (Leverenz et al., 2008).

Clinicopathological Correlations

In LBD, LB density, but not amyloid plaque or NFT burden, is correlated with dementia severity (Haroutunian et al., 2000; Samuel, Galasko, Masliah, & Hansen, 1996). Nevertheless, neurofibrillary pathology seems to affect the clinical characteristics of DLB. In fact, DLB patients with low Braak NFT stages and load show more core clinical features of DLB, while those with higher Braak NFT stages and density show a clinical pattern more similar to AD (Merdes et al., 2003).

There are specific neuropathological findings associated with DLB symptoms. For example, the presence and onset of VH are associated with high LB density in the amygdala, parahippocampus, and the inferior temporal cortex (Harding, Broe, & Halliday, 2002). These structures seem to be implicated in generation of complex visual images, while the occipital lobe is involved in simpler visual processes. The hippocampus is also affected in DLB, but the pattern is different from that seen in AD. The neuronal loss mainly involves the presubiculum and Lewy neurites concentrated in the CA2/3 region, but the CA1 and subiculum regions, affected in AD, are spared. The presubiculum has reciprocal connections with the dorsolateral prefrontal cortex,

TABLE 7.2 Revised Consensus Pathological Guidelines for DLB Diagnosis Assessing the Likelihood That the Pathological Findings Are Associated With a DLB Clinical Syndrome

		AD PATHOLOGY		
		Nia-Reagan Low (Braak Stage 0–II)	Nia-Reagan Intermediate (Braak Stage III–IV)	Nia-Reagan High (Braak Stage V–VI)
LB PATHOLOGY	Brain stem predominant	Low	Low	Low
	Limbic/Transitional	High	Intermediate	Low
	Diffuse neocortical	High	High	Intermediate

AD, Alzheimer's disease; DLB, dementia with Lewy bodies; LB, Lewy body; NIA, National Institute on Aging.

Source: McKeith et al. (2005).

which may explain the working memory problems seen in these subjects (Harding, Lakay, Halliday, 2002).

ETIOLOGY AND PATHOGENESIS

DLB and other entities such as PD and multiple system atrophy (MSA) have been grouped under the term *synucleinopathies* due to the existence of α-synuclein inclusions in the brain. Alpha-synuclein is a normal presynaptic protein implicated in vesicle production and neurotransmitter release, especially dopamine (Schulz-Schaeffer, 2010). This protein is natively unfolded, but if it accumulates it aggregates into soluble oligomers that later could form insoluble fibrils, the main component of LBs. The cause of the presence of α-synuclein aggregates is unknown. A possible explanation is that α-synuclein aggregates because it is abnormally processed; for example, in the case of a damaged or mutated α-synuclein, an overexpression of this protein or a dysfunction in the cellular mechanisms that remove abnormal proteins, such as the ubiquitin-proteasome system and autophagy-lysosome pathway. There is evidence suggesting that soluble α-synuclein oligomers are the pathogenic species that cause neural cell death (Angot, Steiner, Hansen, Li, & Brundin, 2010).

Genetics

Genetics can give us some clues about the pathogenic mechanisms in DLB. This disease occurs sporadically in most cases, but familial forms have been reported. In fact, recent discoveries confirm that genetic determinants of DLB overlap substantially with those of PD, suggesting that both entities share pathophysiological and etiological factors. The first evidence for a genetic basis form of DLB was reached with the discovery of α-synuclein mutations (*SNCA*), a cause of autosomal dominant PD. Some point mutations of this gene are associated with PD, but also with Parkinson's disease dementia (PDD) and DLB (Zarranz et al., 2004). Interestingly, mutated α-synuclein is poorly degraded by the chaperone-mediated autophagy and it also inhibits the degradation of other substrates (Cuervo, Stefanis, Fredenburg, Lansbury, & Sulzer, 2004), resulting in the accumulation of proteins in the cytoplasm. *SNCA* multiplications, triplications more than duplications, have also been associated with PDD and DLB (Bonifati, 2008). In these cases, the overexpression of this protein could explain the formation of cytosolic aggregates (Angot et al., 2010). DLB cases have also been associated with mutations in the dardarin gene (*LRRK2*), a cause of an autosomal dominant familial PD (Bonifati, 2008). Unfortunately, the physiological function of this protein in the nervous system is still unclear. Another, relatively recent advance in the genetic field is the discovery of a locus for autosomal dominant familial DLB at 2q35-q36 in a Belgian family. This region overlaps with the PARK11 locus, linked to autosomal dominant familial PD (Bogaerts et al., 2007). However, more studies will be needed to disentangle the role of these mutations in the genetics of LB disorders.

The genetic risk factors for sporadic DLB such as the ApoE and mutations in the glucocerebrosidase (*GBA*) gene have been investigated. The ε4 allele of the *ApoE* gene, the most important genetic risk factor for AD, also seems to be a risk factor for DLB with AD pathology (Galasko et al., 1994; Singleton, et al., 2002; Tsuang et al., 2005). It does not appear to be a significant effect of *ApoE* ε4 on DLB onset or duration, but survival rates may be similarly reduced in both DLB and AD *ApoE* ε4 carriers (Singleton et al., 2002). Glucocerebrosidase is a lysosomal enzyme that catalyzes the hydrolysis of the cellular membrane glucocerebroside to ceramide and glucose. Homozygous and compound heterozygous mutations in GBA result in a default enzyme that causes an autosomal recessive lysosomal storage disorder called Gaucher's disease. The presence of parkinsonism in some patients with Gaucher's disease and their relatives results in studies to investigate GBA mutations in PD and other parkinsonisms (Velayati, Yu, & Sidransky, 2010). Indeed, recent studies found a strong association between *GBA* mutations and PD and DLB (Clark et al., 2009; Goker-Alpan et al., 2008; Sidransky et al., 2009). The mechanisms underlying this association are unknown, although a dysfunction in the autophagy-lysosomal pathway has been proposed (Velayati et al., 2010).

CLINICAL PRESENTATION

The central feature required for a diagnosis of DLB is the presence of dementia: a progressive cognitive decline of sufficient magnitude to interfere with normal social or occupational function. In most cases, but not all of them, cognitive decline is the presenting feature. The pattern of neuropsychological impairment in DLB differs significantly from that seen in AD and other dementias. DLB patients show greater deficits in attentional-executive and visuospatial function (Calderon et al., 2001; Collerton, Burn, McKeith, & O'Brien, 2003), while AD patients have worse memory and naming (Ferman et al., 2006).

The most common deficits seen in DLB are those associated with attentional-executive processes. In fact, these patients are more impaired on measures of attention and fluctuating attention than AD patients (Ballard et al., 2001a; Bradshaw, Saling, Anderson, Hopwood, & Brodtmann, 2006; Metzler-Baddeley, 2007), as well as in their activities of daily living. Some studies have also shown that patients with DLB performed worse than AD on executive function tests, including working memory, inhibitory control, and set shifting (Calderon et al., 2001; Collerton et al., 2003; Crowell, Luis, Cox, & Mullan, 2007). Interestingly, one study showed that DLB and frontotemporal dementia patients had a similar profile of executive dysfunction (Johns et al., 2009). The neural basis of the attentional impairment in DLB is probably related to cholinergic deficiency owing to the neuronal loss in the nucleus basalis of Meynert. The fact that cholinergic neuronal loss and cortical cholinergic deficiency are seen early in DLB (Tiraboschi et al., 2002), and treatment with cholinesterase inhibitors improve attention in these patients (McKeith et al., 2000) seems to support this hypothesis. The executive dysfunction in DLB may be related to LB pathology in the frontal and cingulate cortices, areas classically associated with executive aspects of attention.

Visuoperceptual and spatial functions have been extensively assessed in DLB patients. The clock drawing test and tests requiring individuals copy geometric figures are more impaired than in AD patients (Ala, Hughes, Kyrouac, Ghobrial, & Elble, 2001; Collerton et al., 2003; Metzler-Baddeley, 2007; Mosimann et al., 2004; Noe et al., 2004). Usually, in AD patients, the visuoconstructional disability is proportionate to global cognitive impairment, as measured with the Mini-Mental State Examination (MMSE), while in DLB there is no significant correlation between MMSE scores and constructional ability (Cormack, Aarsland, Ballard, & Tovée, 2004). DLB subjects also perform worse than AD subjects in simple tasks such as discriminating object size and form and on the overlapping figures tasks. Moreover, visual perception is worse in subjects with VH (Mori et al., 2000; Mosimann et al., 2004), indicating that visual perceptual deficits in patients with DLB predispose them to VH. Hence, the neuropsychological findings show early and pronounced visuoperceptual impairment affecting object and space perception in DLB, and possibly, damage of both the ventral occipitotemporal stream and the dorsal occipitoparietal stream (which mediate object recognition and visuospatial analysis, respectively; Metzler-Baddeley, 2007). Functional neuroimaging studies have shown occipital cortex dysfunction, affecting not only the primary visual area, but also the association cortex in DLB (Albin et al., 1996; Colloby et al., 2002; Higuchi et al., 2000; Ishii et al., 1998, 1999; Minoshima et al., 2001; Perneczky et al., 2008).

Core Symptoms

Core features of DLB are fluctuating cognition, recurrent and persistent VH, and parkinsonism. Fluctuation in cognitive function resembles signs of delirium with no identifiable precipitant and implies a change in cognition, abilities, and arousal that last for minutes, hours, or even days. Fluctuations are described as brief interruptions of consciousness, periods of confusion or diminished attention, or excessive somnolence. But cognitive fluctuations have proven to be difficult to characterize. Moreover, the prevalence of fluctuations in DLB samples ranges from 10% to 80% due to low inter-rater reliability (Ferman & Boeve, 2007; Mega et al., 1996). Some characteristics of cognitive fluctuations can help in distinguishing DLB from AD. For example, the combination of daytime drowsiness and lethargy, daytime sleep, staring into space for long periods of time, and episodes of disorganized speech are highly predictive of DLB (Ferman et al., 2004). These fluctuating symptoms have a great impact on the subject's life, affecting cognitive performance and activities of daily living (Ballard, Walker, O'Brien, Rowan, & McKeith, 2001c).

VH are commonly present early in the course of the DLB, and in early dementia stages they are the best positive predictor of this disease at autopsy (Tiraboschi et al., 2006). VH are typically recurrent, well formed, and complex. Patients frequently report seeing people, animals, and objects (Mosimann et al., 2006). Hallucinations in other sensory modalities can occur, especially auditory, but generally in combination with VH (Ferman & Boeve, 2007). Subjects with DLB and VH show more severe visuoperceptual dysfunction compared to those who do not have them (Mori et al., 2000), and this issue has been related to damage in the occipital lobes shown by functional neuroimaging studies. Nevertheless, VH are also associated with greater deficits in cortical acetylcholine and, in fact, their presence predicts a better clinical response to cholinesterase inhibitors (McKeith, Mintzer et al., 2004; McKeith, Wesnes, Perry, & Ferrara, 2004).

Parkinsonism is reported in up to 75% of patients with DLB at diagnosis, and most of them develop it during the course of the disease (Aarsland, Ballard, McKeith, Perry, & Larsen, 2001; Lopez et al., 2000b). However, in some series, between 25% and 50% of patients have no evidence of parkinsonism (Aarsland et al., 2001; Merdes et al., 2003), making the clinical diagnosis of DLB difficult (McKeith et al., 2000). Parkinsonism in DLB tends to be more symmetric than in PD, has a poorer response to levodopa, a faster motor decline, and rest tremor is less frequently seen than postural or action tremor. There is also a predominance of axial symptoms such as hypomimia, postural instability, and gait difficulty, believed to be mediated by non-dopaminergic mechanisms (Aarsland et al., 2001; Burn et al., 2006; Gnanalingham, Byrne, Thornton, Sambrook, & Bannister, 1997).

Other Symptoms

There is a wide variety of symptoms commonly present in DLB. Severe neuroleptic sensitivity and REM sleep behavioral disorder (RBD) are classified as suggestive features for DLB diagnosis, while others lack sufficient diagnostic specificity. RBD is a parasomnia characterized by vivid and recurrent dreams during REM sleep without muscle atonia. These episodes are often reported by the bed partner and they are described as vocalizations and abnormal and often violent movements when dreaming (Boeve et al., 2007). RBD is recognized to be an early manifestation of synucleinopathies, which may be present years or decades before the onset of parkinsonism or cognitive impairment (Claassen et al., 2010). In some patients with idiopathic RBD, striatal dopaminergic deficits and substantia nigra hyperechogenicity on transcranial sonography can be observed, and this may represent a risk factor for the development of PD, DLB, or MSA (Iranzo et al., 2010). Classically, a severe sensitivity to neuroleptics has been described in DLB patients. Approximately 40% of the patients exposed to typical neuroleptics develop sudden onset or exacerbation of parkinsonism and impaired consciousness with increased risk of mortality (McKeith, Fairbairn, Perry, Thompson, & Perry, 1992). This severe reaction has also been reported with atypical neuroleptics (McKeith et al., 2005). It is not possible to predict severe neuroleptic reactions in a patient before the drug is administrated; therefore, typical antipsychotics are not recommended in DLB management and newer ones must be used with caution.

Severe autonomic dysfunction occurs frequently in DLB, causing carotid-sinus hypersensitivity, orthostatic hypotension, urinary incontinence, constipation, and impotence; it also probably contributes to episodes of loss of consciousness, syncope, and falls (McKeith et al., 2005). Psychiatric symptoms, other than VH, are common in DLB. Hallucinations in other modalities, systematized delusions, apathy, depression, anxiety, and somatoform disorders are also described (McKeith, Mintzer et al., 2004; Onofrj, Bonanni, Manzoli, & Thomas, 2010). Anosmia is another frequent clinical finding in DLB. Nevertheless, it is also characteristic of other LB disorders and it is occasionally present in AD, which limits its value to discriminate between these entities (McShane et al., 2001; Olichney et al., 2005).

CLINICAL DIAGNOSIS

In 1996, the first consensus guidelines for the clinical diagnosis of DLB were published (McKeith et al., 1996). These criteria were based on the main clinical symptoms associated with DLB autopsy proven cases (Perry et al., 1990). The certainty of the clinical diagnosis was graded as "Probable" and "Possible." The term *Probable DLB* indicated that a dementia syndrome was present, and it was associated with at least two of the following signs and symptoms: fluctuating cognition, VH, and parkinsonism (McKeith et al., 1996). *Possible DLB* indicates that the dementia syndrome is associated with one of the signs and symptoms previously described. However, clinicopathological studies showed that these criteria had high specificity but low sensitivity to diagnose DLB (McKeith et al., 2004). A revised version of the criteria was published in 2005 (Table 7.3; McKeith et al., 2005), where there was a modification to the pathological classification, although no major clinical changes were done. One unsolved issue in the operationalization of these criteria is the determination of the onset of the cognitive and motor symptoms. The criteria require that for the diagnosis of DLB the dementia onset should occur within 1 year of the onset of parkinsonism, while for PDD there should be more than 1 year between the onset of motor symptoms and the dementia syndrome. This 1-year rule has been a matter of controversy because it is difficult to determine the exact onset of the cognitive and motor symptoms. In spite of a few clinical differences, there are slight pathological differences between PDD and DLB; indeed, they may represent different points on the continuous spectrum of LB disorders (Lippa et al., 2007).

TABLE 7.3 Revised Criteria for the Clinical Diagnosis of DLB

1. *Central feature* (essential for a diagnosis of Possible or Probable DLB)   • Dementia defined as progressive cognitive decline of sufficient magnitude to interfere with normal social or occupational function   • Prominent or persistent memory impairment may not necessarily occur in the early stages but is usually evident with progression   • Deficit on tests of attention, executive function, and visuospatial ability may be especially prominent
2. *Core features* (two core features are sufficient for a diagnosis of Probable DLB, one for Possible DLB)   • Fluctuating cognition with pronounced variations in attention and alertness   • Recurrent visual hallucinations typically well formed and detailed   • Spontaneous features of parkinsonism
3. *Suggestive features* (If one or more of these is present in addition to one or more core features, a diagnosis of Probable DLB can be made. In the absence of any core features, one or more suggestive features are sufficient for Possible DLB. Probable DLB should not be diagnosed on the basis of suggestive features alone.)   • REM sleep behavior disorders   • Severe neuroleptic sensitivity   • Low dopamine transporter uptake in basal ganglia demonstrated by SPECT or PET imaging
4. *Supportive features* (commonly present but not proven to have diagnostic specificity)   • Repeated falls and syncope   • Transient, unexplained loss of consciousness   • Severe autonomic dysfunction   • Hallucinations in other modalities   • Systematized delusions   • Depression   • Relative preservation of medial temporal lobe on CT/MRI scan   • Generalized low uptake on SPECT/PET scan with reduced occipital activity   • Abnormal (low uptake) MIBG myocardial scintigraphy   • Prominent slow wave activity on EEG with temporal lobe transient sharp waves

DLB, dementia with Lewy bodies; MIBG, ^{123}I-metaiodobenzylguanidine; REM, rapid eye movement; SPECT, single-photon emission computed tomography.

Source: McKeith et al. (2005).

Differential Diagnosis

The most important differential diagnosis of DLB is AD (McKeith et al., 2000). Severity of the dementia syndrome plays an important role in the differential diagnosis, because when fluctuating cognition, VH, and parkinsonism are present early in the dementia course, they highly suggest a diagnosis of DLB, but in more advanced stages, they become less specific for DLB and overlap considerably with AD (Lopez et al., 2000a, 2000b). The neuropsychological profile may be useful for the accurate diagnosis of DLB. One study showed that the lack of visuospatial dysfunction was the best negative predictor for DLB at autopsy (Tiraboschi et al., 2006). Other neurodegenerative disorders with parkinsonian symptoms such as vascular dementia, PDD, frontotemporal dementia with parkinsonism, atypical parkinsonisms (MSA, corticobasal degeneration, or progressive supranuclear palsy), and Creutzfeldt–Jakob disease should be taken into account in the differential diagnosis of DLB (Geser, Wenning, Poewe, & McKeith, 2005).

LABORATORY BIOMARKERS

Clinical studies employ mainly blood (serum or plasma) or cerebrospinal fluid (CSF) to search biochemical markers of neurodegenerative diseases. Typically, the CSF better reflects the situation in the brain, while biochemical values in plasma or serum may be affected by many unrelated factors. In the CSF, the core components of LB, NFT, and amyloid plaques can be detected. Nevertheless, the role of these markers in DLB diagnosis has to be established properly, and none of them is used in the clinical practice for diagnostic purposes.

Monomeric soluble α-synuclein can be measured in the CSF, but the available studies in DLB patients show conflicting results. Elevated, unchanged, and decreased total α-synuclein levels have been reported in these patients compared to AD and control subjects (Mukaetova-Ladinska, Monteith, & Perry, 2010). On the other hand, there are limited data about oligomeric α-synuclein in CSF, but this could be a good potential biomarker for synucleinopathies. Recently, one study found that the levels of oligomeric α-synuclein and the ratio between oligomers and total α-synuclein in CSF were significantly increased in PD patients compared to control subjects (Tokuda et al., 2010). However, new studies replicating this finding are needed and the possible application to DLB has to be tested.

Amyloid plaques are one of the neuropathological hallmarks of AD, but they are also present in DLB. These plaques are formed by Aβ, a 36–43 amino acid peptide originating from proteolysis of the amyloid protein precursor. AD patients have lower levels of Aβ42 in the CSF compared to normal controls (Andreasen et al., 2001; Galasko et al., 1998), and this is also found in DLB (Bibl et al., 2006). The low CSF Aβ42 levels may represent the retention of the proteins into plaques, resulting in reduced availability to diffuse into the CSF. This is supported by the inverse correlation between the amyloid plaque load measured in vivo by amyloid imaging and Aβ42 levels in the CSF of DLB patients (Maetzler et al., 2009). Shorter amyloid peptides (Aβ37, Aβ38, and Aβ40) in the CSF of DLB patients show no difference with respect to controls, but they appear to be slightly more elevated in AD as compared with other dementias (Bibl et al., 2006). Hence, the introduction of ratios, especially Aβ42/Aβ37 and Aβ42/Aβ38 ratios, improves the diagnostic test accuracy to differentiate AD from DLB (Bibl et al., 2006; Mulugeta et al., 2011). On the other hand, an oxidized Aβ40 peptide was found to be significantly higher in DLB than in PDD, and it could be a consistent marker to distinguish these two entities (Bibl et al., 2006).

The NFTs are formed by tau proteins, a microtubule-associated stabilizing protein essential for axonal transport. Tau is hyperphosphorylated in AD, which tends to aggregate, leading to neuronal dysfunction. CSF levels of total tau (t-tau) and phosphorylated tau (p-tau) are increased in AD patients (Andreasen et al., 2001; Galasko et al., 1998). It is believed that this is secondary to neuronal damage, and consequently, tau is released and transported to the CSF. However, p-tau appears to be better than t-tau in the diagnosis of AD (Mitchell, 2009). Tau levels are normal or high in DLB, but most studies showed that the levels are definitely lower than those found in AD (Mukaetova-Ladinska et al., 2010), and this observation could be used to distinguish DLB from AD (Hampel et al., 2004). Possibly, the combination of all these markers will improve the accuracy of DLB diagnosis in the future.

ELECTROPHYSIOLOGY

Occasionally, prominent slow wave activity on EEG with temporal lobe transient sharp waves has been reported in patients with DLB (Briel et al., 1999). In fact, this EEG pattern has been introduced as a supportive feature in the latest revision of clinical diagnostic criteria for DLB (McKeith et al., 2005). However, these findings are rare, and therefore unreliable for diagnosis. On the other hand, one study has found that the presence of slow wave activity in posterior derivations and frequency variation significantly differentiated patients with DLB from those with AD at the earliest stages of dementia. Interestingly, patients with PDD and cognitive fluctuations showed similar EEG changes to the DLB group (Bonanni et al., 2008).

NEUROIMAGING

Structural Neuroimaging

Structural neuroimaging techniques—either CT or MRI—are normally performed during the clinical assessment of patients with cognitive impairment, mainly to rule out entities such as brain tumors, normal pressure hydrocephalus, and vascular lesions. However, these techniques, especially MRI due to its higher sensitivity, also show brain atrophy caused by the neurodegenerative process. Several methods are used to analyze MRI data including visual inspection, region of interest (ROI) analysis, or voxel-based morphometry (VBM). The first two methods depend on the a priori choice of structures, while VBM is an operator-independent analysis. Despite some inconsistent results between MRI studies, a frequent finding has been the relative preservation of the medial temporal lobe volume in DLB subjects when compared to those with AD (Barber et al., 1999; Barber, Ballard, McKeith, Gholkar, & O'Brien, 2000; Burton et al., 2002, 2009; Whitwell et al., 2007), which could be used as support for the diagnosis of DLB (McKeith et al., 2005).

Functional Neuroimaging

Brain functional neuroimaging techniques—PET and single-photon emission computed tomography (SPECT)—allow a broad range of cerebral functions to be assessed in patients currently living with dementia. Actually, brain metabolism, brain perfusion, and different neurotransmitter systems can be measured with a great variety of PET and SPECT tracers. However, brain metabolism with the glucose analog 2-[^{18}F]-fluoro-2-deoxy-D-glucose (^{18}F-FDG) and brain perfusion with technetium-99m hexamethylpropylamine oxime (99mTc-HMPAO) are the two more widely employed techniques in the evaluation of patients with dementia, both in clinical practice and in research. Brain SPECT with 99mTc-HMPAO evaluates the regional cerebral blood flow, an indirect measure of brain metabolism. The most relevant finding on brain perfusion SPECT in DLB subjects is occipital hypoperfusion, which appears to have high sensitivity and specificity to distinguish DLB from other dementias, especially AD (Colloby et al., 2002; Ishii et al., 1999; Lobotesis et al., 2001; Varma et al., 1997). On the other hand, ^{18}F-FDG PET estimates the regional brain rate of glucose consumption, therefore providing information about the pattern of neuronal loss or synapse dysfunction in patients with dementia. The DLB metabolic pattern on ^{18}F-FDG PET is characterized by a parietotemporal, frontal, and occipital hypometabolism (Albin et al., 1996; Higuchi et al., 2000; Ishii et al., 1998; Minoshima et al., 2001), and a relative preservation of metabolic activity in the posterior cingulate cortex ("cingulate island sign"; Figure 7.2; Lim et al., 2009). Only the presence of occipital hypometabolism was able to distinguish DLB from AD with 90% sensitivity and 80% specificity in an autopsy confirmed study (Minoshima et al., 2001). A recent ^{18}F-FDG PET study has correlated the presence of VH in DLB patients with hypometabolism in visual association areas rather than the primary visual cortex (Perneczky et al., 2008).

As previously mentioned, patients with DLB have a reduced striatal dopaminergic innervation due to substantia nigra degeneration (McKeith et al., 1996). The dopaminergic neurotransmitter system can be assessed in vivo in DLB patients using different PET or SPECT radiotracers for striatal presynaptic dopaminergic markers

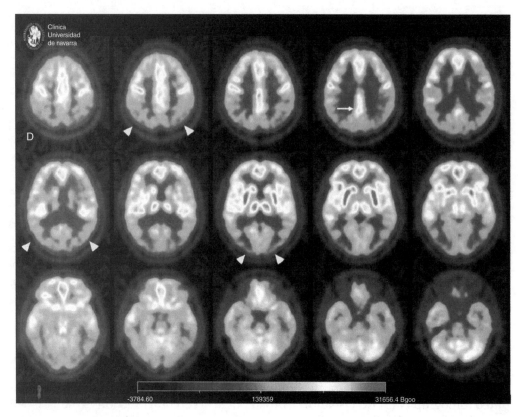

FIGURE 7.2 *(See color insert.)* ^{18}F-FDG PET scan showing parietotemporal and occipital cortices' hypometabolism in a patient with DLB (white head arrows). The white arrow points to the posterior cingulated cortex, demonstrating the cingulate island sign.

DLB, dementia with Lewy bodies.

Courtesy of Dr. Javier Arbizu, Department of Nuclear Medicine, Clínica Universidad de Navarra, Pamplona, Spain.

such as the dopamine transporter (DAT), the vesicular monoamine transporter type 2 (VMAT2), and the aromatic L-amino acid decarboxylase (AADC). The most widely used radioligands for DAT are the SPECT tracers [^{123}I]-2β-carbomethoxy-3β-(4-iodophenyl)-N-(3-fluoropropyl), nortropane (^{123}I-FP-CIT; McKeith et al., 2007; Walker et al., 2002), and [^{123}I]-2β-carbomethoxy-3β-(4-iodophenyl)tropane (^{123}I-β-CIT; Donnemiller et al., 1997); for VMAT2 is the PET tracer ^{11}C-dihydrotetrabenazine (^{11}C-DTBZ; Gilman et al., 2004); and to assess AADC activity is the PET tracer ^{18}F-fluorodopa (FDOPA; Hu et al., 2000). In DLB patients, these dopaminergic neuroimaging techniques often show an asymmetrical reduction in striatal binding or uptake between the two hemispheres, affecting the putamen more than the caudate nucleus; while in AD they are completely normal (Donnemiller et al., 1997; Gilman et al., 2004; Hu et al., 2000; McKeith et al., 2007; Walker et al., 2002). In fact, ^{123}I-FP-CIT SPECT imaging has demonstrated 77.7% sensitivity and 90.4% specificity in the antemortem differentiation of DLB from other causes of dementia, mainly AD (McKeith et al., 2007); and the sensitivity and specificity increased to 88% and 100%, respectively, in autopsy-confirmed cases (Walker et al., 2007). This technique may be useful in patients where the certainty for the diagnosis is low (Possible DLB) or to confirm a diagnosis in cases with Probable DLB, but it is not helpful to differentiate DLB from PDD or atypical parkinsonism syndromes (McKeith et al., 2007).

The brain cholinergic system has also been evaluated in DLB subjects with PET acetylcholine analog tracers as N-[^{11}C]-methyl-4-piperidyl acetate (MP4A; Shimada et al., 2009) and N-[^{11}C]-methyl-4-piperidyl propionate (MP4P; Bohnen et al., 2003). These PET studies have shown a widespread reduction in cortical cholinergic function, especially in the occipital cortex, probably owing to the neuronal loss in the nucleus basalis of Meynert (Bohnen et al., 2003; Klein et al., 2010; Shimada et al., 2009). Surprisingly, the cholinergic deficit in DLB patients is more severe than in AD subjects (Bohnen et al., 2003), as noted in autopsy studies (Hansen et al., 1990; Perry et al., 1994). On the other hand, the degree of cholinergic system dysfunction appears to be similar in DLB and PDD (Shimada et al., 2009). This severe cholinergic deficit associated with DLB may explain why cholinesterase inhibitors markedly improve symptoms in patients (McKeith et al., 2000).

Molecular Neuroimaging

The development of PET radiotracers that bind to brain amyloid has revolutionized the use of neuroimaging techniques in patients with dementing neurodegenerative diseases. These molecules allow the localization of AD pathology in vivo, and have helped to further our understanding of the underlying biology of AD. Actually, the best study tracer is the ^{11}C-labeled Pittsburgh compound B (^{11}C-PIB), a molecule with high affinity and specificity to fibrillar Aβ (Klunk et al., 2003). Nevertheless, several other radiotracers are under investigation for the detection of AD pathology.

A high proportion of patients with DLB shows an increased brain ^{11}C-PIB binding. The pattern of distribution of raised amyloid when present is similar to that seen in AD, affecting association cortical areas—mainly the anterior or posterior cingulate followed by the frontal, parietal, temporal, and occipital cortex—and the striatum (Edison et al., 2008; Gomperts et al., 2008). On the other hand, only a minority of PDD subjects have an increased amyloid burden measured by ^{11}C-PIB PET (Edison et al., 2008; Foster et al., 2010), in line with previous neuropathological findings (Ballard et al., 2006). It seems that amyloid load does not correlate with dementia severity in DLB, but it is likely to accelerate the dementia process (Edison et al., 2008; Fujishiro et al., 2010).

OTHER IMAGING TECHNIQUES

Myocardial Scintigraphy

Myocardial scintigraphy with ^{123}I-metaiodobenzylguanidine (MIBG), an analog of norepinephrine, is used to detect postganglionic cardiac sympathetic denervation in PD and differentiate it from atypical parkinsonism. Recent studies have demonstrated that this technique is also useful for the clinical diagnosis of DLB (Tateno, Kobayashi, & Saito, 2009). Indeed, an abnormal MIBG myocardial scintigraphy has been included in the latest guidelines as a supportive feature for the clinical diagnosis of this entity (McKeith et al., 2005). A recent meta-analysis has demonstrated that MIBG scintigraphy has 98% pooled sensitivity and 94% pooled specificity in patients with DLB; additionally, it is an accurate test for differential diagnosis between DLB and other dementias (Treglia & Cason, 2012).

TREATMENT

Currently, there are no curative interventions for DLB, but symptoms can be treated. The evidence base for making recommendations about DLB treatment is limited and the following suggestions are based mainly on consensus opinions of experts in this field. There is evidence that cholinesterase inhibitors are effective in DLB (Edwards et al., 2004; Kaufer, Catt, Lopez, & Dekosky, 1998; Querfurth, Allam, Geffroy, Schiff, & Kaplan, 2000; Shea, MacKnight, & Rockwood, 1998), but placebo-controlled trials are only available for rivastigmine (McKeith et al., 2000). Cholinesterase inhibitors improved cognitive function of DLB patients, especially attention and memory, as well as behavioral symptoms such as apathy, anxiety, delusions, and hallucinations (McKeith et al., 2000). These drugs also seem to be effective against the fluctuating cognitive impairment with impact on global function and activities of daily living (McKeith et al., 2005). All these data suggest that cholinesterase inhibitors could be recommended as a first-line treatment for the cognitive and psychiatric symptoms of DLB (Ferman & Boeve, 2007). In addition to gastrointestinal side effects, these drugs may exacerbate postural hypotension, as well as cause hypersalivation, lacrimation, and increased frequency of urination (McKeith et al., 2004, 2005). A recent randomized placebo-controlled trial has shown that memantine appears to slightly improve global clinical status and behavioral symptoms of patients with mild to moderate DLB (Emre et al., 2010).

The management of psychotic symptoms in the context of DLB is challenging. When pharmacological intervention is needed, the available options include cholinesterase inhibitors and atypical antipsychotics such as quetiapine, clozapine, ziprasidone, and aripiprazole. Antipsychotics are used when the initial treatment with cholinesterase inhibitors is not effective or a more rapid symptom control is required. Typical antipsychotics are not recommended in DLB mainly due to neuroleptic sensitivity but also because they worsen parkinsonism (Weintraub & Hurtig, 2007). Even with atypical neuroleptics, these reactions have been documented and they should be used with caution (McKeith et al., 2005). The use of atypical antipsychotics has also been associated with a small increased risk of death in demented patients, and this should be taken into consideration within the context of medical need for these drugs (Schneider, Dagerman, & Insel, 2005).

Parkinsonian symptoms in DLB patients can be treated with levodopa, although motor improvement is less impressive than in PD (Lucetti et al., 2010). Medication should be introduced at low doses and increased slowly to avoid the appearance of psychotic symptoms. Other medications used to manage symptoms in PD patients, such as dopaminergic agonists, amantadine, and anticholinergic drugs, should be avoided due to a higher risk of adverse neuropsychiatric effects (Ferman & Boeve, 2007).

Depression is frequent in DLB and generally selective serotonin uptake inhibitors (SSRI) and selective serotonin and noradrenalin reuptake inhibitors (SNRI) are recommended to manage it. On the other hand, tricyclic antidepressants should be avoided because of their anticholinergic effect (McKeith et al., 2005). RBD can be treated with low doses of clonazepam at bedtime, but melatonin also can be effective, either alone or in combination with clonazepam. Excessive daytime sleepiness can improve with cholinesterase inhibitors, but if this approach is not effective, psychostimulants such as modafinil and methylphenidate can be used (Ferman & Boeve, 2007).

PROGNOSIS

Cognitive decline is similar to or faster than that seen in AD and vascular dementia, with an annual impairment of 4 to 5 points on the MMSE (Ballard et al., 2001b; Lopez, Hamilton, et al., 2000; Olichney et al., 1998). However, patients with DLB tend to be institutionalized faster than those with AD; this is probably influenced by the presence of parkinsonism (Lopez, Wisniewski, et al., 2000). Motor disability in DLB seems to progress at a faster rate than in PD (Müller et al., 2000). Mean survival of DLB subjects is estimated at 5 years, although some patients show a more rapid progression. Risk factors for shorter survival include older age of onset, fluctuating cognition, hallucinations at onset, and associated AD pathology (Jellinger, Wenning, & Seppi, 2007).

SUMMARY

DLB is characterized by progressive dementia, cognitive fluctuations, VH, and parkinsonism. While the blending of psychiatric, cognitive, and motor features makes DLB somewhat distinct from other forms of dementia, it can create a challenge when it comes to symptom-based treatment. Failure to recognize DLB as the underlying cause of these clinical symptoms can lead to medicinal interventions that have an adverse effect as discussed previously. As a result, it is imperative that clinicians remain aware of the clinical and neuropathological features of DLB. Moving forward, advances in treatment options are essential.

REFERENCES

Aarsland, D., Ballard, C., McKeith, I., Perry, R. H., & Larsen, J. P. (2001). Comparison of extrapyramidal signs in dementia with Lewy bodies and Parkinson's disease. *The Journal of Neuropsychiatry and Clinical Neurosciences, 13*(3), 374–379.

Ala, T. A., Hughes, L. F., Kyrouac, G. A., Ghobrial, M. W., & Elble, R. J. (2001). Pentagon copying is more impaired in dementia with Lewy bodies than in Alzheimer's disease. *Journal of Neurology, Neurosurgery, and Psychiatry, 70*(4), 483–488.

Albin, R. L., Minoshima, S., D'Amato, C. J., Frey, K. A., Kuhl, D. A., & Sima, A. A. (1996). Fluoro-deoxyglucose positron emission tomography in diffuse Lewy body disease. *Neurology, 47*(2), 462–466.

Andreasen, N., Minthon, L., Davidsson, P., Vanmechelen, E., Vanderstichele, H., Winblad, B., & Blennow, K. (2001). Evaluation of CSF-tau and CSF-Abeta42 as diagnostic markers for Alzheimer disease in clinical practice. *Archives of Neurology, 58*(3), 373–379.

Angot, E., Steiner, J. A., Hansen, C., Li, J. Y., & Brundin, P. (2010). Are synucleinopathies prion-like disorders? *Lancet Neurology, 9*(11), 1128–1138.

Ballard, C., O'Brien, J., Gray, A., Cormack, F., Ayre, G., Rowan, E., . . . Tovee, M. (2001a). Attention and fluctuating attention in patients with dementia with Lewy bodies and Alzheimer disease. *Archives of Neurology, 58*(6), 977–982.

Ballard, C., O'Brien, J., Morris, C. M., Barber, R., Swann, A., Neill, D., & McKeith, I. (2001b). The progression of cognitive impairment in dementia with Lewy bodies, vascular dementia and Alzheimer's disease. *International Journal of Geriatric Psychiatry, 16*(5), 499–503.

Ballard, C., Walker, M., O'Brien, J., Rowan, E., & McKeith, I. (2001c). The characterisation and impact of "fluctuating" cognition in dementia with Lewy bodies and Alzheimer's disease. *International Journal of Geriatric Psychiatry, 16*(5), 494–498.

Ballard, C., Ziabreva, I., Perry, R., Larsen, J. P., O'Brien, J., McKeith, I., . . . Aarsland, D. (2006). Differences in neuropathologic characteristics across the Lewy body dementia spectrum. *Neurology, 67*(11), 1931–1934.

Barber, R., Ballard, C., McKeith, I. G., Gholkar, A., & O'Brien, J. T. (2000). MRI volumetric study of dementia with Lewy bodies: A comparison with AD and vascular dementia. *Neurology, 54*(6), 1304–1309.

Barber, R., Gholkar, A., Scheltens, P., Ballard, C., McKeith, I. G., & O'Brien, J. T. (1999). Medial temporal lobe atrophy on MRI in dementia with Lewy bodies. *Neurology, 52*(6), 1153–1158.

Bibl, M., Mollenhauer, B., Esselmann, H., Lewczuk, P., Klafki, H. W., Sparbier, K.,...Wiltfang, J. (2006). CSF amyloid-beta-peptides in Alzheimer's disease, dementia with Lewy bodies and Parkinson's disease dementia. *Brain: A Journal of Neurology, 129*(Pt 5), 1177–1187.

Boeve, B. F., Silber, M. H., Saper, C. B., Ferman, T. J., Dickson, D. W., Parisi, J. E.,...Braak, H. (2007). Pathophysiology of REM sleep behaviour disorder and relevance to neurodegenerative disease. *Brain: A Journal of Neurology, 130*(Pt 11), 2770–2788.

Bogaerts, V., Engelborghs, S., Kumar-Singh, S., Goossens, D., Pickut, B., van der Zee, J.,... Van Broeckhoven, C. (2007). A novel locus for dementia with Lewy bodies: A clinically and genetically heterogeneous disorder. *Brain: A Journal of Neurology, 130*(Pt 9), 2277–2291.

Bohnen, N. I., Kaufer, D. I., Ivanco, L. S., Lopresti, B., Koeppe, R. A., Davis, J. G.,...DeKosky, S. T. (2003). Cortical cholinergic function is more severely affected in parkinsonian dementia than in Alzheimer disease: An in vivo positron emission tomographic study. *Archives of Neurology, 60*(12), 1745–1748.

Bonanni, L., Thomas, A., Tiraboschi, P., Perfetti, B., Varanese, S., & Onofrj, M. (2008). EEG comparisons in early Alzheimer's disease, dementia with Lewy bodies and Parkinson's disease with dementia patients with a 2-year follow-up. *Brain: A Journal of Neurology, 131*(Pt 3), 690–705.

Bonifati, V. (2008). Recent advances in the genetics of dementia with Lewy bodies. *Current Neurology and Neuroscience Reports, 8*(3), 187–189.

Braak, H., Del Tredici, K., Rüb, U., de Vos, R. A., Jansen Steur, E. N., & Braak, E. (2003). Staging of brain pathology related to sporadic Parkinson's disease. *Neurobiology of Aging, 24*(2), 197–211.

Bradshaw, J. M., Saling, M., Anderson, V., Hopwood, M., & Brodtmann, A. (2006). Higher cortical deficits influence attentional processing in dementia with Lewy bodies, relative to patients with dementia of the Alzheimer's type and controls. *Journal of Neurology, Neurosurgery, and Psychiatry, 77*(10), 1129–1135.

Briel, R. C., McKeith, I. G., Barker, W. A., Hewitt, Y., Perry, R. H., Ince, P. G., & Fairbairn, A. F. (1999). EEG findings in dementia with Lewy bodies and Alzheimer's disease. *Journal of Neurology, Neurosurgery, and Psychiatry, 66*(3), 401–403.

Burn, D. J., Rowan, E. N., Allan, L. M., Molloy, S., O'Brien, J. T., & McKeith, I. G. (2006). Motor subtype and cognitive decline in Parkinson's disease, Parkinson's disease with dementia, and dementia with Lewy bodies. *Journal of Neurology, Neurosurgery, and Psychiatry, 77*(5), 585–589.

Burton, E. J., Barber, R., Mukaetova-Ladinska, E. B., Robson, J., Perry, R. H., Jaros, E.,... O'Brien, J. T. (2009). Medial temporal lobe atrophy on MRI differentiates Alzheimer's disease from dementia with Lewy bodies and vascular cognitive impairment: A prospective study with pathological verification of diagnosis. *Brain: A Journal of Neurology, 132*(Pt 1), 195–203.

Burton, E. J., Karas, G., Paling, S. M., Barber, R., Williams, E. D., Ballard, C. G.,...O'Brien, J. T. (2002). Patterns of cerebral atrophy in dementia with Lewy bodies using voxel-based morphometry. *NeuroImage, 17*(2), 618–630.

Byrne, E. J., Lennox, G., & Goodwin-Austen, L. B. (1991). Dementia associated with cortical Lewy bodies: Proposed diagnostic criteria. *Dementia, 2*, 283–284.

Calderon, J., Perry, R. J., Erzinclioglu, S. W., Berrios, G. E., Dening, T. R., & Hodges, J. R. (2001). Perception, attention, and working memory are disproportionately impaired in dementia with Lewy bodies compared with Alzheimer's disease. *Journal of Neurology, Neurosurgery, and Psychiatry, 70*(2), 157–164.

Claassen, D. O., Josephs, K. A., Ahlskog, J. E., Silber, M. H., Tippmann-Peikert, M., & Boeve, B. F. (2010). REM sleep behavior disorder preceding other aspects of synucleinopathies by up to half a century. *Neurology, 75*(6), 494–499.

Clark, L. N., Kartsaklis, L. A., Wolf Gilbert, R., Dorado, B., Ross, B. M., Kisselev, S., . . . Marder, K. (2009). Association of glucocerebrosidase mutations with dementia with Lewy bodies. *Archives of Neurology, 66*(5), 578–583.

Collerton, D., Burn, D., McKeith, I., & O'Brien, J. (2003). Systematic review and meta-analysis show that dementia with Lewy bodies is a visual-perceptual and attentional-executive dementia. *Dementia and Geriatric Cognitive Disorders, 16*(4), 229–237.

Colloby, S. J., Fenwick, J. D., Williams, E. D., Paling, S. M., Lobotesis, K., Ballard, C., . . . O'Brien, J. T. (2002). A comparison of (99m)Tc-HMPAO SPET changes in dementia with Lewy bodies and Alzheimer's disease using statistical parametric mapping. *European Journal of Nuclear Medicine and Molecular Imaging, 29*(5), 615–622.

Cormack, F., Aarsland, D., Ballard, C., & Tovée, M. J. (2004). Pentagon drawing and neuropsychological performance in dementia with Lewy bodies, Alzheimer's disease, Parkinson's disease and Parkinson's disease with dementia. *International Journal of Geriatric Psychiatry, 19*(4), 371–377.

Crowell, T. A., Luis, C. A., Cox, D. E., & Mullan, M. (2007). Neuropsychological comparison of Alzheimer's disease and dementia with Lewy bodies. *Dementia and Geriatric Cognitive Disorders, 23*(2), 120–125.

Cuervo, A. M., Stefanis, L., Fredenburg, R., Lansbury, P. T., & Sulzer, D. (2004). Impaired degradation of mutant alpha-synuclein by chaperone-mediated autophagy. *Science, 305*(5688), 1292–1295.

Del-Ser, T., Munoz, D. G., & Hachinski, V. (1996). Temporal pattern of cognitive decline and incontinence is different in Alzheimer's disease and diffuse Lewy body disease. *Neurology, 46*(3), 682–686.

Dickson, D. W., Crystal, H., Mattiace, L. A., Kress, Y., Schwagerl, A., Ksiezak-Reding, H., . . . Yen, S. H. (1989). Diffuse Lewy body disease: Light and electron microscopic immunocytochemistry of senile plaques. *Acta Neuropathologica, 78*(6), 572–584.

Dickson, D. W., Davies, P., Mayeux, R., Crystal, H., Horoupian, D. S., Thompson, A., & Goldman, J. E. (1987). Diffuse Lewy body disease. Neuropathological and biochemical studies of six patients. *Acta Neuropathologica, 75*(1), 8–15.

Dickson, D. W., Ruan, D., Crystal, H., Mark, M. H., Davies, P., Kress, Y., & Yen, S. H. (1991). Hippocampal degeneration differentiates diffuse Lewy body disease (DLBD) from Alzheimer's disease: Light and electron microscopic immunocytochemistry of CA2–3 neurites specific to DLBD. *Neurology, 41*(9), 1402–1409.

Donnemiller, E., Heilmann, J., Wenning, G. K., Berger, W., Decristoforo, C., Moncayo, R., . . . Ransmayr, G. (1997). Brain perfusion scintigraphy with 99mTc-HMPAO or 99mTc-ECD and ^{123}I-beta-CIT single-photon emission tomography in dementia of the Alzheimer-type and diffuse Lewy body disease. *European Journal of Nuclear Medicine, 24*(3), 320–325.

Edison, P., Rowe, C. C., Rinne, J. O., Ng, S., Ahmed, I., Kemppainen, N., . . . Brooks, D. J. (2008). Amyloid load in Parkinson's disease dementia and Lewy body dementia measured with [^{11}C]PIB positron emission tomography. *Journal of Neurology, Neurosurgery, and Psychiatry, 79*(12), 1331–1338.

Edwards, K. R., Hershey, L., Wray, L., Bednarczyk, E. M., Lichter, D., Farlow, M., & Johnson, S. (2004). Efficacy and safety of galantamine in patients with dementia with Lewy bodies: A 12-week interim analysis. *Dementia and Geriatric Cognitive Disorders, 17*(Suppl 1), 40–48.

Emre, M., Tsolaki, M., Bonuccelli, U., Destée, A., Tolosa, E., Kutzelnigg, A.,...Jones, R.; 11018 Study Investigators. (2010). Memantine for patients with Parkinson's disease dementia or dementia with Lewy bodies: A randomised, double-blind, placebo-controlled trial. *Lancet Neurology, 9*(10), 969–977.

Ferman, T. J., & Boeve, B. F. (2007). Dementia with Lewy bodies. *Neurologic Clinics, 25*(3), 741–760, vii.

Ferman, T. J., Boeve, B. F., Smith, G. E., Silber, M. H., Kokmen, E., Petersen, R. C., & Ivnik, R. J. (1999). REM sleep behavior disorder and dementia: Cognitive differences when compared with AD. *Neurology, 52*(5), 951–957.

Ferman, T. J., Smith, G. E., Boeve, B. F., Graff-Radford, N. R., Lucas, J. A., Knopman, D. S.,... Dickson, D. W. (2006). Neuropsychological differentiation of dementia with Lewy bodies from normal aging and Alzheimer's disease. *The Clinical Neuropsychologist, 20*(4), 623–636.

Ferman, T. J., Smith, G. E., Boeve, B. F., Ivnik, R. J., Petersen, R. C., Knopman, D.,...Dickson, D. W. (2004). DLB fluctuations: Specific features that reliably differentiate DLB from AD and normal aging. *Neurology, 62*(2), 181–187.

Foster, E. R., Campbell, M. C., Burack, M. A., Hartlein, J., Flores, H. P., Cairns, N. J.,...Perlmutter, J. S. (2010). Amyloid imaging of Lewy body-associated disorders. *Movement Disorders, 25*(15), 2516–2523.

Fujishiro, H., Iseki, E., Higashi, S., Kasanuki, K., Murayama, N., Togo, T.,...Sato, K. (2010). Distribution of cerebral amyloid deposition and its relevance to clinical phenotype in Lewy body dementia. *Neuroscience Letters, 486*(1), 19–23.

Galasko, D., Chang, L., Motter, R., Clark, C. M., Kaye, J., Knopman, D.,...Seubert, P. (1998). High cerebrospinal fluid tau and low amyloid beta42 levels in the clinical diagnosis of Alzheimer disease and relation to apolipoprotein E genotype. *Archives of Neurology, 55*(7), 937–945.

Galasko, D., Saitoh, T., Xia, Y., Thal, L. J., Katzman, R., Hill, L. R., & Hansen, L. (1994). The apolipoprotein E allele epsilon 4 is overrepresented in patients with the Lewy body variant of Alzheimer's disease. *Neurology, 44*(10), 1950–1951.

Geser, F., Wenning, G. K., Poewe, W., & McKeith, I. (2005). How to diagnose dementia with Lewy bodies: State of the art. *Movement Disorders, 20*(Suppl 12), S11–S20.

Gibb, W. R., Luthert, P. J., Janota, I., & Lantos, P. L. (1989). Cortical Lewy body dementia: Clinical features and classification. *Journal of Neurology, Neurosurgery, and Psychiatry, 52*(2), 185–192.

Gilman, S., Koeppe, R. A., Little, R., An, H., Junck, L., Giordani, B.,...Wernette, K. (2004). Striatal monoamine terminals in Lewy body dementia and Alzheimer's disease. *Annals of Neurology, 55*(6), 774–780.

Gnanalingham, K. K., Byrne, E. J., Thornton, A., Sambrook, M. A., & Bannister, P. (1997). Motor and cognitive function in Lewy body dementia: Comparison with Alzheimer's and Parkinson's diseases. *Journal of Neurology, Neurosurgery, and Psychiatry, 62*(3), 243–252.

Goker-Alpan, O., Lopez, G., Vithayathil, J., Davis, J., Hallett, M., & Sidransky, E. (2008). The spectrum of parkinsonian manifestations associated with glucocerebrosidase mutations. *Archives of Neurology, 65*(10), 1353–1357.

Gomperts, S. N., Rentz, D. M., Moran, E., Becker, J. A., Locascio, J. J., Klunk, W. E.,...Johnson, K. A. (2008). Imaging amyloid deposition in Lewy body diseases. *Neurology, 71*(12), 903–910.

Halliday, G., Hely, M., Reid, W., & Morris, J. (2008). The progression of pathology in longitudinally followed patients with Parkinson's disease. *Acta Neuropathologica, 115*(4), 409–415.

Hamilton, R. L. (2000). Lewy bodies in Alzheimer's disease: A neuropathological review of 145 cases using alpha-synuclein immunohistochemistry. *Brain Pathology, 10*(3), 378–384.

Hampel, H., Buerger, K., Zinkowski, R., Teipel, S. J., Goernitz, A., Andreasen, N.,…Blennow, K. (2004). Measurement of phosphorylated tau epitopes in the differential diagnosis of Alzheimer disease: A comparative cerebrospinal fluid study. *Archives of General Psychiatry, 61*(1), 95–102.

Hansen, L., Salmon, D., Galasko, D., Masliah, E., Katzman, R., DeTeresa, R.,…Klauber, M. (1990). The Lewy body variant of Alzheimer's disease: A clinical and pathologic entity. *Neurology, 40*(1), 1–8.

Harding, A. J., Broe, G. A., & Halliday, G. M. (2002). Visual hallucinations in Lewy body disease relate to Lewy bodies in the temporal lobe. *Brain: A Journal of Neurology, 125*(Pt 2), 391–403.

Harding, A. J., Lakay, B., & Halliday, G. M. (2002). Selective hippocampal neuron loss in dementia with Lewy bodies. *Annals of Neurology, 51*(1), 125–128.

Haroutunian, V., Serby, M., Purohit, D. P., Perl, D. P., Marin, D., Lantz, M.,…Davis, K. L. (2000). Contribution of Lewy body inclusions to dementia in patients with and without Alzheimer disease neuropathological conditions. *Archives of Neurology, 57*(8), 1145–1150.

Higuchi, M., Tashiro, M., Arai, H., Okamura, N., Hara, S., Higuchi, S.,…Sasaki, H. (2000). Glucose hypometabolism and neuropathological correlates in brains of dementia with Lewy bodies. *Experimental Neurology, 162*(2), 247–256.

Hu, X. S., Okamura, N., Arai, H., Higuchi, M., Matsui, T., Tashiro, M.,…Sasaki, H. (2000). 18F-fluorodopa PET study of striatal dopamine uptake in the diagnosis of dementia with Lewy bodies. *Neurology, 55*(10), 1575–1577.

Iranzo, A., Lomeña, F., Stockner, H., Valldeoriola, F., Vilaseca, I., Salamero, M.,…Santamaria, J.; Sleep Innsbruck Barcelona (SINBAR) group. (2010). Decreased striatal dopamine transporter uptake and substantia nigra hyperechogenicity as risk markers of synucleinopathy in patients with idiopathic rapid-eye-movement sleep behaviour disorder: A prospective study [corrected]. *Lancet Neurology, 9*(11), 1070–1077.

Ishii, K., Imamura, T., Sasaki, M., Yamaji, S., Sakamoto, S., Kitagaki, H.,…Mori, E. (1998). Regional cerebral glucose metabolism in dementia with Lewy bodies and Alzheimer's disease. *Neurology, 51*(1), 125–130.

Ishii, K., Yamaji, S., Kitagaki, H., Imamura, T., Hirono, N., & Mori, E. (1999). Regional cerebral blood flow difference between dementia with Lewy bodies and AD. *Neurology, 53*(2), 413–416.

Jellinger, K. A., Wenning, G. K., & Seppi, K. (2007). Predictors of survival in dementia with Lewy bodies and Parkinson dementia. *Neuro-Degenerative Diseases, 4*(6), 428–430.

Johns, E. K., Phillips, N. A., Belleville, S., Goupil, D., Babins, L., Kelner, N.,…Chertkow, H. (2009). Executive functions in frontotemporal dementia and Lewy body dementia. *Neuropsychology, 23*(6), 765–777.

Kaufer, D. I., Catt, K. E., Lopez, O. L., & DeKosky, S. T. (1998). Dementia with Lewy bodies: Response of delirium-like features to donepezil. *Neurology, 51*(5), 1512.

Klatka, L. A., Louis, E. D., & Schiffer, R. B. (1996). Psychiatric features in diffuse Lewy body disease: A clinicopathologic study using Alzheimer's disease and Parkinson's disease comparison groups. *Neurology, 47*(5), 1148–1152.

Klein, J. C., Eggers, C., Kalbe, E., Weisenbach, S., Hohmann, C., Vollmar, S.,…Hilker, R. (2010). Neurotransmitter changes in dementia with Lewy bodies and Parkinson disease dementia in vivo. *Neurology, 74*(11), 885–892.

Klunk, W. E., Wang, Y., Huang, G. F., Debnath, M. L., Holt, D. P., Shao, L.,…Mathis, C. A. (2003). The binding of 2-(4′-methylaminophenyl)benzothiazole to postmortem brain homogenates is dominated by the amyloid component. *The Journal of Neuroscience, 23*(6), 2086–2092.

Kosaka, K. (1990). Diffuse Lewy body disease in Japan. *Journal of Neurology, 237*(3), 197–204.

Kosaka, K. (1978). Lewy bodies in cerebral cortex, report of three cases. *Acta Neuropathologica, 42*(2), 127–134.

Kosaka, K., Oyanagi, S., Matsushita, M., & Hori, A. (1976). Presenile dementia with Alzheimer-, Pick- and Lewy-body changes. *Acta Neuropathologica, 36*(3), 221–233.

Kosaka, K., Yoshimura, M., Ikeda, K., & Budka, H. (1984). Diffuse type of Lewy body disease: Progressive dementia with abundant cortical Lewy bodies and senile changes of varying degree—a new disease? *Clinical Neuropathology, 3*(5), 185–192.

Kövari, E., Horvath, J., & Bouras, C. (2009). Neuropathology of Lewy body disorders. *Brain Research Bulletin, 80*(4–5), 203–210.

Leverenz, J. B., Hamilton, R., Tsuang, D. W., Schantz, A., Vavrek, D., Larson, E. B.,…Montine, T. J. (2008). Empiric refinement of the pathologic assessment of Lewy-related pathology in the dementia patient. *Brain Pathology, 18*(2), 220–224.

Lim, S. M., Katsifis, A., Villemagne, V. L., Best, R., Jones, G., Saling, M.,…Rowe, C. C. (2009). The 18F-FDG PET cingulate island sign and comparison to ^{123}I-beta-CIT SPECT for diagnosis of dementia with Lewy bodies. *Journal of Nuclear Medicine, 50*(10), 1638–1645.

Lippa, C. F., Duda, J. E., Grossman, M., Hurtig, H. I., Aarsland, D., Boeve, B. F.,…Wszolek, Z. K.; DLB/PDD Working Group. (2007). DLB and PDD boundary issues: Diagnosis, treatment, molecular pathology, and biomarkers. *Neurology, 68*(11), 812–819.

Lobotesis, K., Fenwick, J. D., Phipps, A., Ryman, A., Swann, A., Ballard, C.,…O'Brien, J. T. (2001). Occipital hypoperfusion on SPECT in dementia with Lewy bodies but not AD. *Neurology, 56*(5), 643–649.

Lopez, O. L., Hamilton, R. L., Becker, J. T., Wisniewski, S., Kaufer, D. I., & DeKosky, S. T. (2000a). Severity of cognitive impairment and the clinical diagnosis of AD with Lewy bodies. *Neurology, 54*(9), 1780–1787.

Lopez, O. L., Wisniewski, S., Hamilton, R. L., Becker, J. T., Kaufer, D. I., & DeKosky, S. T. (2000b). Predictors of progression in patients with AD and Lewy bodies. *Neurology, 54*(9), 1774–1779.

Lucetti, C., Logi, C., Del Dotto, P., Berti, C., Ceravolo, R., Baldacci, F.,…Bonuccelli, U. (2010). Levodopa response in dementia with Lewy bodies: A 1-year follow-up study. *Parkinsonism & Related Disorders, 16*(8), 522–526.

Maetzler, W., Liepelt, I., Reimold, M., Reischl, G., Solbach, C., Becker, C.,…Berg, D. (2009). Cortical PIB binding in Lewy body disease is associated with Alzheimer-like characteristics. *Neurobiology of Disease, 34*(1), 107–112.

McKeith, I., Del Ser, T., Spano, P., Emre, M., Wesnes, K., Anand, R.,…Spiegel, R. (2000). Efficacy of rivastigmine in dementia with Lewy bodies: A randomised, double-blind, placebo-controlled international study. *Lancet, 356*(9247), 2031–2036.

McKeith, I., Fairbairn, A., Perry, R., Thompson, P., & Perry, E. (1992). Neuroleptic sensitivity in patients with senile dementia of Lewy body type. *British Medical Journal, 305*(6855), 673–678.

McKeith, I., Mintzer, J., Aarsland, D., Burn, D., Chiu, H., Cohen-Mansfield, J.,…Reid, W.; International Psychogeriatric Association Expert Meeting on DLB. (2004). Dementia with Lewy bodies. *Lancet Neurology, 3*(1), 19–28.

McKeith, I., O'Brien, J., Walker, Z., Tatsch, K., Booij, J., Darcourt, J.,…Reininger, C.; DLB Study Group. (2007). Sensitivity and specificity of dopamine transporter imaging with

^{123}I-FP-CIT SPECT in dementia with Lewy bodies: A phase III, multicentre study. *Lancet Neurology, 6*(4), 305–313.

McKeith, I. G., Ballard, C. G., Perry, R. H., Ince, P. G., O'Brien, J. T., Neill, D.,…Perry, E. K. (2000). Prospective validation of consensus criteria for the diagnosis of dementia with Lewy bodies. *Neurology, 54*(5), 1050–1058.

McKeith, I. G., Dickson, D. W., Lowe, J., Emre, M., O'Brien, J. T., Feldman, H.,…Yamada, M.; Consortium on DLB. (2005). Diagnosis and management of dementia with Lewy bodies: Third report of the DLB Consortium. *Neurology, 65*(12), 1863–1872.

McKeith, I. G., Galasko, D., Kosaka, K., Perry, E. K., Dickson, D. W., Hansen, L. A.,…Perry, R. H. (1996). Consensus guidelines for the clinical and pathologic diagnosis of dementia with Lewy bodies (DLB): Report of the consortium on DLB international workshop. *Neurology, 47*(5), 1113–1124.

McKeith, I. G., Wesnes, K. A., Perry, E., & Ferrara, R. (2004). Hallucinations predict attentional improvements with rivastigmine in dementia with Lewy bodies. *Dementia and Geriatric Cognitive Disorders, 18*(1), 94–100.

McShane, R. H., Nagy, Z., Esiri, M. M., King, E., Joachim, C., Sullivan, N., & Smith, A. D. (2001). Anosmia in dementia is associated with Lewy bodies rather than Alzheimer's pathology. *Journal of Neurology, Neurosurgery, and Psychiatry, 70*(6), 739–743.

Mega, M. S., Masterman, D. L., Benson, D. F., Vinters, H. V., Tomiyasu, U., Craig, A. H.,… Cummings, J. L. (1996). Dementia with Lewy bodies: Reliability and validity of clinical and pathologic criteria. *Neurology, 47*(6), 1403–1409.

Merdes, A. R., Hansen, L. A., Jeste, D. V., Galasko, D., Hofstetter, C. R., Ho, G. J.,…Corey-Bloom, J. (2003). Influence of Alzheimer pathology on clinical diagnostic accuracy in dementia with Lewy bodies. *Neurology, 60*(10), 1586–1590.

Metzler-Baddeley, C. (2007). A review of cognitive impairments in dementia with Lewy bodies relative to Alzheimer's disease and Parkinson's disease with dementia. *Cortex, 43*(5), 583–600.

Minoshima, S., Foster, N. L., Sima, A. A., Frey, K. A., Albin, R. L., & Kuhl, D. E. (2001). Alzheimer's disease versus dementia with Lewy bodies: Cerebral metabolic distinction with autopsy confirmation. *Annals of Neurology, 50*(3), 358–365.

Mitchell, A. J. (2009). CSF phosphorylated tau in the diagnosis and prognosis of mild cognitive impairment and Alzheimer's disease: A meta-analysis of 51 studies. *Journal of Neurology, Neurosurgery, and Psychiatry, 80*(9), 966–975.

Mori, E., Shimomura, T., Fujimori, M., Hirono, N., Imamura, T., Hashimoto, M.,…Hanihara, T. (2000). Visuoperceptual impairment in dementia with Lewy bodies. *Archives of Neurology, 57*(4), 489–493.

Mosimann, U. P., Mather, G., Wesnes, K. A., O'Brien, J. T., Burn, D. J., & McKeith, I. G. (2004). Visual perception in Parkinson disease dementia and dementia with Lewy bodies. *Neurology, 63*(11), 2091–2096.

Mosimann, U. P., Rowan, E. N., Partington, C. E., Collerton, D., Littlewood, E., O'Brien, J. T.,… McKeith, I. G. (2006). Characteristics of visual hallucinations in Parkinson disease dementia and dementia with Lewy bodies. *The American Journal of Geriatric Psychiatry, 14*(2), 153–160.

Mukaetova-Ladinska, E. B., Monteith, R., & Perry, E. K. (2010). Cerebrospinal fluid biomarkers for dementia with Lewy bodies. *International Journal of Alzheimer's Disease, 2010,* 536–538.

Müller, J., Wenning, G. K., Jellinger, K., McKee, A., Poewe, W., & Litvan, I. (2000). Progression of Hoehn and Yahr stages in Parkinsonian disorders: A clinicopathologic study. *Neurology, 55*(6), 888–891.

Mulugeta, E., Londos, E., Ballard, C., Alves, G., Zetterberg, H., Blennow, K.,...Aarsland, D. (2011). CSF amyloid ß38 as a novel diagnostic marker for dementia with Lewy bodies. *Journal of Neurology, Neurosurgery, and Psychiatry, 82*(2), 160–164.

Nakashima-Yasuda, H., Uryu, K., Robinson, J., Xie, S. X., Hurtig, H., Duda, J. E.,...Trojanowski, J. Q. (2007). Co-morbidity of TDP-43 proteinopathy in Lewy body related diseases. *Acta Neuropathologica, 114*(3), 221–229.

Noe, E., Marder, K., Bell, K. L., Jacobs, D. M., Manly, J. J., & Stern, Y. (2004). Comparison of dementia with Lewy bodies to Alzheimer's disease and Parkinson's disease with dementia. *Movement Disorders, 19*(1), 60–67.

Okazaki, H., Lipkin, L. E., & Aronson, S. M. (1961). Diffuse intracytoplasmic ganglionic inclusions (Lewy type) associated with progressive dementia and quadriparesis in flexion. *Journal of Neuropathology and Experimental Neurology, 20*, 237–244.

Olichney, J. M., Galasko, D., Salmon, D. P., Hofstetter, C. R., Hansen, L. A., Katzman, R., & Thal, L. J. (1998). Cognitive decline is faster in Lewy body variant than in Alzheimer's disease. *Neurology, 51*(2), 351–357.

Olichney, J. M., Murphy, C., Hofstetter, C. R., Foster, K., Hansen, L. A., Thal, L. J., & Katzman, R. (2005). Anosmia is very common in the Lewy body variant of Alzheimer's disease. *Journal of Neurology, Neurosurgery, and Psychiatry, 76*(10), 1342–1347.

Onofrj, M., Bonanni, L., Manzoli, L., & Thomas, A. (2010). Cohort study on somatoform disorders in Parkinson disease and dementia with Lewy bodies. *Neurology, 74*(20), 1598–1606.

Perez, F., Helmer, C., Dartigues, J. F., Auriacombe, S., & Tison, F. (2010). A 15-year population-based cohort study of the incidence of Parkinson's disease and dementia with Lewy bodies in an elderly French cohort. *Journal of Neurology, Neurosurgery, and Psychiatry, 81*(7), 742–746.

Perneczky, R., Drzezga, A., Boecker, H., Förstl, H., Kurz, A., & Häussermann, P. (2008). Cerebral metabolic dysfunction in patients with dementia with Lewy bodies and visual hallucinations. *Dementia and Geriatric Cognitive Disorders, 25*(6), 531–538.

Perry, E. K., Haroutunian, V., Davis, K. L., Levy, R., Lantos, P., Eagger, S.,...McKeith, I. G. (1994). Neocortical cholinergic activities differentiate Lewy body dementia from classical Alzheimer's disease. *Neuroreport, 5*(7), 747–749.

Perry, R. H., Irving, D., Blessed, G., Fairbairn, A., & Perry, E. K. (1990). Senile dementia of Lewy body type. A clinically and neuropathologically distinct form of Lewy body dementia in the elderly. *Journal of the Neurological Sciences, 95*(2), 119–139.

Querfurth, H. W., Allam, G. J., Geffroy, M. A., Schiff, H. B., & Kaplan, R. F. (2000). Acetylcholinesterase inhibition in dementia with Lewy bodies: Results of a prospective pilot trial. *Dementia and Geriatric Cognitive Disorders, 11*(6), 314–321.

Samuel, W., Galasko, D., Masliah, E., & Hansen, L. A. (1996). Neocortical Lewy body counts correlate with dementia in the Lewy body variant of Alzheimer's disease. *Journal of Neuropathology and Experimental Neurology, 55*(1), 44–52.

Schneider, L. S., Dagerman, K. S., & Insel, P. (2005). Risk of death with atypical antipsychotic drug treatment for dementia: Meta-analysis of randomized placebo-controlled trials. *Journal of American Medical Association, 294*(15), 1934–1943.

Schulz-Schaeffer, W. J. (2010). The synaptic pathology of alpha-synuclein aggregation in dementia with Lewy bodies, Parkinson's disease and Parkinson's disease dementia. *Acta Neuropathologica, 120*(2), 131–143.

Shea, C., MacKnight, C., & Rockwood, K. (1998). Donepezil for treatment of dementia with Lewy bodies: A case series of nine patients. *International Psychogeriatrics/IPA, 10*(3), 229–238.

Shimada, H., Hirano, S., Shinotoh, H., Aotsuka, A., Sato, K., Tanaka, N., ... Irie, T. (2009). Mapping of brain acetylcholinesterase alterations in Lewy body disease by PET. *Neurology, 73*(4), 273–278.

Sidransky, E., Nalls, M. A., Aasly, J. O., Aharon-Peretz, J., Annesi, G., Barbosa, E. R., ... Ziegler, S. G. (2009). Multicenter analysis of glucocerebrosidase mutations in Parkinson's disease. *The New England Journal of Medicine, 361*(17), 1651–1661.

Singleton, A. B., Wharton, A., O'Brien, K. K., Walker, M. P., McKeith, I. G., Ballard, C. G., ... Morris, C. M. (2002). Clinical and neuropathological correlates of apolipoprotein E genotype in dementia with Lewy bodies. *Dementia and Geriatric Cognitive Disorders, 14*(4), 167–175.

Tateno, M., Kobayashi, S., & Saito, T. (2009). Imaging improves diagnosis of dementia with Lewy bodies. *Psychiatry Investigation, 6*(4), 233–240.

Tiraboschi, P., Hansen, L. A., Alford, M., Merdes, A., Masliah, E., Thal, L. J., & Corey-Bloom, J. (2002). Early and widespread cholinergic losses differentiate dementia with Lewy bodies from Alzheimer disease. *Archives of General Psychiatry, 59*(10), 946–951.

Tiraboschi, P., Salmon, D. P., Hansen, L. A., Hofstetter, R. C., Thal, L. J., & Corey-Bloom, J. (2006). What best differentiates Lewy body from Alzheimer's disease in early-stage dementia? *Brain: A Journal of Neurology, 129*(Pt 3), 729–735.

Tokuda, T., Qureshi, M. M., Ardah, M. T., Varghese, S., Shehab, S. A., Kasai, T., ... El-Agnaf, O. M. (2010). Detection of elevated levels of α-synuclein oligomers in CSF from patients with Parkinson disease. *Neurology, 75*(20), 1766–1772.

Treglia, G., & Cason, E. (2012). Diagnostic performance of myocardial innervation imaging using MIBG scintigraphy in differential diagnosis between dementia with Lewy bodies and other dementias: A systematic review and a meta-analysis. *Journal of Neuroimaging, 22*(2), 111–117.

Tsuang, D. W., Wilson, R. K., Lopez, O. L., Luedecking-Zimmer, E. K., Leverenz, J. B., DeKosky, S. T., ... Hamilton, R. L. (2005). Genetic association between the APOE*4 allele and Lewy bodies in Alzheimer disease. *Neurology, 64*(3), 509–513.

Tsuboi, Y., Uchikado, H., & Dickson, D. W. (2007). Neuropathology of Parkinson's disease dementia and dementia with Lewy bodies with reference to striatal pathology. *Parkinsonism & Related Disorders, 13*(Suppl 3), S221–S224.

Varma, A. R., Talbot, P. R., Snowden, J. S., Lloyd, J. J., Testa, H. J., & Neary, D. (1997). A 99mTc-HMPAO single-photon emission computed tomography study of Lewy body disease. *Journal of Neurology, 244*(6), 349–359.

Velayati, A., Yu, W. H., & Sidransky, E. (2010). The role of glucocerebrosidase mutations in Parkinson disease and Lewy body disorders. *Current Neurology and Neuroscience Reports, 10*(3), 190–198.

Walker, Z., Costa, D. C., Walker, R. W., Shaw, K., Gacinovic, S., Stevens, T., ... Katona, C. L. (2002). Differentiation of dementia with Lewy bodies from Alzheimer's disease using a dopaminergic presynaptic ligand. *Journal of Neurology, Neurosurgery, and Psychiatry, 73*(2), 134–140.

Walker, Z., Jaros, E., Walker, R. W., Lee, L., Costa, D. C., Livingston, G., ... Katona, C. L. (2007). Dementia with Lewy bodies: A comparison of clinical diagnosis, FP-CIT single photon emission computed tomography imaging and autopsy. *Journal of Neurology, Neurosurgery, and Psychiatry, 78*(11), 1176–1181.

Weintraub, D., & Hurtig, H. I. (2007). Presentation and management of psychosis in Parkinson's disease and dementia with Lewy bodies. *The American Journal of Psychiatry, 164*(10), 1491–1498.

Whitwell, J. L., Weigand, S. D., Shiung, M. M., Boeve, B. F., Ferman, T. J., Smith, G. E.,... Jack, C. R. (2007). Focal atrophy in dementia with Lewy bodies on MRI: A distinct pattern from Alzheimer's disease. *Brain: A Journal of Neurology, 130*(Pt 3), 708–719.

Zaccai, J., McCracken, C., & Brayne, C. (2005). A systematic review of prevalence and incidence studies of dementia with Lewy bodies. *Age and Ageing, 34*(6), 561–566.

Zarranz, J. J., Alegre, J., Gómez-Esteban, J. C., Lezcano, E., Ros, R., Ampuero, I.,... de Yebenes, J. G. (2004). The new mutation, E46K, of alpha-synuclein causes Parkinson and Lewy body dementia. *Annals of Neurology, 55*(2), 164–173.

CHAPTER 8

Neuropsychological Disturbance and Alcoholism: Korsakoff's and Beyond

Lokesh Shahani, Chad A. Noggle, and Jon C. Thompson

Alcohol use is very common in our current society, and alcohol abuse and dependence are unfortunately very common as well. According to the 2008 National Survey on Drug Use and Health, slightly more than half of Americans aged 12 years or older (51.6%) reported being current drinkers of alcohol. This translates to an estimated 129 million Americans. More than 23.3% participated in binge drinking in the 30 days prior to the survey (58.1 million people) and 6.9% (17.3 million) reported heavy drinking (Substance Abuse and Mental Health Services Administration, 2009).

Beyond the potential psychosocial ramifications of alcoholism, alcohol is also a known neurotoxin when consumed at excessive levels (Harper, 1998; Oscar-Berman, Shagrin, Evert, & Epstein, 1997). Furthermore, it has long been known that when alcohol is chronically consumed in excess, it can cause structural and functional abnormalities of the brain and other organs (Chanraud et al., 2010; Courville, 1955; Dreyfus & Victor, 1961; Oscar-Berman & Marinkovic, 2007).

The neurological impact of chronic alcohol consumption, especially on cognitive functioning, has been studied for more than 130 years, dating back to the works of Wernicke (1881) and Korsakoff (1887). Fitzhugh, Fitzhugh, and Reitan (1960, 1965) may well be credited with first introducing a neuropsychological model to the systematic study of alcoholism. Since this time, the literature has swelled, increasing our knowledge of the subject matter, and improving our understanding of the dementia syndrome(s) associated with chronic alcohol abuse (American Psychiatric Association [APA], 1994; Oslin, Atkinson, Smith, & Hendrie, 1998).

Prevalence rates of alcohol-related dementias vary across studies, oftentimes based on the criteria used. Prevalence rates have been reported from approximately 2% (Schoenberg, Kokmen, & Okazaki, 1987) to 24% (Carlen et al., 1994). The significant variability in reported prevalence rates is likely due in part to the differing terminology used to describe these neurological manifestations of chronic alcohol use and abuse. The most commonly reported terms found in the literature include alcohol-induced persisting dementia (APA, 1994), alcohol-related dementia (Oslin et al., 1998), and Korsakoff's syndrome (KS; Butters, 1981; Butters & Brandt, 1985;

Oscar-Berman, Kirkley, Gansler, & Couture, 2004). Moreover, each term can have slightly different diagnostic criteria. As a result of the use of different criteria to identify clinical groupings, variations are also found across studies of neuropsychological performance and neuropathology (e.g., Albert, Butters, & Brandt, 1981; Delin & Lee, 1992; Hunkin & Parkin, 1993; Jernigan et al., 1991; Moriyama et al., 2002; Moss, Albert, Butters, & Payne, 1986; Noël et al., 2001; Reed et al., 2003; Shear, Jernigan, & Butters, 1994).

Despite significant clinical focus on the complications of chronic alcohol use and abuse, alcohol may be beneficial when consumed in moderation. In fact, moderate alcohol consumption has demonstrated protective effects against both cardiovascular and cerebrovascular disease, with red wine demonstrating the greatest benefit (Klatsky, 1994; Korsten & Wilson, 1999; Thun et al., 1997). Some have even reported lower risks of dementia secondary to modest alcohol consumption (Ruitenberg et al., 2002). Consequently, it is important for clinicians to clarify the amount and type of alcohol being consumed and the frequency of this consumption when considering its potential role in any neuropsychological profile.

In this chapter, we seek to offer some synthesis of this literature to offer some clarity on cognitive dysfunction as it relates to alcohol and the manifestation of dementia as a result of chronic use, including discussion of the classic KS and related presentations.

NEUROPATHOLOGICAL CHANGES IN RELATION TO ALCOHOLISM

Alcohol consumed at greater than modest levels has been linked to an array of neuropathological changes. Harding, Halliday, Ng, Harper, and Kril (1996) found that excessive alcohol consumption corresponded to volumetric reductions in the brain. Specifically, Harding et al. (1996) found individuals diagnosed with alcoholism had reduced brain weight compared to controls and the degree of brain atrophy correlated with the rate and amount of alcohol consumed over a lifetime. This may correspond to the amount of alcohol consumed, as de Bruin et al. (2005) showed that neither current alcohol intake nor lifetime alcohol intake was associated with decreases in brain volume in males or females who consume moderate levels of alcohol. Although most studies on individuals diagnosed with alcoholism associate brain volume loss with volumetric reductions in the gray matter (e.g., Mann et al., 2001) others have found reductions in white matter volume to account for the majority of brain mass lost (De la Monte, 1988). White matter loss has also been noted in more chronic cases of KS, in which the prefrontal white matter is most severely affected. There appears to be a significant negative correlation between this white matter loss and maximum daily alcohol consumption (Kril, Halliday, Svoboda, & Cartwright, 1997). In fact, postmortem neuropathological studies of individuals with non-Korsakoff alcoholism indicate that the most apparent cortical abnormalities occur in the frontal lobes, with concurrent thinning of the corpus callosum (Pfefferbaum, Lim, Desmond, & Sullivan, 1996), and concomitant compromise of pontocerebellar and cerebello-thalamocortical systems (Sullivan, 2003).

Neuronal loss has also been documented in specific regions of the cerebral cortex (superior frontal association cortex), hypothalamus, and cerebellum in patients with alcoholism (Baker, Harding, Halliday, Kril, & Harper, 1999; Harding et al., 1996; Harper, Kril, & Daly, 1987). Atrophy of the cerebellum, in particular, has been commonly associated with alcoholism (Sullivan, Deshmukh, Desmond, Lim, & Pfefferbaum, 2000), particularly in the area of anterior superior cerebellar vermis. Quantitative pathological studies have further shown that there is a loss of Purkinje cells in the vermis (reduced on average by 43%) that correlates with clinical ataxia/unsteadiness (Baker et al., 1999).

The neurological damage done by chronic alcohol abuse does not necessarily lead to irreversible impairment. With abstinence, recovery is not only found in some functional domains, but research has also suggested neuropathological reversal. Specifically, research has found that metabolic and neuropsychological recovery with abstinence corresponded to volumetric brain gains (Bartsch et al., 2007). Significant increases of cerebellar choline and frontomesial N-acetylaspartate levels have also been reported, suggesting metabolic as well as regionally distinct morphological capacities for partial brain recovery resulting from chronic alcoholism (Bartsch et al., 2007)

EFFECTS OF ALCOHOL DETOXIFICATION/ABSTINENCE

Alcohol intoxification brings with it numerous acute alterations in cognitive functioning and perception. However, for chronic users (i.e., alcoholics), cognitive impairments do not necessarily subside when the acute intoxication does. Research has demonstrated that cognitive deficits in abstinent alcoholics remain across genders and ethnicities (Berglund, Leijonquist, & Hörlén, 1977; Guthrie & Elliott, 1980; Hill & Mikhale, 1979; Hochla, Fabian, & Parsons, 1982; Lee, Jensen, & Bech, 1982; Løberg, 1980; Parsons & Farr, 1981; Wilkinson & Carlen, 1980). Parsons (1986) previously noted that in the first months of abstinence, the deficits are widespread, with between one half and two thirds of abstinent alcoholic persons exhibiting cognitive impairments after acute detoxification. Although research has indicated that many of the cognitive deficits associated with alcoholism are reversible following sustained abstinence, chronic residual deficits are common. Much of this variability can be attributed to a number of factors including the chronicity (i.e., how long has the problem existed) and severity (i.e., how much and what type of alcohol is commonly consumed) of the alcoholism; other dietary practices; the patient's age (De Renzi, Faglioni, Nichelli, & Pignattari, 1984; Ryan & Butters, 1986; Ryan & Lewis, 1988); and possibly other factors such as genetics and psychiatric status. The most significant determinant of the presence of cognitive deficits in persons recovering from alcoholism is the time elapsed since their last drink (Fein, Bachman, Fisher, & Davenport, 1990).

Acute alcohol ingestion has an inhibitory effect at N-methyl-D-aspartate (NMDA) receptors, reducing excitatory glutamatergic transmission; this has an agonistic effect at gamma-aminobutyric acid type-A (GABAA) receptors. During prolonged exposure to alcohol, NMDA receptors are upregulated and GABAA receptors are downregulated, leading to tolerance. The roles are reversed during abstinence, with enhanced NMDA receptor function, reduced GABAergic transmission, and dysregulation of the dopaminergic system, leading to many of the symptoms and signs of withdrawal (McKeon, Frye, & Delanty, 2008).

Alcohol withdrawal is seen following cessation or reduction of alcohol use that has been heavy or prolonged. Symptoms of alcohol withdrawal usually appear within hours and include tremors, insomnia, anxiety, vivid dreams, irritability, nausea, vomiting, headache, and sweating. Most symptoms usually resolve on their own within several hours to days; however, at times, the withdrawal progresses to severe manifestations such as hallucinosis, seizures, and delirium tremens.

Hallucinosis usually occurs within 1 or 2 days of abstaining or decreasing alcohol intake and is distinct from delirium tremens. Hallucinosis is characterized by auditory, visual, or most often tactile hallucinations in the presence of patients' full consciousness and awareness of their surroundings. It is not usually preceded by autonomic signs.

Delirium tremens, commonly known as "DTs," is characterized by a fluctu-ating disturbance of consciousness and change in cognition occurring over a short period of time. It is accompanied by a further exacerbation of autonomic symptoms (sweating, nausea, palpitations, and tremor) and an exacerbation of psychological symptoms including anxiety. Complications may arise as a sequelae of the delirium (injury to patient or staff) or due to medical complications (aspiration pneumonia, arrhythmia, or myocardial infarction), which may lead to death. Mortality associated with DTS has improved from 37% to up to 5% in recent studies (Mayo-Smith et al., 2004; Pristach, Smith, & Whitney, 1983). The improved mortality rate is probably due to earlier identification and improved supportive and pharmacological therapy in addition to advancements in medical care for the medical comorbidities.

Benzodiazepines are the cornerstone of management for alcohol withdrawal and delirium tremens. Lorazepam may be a reasonable choice for the treatment of alcohol withdrawal symptoms from the onset, and also effective therapy for delirium tremens. Neuroleptic agents play a role as an adjunct to benzodiazepines when agita-tion, thought disorder, or perceptual disturbances are not sufficiently controlled by benzodiazepines. In extreme cases, intubation and ventilation in an intensive care setting are required to facilitate adequate sedation.

NEUROPSYCHOLOGICAL FUNCTIONING IN DETOXIFICATION AND ABSTINENCE

Alcohol dependency is commonly associated with a number of neurological impair-ments including deficits in abstract problem solving, visuospatial and verbal learning, memory function, perceptual–motor skills, and even motor function (Oscar-Berman & Hutner, 1993; Sullivan, Rosenbloom, Lim, & Pfefferbaum, 2000). Outcomes related to neuropsychological functioning following detoxification are dependent on the amount of time since the last drink. In this regard, detoxification envelopes three periods: acute detoxification (up to 2 weeks of abstinence), intermediate abstinence (2 weeks to 2 months), and long-term abstinence (greater than 2 months). Across these time periods, individuals may experience a relative change in different domains of neuropsychological functioning in which the most prominent impairment is observed during acute detoxification and slowly resolves as the period of abstinence lengthens. However, not all deficits resolve. As noted in the research, in the first 2 weeks of abstinence (i.e., detoxification), most alcoholics exhibit a variety of neuro-psychological deficits involving just about every cognitive function; yet, during these same initial weeks, individuals also demonstrate the return of cognitive functioning (Ryan & Butters, 1986). The rate of return is most rapid in the first few weeks, pla-teauing off at around 6 weeks (Hannay, Howieson, Loring, Fischer, & Lezak, 2004).

Differences are found across neuropsychological domains. For example, while the verbal and full-scale outcomes on intelligence measures are often relatively normal in patients who recently went through detoxification, performance scales often show a significant weakness. This finding was noted by Grant (1987), among others. When considering the individual domains of intelligence, attention, learning and memory, visuospatial functioning, and executive functioning, mixed results have emerged.

Intelligence

Due to the influence of poor attention, concentration, reaction time, and other acute manifestations of withdrawal, assessment of intelligence during acute detoxification may be of limited utility and one could clearly question the validity and reliability of any such assessment as it relates to establishing chronic impairment or predicting prognosis. As abstinence stretches into the intermediate phases, following detoxification, overall intellectual functioning as well as verbal comprehension abilities of alcoholics oftentimes return to normal ranges. In comparison, perceptual reasoning weaknesses persist during the intermediate-term abstinence period in most recovering alcoholics, as evidenced by lower Performance IQ subtest scores relative to Verbal IQ subtest scores on the Wechsler Adult Intelligence Scale (WAIS) (Fitzhugh et al., 1965; Kleinknecht & Goldstein, 1972; Løberg, 1980; Løberg & Miller, 1986). A core deficit at this point in the recovery process appears to be impairment in higher cognitive functions of perceptual analysis and synthesis. Not surprisingly, during this same phase of recovery, patients commonly demonstrate impairment in other visuospatial and constructional tasks as discussed in the following text.

Attention

In the acute detoxification period, deficits in attention, concentration, and reaction time are the most prominent with less severe but notable deficits in motor coordination, motor speed, judgment, problem solving, learning, and short-term memory (Allen, Faillace, & Reynolds, 1971; Allen, Faillace, & Wagman, 1971; Clarke & Haughton, 1975; Farmer, 1973; Long & McLachlan, 1974; Page & Linden, 1974; Tarter & Jones, 1971; Weingartner, Faillace, & Markley, 1971). During acute withdrawal or in the presence of withdrawal hallucinosis or delirium tremens, attention and concentration are profoundly impacted. Although this domain can be most severely impacted in the acute detoxification period, clinical assessment of individuals during this period may be of limited use. However, as individuals move into the intermediate abstinence period, deficits can still at times be noted in attention and concentration.

On lower-level attention tasks such as directed and sustained attention, outcomes can be quite mixed though the consensus is that general attention is globally spared (Rourke & Løberg, 1996). However, as tasks demand higher-level processing, including sustained attention and working memory, deficits are revealed in the majority of patients (Bartsch et al., 2007). In fact, working memory impairment is consistently reported in relation to alcoholism (e.g., Cairney, Clough, Jaragba, & Maruff, 2007).

Learning and Memory

Research investigating the impact on learning and memory in patients diagnosed with alcoholism has also produced mixed results. Much of the discrepancies found may be attributed to the nature of the tasks participants are required to complete. Similar to outcomes in attention and concentration, as tests become more complex, greater impairment is more commonly noted (Ryan & Butters, 1980). For example, Tarter and Edwards reported that learning and memory deficits were not observed when standard clinical tests were employed at a point of intermediate abstinence, but deficits were elicited by more challenging laboratory tasks (Tarter & Edwards, 1985). At the point of intermediate abstinence, a number of studies have reported short-term impairment and learning deficits in both verbal and nonverbal tasks (Becker, Butters, Hermann, & D'Angelo, 1983; Brandt, Butters, Ryan, & Bayog, 1983; Cutting, 1978; Ron, Acker, & Lishman, 1980; Ryan & Butters, 1980). Individuals diagnosed with alcoholism have a tendency to recall less verbal and figural information during immediate and delayed recall, with no notable difference between verbal and visual learning (Nixon, Kujawski, Parsons, & Yohman, 1987). However, there was no difference between individuals diagnosed with alcoholism and controls with regard to their retention of information that was successfully registered and consolidated.

The authors noted that these indicated deficits were attributable to impairment in acquisition and encoding, with possible retrieval deficits as well (Nixon et al., 1987). A similar pattern was noted by Sherer, Nixon, Parsons, and Adams (1992), in which they found intact retention abilities comparable to controls, although overall performance on a word test was significantly lower in patients diagnosed with alcoholism due to deficits in acquisition and encoding. Ryan (1980) found that abstinent alcoholics took substantially longer than controls to learn a word list. However, the observed differences may be related to task approach

On learning tasks, individuals with alcoholism often employ rote rehearsal strategies at a significantly higher rate than controls and exhibit a proneness to retrograde memory impairment (Butters & Brandt, 1985). Not surprisingly, when it comes to auditory verbal memory, alcoholics tend to do worse on tasks of narrative memory, because they do not lend themselves to a rote rehearsal strategy (Grant & Reed, 1985; Jones & Parsons, 1971). In another study (Ellenberg, Rosenbaum, Goldman, & Whitman, 1980), visuospatial learning abilities were found to recover more slowly than verbal. Of interest, Ryan (1980) found that while abstinent alcoholics took substantially longer than controls to learn a word list, when individuals diagnosed with alcoholism were offered mnemonic strategies for learning and remembering, they did just as well as the control groups.

Although deficits in learning and memory of both verbal and visual information are frequently reported, they oftentimes are mild in nature in younger individuals who are at an intermediate stage of abstinence (Nixon et al., 1987). Furthermore, studies on the reversibility of cognitive deficits in younger populations have suggested that scores on short-term memory tasks can improve relative to the length of abstinence (Allen, Falliace, & Reynolds, 1971; Allen, Faillace, & Wagman, 1971; Weingartner et al., 1971), although discrepancies have been noted across the literature. Some studies have indicated recovery of new verbal learning abilities in the first 2 weeks of abstinence (e.g., Sharp, Rosenbaum, Goldman, & Whitman, 1977), whereas others reported sustained impairment in the past 1 month's time (Ryan, 1980; Weingartner et al., 1971). Some having reported memory deficits tend to improve first but less than completely in the initial weeks of abstinence (Goldman, 1983).

As individuals reach long-term abstinence, deficits in learning and memory are still present in some individuals, but additional recovery remains possible. Leber, Jenkins, and Parsons (1981) compared two groups of individuals diagnosed with alcoholism to controls. The first group had been abstinent for 3 weeks while the second had been abstinent for 11 weeks. The researchers found no significant difference among the three groups in verbal learning and memory. In comparison, those that had been abstinent for 3 weeks performed more poorly than those abstinent for 11 weeks on both a visuospatial learning task and on memory of designs. The 11-week abstinence group performed more poorly than the controls on these same tasks. A study by Yohman, Parsons, and Leber (1985) looked at individuals diagnosed with alcoholism who had abstained from alcohol for 13 months, those who were initially abstinent but then resumed drinking, and controls. Individuals were assessed at baseline and then at the aforementioned 13-month mark. They found that those who abstained for the full 13 months demonstrated improvements in learning, memory, abstracting, problem solving, and verbal abilities. In comparison, those who resumed drinking improved only in verbal abilities. Of note, even after abstaining for 13 months, the abstainers still performed significantly worse than controls on perceptual–motor tasks. The authors suggest the findings indicated that alcoholics who resume drinking, even at a reduced level, do not achieve the same gains in cognitive function as their abstinent peers and that even those who maintain abstinence do not fully recover their cognitive abilities after 13 months in some cognitive domains.

Visuospatial and Perceptual–Motor Functioning

Alcoholism has commonly been associated with deficits in visuospatial and perceptual–motor functioning. In fact, deficits in these areas may be some of the most common residuals of alcoholism, and the most likely to demonstrate chronic impairment even following abstinence. As previously noted, Yohman et al. (1985) found that even after 13 months of abstinence, abstainers still performed significantly worse than controls on perceptual–motor tasks. Many studies have demonstrated an association between alcoholism and deficits in complex visuospatial abilities, whether the tests used incorporate a motor component or not (e.g., Bertera & Parsons, 1978; Brandt et al., 1983; Ryan & Butters, 1986). Parsons and Leber (1981) reported that across eight studies, Block Design, Object Assembly, and Digit Symbol subtest scores on the WAIS were significantly lower in individuals with alcoholism compared to controls. Ryan and Butters (1986) noted that individuals with alcoholism exhibited poor performance on tests that require visuospatial organization, whereas Bowden (1988) did not find the same. Individuals abstinent from alcohol have also shown impairment on visuospatial and constructional tasks involving visuomotor speed, coordination, visual scanning, and disembedding figures from a complex design (Bergman & Agren, 1974; Goldstein & Shelly, 1971; Grant, 1987; Parsons & Leber, 1981; Sugerman & Schneider, 1976). These deficits have been associated with impairment in higher cognitive functions of perceptual analysis and synthesis (Ryan & Butters, 1983; Tarter, 1975) and slowed visual organization and integration (Akshoomoff, Delis, & Kiefner, 1989).

Executive Functioning and Problem Solving

Executive functioning and related abilities are commonly impaired in individuals diagnosed with alcoholism. In fact, deficits are frequently noted on tasks associated with frontal lobe functioning (Rourke & Løberg, 1996; Ryan & Butters, 1986). Parsons and Leber (1981) suggested that executive dysfunction was among the most consistent findings in those diagnosed with alcoholism. For example, they noted that 17 out of 19 studies reviewed found impairment on the Category Test in relation to alcoholism. Rourke and Grant (1999) have reported that the degree of impairment on this test is related to the length of abstinence. Individuals diagnosed with alcoholism reportedly exhibit the greatest difficulty on the subtest that heavily relies on spatial discrimination (i.e., subtest 4; Jones & Parsons, 1972). At the point of intermediate-term abstinence, alcoholics also perform more poorly than nonalcoholic persons on tests of problem-solving and abstracting abilities. Difficulties in maintaining a cognitive set, poor persistence, decreased flexibility in thinking, motor inhibition, perseveration, loss of spatial and temporal orientation, and an impaired ability to organize perceptual–motor responses and poor ability to synthesize spatial elements characterize the test patterns of individuals diagnosed with alcoholism (Hannay et al., 2004).

The Category Test from the Halstead–Reitan battery commonly demonstrates deficits during intermediate abstinence. Roughly 75% of abstinent individuals perform in the impaired range on this test (Grant & Reed, 1985; Jones & Parsons, 1971, 1972; Kleinknecht & Goldstein, 1972; Løberg, 1980; Long & McLachlan, 1974; Parsons & Leber, 1981; Svanum & Schladenhauffen, 1986). Similarly, individuals at the intermediate stage commonly demonstrate impairment on part B of the Trail Making Test, suggesting difficulties in cognitive flexibility (Chelune & Parker, 1981).

Abstinent individuals also perform more poorly than controls on verbal reasoning tests (Jonsson, Cronholm, & Izikowitz, 1962; Yohman & Parsons, 1987).

Sensorimotor Functioning

Beyond cognitive domains, motor deficits are also commonly seen in conjunction with alcoholism. In a study, abstinent alcoholics were evaluated at 2 and 8 weeks after detoxification. At 2 weeks, all individuals performed significantly worse than controls on motor speed, muscle strength, and visuomotor coordination. At 8 weeks, abstinent alcoholics with drinking histories of greater than 10 years remained impaired on motor functioning whereas those who had been drinking for a shorter period performed as well as the controls. The authors concluded that motor functioning does become impaired after chronic alcohol abuse and that the shorter the period of abuse, the greater the potential for recovery with abstinence (Tarter & Jones, 1971). Impairment has also been noted in the efficiency by which patients perform visual search and scanning tasks (Ryan & Butters, 1986). Individuals diagnosed with alcoholism also demonstrate a general slowing in performance, including on manual dexterity tests among others (Rourke & Løberg, 1996).

DEMENTIA AND ALCOHOLISM

Clearly not every individual diagnosed with alcoholism is able to maintain abstinence. For some, their alcoholism becomes increasingly severe, disrupting all aspects of their life. In some cases, the alcoholism persists and more severe neurological damage occurs, leading to a persisting dementia. Significant mental and personality deterioration occurring after years of alcohol abuse can manifest as an alcoholic dementia that may involve a multitude of neurocognitive deficits without the profound amnesia corresponding to KS (Rourke & Løberg, 1996; Ryan & Butters, 1986). In these cases, there is often an expansion of the deficits and neuropathological findings previously discussed. When symptoms of profound cognitive and motor deficits are observed, acutely or chronically, patients are typically diagnosed with Wernicke's Encephalopathy (WE) and KS.

WERNICKE–KORSAKOFF'S SYNDROME: HISTORICAL CONTEXT

In 1881, the German neurologist Carl Wernicke published three case reports describing a fatal encephalopathy that afflicted two alcoholic men and a woman who developed persistent vomiting due to pyloric stenosis secondary to sulfuric acid ingestion. Wernicke noted that all three patients exhibited the same triad of symptoms, acute mental confusion, ataxia, and ophthalmoplegia, and all three died. Wernicke conducted brain autopsies identifying punctate hemorrhages in the gray matter surrounding the third and fourth ventricles and the aqueduct. The disorder associated with clinical and pathological findings described by Wernicke came to be known as WE.

WERNICKE'S ENCEPHALOPATHY

WE is an acute, neuropsychiatric syndrome characterized by nystagmus and ophthalmoplegia, mental-status changes, and unsteadiness of gait (Scolding & Marsden, 2003). However, the simultaneous presentation of all three symptoms is seen in only 16% of patients (Harper, Giles, & Finlay-Jones, 1986; Victor et al., 1971). These changes largely result from an involvement of thalamic or mamillary bodies and range from a confusional state to mental sluggishness, apathy, impaired awareness of the immediate situation, inability to concentrate, and, if left untreated, coma and death (Harper et al., 1986; Sechi & Serra, 2007; Victor et al., 1989). Some patients may present with confusion or agitation, hallucinations, and behavioral disturbances, mimicking an acute psychotic disorder (Jiang et al., 2006; Kulkarni, Lee, Holstein, & Warner, 2005; Sechi & Serra, 2007; Worden & Allen, 2006). Ocular abnormalities, occurring in about 29% of patients, include nystagmus, symmetrical or asymmetrical palsy of both lateral recti and other ocular muscles, and conjugate-gaze palsies, which result from lesions of the pontine tegmentum and of the abducens and oculomotor nuclei (Victor et al., 1989). A few patients have a sluggish reaction of the pupils to light, anisocoria, and light-near dissociation (Cooke, Hicks, Page, & McKinstry, 2006; Sechi & Serra, 2007). Bilateral visual disturbances with optic disk edema, sometimes with retinal hemorrhages, may be the presenting features of WE (Ghez, 1969; Sechi & Serra, 2007). Loss of equilibrium with incoordination of gait and trunk ataxia affect about 23% of patients and result from an involvement of cerebellar vermis and vestibular dysfunction (Sechi et al., 1996; Sechi & Serra, 2007). The coexistence of polyneuropathy may be a contributing factor.

WE results from a deficiency in vitamin B_1 (thiamine), which in its biologically active form, thiamine diphosphate, is an essential coenzyme in several biochemical pathways in the brain (Manzo, Locatelli, Candura, & Costa, 1994; Sechi & Serra, 2007). Thiamine in the central nervous system is particularly key in glucose metabolism. Thiamine deficiency diminishes thiamine-dependent enzyme activity, alters mitochondrial function, impairs oxidative metabolism, and causes selective neuronal death (Gibson & Zhang, 2002; Hazell, Todd, & Butterworth, 1998; Ke, DeGiorgio, Volpe, & Gibson, 2003). Thiamine deficiency in both humans and rodent models, corresponds with acute and chronic neuronal damage with evidence of hemorrhages, demyelinization, gliosis, and neuronal loss localized to the mamillary bodies, thalamic nuclei, and cerebellum with relative sparing of cerebral cortical structures (Harper, Dixon, Sheedy, & Garrick, 2003). In individuals diagnosed with alcoholism, thiamine deficiency may result from an inadequate dietary intake, an impaired thiamine absorption in the gastrointestinal tract, a reduced liver storage, and a decrease in the transformation of thiamine into its active form (Butterworth, 1995). However, WE is not necessarily diagnostic of alcoholism.

In recent years, there has been an increase in the number of clinical settings in which WE is observed possibly due to dietary practices and food production. For example, rice is a staple diet for a large population. The husk of the rice is rich in thiamine; however, milling results in removal of husk and hence consumption of polished rice has resulted in an increased risk of thiamine deficiency in regions where this rice makes up a majority of individuals' diets.

Chronic alcohol misuse does not result in WE if the dietary intake of thiamine is adequate. However, self neglect of the low content of vitamins and minerals in alcoholic beverages, the decreased transport of thiamine across intestinal mucosa, the low capacity of the liver to store the vitamins, and the impaired conversion of thiamine to the active compound thiamine pyrophosphate results in thiamine deficiency in people with alcohol-related disorders. Moreover, the metabolism of alcohol raises the demand for thiamine; therefore, alcohol-dependent people typically require more of the vitamin than nonalcoholic people do (Sechi & Serra, 2007).

Gastrointestinal surgeries, especially the very popular gastric bypass surgery for weight reduction, has been associated with cases of WE (Sechi & Serra, 2007; Singh & Kumar, 2007). The mechanisms responsible for WE after gastrointestinal surgery include the occurrence of vomiting, poor compliance with an adequate dietary intake, the limited amount of food ingested, poor digestion of food with consequent malabsorption, and the reduced area of the gastric and duodenal mucosa useful for absorbing thiamine (Sechi & Serra, 2007; Shuster & Vázquez, 2005).

About 19% of patients have none of the symptoms of the classic triad at the presentation of WE (Harper et al., 1986), although usually one or more symptoms appear later in the course of the disease (Reuler, Girard, & Cooney, 1985; Sechi & Serra, 2007). This makes the diagnosis of the syndrome difficult in the acute stage. As WE is a medical emergency, appropriate identification and treatment are most essential. No particular laboratory or radiological study has been recommended, per se, for diagnosis of the WE; hence, diagnosis is based on clinical symptoms. However, pathologically, WE mainly affects the mamillary bodies, thalamus, and periventricular regions around the third and fourth ventricles, and aqueduct (Scolding & Marsden, 2003). The cerebral cortex is also commonly involved (D'Aprile, Tarantino, Santoro, & Carella, 2000; Doss, Mahad, & Romanowski, 2003; Kinoshita, Inoue, Tsuru, Yasukouchi, & Yokota, 2001; Liu et al., 2006; Victor, Adams, & Collins, 1973; Yamashita & Yamamoto, 1995; Zhong, Jin, & Fei, 2005). When it comes to imaging, MRI is most effective in viewing pathological markers (Antunez et al., 1998; Osborn, 2005). The typical MRI findings, such as high-intensity areas in the thalamus, periventricular regions surrounding the third and fourth ventricles, and the aqueduct on T2-weighted imaging (T2WI), perfusion-weighted imaging (PWI), diffusion-weighted imaging (DWI), and fluid attenuation inversion recovery (FLAIR), as well as enhancement of the mamillary bodies, are considered to reflect these pathological changes (Antunez et al., 1998; Halavaara, Brander, Lyytinen, Setälä, & Kallela, 2003; Osborn, 2005; Shogry & Curnes, 1994). These pathological markers are not consistently seen, which is why, if the diagnosis is suspected, the patient should be started on thiamine intravenously or intramuscularly to ensure adequate absorption. Patients should be treated empirically with a minimum of 500 mg thiamine hydrochloride (dissolved in 100 mL of normal saline), given by infusion over a period of 30 minutes, 3 times per day for 2 to 3 days. Where there is no response, supplementation may be discontinued after 2 to 3 days. Where an effective response is observed, 250 mg thiamine given intravenously or intramuscularly daily for 3 to 5 days, or until clinical improvement ceases, should be continued (Sechi & Serra, 2007). It is mandatory that thiamine is given before or concomitantly with intravenous administration of glucose when a diagnosis of WE is suspected, because glucose alone can precipitate the disorder in thiamine-deficient individuals (Sechi & Serra, 2007).

Victor found that recovery from the ophthalmoplegia was complete after a few hours, except for a residual, fine, horizontal nystagmus in 60% of patients. Recovery from ataxia occurred after a few days, although in some cases it was incomplete. The changes in mental status tended to improve after 2 to 3 weeks of therapy (Sechi & Serra, 2007; Victor et al., 1989).

KORSAKOFF'S SYNDROME

KS has been defined by Victor et al. (1971) as "an abnormal mental state in which memory and learning are affected out of all proportion to other cognitive functions in an otherwise alert and responsive patient." WE, as previously mentioned, is reversible if treated with a timely and adequate dose of parenteral thiamine. If it is undiagnosed or inadequately treated, it is likely to proceed to the chronic state, KS. Evidence that WE can progress to the chronic neurologic condition known as

KS comes from cohort studies that followed individuals' clinical trajectories as the acute signs of WE resolved following treatment with thiamine. Victor et al. (1971, 1989) prospectively followed 245 patients over 11 years and reported that 84% of the WE alcoholic individuals in their cohort progressed to KS. Victor et al. (1989) noted that memory and amnesia were challenging to assess accurately amid the acute mental status changes associated with WE. Recovery to where memory could be accurately assessed took from 1 week to 2 months (Lough, 2012). It is important for clinicians to understand the difference among WE, KS, and Wernicke–Korsakoff's syndrome.

Because KS often follows WE, and both appear to share common pathological substrates, a number of researchers describe this continuum as Wernicke–Korsakoff's syndrome (Kato, 1999; Victor, 1994). Consequently, some only use the term *Wernicke–Korsakoff's syndrome* when alcohol is seen as the causal factor. When the onset of the chronic state appears more insidious and not necessarily linked to alcoholism or preceded by WE, oftentimes it will be merely termed *Korsakoff's syndrome*. Still others use the specifier of alcoholic KS. Caine, Halliday, Kril, and Harper (1997) offered an operational definition of Wernicke–Korsakoff's syndrome, suggesting that the term stipulates an unremitting anterograde amnesia and "disorientation in the absence of an acute confusional state," and two of the following: dietary deficiency, occulomotor abnormalities, cerebellar dysfunction, and "either an altered mental state or mild memory impairment" (p. 54).

Neuropsychological assessments have demonstrated deficits in memory for new materials and in gait and balance despite sparing of general intelligence, adequate immediate recall and well preserved visuoperceptual implicit learning. Additionally, deficits have been noted in the prefrontal neural circuitry with weaknesses indicated on tests of problem solving, working memory, cognitive flexibility, perseveration, and self-regulation (Zahr, Kaufman, & Harper, 2011). Alcohol in the absence of KS has been known to cause some mild executive dysfunction. Pitel et al. (2008) compared domains of episodic and working memory for patients with alcohol use disorders and KS and demonstrated that patients with KS had greater impairment in the episodic memory as compared to the working memory.

Korsakoff characterized the memory disorder as occurring in a setting of clear consciousness but with a severe impairment of current and recent memory. Current and recent memory was affected more than remote memory, but the impairment could involve memories from up to 30 years earlier. Defective encoding of new information has been noted as the common component of the Korsakoff memory dysfunction (Butters & Brandt, 1985; Ryan & Butters, 1986). The learning deficits are not modality specific, but extend to all types of information (O'Connor & Verfailie, 2002). The disorder was also associated with confabulations and these false recollections often represented real memories that were recalled out of temporal sequence (Kopelman, Thomson, Guerrini, & Marshall, 2009).

KS is qualitatively characterized by a chronic and striking loss of working memory with relatively little loss of reference memory. Immediate recall also shows little difference between Korsakoff patients and normal controls (Kopelman, 1985, 1986). Attention oftentimes appears relatively spared, with patients performing well on digit span, serial sevens, and other simple attention tasks (Kopelman, 1985). On more complex aspects of attention such as shifting and dividing attention (Oscar-Berman, 1980, 1984) and working memory (O'Connor & Verfaellie, 2002), Korsakoff patients demonstrate significant impairment. In addition, emotional changes may develop, including apathy, blandness, or mild euphoria, with little or no reaction to events

(Sechi & Serra, 2007). Patients are also particularly prone to confabulation in the early stages of the disease (De Rinzi, 2000).

KS does not always manifest itself following a distinct WE. Some patients are initially comatose or semiconscious, and upon resolution of the acute disorder it is realized that the patient has an underlying KS, resulting in delayed or inadequate treatment. Other patients have a more insidious onset where there may have been either no known history of previous WE or only a transient period of encephalopathy (Kopelman et al., 2009).

The classical neuropathological changes described by Victor and Adams in early 1970s include lesions in the periventricular region around the third and the fourth ventricle and atrophy of the mamillary bodies (Victor et al., 1971). More recent studies have demonstrated a broader impact of alcoholism involving both cortical and subcortical structures including periaquaeductal and periventricular gray matter, dorsolateral prefrontal, ventral/orbitofrontal, anterior cingulated, hippocampal regions, the insula, hypothalamus, middle cingulate cortex, cerebellum, basal forebrain, sublenticular extended amygdala, and a large portion of the ventral tegmentum (Barbas 2007; Barrett, Mesquita, Ochsner, & Gross, 2007; Makris et al., 2008; Pitel et al., 2009; Vetreno, Ramos, Anzalone, & Savage, 2012; Yeterian, Pandya, Tomaiuolo, & Petrides, 2012; Zahr et al., 2011; Zahr, Pitel, Chanraud, & Sullivan, 2010). This is in addition to the hallmark involvement of the mamillary bodies and the region enclosed by the anterior and mediodorsal thalamic nuclei, including the paratae-nial nucleus (Caulo et al., 2005; Vetreno et al., 2012). A gross morphological view of the brains of KS patients reveals cortical thinning, sulcal widening, and ventricular enlargement (Jung, Chanraud, & Sullivan, 2012). Neuronal loss in the areas of medial and anterior thalamus, as well as the basal forebrain, and reduction in Purkinje cell density noted in the cerebellum, suggests that this brain region is highly sensitive to thiamine deficiency (Zahr et al., 2011). In autopsy studies, cell counting has shown that KS could be associated with a reduction of basal forebrain cholinergic neurons (BFCNs), including the nucleus basalis of Meynert, the major source of cortical acetylcholine (Arendt et al., 1988). Mayes et al. (1988) found a decrease in the number or nucleolar volume of magnocellular neurons in the nucleus basalis of Meynert in two cases of KS when doing morphometric measurement of BFCNs. However, Cullen, Halliday, Caine, and Kril (1997) noted that cell loss in the cholinergic nucleus basalis is only minor and would not appear to account for the extent of memory issues demonstrated by patients.

As noted previously, MRI is helpful in some cases for acute detection of WE. Cytotoxic edema and vasogenic edema are typical neuroimaging findings of WE, presenting as bilateral symmetrical hyperintense signals on T2-weighted MR images. During the acute symptomatic stage, thiamine-related glucose and oxidative cellular energy metabolism are disturbed; this results in an imbalance of ionic gradients across the cell membrane, which leads to intracellular water shift and cell injury (cytotoxic edema), and the breakdown of the blood–brain barrier permeability, allowing intravascular fluid to penetrate into the cerebral parenchymal extracellular space (vasogenic edema). The most frequently affected regions are the medial thalamus and periventricular region of the third ventricle, periaqueductal area, mamillary bodies, and midbrain tectum (Jung et al., 2012). Neuropathological studies have reported that neuronal loss in the anterior thalamic nuclei is the best predictor of memory impairment in KS (Harding, Halliday, Caine, & Kril, 2000).

Following the resolution of edema and inflammation of acute WE, typical neuroimaging findings of KS are presented as volume deficits in affected brain regions

(Sullivan & Pfefferbaum, 2009). Accordingly, hyperintensities observed in the periventricular and periaqueductal areas at the acute stage are replaced by ventricle enlargement and aqueductal dilatation when reexamined 6 to 12 months later in the chronic KS (Gallucci, Bozzao, Splendiani, Masciocchi, & Passariello, 1990). The volume of the mamillary bodies, thalamus, pons, hippocampus, cerebellar hemispheres, and anterior superior vermis, after adjusting for age and intracranial volume, were 1.0 to 2.0 standard deviations below healthy controls in those with KS (Sullivan & Pfefferbaum, 2009).

Degradation of the dorsomedial thalamus has also been linked to the persistent memory impairment in patients with KS. The role of the anterior thalamus in KS is supported by neuroimaging studies demonstrating that a structural lesion in the mamillothalamic tract—white matter projections from the mamillary body to the anterior thalamus—results in this syndrome (Josseaume et al., 2007). PET studies also have reported that permanent amnesia was associated with hypometabolism in the thalamus (Reed et al., 2003).

Alcohol rehabilitation and early recognition and treatment of WE remain the most effective methods to prevent KS. Specifically, timely and adequate treatment of thiamine deficits is critical to prevent progression of the disease (Thomson, Cook, Touquet, & Henry; Royal College of Physicians, London, 2002). The optimal treatment strategy for patients with an established KS is not clear, although treatment of thiamine deficits is often still suggested. These patients are at increased risk of developing other psychiatric disorders such as anxiety, depression, and psychosis. Patients with KS are capable of new learning, particularly if the information is cued and visuoperceptual or procedural in nature. Patients with KS are also better able to recall new information over a longer period of time if they are not allowed to guess (Baddeley & Wilson, 1994). New learning is facilitated if patients live in a calm and well-structured environment and have the support of a psychologist. The nutrition of patients with KS should be considered as well. Nutritional evaluation and planning is often inadequate and not designed to optimize brain function. With abstinence from alcohol and adequate rehabilitation, patients with KS often have a normal life expectancy (Kopelman et al., 2009).

SUMMARY

Chronic alcohol use has been related to various linked disorders when used in excess, particularly when this excessive use becomes chronic. Chronic alcohol abuse has also been shown to give rise to various persistent cognitive deficits. With the rise in the geriatric population it is likely that there will be a corresponding and significant increase in the number of individuals diagnosed with dementia, leading to an associated increase in the social and health care burden on an already taxed system. Identifying the relative contribution of alcohol toward degenerative cognitive diseases will become increasingly important. Identifying and appropriately treating reversible causes of cognitive dysfunction should be prioritized. Practicing clinicians must be aware of the potential contributions of alcohol or any other substance to the functional profile of patients seen in consultation. This is particularly true given the relative impact that effective intervention can have in patients whose deficits stem from alcohol abuse as the reversal of deficits and even neuropathological changes are possible if supplied in a timely manner. While full recovery may not always be possible even with timely diagnosis and intervention, it is clear that if intervention is not provided, patients may reach a point where impairment is of such severity and chronicity that little to no recovery may be achieved.

REFERENCES

Akshoomoff, N. A., Delis, D. C., & Kiefner, M. G. (1989). Block constructions of chronic alcoholic and unilateral brain-damaged patients: A test of the right hemisphere vulnerability hypothesis of alcoholism. *Archives of Clinical Neuropsychology, 4*(3), 275–281.

Albert, M. S., Butters, N., & Brandt, J. (1981). Patterns of remote memory in amnesic and demented patients. *Archives of Neurology, 38*(8), 495–500.

Allen, R. P., Faillace, L. A., & Reynolds, D. M. (1971). Recovery of memory functioning in alcoholics following prolonged alcohol intoxication. *The Journal of Nervous and Mental Disease, 153*(6), 417–423.

Allen, R. P., Faillace, L. A., & Wagman, A. (1971). Recovery time for alcoholics after prolonged alcohol intoxication. *The Johns Hopkins Medical Journal, 128*(3), 158–164.

American Psychiatric Association (APA). (1994). *Diagnostic and Statistical Manual of Mental Disorders* (4th ed). Washington, DC: American Psychiatric Association.

Antunez, E., Estruch, R., Cardenal, C., Nicolas, J. M., Fernandez-Sola, J., & Urbano-Marquez, A. (1998). Usefulness of CT and MR imaging in the diagnosis of acute Wernicke's encephalopathy. *American Journal of Roentgenology, 171*(4), 1131–1137.

Arendt, T., Allen, Y., Sinden, J., Schugens, M. M., Marchbanks, R. M., Lantos, P. L., & Gray, J. A. (1988). Cholinergic-rich brain transplants reverse alcohol-induced memory deficits. *Nature, 332*(6163), 448–450.

Baddeley, A., & Wilson, B. A. (1994). When implicit learning fails: Amnesia and the problem of error elimination. *Neuropsychologia, 32*(1), 53–68.

Baker, K. G., Harding, A. J., Halliday, G. M., Kril, J. J., & Harper, C. G. (1999). Neuronal loss in functional zones of the cerebellum of chronic alcoholics with and without Wernicke's encephalopathy. *Neuroscience, 91*(2), 429–438.

Barbas, H. (2007). Flow of information for emotions through temporal and orbitofrontal pathways. *Journal of Anatomy, 211*(2), 237–249.

Barrett, L. F., Mesquita, B., Ochsner, K. N., & Gross, J. J. (2007). The experience of emotion. *Annual Review of Psychology, 58*, 373–403.

Bartsch, A. J., Homola, G., Biller, A., Smith, S. M., Weijers, H. G., Wiesbeck, G. A.,...Bendszus, M. (2007). Manifestations of early brain recovery associated with abstinence from alcoholism. *Brain: A Journal of Neurology, 130*(Pt 1), 36–47.

Becker, J. T., Butters, N., Hermann, A., & D'Angelo, N. (1983). A comparison of the effects of long-term alcohol abuse and aging on the performance of verbal and nonverbal divided attention tasks. *Alcoholism, Clinical and Experimental Research, 7*(2), 213–219.

Berglund, M., Leijonquist, H., & Hörlén, M. (1977). Prognostic significance and reversibility of cerebral dysfunction in alcoholics. *Journal of Studies on Alcohol, 38*(9), 1761–1770.

Bergman, H., & Agren, G. (1974). Cognitive style and intellectual performance in relation to the progress of alcoholism. *Quarterly Journal of Studies on Alcohol, 35*, 1242–1255.

Bertera, J. H., & Parsons, O. A. (1978). Impaired visual search in alcoholics. *Alcoholism, Clinical and Experimental Research, 2*(1), 9–14.

Bowden, S. C. (1988). Learning in young alcoholics. *Journal of Clinical and Experimental Neuropsychology, 10*(2), 157–168.

Brandt, J., Butters, N., Ryan, C., & Bayog, R. (1983). Cognitive loss and recovery in long-term alcohol abusers. *Archives of General Psychiatry, 40*(4), 435–442.

Butters, N. (1981). The Wernicke-Korsakoff syndrome: A review of psychological, neuropathological and etiological factors. *Currents in Alcoholism, 8*, 205–232.

Butters, N., & Brandt, J. (1985). The continuity hypothesis: The relationship of long-term alcoholism to the Wernicke-Korsakoff syndrome. *Recent Developments in Alcoholism, 3*, 207–226.

Butterworth, R. F. (1995). Pathophysiology of alcoholic brain damage: Synergistic effects of ethanol, thiamine deficiency and alcoholic liver disease. *Metabolic Brain Disease, 10*(1), 1–8.

Caine, D., Halliday, G. M., Kril, J. J., & Harper, C. G. (1997). Operational criteria for the classification of chronic alcoholics: Identification of Wernicke's encephalopathy. *Journal of Neurology, Neurosurgery, and Psychiatry, 62*(1), 51–60.

Cairney, S., Clough, A., Jaragba, M., & Maruff, P. (2007). Cognitive impairment in Aboriginal people with heavy episodic patterns of alcohol use. *Addiction, 102*(6), 909–915.

Carlen, P. L., McAndrews, M. P., Weiss, R. T., Dongier, M., Hill, J. M., Menzano, E.,... Eastwood, M. R. (1994). Alcohol-related dementia in the institutionalized elderly. *Alcoholism, Clinical and Experimental Research, 18*(6), 1330–1334.

Caulo, M., Van Hecke, J., Toma, L., Ferretti, A., Tartaro, A., Colosimo, C.,...Uncini, A. (2005). Functional MRI study of diencephalic amnesia in Wernicke-Korsakoff syndrome. *Brain: A Journal of Neurology, 128*(Pt 7), 1584–1594.

Chanraud, S., Pitel, A. L., & Sullivan, E. V. (2010). Structural imaging of alcoholic abuse. In M. E. Shenton & B. I. Turetsky (Eds.), *Understanding neuropsychiatric disorders*. New York, NY: Cambridge University Press.

Chelune, G. J., & Parker, J. B. (1981). Neuropsychological deficits associated with chronic alcohol abuse. *Clinical Psychology Review, 1*, 181–195.

Clarke, J., & Haughton, H. (1975). A study of intellectual impairment and recovery rates in heavy drinkers in Ireland. *The British Journal of Psychiatry, 126*, 178–184.

Cooke, C. A., Hicks, E., Page, A. B., & McKinstry, S. (2006). An atypical presentation of Wernicke's encephalopathy in an 11-year-old child. *Eye, 20*(12), 1418–1420.

Courville, C. B. (1955). *Effects of alcohol on the nervous system of man*. Los Angeles: San Lucas Press.

Cullen, K. M., Halliday, G. M., Caine, D., & Kril, J. J. (1997). The nucleus basalis (Ch4) in the alcoholic Wernicke-Korsakoff syndrome: Reduced cell number in both amnesic and non-amnesic patients. *Journal of Neurology, Neurosurgery, and Psychiatry, 63*(3), 315–320.

Cutting, J. (1978). Specific psychological deficits in alcoholism. *The British Journal of Psychiatry, 133*, 119–122.

D'Aprile, P., Tarantino, A., Santoro, N., & Carella, A. (2000). Wernicke's encephalopathy induced by total parenteral nutrition in patient with acute leukaemia: Unusual involvement of caudate nuclei and cerebral cortex on MRI. *Neuroradiology, 42*(10), 781–783.

de Bruin, E. A., Hulshoff Pol, H. E., Bijl, S., Schnack, H. G., Fluitman, S., Böcker, K. B.,...Verbaten, M. N. (2005). Associations between alcohol intake and brain volumes in male and female moderate drinkers. *Alcoholism, Clinical and Experimental Research, 29*(4), 656–663.

De la Monte, S. M. (1988). Disproportionate atrophy of cerebral white matter in chronic alcoholics. *Archives of Neurology, 45*, 990–992.

Delin, C. R., & Lee, T. H. (1992). Drinking and the brain: Current evidence. *Alcohol and Alcoholism, 27*(2), 117–126.

De Rinzi, E. (2000). Disorders of visual recognition. *Seminars in Neurology, 20*, 479–485.

De Renzi, E., Faglioni, P., Nichelli, P., & Pignattari, L. (1984). Intellectual and memory impairment in moderate and heavy drinkers. *Cortex, 20*(4), 525–533.

Doss, A., Mahad, D., & Romanowski, C. A. (2003). Wernicke encephalopathy: Unusual findings in nonalcoholic patients. *Journal of Computer Assisted Tomography, 27*(2), 235–240.

Dreyfus, P. M., & Victor, M. (1961). Effects of thiamine deficiency on the central nervous system. *The American Journal of Clinical Nutrition, 9*, 414–425.

Ellenberg, L., Rosenbaum, C., Goldman, M. S., & Whitman, R. D. (1980). Recoverability of psychological functioning following alcohol abuse: Lateralization effects. *Journal of Consulting and Clinical Psychology, 48*(4), 503–510.

Farmer, R. H. (1973). Functional changes during early weeks of abstinence, measured by the Bender-Gestalt. *Quarterly Journal of Studies on Alcohol, 34*(3), 786–796.

Fein, G., Bachman, L., Fisher, S., & Davenport, L. (1990). Cognitive impairments in abstinent alcoholics. *The Western Journal of Medicine, 152*(5), 531–537.

Fitzhugh, L. C., Fitzhugh, K. B., & Reitan, R. M. (1960). Adaptive abilities and intellectual functioning in hospitalized alcoholics. *Quarterly Journal of Studies on Alcohol, 21,* 414–423.

Fitzhugh, L. C., Fitzhugh, K. B., & Reitan, R. M. (1965). Adaptive abilities and intellectual functioning of hospitalized alcoholics: Further considerations. *Quarterly Journal of Studies on Alcohol, 26*(3), 402–411.

Gallucci, M., Bozzao, A., Splendiani, A., Masciocchi, C., & Passariello, R. (1990). Wernicke encephalopathy: MR findings in five patients. *American Journal of Roentgenology, 155*(6), 1309–1314.

Ghez, C. (1969). Vestibular paresis: A clinical feature of Wernicke's disease. *Journal of Neurology, Neurosurgery, and Psychiatry, 32*(2), 134–139.

Gibson, G. E., & Zhang, H. (2002). Interactions of oxidative stress with thiamine homeostasis promote neurodegeneration. *Neurochemistry International, 40*(6), 493–504.

Goldman, M. S. (1983). Cognitive impairment in chronic alcoholics. Some cause for optimism. *The American Psychologist, 38*(10), 1045–1054.

Goldstein, G., & Shelly, C. H. (1971). Field dependence and cognitive, perceptual and motor skills in alcoholics. A factor-analytic study. *Quarterly Journal of Studies on Alcohol, 32*(1), 29–40.

Grant, I. (1987). Alcohol and the brain: Neuropsychological correlates. *Journal of Consulting and Clinical Psychology, 55*(3), 310–324.

Grant, I., & Reed, R. (1985). Neuropsychology of alcohol and drug abuse. In A. L. Alterman (Ed.), *Substance abuse and psychopathology* (Chapter 11, pp. 298–341). New York, NY: Plenum Press.

Guthrie, A., & Elliott, W. A. (1980). The nature and reversibility of cerebral impairment in alcoholism; treatment implications. *Journal of Studies on Alcohol, 41*(1), 147–155.

Halavaara, J., Brander, A., Lyytinen, J., Setälä, K., & Kallela, M. (2003). Wernicke's encephalopathy: Is diffusion-weighted MRI useful? *Neuroradiology, 45*(8), 519–523.

Hannay, H. J., Howieson, D. B., Loring, D. W., Fischer, J. S., & Lezak, M. D. (2004). Neuropathology for neuropsychologists. In M. D. Lezak, D. B. Howieson, & D. W. Loring (Eds.), *Neuropsychological assessment* (4th ed., pp. 157–285). New York, NY: Oxford University Press.

Harding, A. J., Halliday, G. M., Ng, J. L., Harper, C. G., & Kril, J. J. (1996). Loss of vasopressin-immunoreactive neurons in alcoholics is dose-related and time-dependent. *Neuroscience, 72*(3), 699–708.

Harding, A., Halliday, G., Caine, D., & Kril, J. (2000). Degeneration of anterior thalamic nuclei differentiates alcoholics with amnesia. *Brain: A Journal of Neurology, 123*(Pt 1), 141–154.

Harper, C. (1998). The neuropathology of alcohol-specific brain damage, or does alcohol damage the brain? *Journal of Neuropathology and Experimental Neurology, 57*(2), 101–110.

Harper, C., Dixon, G., Sheedy, D., & Garrick, T. (2003). Neuropathological alterations in alcoholic brains. Studies arising from the New South Wales Tissue Resource Centre. *Progress in Neuro-Psychopharmacology & Biological Psychiatry, 27*(6), 951–961.

Harper, C. G., Giles, M., & Finlay-Jones, R. (1986). Clinical signs in the Wernicke-Korsakoff complex: A retrospective analysis of 131 cases diagnosed at necropsy. *Journal of Neurology, Neurosurgery, and Psychiatry, 49*(4), 341–345.

Harper, C., Kril, J., & Daly, J. (1987). Are we drinking our neurones away? *British Medical Journal, 294*(6571), 534–536.

Hazell, A. S., Todd, K. G., & Butterworth, R. F. (1998). *Mechanisms of neuronal cell death in Wernicke's encephalopathy. Metabolic Brain Disease, 13,* 97–122.

Hill, S., & Mikhale, M. (1979). Computerized transaxial tomographic and neuropsychological evaluations in chronic alcoholics and heroin abusers. *American Journal of Psychiatry, 136,* 598–602.

Hochla, N. A., Fabian, M. S., & Parsons, O. A. (1982). Brain-age quotients in recently detoxified alcoholic, recovered alcoholic and nonalcoholic women. *Journal of Clinical Psychology, 38*(1), 207–212.

Hunkin, N. M., & Parkin, A. J. (1993). Recency judgements in Wernicke-Korsakoff and post-encephalitic amnesia: Influences of proactive interference and retention interval. *Cortex, 29*(3), 485–499.

Jiang, W., Gagliardi, J. P., Raj, Y. P., Silvertooth, E. J., Christopher, E. J., & Krishnan, K. R. (2006). Acute psychotic disorder after gastric bypass surgery: Differential diagnosis and treatment. *The American Journal of Psychiatry, 163*(1), 15–19.

Jernigan, T. L., Butters, N., DiTraglia, G., Schafer, K., Smith, T., Irwin, M.,...Cermak, L. S. (1991). Reduced cerebral grey matter observed in alcoholics using magnetic resonance imaging. *Alcoholism, Clinical and Experimental Research, 15*(3), 418–427.

Jones, B., & Parsons, O. A. (1971). Impaired abstracting ability in chronic alcoholics. *Archives of General Psychiatry, 24*(1), 71–75.

Jones, B., & Parsons, O. A. (1972). Specific vs generalized deficits of abstracting ability in chronic alcoholics. *Archives of General Psychiatry, 26*(4), 380–384.

Jonsson, C. O., Cronholm, B., & Izikowitz, S. (1962). Intellectual changes in alcoholics. Psychometric studies on mental sequels of prolonged intensive abuse of alcohol. *Quarterly Journal of Studies on Alcohol, 23,* 221–242.

Josseaume, T., Auffray Calvier, E., Daumas Duport, B., Lebouvier, T., Pouliquen Mathieu, G.... Desal, H. (2007). [Acute anterograde amnesia by infarction of the mamillothalamic tracts]. *Journal of Neuroradiology, 34*(1), 59–62.

Jung, Y. C., Chanraud, S., & Sullivan, E. V. (2012). Neuroimaging of Wernicke's encephalopathy and Korsakoff's syndrome. *Neuropsychology Review, 22*(2), 170–180.

Kato, M. (1999). Korsakoff syndrome. In M. Matsusita (Ed.), *Encyclopedia of clinical psychiatry S2* (pp. 175–193). Tokyo: Nakayama Shotenn.

Ke, Z. J., DeGiorgio, L. A., Volpe, B. T., & Gibson, G. E. (2003). Reversal of thiamine deficiency-induced neurodegeneration. *Journal of Neuropathology and Experimental Neurology, 62*(2), 195–207.

Kinoshita, Y., Inoue, Y., Tsuru, E., Yasukouchi, H., & Yokota, A. (2001). [Unusual MR findings of Wernicke encephalopathy with cortical involvement]. *Brain and Nerve, 53*(1), 65–68.

Klatsky, A. L. (1994). Epidemiology of coronary heart disease—influence of alcohol. *Alcoholism, Clinical and Experimental Research, 18*(1), 88–96.

Kleinknecht, R. A., & Goldstein, S. G. (1972). Neuropsychological deficits associated with alcoholism. A review and discussion. *Quarterly Journal of Studies on Alcohol, 33*(4), 999–1019.

Kopelman, M. D. (1985). Rates of forgetting in Alzheimer-type dementia and Korsakoff's syndrome. *Neuropsychologia, 23*(5), 623–638.

Kopelman, M. D. (1986). Recall of anomalous sentences in dementia and amnesia. *Brain and Language, 29*(1), 154–170.

Kopelman, M. D., Thomson, A. D., Guerrini, I., & Marshall, E. J. (2009). The Korsakoff syndrome: Clinical aspects, psychology and treatment. *Alcohol and Alcoholism, 44*(2), 148–154.

Korsakoff, S. (1887). Disturbance of psychic activity in alcoholic paralysis. *Vestin Kline Psichiatra Neurologia, 4,* 1–102.

Korsten, M. A. & Wilson, J. S. (1999). Health effects of alcohol. In R. T. Ammerman, P. J. Ott, & R. E. Tarter (Eds.), *Prevention and societal impact of drug and alcohol abuse.* Mahwah, NJ: Erlbaum.

Kril, J. J., Halliday, G. M., Svoboda, M. D., & Cartwright, H. (1997). The cerebral cortex is damaged in chronic alcoholics. *Neuroscience, 79*(4), 983–998.

Kulkarni, S., Lee, A. G., Holstein, S. A., & Warner, J. E. (2005). You are what you eat. *Survey of Ophthalmology, 50*(4), 389–393.

Leber, W. R., Jenkins, R. L., & Parsons, O. A. (1981). Recovery of visual-spatial learning and memory in chronic alcoholics. *Journal of Clinical Psychology, 37*(1), 192–197.

Lee, K., Jensen, E., & Bech, P. (1982). Neuropsychological and computerized tomographic evaluations of young alcoholics. *The British Journal of Psychiatry, 141*, 282–285.

Liu, Y. T., Fuh, J. L., Lirng, J. F., Li, A. F., Ho, D. M., & Wang, S. J. (2006). Correlation of magnetic resonance images with neuropathology in acute Wernicke's encephalopathy. *Clinical Neurology and Neurosurgery, 108*(7), 682–687.

Løberg, T. (1980). Alcohol misuse and neuropsychological deficits in men. *Journal of Studies on Alcohol, 41*(1), 119–128.

Løberg, T., & Miller, W. R. (1986). Personality, cognitive, and neuropsychological correlates of harmful alcohol consumption: A cross-national comparison of clinical samples. *Annals of the New York Academy of Sciences, 472*, 75–97.

Long, J. A., & McLachlan, J. F. (1974). Abstract reasoning and perceptual-motor efficiency in alcoholics. Impairment and reversibility. *Quarterly Journal of Studies on Alcohol, 35*(4 Pt A), 1220–1229.

Lough, M. E. (2012). Wernicke's encephalopathy: Expanding the diagnostic toolbox. *Neuropsychology Review, 22*(2), 181–194.

Makris, N., Oscar-Berman, M., Jaffin, S. K., Hodge, S. M., Kennedy, D. N., Caviness, V. S., … Harris, G. J. (2008). Decreased volume of the brain reward system in alcoholism. *Biological Psychiatry, 64*(3), 192–202.

Mann, K., Agartz, I., Harper, C., Shoaf, S., Rawlings, R. R., Momenan, R.,… Heinz, A. (2001). Neuroimaging in alcoholism: Ethanol and brain damage. *Alcoholism, Clinical and Experimental Research, 25*(5 Suppl ISBRA), 104S–109S.

Manzo, L., Locatelli, C., Candura, S. M., & Costa, L. G. (1994). Nutrition and alcohol neurotoxicity. *Neurotoxicology, 15*(3), 555–565.

Mayes, A. R., Meudell, P. R., Mann, D., & Pickering, A. (1988). Location of lesions in Korsakoff's syndrome: Neuropsychological and neuropathological data on two patients. *Cortex, 24*(3), 367–388.

Mayo-Smith, M. F., Beecher, L. H., Fischer, T. L., Gorelick, D. A., Guillaume, J. L., Hill, A.,…Melbourne, J.; Working Group on the Management of Alcohol Withdrawal Delirium, Practice Guidelines Committee, American Society of Addiction Medicine. (2004). Management of alcohol withdrawal delirium. An evidence-based practice guideline. *Archives of Internal Medicine, 164*(13), 1405–1412.

McKeon, A., Frye, M. A., & Delanty, N. (2008). The alcohol withdrawal syndrome. *Journal of Neurology, Neurosurgery, and Psychiatry, 79*(8), 854–862.

Moriyama, Y., Mimura, M., Kato, M., Yoshino, A., Hara, T., Kashima, H.,…Watanabe, A. (2002). Executive dysfunction and clinical outcome in chronic alcoholics. *Alcoholism, Clinical and Experimental Research, 26*(8), 1239–1244.

Moss, M. B., Albert, M. S., Butters, N., & Payne, M. (1986). Differential patterns of memory loss among patients with Alzheimer's disease, Huntington's disease, and alcoholic Korsakoff's syndrome. *Archives of Neurology, 43*(3), 239–246.

Nixon, S. J., Kujawski, A., Parsons, O. A., & Yohman, J. R. (1987). Semantic (verbal) and figural memory impairment in alcoholics. *Journal of Clinical and Experimental Neuropsychology, 9*, 311–322.

Noël, X., Van der Linden, M., Schmidt, N., Sferrazza, R., Hanak, C., Le Bon, O.,...Verbanck, P. (2001). Supervisory attentional system in nonamnesic alcoholic men. *Archives of General Psychiatry, 58*(12), 1152–1158.

O'Connor, M. G., & Verfaellie, M. (2002). The amnesic syndrome: Overview and subtypes. In A. D. Baddeley, B. Wilson, & M. Kopelman (Eds.), *The handbook of memory disorders*. Chichester, UK: Wiley.

Osborn, A. G. (2005). Alcoholic encephalopathy. In A. G. Osborn , K. L. Salzman, G. Katzman, J. Provenzale, M. Castillo, G. Hedlund, . . . B. Hamilton (Eds.), *Diagnostic imaging: Brain* (1st ed., Part I, Section 10, pp. 20–23). Salt Lake City: AMIRSYS.

Oscar-Berman, M. (1980). Neuropsychological consequences of long-term chronic alcoholism. *American Scientist, 68*, 410–419.

Oscar-Berman, M. (1984). Comparative neuropsychology and alcoholic Korsakoff disease. In L. R. Squire & N. Butters (Eds.), *Neuropsychology of memory*. New York, NY: Guilford.

Oscar-Berman, M., & Hutner, N. (1993). Frontal lobe changes after chronic alcohol ingestion. In W. A. Hunt & S. J. Nixon (Eds.), *Alcohol induced brain damage* (pp. 121–156). Rockville, MD: NIH Publications.

Oscar-Berman, M., Kirkley, S. M., Gansler, D. A., & Couture, A. (2004). Comparisons of Korsakoff and non-Korsakoff alcoholics on neuropsychological tests of prefrontal brain functioning. *Alcoholism, Clinical and Experimental Research, 28*(4), 667–675.

Oscar-Berman, M., & Marinkovic, K. (2007). Alcohol: Effects on neurobehavioral functions and the brain. *Neuropsychology Review, 17*(3), 239–257.

Oscar-Berman, M., Shagrin, B., Evert, D. L., & Epstein, C. (1997). Impairments of brain and behavior: The neurological effects of alcohol. *Alcohol Health and Research World, 21*(1), 65–75.

Oslin, D., Atkinson, R. M., Smith, D. M., & Hendrie, H. (1998). Alcohol related dementia: Proposed clinical criteria. *International Journal of Geriatric Psychiatry, 13*(4), 203–212.

Page, R. D., & Linden, J. D. (1974). "Reversible" organic brain syndrome in alcoholics. A psychometric evaluation. *Quarterly Journal of Studies on Alcohol, 35*(1), 98–107.

Parsons, O. A. (1986). Alcoholics' neuropsychological impairment: Current findings and conclusions. *Annals of Behavavioral Medicine, 8*, 13–19.

Parsons, O. A. & Farr, S. (1981). The neuropsychology of alcohol and drug use, chap 10. In S. Filskov & T. Boll (Eds.), *Handbook of clinical neuropsychology* (pp. 320–365). New York, NY: Wiley.

Parsons, O. A., & Leber, W. R. (1981). The relationship between cognitive dysfunction and brain damage in alcoholics: Causal, interactive, or epiphenomenal? *Alcoholism, Clinical and Experimental Research, 5*(2), 326–343.

Pfefferbaum, A., Lim, K. O., Desmond, J. E., & Sullivan, E. V. (1996). Thinning of the corpus callosum in older alcoholic men: A magnetic resonance imaging study. *Alcoholism, Clinical and Experimental Research, 20*(4), 752–757.

Pitel, A. L., Aupée, A. M., Chételat, G., Mézenge, F., Beaunieux, H., de la Sayette, V.,... Desgranges, B. (2009). Morphological and glucose metabolism abnormalities in alcoholic Korsakoff's syndrome: Group comparisons and individual analyses. *PloS One, 4*(11), e7748.

Pitel, A. L., Beaunieux, H., Witkowski, T., Vabret, F., de la Sayette, V., Viader, F.,...Eustache, F. (2008). Episodic and working memory deficits in alcoholic Korsakoff patients:

The continuity theory revisited. *Alcoholism, Clinical and Experimental Research, 32*(7), 1229–1241.

Pristach, C. A., Smith, C. M., & Whitney, R. B. (1983). Alcohol withdrawal syndromes—prediction from detailed medical and drinking histories. *Drug and Alcohol Dependence, 11*(2), 177–199.

Reed, L. J., Lasserson, D., Marsden, P., Stanhope, N., Stevens, T., Bello, F.,…Kopelman, M. D. (2003). FDG-PET findings in the Wernicke-Korsakoff syndrome. *Cortex, 39*(4–5), 1027–1045.

Reuler, J. B., Girard, D. E., & Cooney, T. G. (1985). Current concepts. Wernicke's encephalopathy. *The New England Journal of Medicine, 312*(16), 1035–1039.

Ron, M. A., Acker, W., & Lishman, W. A. (1980). Morphological abnormalities in the brains of chronic alcoholics—a clinical psychological and computerized axial tomographic study. *Acta Psychiatrica Scandinavica. Supplementum, 286*, 41–46.

Rourke, S. B., & Grant, I. (1999). The interactive effects of age and length of abstinence on the recovery of neuropsychological functioning in chronic male alcoholics: A 2-year follow-up study. *Journal of the International Neuropsychological Society, 5*(3), 234–246.

Rourke, S. B., & Løberg, T. (1996). Neurobehavioral correlates of alcoholism. In I. Grant & K. M. Adams (Eds.), *Neuropsychological assessment of neuropsychiatric disorders* (pp. 423–485). New York, NY: Oxford University Press.

Ruitenberg, A., van Swieten, J. C., Witteman, J. C., Mehta, K. M., van Duijn, C. M., Hofman, A., & Breteler, M. M. (2002). Alcohol consumption and risk of dementia: The Rotterdam Study. *Lancet, 359*(9303), 281–286.

Ryan, C. (1980). Learning and memory deficits in alcoholics. *Journal of Studies on Alcohol, 41*(5), 437–447.

Ryan, C., & Butters, N. (1980). Learning and memory impairments in young and old alcoholics: Evidence for the premature-aging hypothesis. *Alcoholism, Clinical and Experimental Research, 4*(3), 288–293.

Ryan, C., & Butters, N. (1983). Cognitive deficits in alcoholics. In B. Kissin & H. Begleiter (Eds.), *The pathogenesis of alcoholism-Vol 7, biological factors* (Chapter 12, pp. 485–538). New York, NY: Plenum Press.

Ryan, C., & Butters, N. (1986). Neuropsychology of alcoholism. In D. Weddings, A. M. Horton Jr., & J. S. Webster (Eds.), *The neuropsychology handbook*. New York, NY: Springer.

Ryan, J. J., & Lewis, C. V. (1988). Comparison of normal controls and recently detoxified alcoholics on the Wechsler Memory Scale-Revised. *The Clinical Neuropsychologist, 2*, 173–180.

Schoenberg, B. S., Kokmen, E., & Okazaki, H. (1987). Alzheimer's disease and other dementing illnesses in a defined United States population: Incidence rates and clinical features. *Annals of Neurology, 22*(6), 724–729.

Scolding, N., & Marsden, C. D. (2003). Metabolic disorders and the nervous system. In D. A. Warrell, T. M. Cox, J. D. Firth , & E. J. Benz Jr. (Eds.), *Oxford textbook of medicine* (4th ed., vol. 3, pp. 1149–1155). New York, NY: Oxford University Press.

Sechi, G. P., Bosincu, L., Cossu Rocca, P., Deiana, G. A., Correddu, P., & Murrighile, R. M. (1996). Hyperthermia, choreic dyskinesias and increased motor tone in Wernicke's encephalopathy. *European Journal of Neurology, 3*(Suppl. 5), 133.

Sechi, G., & Serra, A. (2007). Wernicke's encephalopathy: New clinical settings and recent advances in diagnosis and management. *Lancet Neurology, 6*(5), 442–455.

Sharp, J. R., Rosenbaum, G., Goldman, M. S., & Whitman, R. D. (1977). Recoverability of psychological functioning following alcohol abuse: Acquisition of meaningful synonyms. *Journal of Consulting and Clinical Psychology, 45*(6), 1023–1028.

Shear, P. K., Jernigan, T. L., & Butters, N. (1994). Volumetric magnetic resonance imaging quantification of longitudinal brain changes in abstinent alcoholics. *Alcoholism, Clinical and Experimental Research, 18*(1), 172–176.

Sherer, M., Nixon, S. J., Parsons, O. A., & Adams, R. L. (1992). Performance of alcoholic and brain-damaged subjects on the Luria Memory Words test. *Archives of Clinical Neuropsychology, 7*(6), 499–504.

Shogry, M. E., & Curnes, J. T. (1994). Mamillary body enhancement on MR as the only sign of acute Wernicke encephalopathy. *American Journal of Neuroradiology, 15*(1), 172–174.

Shuster, M. H., & Vázquez, J. A. (2005). Nutritional concerns related to Roux-en-Y gastric bypass: What every clinician needs to know. *Critical Care Nursing Quarterly, 28*(3), 227–260; quiz 261.

Singh, S., & Kumar, A. (2007). Wernicke encephalopathy after obesity surgery: A systematic review. *Neurology, 68*(11), 807–811.

Substance Abuse and Mental Health Services Administration. (2009). *Results from the 2008 National Survey on Drug Use and Health: National Findings (Office of Applied Studies, Substance NSDUH Series H-36, HHS Publication No. SMA 09–4434).* Rockville, MD.

Sugerman, A., & Schneider, D. (1976). Cognitive styles in alcoholism. In R. Tarter & A. Sugerman (Eds.), *Alcoholism: Interdisciplinary approaches to an enduring problem* (Chapter 11, pp. 395–433). Reading, MA: Addison-Wesley.

Sullivan, E. V. (2003). Compromised pontocerebellar and cerebellothalamocortical systems: Speculations on their contributions to cognitive and motor impairment in nonamnesic alcoholism. *Alcoholism, Clinical and Experimental Research, 27*(9), 1409–1419.

Sullivan, E. V., Deshmukh, A., Desmond, J. E., Lim, K. O., & Pfefferbaum, A. (2000). Cerebellar volume decline in normal aging, alcoholism, and Korsakoff's syndrome: Relation to ataxia. *Neuropsychology, 14*(3), 341–352.

Sullivan, E. V., & Pfefferbaum, A. (2009). Neuroimaging of the Wernicke-Korsakoff syndrome. *Alcohol and Alcoholism, 44*(2), 155–165.

Sullivan, E. V., Rosenbloom, M. J., Lim, K. O., & Pfefferbaum, A. (2000). Longitudinal changes in cognition, gait, and balance in abstinent and relapsed alcoholic men: Relationships to changes in brain structure. *Neuropsychology, 14*(2), 178–188.

Svanum, S., & Schladenhauffen, J. (1986). Lifetime and recent alcohol consumption among male alcoholics. Neuropsychological implications. *The Journal of Nervous and Mental Disease, 174*(4), 214–220.

Tarter, R. E. (1975). Psychological deficit in chronic alcoholics: A review. *The International Journal of the Addictions, 10,* 327–368.

Tarter, R. E., & Edwards, K. L. (1985). Neuropsychology of alcoholism. In R. E. Tarter & D. H. Van Thiel (Eds.), *Alcohol and the brain: Chronic effects* (Chapter 8, pp. 217–244). New York, NY: Plenum Press.

Tarter, R. E., & Jones, B. M. (1971). Motor impairment in chronic alcoholics. *Diseases of the Nervous System, 32*(9), 632–636.

Thomson, A. D., Cook, C. C., Touquet, R., & Henry, J. A.; Royal College of Physicians, London. (2002). The Royal College of Physicians report on alcohol: Guidelines for managing Wernicke's encephalopathy in the accident and Emergency Department. *Alcohol and Alcoholism, 37*(6), 513–521.

Thun, M. J., Peto, R., Lopez, A. D., Monaco, J. H., Henley, S. J., Heath, C. W., & Doll, R. (1997). Alcohol consumption and mortality among middle-aged and elderly U.S. adults. *The New England Journal of Medicine, 337*(24), 1705–1714.

Vetreno, R. P., Ramos, R. L., Anzalone, S., & Savage, L. M. (2012). Brain and behavioral pathology in an animal model of Wernicke's encephalopathy and Wernicke-Korsakoff Syndrome. *Brain Research, 1436,* 178–192.

Victor, M. (1994). Alcoholic dementia. *The Canadian Journal of Neurological Sciences, 21*(2), 88–99.

Victor, M., Adams, R. D., & Collins, G. H. (1971). The Wernicke-Korsakoff syndrome. A clinical and pathological study of 245 patients, 82 with post-mortem examinations. *Contemporary Neurology Series, 7*, 1–206.

Victor, M., Adams, R. D., & Collins, G. H. (1973). *The Wernicke-Korsakoff syndrome* (2nd ed., pp. 94–95). Philadelphia, PA: Davis.

Victor, M., Adams, R. D., & Collins, G. H. (1989). *The Wernicke-Korsakoff syndrome and related neurologic disorders due to alcoholism and malnutrition* (2nd ed.). Philadelphia, PA: F.A. Davis.

Weingartner, H., Faillace, L. A., & Markley, H. G. (1971). Verbal information retention in alcoholics. *Quarterly Journal of Studies on Alcohol, 32*(2), 293–303.

Wernicke, C. (1881). *Die acute, haemorrhagische Poliencephalitis superior. Lehrbuch der Gehirnkrankheiten für Ärzte und Studirende, Band II* (pp. 229–242). Kassel: Theodor Fischer.

Wilkinson, D. A., & Carlen, P. L. (1980). Neuropsychological and neurological assessment of alcoholism; discrimination between groups of alcoholics. *Journal of Studies on Alcohol, 41*(1), 129–139.

Worden, R. W., & Allen, H. M. (2006). Wernicke's encephalopathy after gastric bypass that masqueraded as acute psychosis: A case report. *Current Surgery, 63*(2), 114–116.

Yamashita, M., & Yamamoto, T. (1995). Wernicke encephalopathy with symmetric pericentral involvement: MR findings. *Journal of Computer Assisted Tomography, 19*(2), 306–308.

Yeterian, E. H., Pandya, D. N., Tomaiuolo, F., & Petrides, M. (2012). The cortical connectivity of the prefrontal cortex in the monkey brain. *Cortex, 48*(1), 58–81.

Yohman, J. R., & Parsons, O. A. (1987). Verbal reasoning deficits in alcoholics. *The Journal of Nervous and Mental Disease, 175*(4), 219–223.

Yohman, J. R., Parsons, O. A., & Leber, W. R. (1985). Lack of recovery in male alcoholics' neuropsychological performance one year after treatment. *Alcoholism, Clinical and Experimental Research, 9*(2), 114–117.

Zahr, N. M., Kaufman, K. L., & Harper, C. G. (2011). Clinical and pathological features of alcohol-related brain damage. *Nature Reviews. Neurology, 7*(5), 284–294.

Zahr, N. M., Pitel, A. L., Chanraud, S., & Sullivan, E. V. (2010). Contributions of studies on alcohol use disorders to understanding cerebellar function. *Neuropsychology Review, 20*(3), 280–289.

Zhong, C., Jin, L., & Fei, G. (2005). MR Imaging of nonalcoholic Wernicke encephalopathy: A follow-up study. *American Journal of Neuroradiology, 26*(9), 2301–2305.

CHAPTER 9

Frontotemporal Dementias

Dong (Dan) Y. Han, Benjamin A. Pyykkonen,
Anne L. Shandera-Ochsner, and Frederick A. Schmitt

Dementia is an umbrella term for conditions such as Alzheimer's disease (AD), dementia with Lewy bodies (DLB), vascular dementia (VaD), and frontotemporal dementia (FTD). Under that umbrella, FTD, also known as frontotemporal lobar degeneration (FTLD), can be further categorized to define a group of neurodegenerative disorders resulting from a progressive deterioration of the cells in the anterior temporal and/or frontal lobes of the brain. More specifically, ventromedialfrontopolar cortex is identified with metabolic impairment in FTD (Salmon et al., 2003). The clinical features include progressive behavioral, language, and/or motor deteriorations, which inevitably result in significant functional decline.

These symptom patterns were first described in a case study by Arnold Pick (1892), in which he identified elderly patients with progressive language decline and atrophy of the brain. His case study, "On the Relationship Between Aphasia and Senile Atrophy of the Brain," continues to serve as a frame of reference for focal neurological deficits in diffuse neurodegenerative disorders (Kirshner, 2010; Takeda, Kishimoto, & Yokota, 2012). Then, throughout the 1980s and 1990s, two parallel data streams accumulated data regarding focal neural degeneration; that is, primarily language-centered versus primarily behavior-centered symptomatology. While the European literature primarily focused on behavioral symptom patterns (i.e., frontal dementia), the North American literature primarily focused on the degenerative language condition described as primary progressive aphasia (PPA). In recent years, these conditions have merged under the umbrella terms FTD or FTLD (Kirshner, 2010).

This chapter elaborates on the history, epidemiology, pathophysiology, clinical features, treatment, and outcomes of FTD. The history and background section of each of the FTD categories highlights the evolution of the disease conceptualization.

The FTD subtypes are conceptualized in three categories: neurobehavioral variant, motor variant, and language variant. First, the neurobehavioral variant of FTD includes the classic identification of Pick's disease or behavioral variant of FTD (bvFTD). Second, the motor variant of FTD includes progressive supranuclear palsy (PSP), corticobasal degeneration (CBD), and FTD with motor neuron disease (FTD-MND). Third, the language variant of FTD consists of PPA, which can be

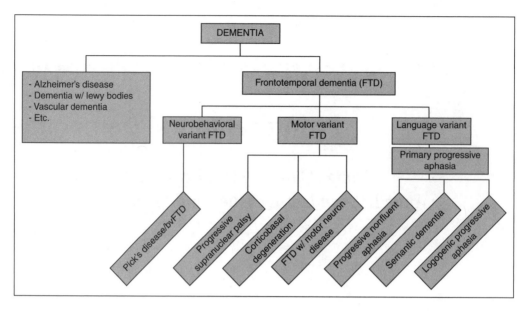

FIGURE 9.1 Frontotemporal dementia (FTD) categories and subtypes, under the "dementia" umbrella.

further divided into progressive nonfluent aphasia (PNFA), semantic dementia, and logopenic progressive aphasia. The categories are largely identified by their respective primary lesion location and differ in their clinical features and subsequent treatment options (see Figure 9.1).

The majority of this chapter illustrates the features of all three categories of FTD, while further details are expanded for the language category of FTD in additional chapters of this book.

NEUROBEHAVIORAL VARIANT OF FTD

History

The first diagnostic guidelines for bvFTD (also known as Pick's disease or the frontal variant) were the Lund and Manchester Groups (1994) criteria. At that time, the term *frontotemporal dementia* was coined to refer exclusively to what is now known as bvFTD. While the term FTD was perhaps an appropriate descriptor of the disorder due to the hallmark atrophy of both the frontal and temporal lobes (Neary, Snowden, & Mann, 2005), FTD is now more commonly used to describe the group of dementias (detailed in this chapter) involving varying degrees of frontal and/or temporal lobe degeneration. In 1998, Neary et al. provided expanded criteria that included "core" and "supportive" features of the disease. The Neary et al. criteria have been widely accepted. Since then, other groups have proposed updated criteria. For instance, Rascovsky et al. (2007) suggested revisions to the Neary criteria via expert consensus, and researchers at the University of California San Francisco provide what appear to be these updated criteria for bvFTD on their website (http://memory.ucsf.edu/ftd), noting that they were derived in 2010. Neary and Snowden (2013) also furthered an update, abandoning Pick-related terminologies from their criteria.

Epidemiology

The bvFTD occurs more often than the motor or language variants of FTD (Seeley et al., 2007). Epidemiological studies in the United Kingdom identified that, after AD, FTD is the second most common cause of early-onset dementia—occurring at a rate of approximately 15 per 100,000 in adults aged 45 to 64 years (Piguet, Hornberger, Mioshi, & Hodges, 2011). The ratio of bvFTD to AD varies from roughly 1 to 4 in cases in Sweden and Japan to 1 to 3 in the United Kingdom. When consideration is restricted to cases with onset prior to age 50 years, the ratio narrows to 1 to 1.7 in the U.K. sample. In a sample of 85-year-olds in Sweden, a 3% prevalence of bvFTD was found (Neary et al., 2005). The disorder was once thought to afflict women and men equally, but the results of more recent work (including a large-scale demographic study) show that it is more common in men (Johnson et al., 2005; Rabinovici & Miller, 2010). Median survival rates for bvFTD reported in recent reviews range from 3 to 4.5 years (Piguet et al., 2011) to 6 to 8 years (Neary et al., 2005) to just more than 8 years (Rabinovici & Miller, 2010).

Neuropathology/Pathophysiology

The microtubule-binding protein tau has been implicated in the pathophysiology of several neurodegenerative disorders. In the healthy brain, the human tau gene (*17q21*) serves to promote stability of microtubules (mostly in neurons) by interacting with tubulin. In the diseased brain, mutated tau protein can affect the integrity of microtubules and produce toxic inclusions (Rabinovici & Miller, 2010). Many of the bvFTD cases with abnormal tau can be classified pathologically as Pick's disease. Pick's disease (always caused by tauopathy) involves hallmark argyrophilic, circular inclusions, called Pick bodies, or balloon-like Pick cells located in neuronal cytoplasm (see Figure 9.2). The amygdala, frontal and temporal neocortex, and dentate gyrus of the hippocampus are locations where Pick bodies are commonly found. Patients with bvFTD who have tauopathy not due to Pick's disease have a mutation of the microtubule-associated protein tau (*MAPT*) gene located on chromosome 17 (Rabinovici & Miller, 2010).

The majority of individuals who do not show evidence of tau abnormalities (i.e., tau negative) have ubiquitin-positive inclusions. Individuals with ubiquitin-positive inclusions not showing evidence of tau abnormalities is likely due to an immunoreactive response to ubiquitin, an enzyme responsible for recycling proteins. The ubiquitinated protein is typically the 43 kDa TAR DNA-binding protein (TDP-43; Piguet et al., 2011; Rabinovici & Miller, 2010). These TDP-43 inclusions are usually found in the dentate gyrus of the hippocampus and in the frontotemporal cortex (Rabinovici & Miller, 2010). TDP-43 inclusions are associated with progranulin gene (*PGRN*) mutations. TDP-43 inclusions can be found in individuals with Pick's disease as well (Rabinovici & Miller, 2010).

The majority of bvFTD cases show either tau or TDP-43 pathology with equal distribution between the two. Familial bvFTD is linked to chromosome 17q21–22 (Rabinovici & Miller, 2010). A minority of familial cases show inclusions of RNA-binding proteins fused in sarcoma (FUS; Piguet et al., 2011). These cases with FUS-positive inclusions have been associated with younger age of onset (mean age of 38 years), pronounced atrophy of the caudate, and major behavioral disruption (Rabinovici & Miller, 2010).

Several studies have suggested that bvFTD may involve altered metabolism of the neurotransmitter serotonin. Lower levels of cerebrospinal fluid (CSF) dopamine

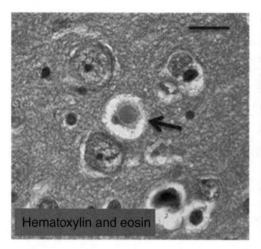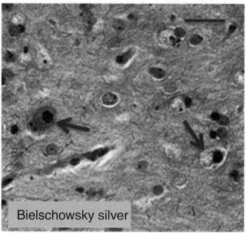

FIGURE 9.2 Histopathological confirmation of Pick's disease. A 2 × 2 × 0.5 cm portion of the right frontal lobe was examined. Hematoxylin and eosin stain (left) shows cytoplasmic inclusions (arrow) and sporadic "balloon cells." Congo red stain was negative for amyloid plaques (not shown). Bielschowsky silver stain showed intracytoplasmic inclusions consistent with Pick bodies (arrows). Electron microscopy was performed that showed discrete regions with filaments compatible with Pick bodies (not shown). Scale bars are 20μ (left) and 30μ (right).

have also been found in some studies of bvFTD and Pick's disease patients. Unlike in AD, the cholinergic system appears to function normally (Huey, Putnam, & Grafman 2006). Accordingly, the efficacy of acetylcholinesterase inhibitors (AChEIs) may be limited in these patients compared to their use with AD patients.

Although a normal structural MRI does not rule out the possibility of the disease early on, scans of bvFTD patients typically show atrophy of the orbitofrontal, mesial frontal, and anterior insula cortices. Degradation of the anterior cingulate–frontal insular network appears to be linked to impaired social cognition (Piguet et al., 2011). Subcortical areas of atrophy include the hippocampus, caudate, putamen, striatum, thalamus, and amygdala. Atrophy of the amygdala discriminates between bvFTD and AD (Piguet et al., 2011). Repeat MRIs reveal increased atrophy as the disease progresses.

Structural changes in the brain have been linked with behavioral deficits. For instance, dorsomedial frontal atrophy is associated with apathy and motor problems, while orbitofrontal atrophy is linked to disinhibition. Bilateral dorsolateral prefrontal atrophy is associated with Pick's disease (Piguet et al., 2011).

Functional neuroimaging shows frontal hypoperfusion on single-photon emission computed tomography (SPECT; different from posterior cingulate and temporoparietal patterns seen in AD) and frontal hypometabolism on FDG-PET (again, different from temporoparietal decreases in AD; Ashford et al., 2000; Piguet et al., 2011; Rabinovici & Miller, 2010; Schmitt, Shih, & DeKosky, 1992). Furthermore, SPECT studies have demonstrated posterotemporal and inferioparietal association with AD severity, whereas prefrontal perfusion showed less association with severity, differentiating this pattern from bvFTD (Ashford et al., 2000). FDG-PET hypometabolism is detectable very early in the disease process (before structural MRI changes) and is another good differentiator of bvFTD from AD (Piguet et al., 2011).

Clinical Features

Course

The disease is characterized by an insidious onset. As lack of insight is a common early feature of bvFTD, the patient's symptoms may first be brought to the attention of health care providers by a spouse or other family member. The age of onset is usually between 45 and 64 years. Individuals with bvFTD commonly have a family history of FTD (Rabinovici & Miller, 2010). The average length of time from onset to death is 6 to 8 years (Neary et al., 2005), and bvFTD patients die on average 5 years earlier than those with the language variant of FTD (approximately 7 vs. 12 years after disease onset; Piguet et al., 2011).

Clinical Presentation

As the name implies, behavioral changes are the most dramatic feature of this variant of FTD. The Neary et al. (1998, 2005) criteria designate "core" features of bvFTD as insidious onset and gradual progression with early impairment of social conduct, regulation of personal conduct, insight, and emotional blunting. Significant personality changes occur: a blend of apathy (disinterest in responsibilities and social life) and disinhibition (in conversation and behavior), and uncaring/lack of empathy toward family and friends. Impaired insight is also present; the patient may admit to mild memory problems or deny cognitive problems altogether. Impaired insight is accompanied by changes in religious or political beliefs and social mannerisms. Repetitive motor behaviors (e.g., throat clearing), overeating, and hoarding/collecting behaviors are often present. Neary et al. (2005) described three possible "phenotypic variations" of bvFTD clinical presentation: (a) social disinhibition, (b) apathy/ withdrawal, and (c) stereotyped motor behaviors. Functional impairment is prominent even in early bvFTD and is more dramatic in terms of decreased ability to perform activities of daily living (ADL) and to drive than other FTD variants or AD (Piguet et al., 2011).

Neuropsychological Performance

Mini-Mental State Examination (MMSE) scores may be relatively unaffected (above suggested "dementia" cutoff) despite significant social and functional decline (Gregory & Hodges, 1996; Gregory, Serra-Mestres, & Hodges, 1999). In patients with impaired cognitive test performance, executive function is the most common domain affected (i.e., deficits in judgment, attention, planning, and organization). Letter fluency scores are worse in patients with bvFTD than in those with AD (Thompson, Stopford, Snowden, & Neary, 2005). Poor performance on the Iowa Gambling Task (a measure of executive skills) may be a reliable discriminator of bvFTD (Piguet et al., 2011). Atrophy of the dorsolateral prefrontal cortex is associated much more highly with executive task difficulty than atrophy limited to the orbitomedial frontal cortex.

Episodic memory impairments may not be as uncommon as previously believed (Piguet et al., 2011). Performance on memory tasks may be poor due to impaired attention. Visuospatial impairment is extremely rare even in advanced stages of the disease (Neary et al., 2005; Rabinovici & Miller, 2010). Tasks involving drawing may reflect impaired planning ability or perseveration but intact spatial orientation (Neary et al., 2005). Patients in later-stage bvFTD tend to show increased range and severity of cognitive deficits, consistent with advancing cortical atrophy of the frontal and temporal lobes (Piguet et al., 2011). Tests of emotion detection may be sensitive to early deficits and should be included in the assessment of suspected bvFTD patients (Piguet et al., 2011).

The neuropsychological examination provides a rich context for behavioral observations specific to bvFTD. For example, Thompson et al. (2005) observed that 91% of patients with AD displayed appropriate behavior and cooperation during neuropsychological testing compared with only 30% of patients with bvFTD. Furthermore, perseverative errors, task rule violations, impulsivity, and confabulations during neuropsychological testing are more common in bvFTD patients than in patients with other disorders (Neary et al., 2005; Rabinovici & Miller, 2010).

Neurological Findings

Early-stage bvFTD patients oftentimes have normal neurological examination results. With time, parkinsonian features such as muscle rigidity and akinesia are often present (Neary et al., 2005). Approximately half of bvFTD patients have amyotrophic lateral sclerosis (ALS) and half of ALS patients have bvFTD; thus, a neuromuscular evaluation is recommended for all bvFTD patients (Rabinovici & Miller, 2010).

Possible bvFTD Subtypes

Hu et al. (2007) examined neuropathological and clinical characteristics of bvFTD patients to determine whether the underlying pathology of the cases made a difference in the clinical expression of the disease. They found that patients with tau-positive pathology (most had Pick's disease) were significantly more likely to exhibit deficits in judgment and/or planning. On the other hand, patients with non-tau pathology had significantly greater likelihood of dysregulated personal conduct and poor hygiene. The observed differences between the two groups could not be explained by disease duration, but the authors cautioned that it is possible that the clinical characteristics of the groups become more similar over time.

Over the past few years, attention has been paid to the possible existence of bvFTD phenocopy syndrome—a label applied to cases that present with bvFTD clinical features but fail to show atrophy at onset and do not progress in the typical fashion. These patients have been noted to have much longer mortality rates (10 vs. 3 years) and do not show FTD neuropathology at autopsy. In a review of the research on this topic, Kipps, Hodges, and Hornberger (2010) concluded that the "phenocopy" group is unlikely to have a progressive neurodegenerative disorder. However, the current diagnostic criteria are unable to discriminate between true and phenocopy bvFTD; therefore, Kipps et al. suggested that clinicians incorporate information about patients' performance of ADL, executive tasks, and social cognition into their diagnostic reasoning (Kipps et al., 2010).

Differential Diagnoses

The symptom profile, low base rate, and relatively young age of onset of bvFTD present challenges as many patients may appear to have a "purely psychiatric" condition. A positive history of psychological distress warrants consideration but by no means excludes the possibility of bvFTD. Obtaining a detailed medical history and laboratory testing can help discriminate possible bvFTD from nondegenerative conditions such as substance abuse, infection, and vascular disease.

As described earlier, bvFTD can be differentiated from AD through patterns of atrophy and through hypoperfusion and hypometabolism on neuroimaging. Neuropsychological test score profiles may also be useful in discriminating bvFTD from AD, as AD patients often present with memory impairments and do not show the same preservation of visuospatial ability seen in bvFTD patients. One study (Rascovsky, Salmon, Hansen, & Galasko, 2008) found that bvFTD patients produce profiles different from AD patients on the Mattis Dementia Rating Scale (DRS), with better memory subscale and poorer conceptualization subscale scores. Patients with bvFTD may also be distinguished from those with VaD or AD by their striking poverty of appropriate emotion and insight, and engagement in repetitive movements or gluttonous eating habits (Neary et al., 2005).

Treatment and Intervention

The unfortunate reality, according to the authors of the most recent review of the literature (Jicha & Nelson, 2011; Piguet et al., 2011), is that no specific treatment has been developed for bvFTD. Therefore, the options described in this section are primarily symptom management and/or palliative in nature.

Medical

Only a handful of studies of pharmacological treatments for bvFTD have been published—very few of them blinded, placebo-controlled trials—and results have been inconsistent. As noted earlier, some studies suggest that bvFTD patients may have dysfunctional metabolism of serotonin. This possibility has led to the use of SSRI medications, but the evidence for this practice is largely based on a single meta-analysis that included several non-placebo-controlled studies (Rabinovici & Miller, 2010). Nonetheless, selective serotonin reuptake inhibitors (SSRIs)/serotonin-norepinephrine reuptake inhibitors (SNRIs) are currently the "first-line" pharmacotherapy for bvFTD. Evidence from a randomized placebo-controlled trial indicates that trazodone may also be helpful in treating behavioral problems associated with bvFTD, but the rate of undesirable side effects, such as drowsiness, makes this a less attractive option (Rabinovici & Miller, 2010).

Other drugs sometimes used (with variable efficacy) to target bvFTD symptoms are atypical antipsychotics and AChEIs (Huey et al., 2006; Piguet et al., 2011). However, extreme caution must be taken when considering the use of atypical antipsychotics as these drugs are associated with increased risk of death in elderly patients with dementia (Rabinovici & Miller, 2010). Also, because the cholinergic system may function more normally in contrast to that of AD patients, AChEIs may not show significant efficacy as desired. Efforts are underway to create drugs to target the underlying pathologies of bvFTD (Jicha & Nelson, 2011; Piguet et al., 2011); hopefully this line of research will yield more effective pharmacotherapies.

Behavioral

Given the relatively weak evidence for the efficacy of the current pharmacotherapeutic approaches, nondrug interventions are considered the primary avenue for targeting bvFTD symptoms. Education (for the patient and caregiver) is important and can be accomplished in office visits with health care providers as well as in support group settings. Establishment of a physical exercise routine may slow the progression of motor symptoms. Modification plans may be devised for the home or other environments to assist with targeting inappropriate behaviors (Rabinovici & Miller, 2010). Behavior modification might include a model involving education of caregivers on antecedent-behavior-consequence patterns with clinician recommendations for targeting undesired behaviors, but this system still needs to be validated (Piguet et al., 2011).

Social

Provision of support to the caregivers of patients with bvFTD is a critical component of treatment due to the significant strain the disease imposes on the patient's support network (Neary et al., 2005). Caregivers of patients with bvFTD report higher stress than those who care for patients with AD and thus are in great need of education and encouragement to pursue self-care (Piguet et al., 2011).

Discussion of end-of-life planning is important given the relatively rapid progression of the disease (Rabinovici & Miller, 2010). As the patient's functional abilities decline, transition to a skilled nursing facility is usually necessary (Neary et al., 2005).

Cognitive

No formal cognitive rehabilitative programs have been proposed. Due to the progressive nature of the disease, the clinician may serve the patient's needs best by educating caregivers about the patient's cognitive limitations and encouraging acceptance. The neuropsychological evaluation and detailed interview will provide detailed information about the patient's areas of cognitive strength and weakness. Given common executive deficits and relatively early impairment of the bvFTD patient's driving ability (Piguet et al., 2011), a formal driving assessment may be recommended. Because of the lack of awareness of cognitive deficits by patients with bvFTD, compensatory rehabilitative strategies are usually of little value.

Prognosis and Long-Term Outcomes

Factors associated with a more rapid decline in functional ability are (a) more severe frontal lobe volume loss, (b) older age of onset of bvFTD, (c) early impairment on neuropsychological testing, and, interestingly, (d) *less* severe behavioral impairment (Josephs et al., 2011). PGRN mutation is associated with functional decline that occurs at a rate that is twice as fast as that typical of patients with bvFTD (Josephs et al., 2011). Patients with bvFTD demonstrate greater severity of symptoms and rapidity of progression than patients with AD or language variants of FTD. Those with bvFTD and ALS or MND have shorter survival rates (Piguet et al., 2011).

MOTOR VARIANT OF FTD

History and Background

As mentioned earlier, Arnold Pick (1892) first described the clinical features of "Pick's disease," and this syndrome later came to be incorporated under the term FTD. This syndrome described by Pick included progressive aphasia, apraxia, and behavioral disruption noted in the context of frontotemporal atrophy (Kertesz, McMonagle, Blair, Davidson, & Munoz, 2005). Then in 1926, Onari and Spatz discovered that "Pick body" inclusions were characteristic of the disorder. Subsequent additions to this diagnostic grouping included pathological conditions that included ubiquitin, tau, and synuclein negative inclusions as well as MND-type inclusions. These inclusions are characteristic of PSP, CBD, and FTD-MND. Each of these motor variant lobar atrophies is described in detail in the following text.

PROGRESSIVE SUPRANUCLEAR PALSY

History

PSP, previously known as *Steele–Richardson–Olszewski syndrome*, is the most common of the motor variants. This condition was first described by Steele, Richardson, and Olszewski in 1964 and further conceptualized as a "subcortical dementia" by Albert, Feldman, and Willis in 1974. PSP is characterized by a cluster of symptoms.

The hallmark features of this syndrome include bradykinesia, rigidity, falls, and supranuclear vertical gaze palsy (Hauw et al., 1994; Litvan et al., 1997). Vertical gaze palsy is characterized by impaired vertical movement of the eyes. More specifically, the downward gaze is impaired. Additionally, early falls (above and beyond that of Parkinson's disease [PD]) are often a leading indicator of this condition (Nath, Ben-Shlomo, Thomson, Lees, & Burn, 2003). In addition to this behavioral presentation, these individuals often have a diminished response to dopaminergic medications (Litvan et al., 1997). The similarity of these symptoms to those of PD resulted in this condition being described as a parkinsonian or parkinsonian plus syndrome; this symptom-based classification stood until more recent developments revealed that PSP was biologically and pathologically more closely related to FTD (Kertesz & McMonagle, 2010).

Epidemiology

Although PSP is the most common motor variant of FTD, this syndrome is still generally rare. Estimates regarding the incidence of PSP vary according to the method of data collection. The variability in estimates is considerable, ranging from 1.0 to 6.4 per 100,000. In a review of 800,000 participants in a large epidemiological study in the United Kingdom, lifetime prevalence was 1.0 per 100,000 (Nath et al., 2001). This study employed passive referral mechanisms, which, from a methodological standpoint, may lead to an underestimation of true prevalence. In a similar epidemiological study in the United States, again employing passive participant acquisition and age adjustment, prevalence was estimated to be 1.39 per 100,000 (Golbe, Davis, Schoenberg, & Duvoisin, 1988). However, when more active community-based recruitment strategies were employed, the lifetime prevalence rates considerably increased. When employing such a community-based recruitment strategy, an age-adjusted prevalence of 6.5 to 5.0 per 100,000 was noted in the United Kingdom (Nath et al., 2001). Given the nature of the syndrome's presenting symptoms and underlying pathology, it is rather surprising that not all subjects were referred to a neurologist.

The symptoms and pathology of PSP leading to most of these cases being referred for neurological consultation has been a major operating assumption in previous attempts to estimate the lifetime incidence of PSP. Therefore, estimates not drawing beyond neurological practice may underestimate the actual prevalence. Consistent with the community-based estimates, a review of epidemiological data from a large community-based study in Olmstead County, Minnesota, identified 5.3 cases per 100,000 for ages 50 to 99 years (Bower, Maraganore, McDonnell, & Rocca, 1997), and a community-based study conducted in London revealed a prevalence of 6.4 per 100,000 (Schrag, Ben-Shlomo, & Quinn, 1999). Community studies, although prone to sampling bias due to the smaller number of overall participants, are more sensitive and better able to identify individuals who have the syndrome. Additionally, men are affected slightly more often than women, but this gender discrepancy has not been present in all studies. Although sporadic cases of familial PSP have been reported (Gazeley & Maguire, 1996), PSP does not appear to run in families, and the etiology of this underlying syndrome remains unclear.

Neuropathology/Pathophysiology

The formation of astrocytic lesions, tau-positive neurofibrillary tangles, and neuropil threads within the brain stem and basal ganglia is characteristic of the neuropathology/pathophysiology of PSP (Dickson, 1999; Litvan et al., 1997). This presentation is unique from other disorders such as Alzheimer's and Pick's diseases due to the presence of the tau pathology predominantly within the basal ganglia. Therefore, the diagnosis of PSP is excluded in the presence of "large or numerous infarcts, marked diffuse or focal atrophy, Lewy bodies, changes diagnostic of AD, oligodendroglial argyrophilic inclusions, Pick bodies, diffuse spongiosis, and prion protein-positive amyloid plaques. The diagnosis of combined PSP is proposed when other neurological disorders exist concomitantly with PSP (Hauw et al., 1994).

Additionally, intracellular neurofibrillary tangles and glial tangles in the caudal intralaminar nuclei of the thalamus have been demonstrated in PSP, which may in part account for the differences in presentation from PD (Henderson, Carpenter, Cartwright, & Halliday, 2000). Additionally, diffuse basal ganglia degeneration is evident in PSP and is not localized to particular regions (Henderson et al., 2000). Diffuse basal ganglia involvement may be a factor in poorer treatment outcomes when compared to PD. In a comparison to individuals with PD ($N = 17$), participants with PSP ($N = 21$) were distinguished from both PD and controls ($N = 23$) by whole-brain volume loss, ventricular dilation, and disproportionate atrophy of the frontal cortex (Cordato et al., 2002). Additional differences were noted by these researchers in caudate volume, but this difference was not deemed clinically significant as it was proportionate to overall volume loss. Previous postmortem work by this same group demonstrated an association between frontal atrophy and cognition in PSP, but did not demonstrate an association between subcortical atrophy and cognition (Cordato, Halliday, Harding, Hely, & Morris, 2000).

Clinical Features

Course

PSP is most commonly evident by the seventh decade of life. This condition often first presents with 1 year of hard falls followed by stiffness, vertical gaze palsy, and swallowing difficulties (Nath et al., 2003). Mean life expectancy after diagnosis is 5 years (Bower et al., 1997). Cause of death is generally due to complications with the condition itself, including pneumonia and pulmonary embolism. The median time of the first onset of significant motor impairment is 4 years following disease onset (Goetz, Leurgans, Lang, & Litvan, 2003).

Neuropsychological Performance

As much as 52% of individuals with PSP present with behavioral and cognitive changes, often early in the disease process (Bak, Crawford, Hearn, Mathuranath, & Hodges, 2005). In individuals with PSP, frontal/executive function was the domain of particular impairment (Kertesz & McMonagle, 2010), which may be related to frontal volume loss (Cordato et al., 2002). In their review of cognitive performance in PSP and CBD, Kertesz and McMonagle (2010) described this frontal/executive impairment as "early and pervasive in PSP." In their 2002 study, Cordato et al. identified greater endorsement of frontal symptoms by individuals with PSP than normal controls and individuals with PD on the frontal behavioral inventory (FBI). Additionally, significant impairment on the DRS was shown in 57% of subjects, and up to 62% demonstrated impairment on the Frontal Systems Battery in a large sample of individuals with PSP (Brown et al., 2010). On the DRS, impairment was primarily evident on the initiation and perseveration subtest.

Although additional deficits are evident in other domains, it is often difficult to identify the contribution that frontal/executive deficits might have on the performance in other domains of neuropsychological functioning. Additionally, profound deficits in cognitive processing speed are often evident in PSP, especially in more advanced cases (Dubois et al., 2005). In some cases, response latencies of up to 5 minutes have been reported (Kertesz & McMonagle, 2010). Deficits in visuospatial ability (Bak, Caine, Hearn, & Hodges, 2006; Borroni et al., 2008); complex attention (Robbins et al., 1994); memory (Esmonde, Giles, Gibson, & Hodges, 1996; Grafman, Litvan, & Stark, 1995); language (Cotelli et al., 2006: Rosser & Hodges, 1994); and emotion are evident in this population (Ghosh, Rowe, Calder, Hodges, & Bak, 2009). As for speech and language performance, there is a progression leading to profound deficits in speech late in the disorder, as "unintelligible speech occurred at a median disease duration of 71 months" (Goetz et al., 2003). However, it should be noted that this level of speech impairment is not unique to PSP in the later stages of the dementing process, as all aspects of cognition are impaired by these stages of the dementing process. With regard to course and development of cognitive symptoms, a faster pace of decline in cognitive function is noted in individuals diagnosed with PSP when compared to those with PD and MSA (multisystem atrophy/striatonigral degeneration) at 21-month follow-up (Soliveri et al., 2000).

Significant numbers of individuals also endorse clinically significant emotional distress; 40% of individuals with PSP endorsed clinically significant levels of depressive- or anxiety-related symptomatology (Borroni et al., 2008). This pattern of emotional distress characterized by anxiety and depression is not inconsistent with disruption of fronto-subcortical networks (Aarsland, Litvan, & Larsen, 2001). Overall, individuals with PSP demonstrate significant cognitive and emotional deficits, with particular impairment in executive functioning, visuospatial ability, and inhibition. Individuals also commonly exhibit apathy. Furthermore, these diffuse cognitive deficits appear to be at least in part mediated by deficits in executive functioning. This impairment in executive functioning is of particular interest as this domain has been demonstrated as the strongest predictor of a patient's functional status and quality of life (Cahn-Weiner et al., 2007). Finally, not only do individuals with PSP present with significant cognitive deficits, individuals with PSP demonstrate reduced awareness of their cognitive deficits (O'Keeffe et al., 2007).

Neurological Findings

The hallmark features of PSP include gait impairment with multiple falls (particularly backwards), bradykinesia, rigidity, and vertical gaze palsy (Hauw et al., 1994; Litvan et al., 1997). The vertical gaze palsy in particular is indicative of PSP. The prominence of this symptom has led to what has been colloquially termed the "dirty tie" sign in individuals with PSP. This "dirty tie" term is based on the patient's lack of downward vertical gaze; that is, the vertical gaze palsy results in impaired awareness of spills on the chest and torso area. Although more accurately classified as a variant of frontal temporal dementia, additional neurological symptoms are consistent with multiple parkinsonian symptoms, including difficulty swallowing, speech difficulties, and slowed speech, but tremor is less likely to be evident in PSP. Additionally, individuals with PSP often demonstrate truncal rigidity.

Possible PSP Subtypes

Williams et al. (2005) proposed two different clinical phenotypes of PSP: Richardson's syndrome and PSP-parkinsonism. Richardson's syndrome is characterized by early onset of postural instability and falls, supranuclear vertical gaze palsy, and cognitive dysfunction, while PSP-parkinsonism is characterized by an asymmetric onset of motor symptoms, tremor, a moderate initial therapeutic response to levodopa, and frequent confusion with PD (Williams et al., 2005).

Differential Diagnoses

PSP has many parkinsonian features, similar to the neurological findings in PD. This similarity is evident in the commonality of overt signs and symptoms of both conditions, including gait instability, rigidity, and bradykinesia. The similarities between the symptom profiles of PD and PSP resulted in the identification of the latter as a parkinsonian syndrome until relatively recently (Kertesz & McMonagle, 2010). Despite the presence of parkinsonian signs, biologically, the relationship between PSP and FTD is much stronger. Nevertheless, there are a few hallmark characteristics of PSP that help provide diagnostic clarity with regard to PD (Litvan et al., 1997). That is, having had falls during the first year of symptom expression, increased postural instability early in the course of the disease, absence of response to levodopa, absence of tremor-dominant disease presentation, and supranuclear gaze palsy are points of divergence in symptom expression in these conditions (Litvan et al., 1997). Additionally, preliminary examination has suggested that a simple test of motor control called an "applause sign" might also be helpful in this differential diagnosis (Dubois et al., 2005; Kuniyoshi et al., 2002). Nevertheless, misdiagnosis with PD is common (Bak et al., 2005; Litvan et al., 2003; Nath et al., 2003).

Additional conditions with similar symptoms posing difficult differentials include MSA, DLB, and CBD. MSA has significant overlap of symptoms with both PD and PSP, namely gait ataxia and rigidity. In statistical analysis, PSP is successfully differentiated from MSA based on later age of onset and lack of supranuclear gaze palsy in MSA (Litvan et al., 1997). DLB is adequately differentiated from PSP based on the presence of supranuclear gaze palsy and gait instability (Litvan et al., 1997). Additional diagnostic differences include the presence of symptoms consistent with a formal thought disorder (i.e., formed hallucinations) and an adverse response to traditional antipsychotic medications. The differential between PSP and CBD is described in the following sections.

Treatment and Intervention

PSP is a progressive condition, with few, if any, treatment options available at this time. There is limited support for treatments designed to reverse or halt the underlying dementia process. No clear benefit from medication has been demonstrated. Trials of riluzole (Bensimon et al., 2009), donepezil (Litvan et al., 2001), physostigmine (Frattali, Sonies, Chi-Fishman, & Litvan, 1999), zolpidem (Daniele, Moro, & Bentivoglio, 1999), and pramipexole were demonstrated to have little effect (Weiner, Minagar, & Shulman, 1999). Some preliminary support for agents addressing mitochondrial function have "shown positive effect" in a Phase II study, and ongoing efforts to address tau dysfunction are in earlier states of preparation (Stamelou et al., 2010). However, pharmacological interventions, as of yet, have not been proven to be particularly beneficial in the treatment of PSP, although some medications might be helpful in addressing select symptoms of PSP. As such, all treatments of PSP are supportive in nature.

Efforts made to remediate physical deficits with balance and eye movement training have been effective in enhancing stance time and walking speed (Zampieri & Di Fabio, 2008). An additional report indicated some improvement in gait following therapies focused on limb coordination activities, tilt-board balancing, ambulation activities, and activities to improve route finding and visual scanning ability (Izzo, DiLorenzo, & Roth, 1986). Despite the limited potential for enhancing physical function, the benefit from this remediation is likely to be rather short lived given the rapid progression of the disease process. Therefore, interventions designed to support caregivers are most likely to enhance the patient's functional capacity. This emphasis on caregiver support is especially valuable given the impact of the patient's executive dysfunction on caregiver burden.

CORTICOBASAL DEGENERATION

History

First described by Rebeiz, Kolodny, and Richardson (1967), CBD was identified in three patients presenting with a unique neuropathological distribution and pattern of physical symptoms, including clumsiness and slowed movements of the left arm and leg, with a progression of impairment to contralateral limbs and profoundly impaired voluntary movement. Six additional cases with similar symptomatology were described by Watts et al. (1985). They termed this cluster of symptoms *corticobasal ganglionic degeneration*. Three additional cases with similar pathology were identified by Gibb, Luthert, and Marsden in 1989. This group shortened the term to its present form, *corticobasal degeneration*.

Epidemiology

To date, no systematic examination of the prevalence/incidence of CBD has been performed. Nevertheless, the condition is understood to be rather rare and perhaps less common than PSP, which as previously noted demonstrates prevalence rates as high as 6.4 cases per 100,000 (Schrag et al., 1999). In this same community-based study of 121,628 participants, Schrag et al. did not identify a single case of CBD. Although not evident in community-based studies, estimates based on the percentage of cases of parkinsonism that are accounted for by CBD (4%–6%) suggest that the prevalence of CBD is estimated to be 4.9 to 7.3 per 100,000.

Neuropathology/Pathophysiology

CBD is a progressive extrapyramidal disorder with a characteristic cluster of neurological, cognitive, and behavioral signs. Neuroanatomic studies demonstrate an asymmetrical pattern of brain atrophy of the bilateral premotor cortex, superior parietal lobules, and striatum (Boxer et al., 2006). Frontal involvement, in particular superiofrontal, has been demonstrated in CBD, with relative sparing of the occipital and temporal lobes (Belfor et al., 2006). In addition, "the anterior limb of the internal capsule is attenuated; caudate and thalamus are atrophic and the substantia nigra is pale" (Belfor et al., 2006).

Despite some neuropathological overlap of tau-immunoreactive inclusions among Pick's disease, PSP, and CBD, their glial inclusions vary between the disorders, suggesting that each is a distinct pathophysiological entity (Feany, Mattiace, & Dickson, 1996). Also, when compared to patients with Pick's disease, patients with CBD demonstrate greater globus pallidus involvement (Dickson et al., 2002).

In addition to these findings, the presence of CSF tau has been shown to reliably differentiate CBD from AD, but was unable to reliably differentiate CBD from other tauopathies (Shoji et al., 2002). Belfor et al. (2006) reported pathological diagnostic criteria to include "thread like lesions in gray and white matter and astrocytic plaques positive on Gallyas stain." Additionally, ballooned neurons, which are characteristic of PSP and other neurodegenerative diseases, are not seen in CBD (Dickson, 1999).

Both PSP and CBD present with astrocytic lesions; however, the dispersion characteristic of each disorder is unique; with PSP, the lesions are found in the basal ganglia, diencephalon, and brain stem, while the majority of pathology in CBD is evident in the cerebrum (Dickson, 1999). Focal short waves on EEG have also been reported as "useful supplementary information to distinguish between [CBD and PSP] at early stages" (Tashiro et al., 2006).

Clinical Features

Course

The small number of cases presents a barrier to identifying accurate prevalence and incidence data. Although some investigators report rare cases of early onset, CBD typically presents late in life, generally between the sixth and eighth decades (Mahapatra, Edwards, Schott, & Bhatia, 2004).

Neurological Findings/Clinical Presentation

CBD is characterized by its clinical presentation of limb apraxia (asymmetric presentation initially), alien limb syndrome, cortical reflex myoclonus, and cortical sensory impairment (Tashiro et al., 2006). There is significant overlap between the symptoms of CBD and those of PSP. Both conditions demonstrate a number of parkinsonian signs, including bradykinesia, rigidity, and gait disturbance. Additional similarities include some degree of vertical gaze palsy (not as severe as in PSP) and significant impairment of executive functioning (Rinne, Lee, Thompson, & Marsden, 1994). Asymmetric limb involvement, with occasional gait and speech disturbances, is often present in cases of CBD (Belfor et al., 2006). Similar to PSP, there is poor response to levodopa in patients with CBD (Belfor et al., 2006). Rigid dystonic jerking of the hands has also been noted (Thompson et al., 1994). Frontal release signs are also common in CBD (Mahapatra et al., 2004). Cortical sensory deficits, including agraphesthesia, astereoagnosia, or extinction to simultaneous stimulation, are often present (Belfor et al., 2006).

However, the most distinctive neurological features of CBD include the presence of ideomotor apraxia and the alien hand phenomenon, present in approximately 60% of individuals with CBD (Belfor et al., 2006). Compared to PSP, CBD may be differentiated by considering the presence of abnormal gait, moderate to severe vertical gaze palsy, and bilateral bradykinesia, with PSP demonstrating greater levels of impairment on these signs (Litvan et al., 1997). Although occulomotor impairment is common in CBD, the most reliable diagnostic features of CBD include asymmetric parkinsonism, limb dystonia, ideomotor apraxia, and gait disturbance (Belfor et al., 2006; Litvan, 1997; Litvan et al., 1997).

Neuropsychological Performance

Although initially believed to be rare, significant cognitive impairment and dementia are common features of CBD (Mahapatra et al., 2004). This increased awareness of cognitive impairment in CBD is largely a function of the use of measures that are more sensitive to cognitive dysfunction, as early studies generally employed limited screening measures such as the MMSE. Although increased attention has been given to other aspects of cognitive performance in CBD, psychomotor performance has long been identified as a domain of significant impairment (Mahapatra et al., 2004).

Individuals with CBD generally demonstrate asymmetric ideomotor and limb kinetic apraxia (Peigneux et al., 2001). This apraxia is characterized by deficits in spatial organization, timing, and sequencing. Following motor impairment, executive dysfunction is the most prominent feature of CBD (Kertesz, Martinez-Lage, Davidson, & Munoz, 2000). Within this general executive impairment, deficits in inhibition are prominent in CBD (Kertesz & McMonagle, 2010). Kertesz and McMonagle (2010) described the pattern of behavioral impairment in CBD as having significant "overlap" with that of bvFTD, including symptoms of disinhibition, apathy, perseveration, and inattention.

Memory impairment is also a common neuropsychological feature in CBD. This impairment is increasingly evident in pathologically confirmed cases, where hippocampal damage is particularly prominent (Bergeron, Pollanen, Weyer, Black, & Lang, 1996). Deficits in language performance are also often present and appear to be secondary to impairment of motor components of speech; however, deficits in naming have also been demonstrated. Additionally, deficits in visuospatial ability are often present in CBD (Frattali, Grafman, Patronas, Makhlouf, & Litvan, 2000; Graham, Bak, & Hodges, 2003; Kertesz et al., 2000).

Problems with emotional functioning have also been reported. As many as 73% of individuals endorse depression, and as many as 20% of individuals with CBD endorse symptoms of irritability and depression (Cummings & Litvan, 2000).

Differential Diagnoses

Ideomotor and ideational apraxia is a hallmark feature of the disorder, and serves as a significant component of the differential diagnostic process when considering disorders with symptom profiles similar to those of CBD. However, differential diagnoses continue to be difficult. Despite a specificity of nearly 100% in the diagnosis of CBD, sensitivity approaches only half the value (Mahapatra et al., 2004).

Despite this limited sensitivity, cases of CBD can be successfully differentiated from those of PSP on the basis of the presence of alien limb syndrome, the lack of severe vertical gaze palsy, and the presence of unilateral bradykinesia (Litvan et al., 1997). Significant cognitive impairment meeting criteria for dementia is not uncommon in CBD; so other progressive dementing conditions such as AD, DLB, and PNFA may also present as potential diagnostic considerations. However, these conditions rarely present with the characteristic motor features of CBD (Mahapatra et al., 2004). Finally, differentiating CBD from other conditions with significant parkinsonian features remains difficult, as many of these conditions may have atypical presentations that can mimic CBD. Diagnosis based on clinical features remains difficult, and it appears that neuropathological investigation continues to be the definitive diagnosis.

Treatment and Intervention

Treatment is limited to symptom management, as no intervention has been shown to halt or reverse the underlying pathology characteristic of CBD. Pharmacological interventions to address specific symptoms such as dystonia, rigidity, and tremor have shown limited success (Mahapatra et al., 2004). As in the other motor variants of FTD, symptom management and caregiver support present as the primary domains of interventions.

FRONTOTEMPORAL DEMENTIA–MOTOR NEURON DISEASE

History

It has been speculated for a number of years that MND, FTD-MND, and FTLD represent a clinical continuum rather than three discrete diagnostic entities (Al-Sarraj, 2008; Talbot et al., 1995). This possibility is supported by clinical and histopathological research, which increasingly suggests that MND represents one end of a spectrum, FTLD represents the other, and FTD-MND falls somewhere in between. Recent pathological studies have identified significant ubiquitin-positive inclusions in cases of MND that were previously believed to be relatively free of cortical involvement (Mitsuyama & Inoue, 2009). This finding is consistent with research identifying the correlation between MND and cognitive impairment. Talbot et al. (1995) describe MND as "a degenerative disorder...that manifests progressive weakness of bulbar, limb thoracic, and abdominal musculature."

Epidemiology

In a review of the incidence and prevalence of multiple neurological conditions, the incidence of MND ranged from 1.06 to 2.4 per 100,000 person-years, and a prevalence of 4.02 to 4.91 per 100,000 (Hoppitt et al., 2011). In another study, 15% of patients with ALS met criteria for dementia, with the expression of this cognitive impairment being consistent with FTD (Ringholz et al., 2005).

Neuropathology/Pathophysiology

The recent identification of a biological marker for the major constituent component of ubiquitin-positive inclusions has prompted a reconceptualization of MND and its relationship with FTD (Mitsuyama & Inoue, 2009). Following the identification of "TAR DNA-binding protein of 43 kDa (TDP-43) as the major constituent of the ubiquitin-positive inclusions" it has been clearly demonstrated that all cases of MND "share the occurrence of ubiquitinated TDP-43-positive inclusions" (Mitsuyama & Inoue, 2009). Additionally, neuroimaging studies identified frontotemporal lobar atrophy in cases of FTD-MND (Mitsuyama & Inoue, 2009).

More specifically, in a postmortem examination of 65 brains, Snowden, Neary, and Mann (2007) identified a distinct neuropathological pattern that was correlated with clinical presentation in FTD-MND. This pattern suggested a "relatively circumscribed frontal lobe pathology," which was in contrast to that of bvFTD and semantic dementia, in which frontal lobe pathology was accompanied by atrophy of the anterior temporal lobe and temporal lobe pathology, respectively. Additionally, FTD-MND is not associated with tau pathology, but is instead characterized by uniquitin-based pathology (Snowden et al., 2007). Additional findings often associated with FTD-MND include anterior root atrophy in the spinal cord, degeneration of the corticospinal tract, and distinctive atrophy of the precentral gyrus (Al-Sarraj, 2008).

Clinical Features

Course

The clinical course of FTD-MND is rather uniform, with relatively consistent age of onset, cognitive course, and noncognitive neuropsychiatric symptoms (Mitsuyama & Inoue, 2009). In their review of FTD-MND, Mitsuyama and Inoue (2009) reported an equal male to female ratio, a mean age of onset of 55.5 years (range = 38–78 years), and the late 50s as the mean age of death. Therefore, the course of this condition is characterized by rather rapid progression from diagnosis to death. In cases of MND, the disease quickly progresses, with mean survival of 26.8 months (Rusina et al., 2010). Individuals with FTD-MND demonstrate an even more rapid course (Olney et al., 2005; Phukan, Pender, & Hardiman, 2007).

Clinical Presentation

In individuals with FTD-MND, the most common presenting symptoms include dementia with significant disinhibition and personality changes (Mitsuyama & Inoue, 2009). According to this same review, clinical MND symptoms, namely neurological signs (please see the section Neurological Findings that follows), emerge 6 to 12 months after the onset of cognitive and psychiatric symptoms. Additionally, these patients may present with retrieval-based memory dysfunction and impaired speech production. This pattern of cognitive dysfunction is consistent with bilateral frontal involvement, and related to the disruptions of diverse frontal networks including medial-frontal, dorsolateral, and orbitofrontal networks. Global intellectual impairment may also occur, which can present in relation to such bilateral frontal involvement, although it is not specific to this anatomical origin.

Neuropsychological Performance

Even in nondemented individuals with MND, neuropsychological performance demonstrates deficits consistent with executive dysfunction (Al-Sarraj, 2008; Bak & Hodges, 1999). Deficits on measures of verbal fluency are not uncommon (Abrahams, Leigh, & Goldstein, 2005; Lepow et al., 2010). Other general language impairment has also been noted (Bak & Hodges, 2004). Even in cases of MND not meeting criteria for FTD or dementia of any type, significant memory deficits have been noted (Mantovan et al., 2003).

Neurological Findings

The presence of slowed vertical saccades is a relatively common symptom in FTD-MND (Moon, Lee, Seo, Kang, & Na, 2008). Motor symptoms related to MND in FTD-MND include muscle weakness, clumsiness, tripping or falling due to weak or stiff legs, weak respiratory muscles, muscle atrophy, fasciculations, muscle cramps, dysphagia, dysarthria spasticity, and hyperreflexia. Behavioral disinhibition consistent with frontal executive impairment may also be present.

Differential Diagnoses

Behavioral signs consistent with frontal executive impairment such as hyperorality, disinhibition, perseverative behaviors, stimulus boundedness, and progressively reduced spontaneous speech may all be helpful in differentiating FTD-MND from progressive dementias such as AD and DLB. When considering additional differentials, the presence of motor neuron signs moving from distal to proximal motor involvement and a rapid course are characteristic of MND (Holland, McBurney, Moossy, & Reinmuth, 1985).

Treatment and Intervention

Given the aggressive nature and rapid course of FTD-MND, treatment options are largely limited to palliative care, which may include respiratory support. The drug riluzole is the only drug approved by the Food and Drug Administration (FDA) for the treatment of ALS (Miller, Mitchell, Lyon, & Moore, 2007). This treatment was shown to extend life by an average of 2 months. Currently, no additional treatment options beyond palliative care have been developed. Again, as with other motor variants of frontal temporal dementia, symptom management and caregiver support present as the primary domains of interventions.

LANGUAGE CATEGORY OF FTD

In 1985, Holland et al. presented a case study of language deterioration in Pick's disease with neurofibrillary tangles. Throughout the 20th century, sporadic cases were presented where patients would suffer language deterioration with comparatively normal cognition and without typical Pick's disease features. M. Marsel Mesulam named this syndrome *primary progressive aphasia* in 1982 (Mesulam, 1982). Many patients with PPA who do not depend on their verbal skills can continue to function well at work, as they do not exhibit memory decline in the same fashion as in other types of FTD. Some do however, especially in the later stages of disease progression, show behavioral changes described under FTD (Kirshner, 2010).

The most common symptom of PPA is word-finding difficulty. This deficit is also commonly accompanied by reduced verbal fluency/hesitancy, verbal comprehension deficit, and dysarthria. Initially, PPA was identified with two subtypes: PNFA and fluent aphasia with anomia. More recently, PPA was further divided into three subtypes: (a) PNFA, (b) semantic dementia or temporal variant FTD, and (c) logopenic progressive aphasia or the logopenic/phonological variant PPA (Kirshner, 2010).

PROGRESSIVE NONFLUENT APHASIA

In PNFA, speech production is effortful, hesitant, and halting. Phonemic paraphasic errors are common, as is syntax-related comprehension. However, single-word comprehension and object knowledge are comparatively spared. Language production is simplified and agrammatic. Hence, holophrastic speech is common (e.g., single-word expressions such as "Go" or "This"). This deficit is also accompanied by weakness or incoordination of speech production. In short, PNFA can be conceptualized as Broca's-like aphasia, commonly accompanied by dysarthria and phonemic verbal fluency deficit. Pathologically, it differs from an Alzheimer's pathology, and is commonly a *MAPT* gene mutation, or other tau-based disorder (Kirshner, 2010). Patients with PNFA may eventually become mute.

The Association for Frontotemporal Degeneration (2011) also notes that difficulty swallowing is common in these patients, and that reading and writing abilities are preserved longer than speech production. However, reading and writing abilities also eventually decline. Further details are provided in Chapter 11 of this textbook, titled "Primary Progressive Aphasia."

SEMANTIC DEMENTIA OR TEMPORAL VARIANT FTD

Semantic dementia or temporal variant FTD was first named by Snowden, Goulding, and Neary in 1989 and further operationalized by Hodges et al. in the 1990s (Hodges & Patterson, 2007; Hodges, Patterson, Oxbury, & Funnell, 1992). Semantic dementia, in contrast to PNFA, is a fluent aphasia with impaired naming, word comprehension (especially nouns), and object recognition. Repetition and motor speech production are comparatively spared, as are other cognitive faculties (Kirshner, 2010). According to the Association for Frontotemporal Degeneration (2011), the hallmark of semantic dementia is difficulty generating or recognizing familiar words; for example, when a patient is shown a picture of a cat, he or she can neither come up with the word *cat* nor recognize the word *cat* when provided. Some cases also have problems recognizing familiar objects and faces. Imaging studies typically demonstrate temporal atrophy. Later stages can often include typical behavioral abnormalities of FTD.

The pathology can be variable. Most cases have ubiquitin immunoreactive inclusions in the cytoplasm or nucleus, or ubiquitin immunoreactive neurites. Others have progranulin mutations, and a few have even been associated with AD (Kirshner, 2010). Further details are provided in Chapter 10 of this textbook, titled "Semantic Dementia."

LOGOPENIC PROGRESSIVE APHASIA OR
LOGOPENIC/PHONOLOGICAL VARIANT PPA

Logopenic progressive aphasia (LPA) or the logopenic/phonological variant of PPA was operationalized by Gorno-Tempini et al. as recently as 2008 (Gorno-Tempini et al., 2008). In LPA, patients display decreased/slowed speech rate with long word-finding pauses. Grammar and articulation are comparatively spared. Phonemic paraphasic errors can be present, accompanied by impaired repetition and verbal comprehension for sentences. However, repetition and comprehension may be spared for singular words. Naming ability is moderately affected. Atrophy of the posterior left superior and middle temporal gyri and the inferior parietal lobule can be found in LPA. Cognitive and neuroimaging data indicate that a deficit in phonological loop functions may be the core mechanism underlying the LPA clinical syndrome. LPA is usually associated with a focal presentation of AD (Gorno-Tempini et al., 2008; Kirshner, 2010).

CASE REPORT: BIOPSY-PROVEN PICK'S DISEASE

The following is one of the earliest cases of biopsy-proven Pick's disease in documentation:A 55-year-old Caucasian woman with 8 years of formal education presented to her local neurologist in 1984 with symptoms of anxiety, depression (with a history of electroconvulsive therapy [ECT] treatments at age 41 years), very mild difficulties with word finding, and difficulties with immediate memory. No hallucinations or delusions were documented. Her past medical history reflected cholecystectomy, hysterectomy, and urinary bladder repair, but was otherwise unremarkable. Memory and language symptoms had been present for 2 years prior to her visit to the neurologist. Family history was significant for heart disease and diabetes, but had no neurological or psychiatric disorders. Mental status examination showed that she was oriented, alert, and generally cognitively intact, with very mild paraphasias and hesitancy in speech along with a very mild clumsiness in gait. Her first formal cognitive assessment showed average IQ (SS = 94) with impaired verbal abstraction, reduced mental calculations, dysnomia, and moderately impaired immediate memory with only mild impairment in delayed recall. Performances on Trail Making Tests showed average ability for simple scanning and sequencing, but severely impaired ability for alternation of sets. A repeated cognitive evaluation 1 year later showed a notable decline in IQ (70) with impairments in vocabulary, verbal, and visual abstraction; problem solving; and impaired recent and remote memory. In addition, behavior reflected a high degree of anxiety. Additional medical evaluation showed diverticulitis with iron deficiency, and her CT scan was interpreted as being within normal limits even though mild atrophic changes were appreciated, and her repeat EEG was unremarkable. She was treated with Xanax (0.5 mg three times per day), and her behavioral symptoms improved. At that time, her diagnosis was considered to reflect an acute dementia of an unknown origin.

Consultation was sought 18 months later at a university setting Alzheimer's Disease Center. At that point, her family reported an increase in inappropriate behavior, impaired orientation, and reduced expressive language (oral and written), along with evolving memory impairment. Her neurological examination was generally unremarkable with the exception of prominent snout, grasp, and suck reflexes. MRI showed moderate bifrontal atrophy (see Figure 9.3; actual patient MRI), and a SPECT study showed bilaterally reduced perfusion in the frontal lobes. Formal testing was limited to the MMSE (5 of 30 correct) and the Alzheimer's Disease Assessment Scale (59/70); both reflected severe impairment. Prominent findings included expressive and receptive aphasia, ideational and constructional dyspraxia, left/right confusion, and visual agnosia.

As a result, she was referred to the neurosurgery team for a right frontal biopsy (see Figure 9.2; actual patient biopsy). The results reflected cortical Pick bodies and balloon cells, as well as astrocytosis in the subcortical white matter. Neuritic plaques and neurofibrillary tangles were not seen in the biopsy specimen. In addition, electron microscopy analysis showed that mitochondria surrounding the Pick bodies were swollen and had lost their cristae. The neuronal inclusions also appeared to be loosely arranged and organized filaments measuring 130 Å in width, and the majority of these filaments appeared to be straight and nonpaired.

At that point, the patient was diagnosed with Pick's disease. Follow-up evaluations reflected worsening of her cognition, and she eventually became mute but was able to follow simple commands. Her neurological examination continued to reflect only abnormal frontal reflexes until she died in 1990. No postmortem examination was completed as per her family's wishes.

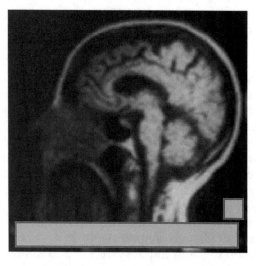

FIGURE 9.3 Imaging slide demonstrating significant frontal lobe atrophy.

SUMMARY

FTD actually represents a group of neurodegenerative disorders. These disorders are grouped as such, as they result from a progressive deterioration of the cells in the anterior temporal and/or frontal lobes of the brain. The clinical features include progressive behavioral, language, and/or motor deteriorations, which inevitably result in significant functional decline. Consequently, the FTD subtypes are conceptualized in three categories (neurobehavioral variant, motor variant, and language variant) based on the primary clinical features, and in the case of the motor and language variants, are further divided into individual disorders. Although there is some commonality in the regional origin of the FTDs, specific discrepancies in the pathophysiology of each disorder corresponds to resulting differences in symptomatology. Understanding these differences is crucial for both diagnostic and treatment reasons.

ACKNOWLEDGMENTS

Special acknowledgments to Dr. Stephen DeKosky for neurological examinations, Drs. Wei-Jen Shih and Jack Coupal for imaging studies, and Drs. Donita Lightner and Amelia Anderson, and Ms. Gina Mullin for their respective contributions. Neuropathological samples and analyses are courtesy of Drs. Philip Tibbs, Diane Wilson, Peter Nelson, and William Markesbery. The authors would also like to gratefully acknowledge support from the National Institutes of Health, Bethesda, MD (5 R01 HD064993; 5 R01 AG019241; 5 R01 AG027219; 5 P30 AG028383).

REFERENCES

Aarsland, D., Litvan, I., & Larsen, J. P. (2001). Neuropsychiatric symptoms of patients with progressive supranuclear palsy and Parkinson's disease. *The Journal of Neuropsychiatry and Clinical Neurosciences, 13*(1), 42–49.

Abrahams, S., Leigh, P. N., & Goldstein, L. H. (2005). Cognitive change in ALS: A prospective study. *Neurology, 64*(7), 1222–1226.

Albert, M. L., Feldman, R. G., & Willis, A. L. (1974). The "subcortical dementia" of progressive supranuclear palsy. *Journal of Neurology, Neurosurgery, and Psychiatry, 37*(2), 121–130.

Al-Sarraj, S. (2008). Dementia and motor neuron disease. *Handbook of Clinical Neurology, 89,* 431–441.

Ashford, J. W., Shih, W. J., Coupal, J., Shetty, R., Schneider, A., Cool, C.,…Schmitt, F. A. (2000). Single SPECT measures of cerebral cortical perfusion reflect time-index estimation of dementia severity in Alzheimer's disease. *Journal of Nuclear Medicine, 41*(1), 57–64.

Association for Frontotemporal Degeneration. (2011). Retrieved from http://www.theaftd.org/

Bak, T. H., Caine, D., Hearn, V. C., & Hodges, J. R. (2006). Visuospatial functions in atypical parkinsonian syndromes. *Journal of Neurology, Neurosurgery, and Psychiatry, 77*(4), 454–456.

Bak, T. H., Crawford, L. M., Hearn, V. C., Mathuranath, P. S., & Hodges, J. R. (2005). Subcortical dementia revisited: Similarities and differences in cognitive function between progressive supranuclear palsy (PSP), corticobasal degeneration (CBD) and multiple system atrophy (MSA). *Neurocase, 11*(4), 268–273.

Bak, T. H., & Hodges, J. R. (1999). Cognition, language and behaviour in motor neurone disease: Evidence of frontotemporal dysfunction. *Dementia and Geriatric Cognitive Disorders, 10*(Suppl 1), 29–32.

Bak, T. H., & Hodges, J. R. (2004). The effects of motor neurone disease on language: Further evidence. *Brain and Language, 89*(2), 354–361.

Belfor, N., Amici, S., Boxer, A. L., Kramer, J. H., Gorno-Tempini, M. L., Rosen, H. J., & Miller, B. L. (2006). Clinical and neuropsychological features of corticobasal degeneration. *Mechanisms of Ageing and Development, 127*(2), 203–207.

Bensimon, G., Ludolph, A., Agid, Y., Vidailhet, M., Payan, C., & Leigh, P. N.; NNIPPS Study Group. (2009). Riluzole treatment, survival and diagnostic criteria in Parkinson plus disorders: The NNIPPS study. *Brain: A Journal of Neurology, 132*(Pt 1), 156–171.

Bergeron, C., Pollanen, M. S., Weyer, L., Black, S. E., & Lang, A. E. (1996). Unusual clinical presentations of cortical-basal ganglionic degeneration. *Annals of Neurology, 40*(6), 893–900.

Borroni, B., Turla, M., Bertasi, V., Agosti, C., Gilberti, N., & Padovani, A. (2008). Cognitive and behavioral assessment in the early stages of neurodegenerative extrapyramidal syndromes. *Archives of Gerontology and Geriatrics, 47*(1), 53–61.

Bower, J. H., Maraganore, D. M., McDonnell, S. K., & Rocca, W. A. (1997). Incidence of progressive supranuclear palsy and multiple system atrophy in Olmsted County, Minnesota, 1976 to 1990. *Neurology, 49*(5), 1284–1288.

Boxer, A. L., Geschwind, M. D., Belfor, N., Gorno-Tempini, M. L., Schauer, G. F., Miller, B. L.,...Rosen, H. J. (2006). Patterns of brain atrophy that differentiate corticobasal degeneration syndrome from progressive supranuclear palsy. *Archives of Neurology, 63*(1), 81–86.

Brown, R. G., Lacomblez, L., Landwehrmeyer, B. G., Bak, T., Uttner, I., Dubois, B.,...Leigh, N. P.; NNIPPS Study Group. (2010). Cognitive impairment in patients with multiple system atrophy and progressive supranuclear palsy. *Brain: A Journal of Neurology, 133*(Pt 8), 2382–2393.

Cahn-Weiner, D. A., Farias, S. T., Julian, L., Harvey, D. J., Kramer, J. H., Reed, B. R.,...Chui, H. (2007). Cognitive and neuroimaging predictors of instrumental activities of daily living. *Journal of the International Neuropsychological Society, 13*(5), 747–757.

Cordato, N. J., Halliday, G. M., Harding, A. J., Hely, M. A., & Morris, J. G. (2000). Regional brain atrophy in progressive supranuclear palsy and Lewy body disease. *Annals of Neurology, 47*(6), 718–728.

Cordato, N. J., Pantelis, C., Halliday, G. M., Velakoulis, D., Wood, S. J., Stuart, G. W.,...Morris, J. G. (2002). Frontal atrophy correlates with behavioural changes in progressive supranuclear palsy. *Brain: A Journal of Neurology, 125*(Pt 4), 789–800.

Cotelli, M., Borroni, B., Manenti, R., Alberici, A., Calabria, M., Agosti, C.,...Cappa, S. F. (2006). Action and object naming in frontotemporal dementia, progressive supranuclear palsy, and corticobasal degeneration. *Neuropsychology, 20*(5), 558–565.

Cummings, J. L., & Litvan, I. (2000). Neuropsychiatric aspects of corticobasal degeneration. *Advances in Neurology, 82*, 147–152.

Daniele, A., Moro, E., & Bentivoglio, A. R. (1999). Zolpidem in progressive supranuclear palsy. *The New England Journal of Medicine, 341*(7), 543–544.

Dickson, D. W. (1999). Neuropathologic differentiation of progressive supranuclear palsy and corticobasal degeneration. *Journal of Neurology, 246*(Suppl 2), II6–II15.

Dickson, D. W., Bergeron, C., Chin, S. S., Duyckaerts, C., Horoupian, D., Ikeda, K.,...Litvan, I.; Office of Rare Diseases of the National Institutes of Health. (2002). Office of Rare Diseases neuropathologic criteria for corticobasal degeneration. *Journal of Neuropathology and Experimental Neurology, 61*(11), 935–946.

Dubois, B., Slachevsky, A., Pillon, B., Beato, R., Villalponda, J. M., & Litvan, I. (2005). "Applause sign" helps to discriminate PSP from FTD and PD. *Neurology, 64*(12), 2132–2133.

Esmonde, T., Giles, E., Gibson, M., & Hodges, J. R. (1996). Neuropsychological performance, disease severity, and depression in progressive supranuclear palsy. *Journal of Neurology, 243*(9), 638–643.

Feany, M. B., Mattiace, L. A., & Dickson, D. W. (1996). Neuropathologic overlap of progressive supranuclear palsy, Pick's disease and corticobasal degeneration. *Journal of Neuropathology and Experimental Neurology, 55*(1), 53–67.

Frattali, C. M., Grafman, J., Patronas, N., Makhlouf, F., & Litvan, I. (2000). Language disturbances in corticobasal degeneration. *Neurology, 54*(4), 990–992.

Frattali, C. M., Sonies, B. C., Chi-Fishman, G., & Litvan, I. (1999). Effects of physostigmine on swallowing and oral motor functions in patients with progressive supranuclear palsy: A pilot study. *Dysphagia, 14*(3), 165–168.

Gazeley, S., & Maguire, J. A. (1996). Familial progressive supranuclear palsy. *Clinical Neuropathology, 15*(4), 215–220.

Ghosh, B. C., Rowe, J. B., Calder, A. J., Hodges, J. R., & Bak, T. H. (2009). Emotion recognition in progressive supranuclear palsy. *Journal of Neurology, Neurosurgery, and Psychiatry, 80*(10), 1143–1145.

Gibb, W. R., Luthert, P. J., & Marsden, C. D. (1989). Corticobasal degeneration. *Brain: A Journal of Neurology, 112*(Pt 5), 1171–1192.

Goetz, C. G., Leurgans, S., Lang, A. E., & Litvan, I. (2003). Progression of gait, speech and swallowing deficits in progressive supranuclear palsy. *Neurology, 60*(6), 917–922.

Golbe, L. I., Davis, P. H., Schoenberg, B. S., & Duvoisin, R. C. (1988). Prevalence and natural history of progressive supranuclear palsy. *Neurology, 38*(7), 1031–1034.

Gorno-Tempini, M. L., Brambati, S. M., Ginex, V., Ogar, J., Dronkers, N. F., Marcone, A.,... Miller, B. L. (2008). The logopenic/phonological variant of primary progressive aphasia. *Neurology, 71*(16), 1227–1234.

Grafman, J., Litvan, I., & Stark, M. (1995). Neuropsychological features of progressive supranuclear palsy. *Brain and Cognition, 28*(3), 311–320.

Graham, N. L., Bak, T. H., & Hodges, J. R. (2003). Corticobasal degeneration as a cognitive disorder. *Movement Disorders, 18*(11), 1224–1232.

Gregory, C. A., & Hodges, J. R. (1996). Frontotemporal dementia: Use of consensus criteria and prevalence of psychiatric features. *Neuropsychiatry, Neuropsychology, & Behavioral Neurology, 9*(3), 145–153.

Gregory, C. A., Serra-Mestres, J., & Hodges, J. R. (1999). Early diagnosis of the frontal variant of frontotemporal dementia: How sensitive are standard neuroimaging and neuropsychologic tests? *Neuropsychiatry, Neuropsychology, and Behavioral Neurology, 12*(2), 128–135.

Hauw, J. J., Daniel, S. E., Dickson, D., Horoupian, D. S., Jellinger, K., Lantos, P. L.,...Litvan, I. (1994). Preliminary NINDS neuropathologic criteria for Steele-Richardson-Olszewski syndrome (progressive supranuclear palsy). *Neurology, 44*(11), 2015–2019.

Henderson, J. M., Carpenter, K., Cartwright, H., & Halliday, G. M. (2000). Loss of thalamic intralaminar nuclei in progressive supranuclear palsy and Parkinson's disease: Clinical and therapeutic implications. *Brain: A Journal of Neurology, 123*(Pt 7), 1410–1421.

Hodges, J. R., & Patterson, K. (2007). Semantic dementia: A unique clinicopathological syndrome. *Lancet Neurology, 6*(11), 1004–1014.

Hodges, J. R., Patterson, K., Oxbury, S., & Funnell, E. (1992). Semantic dementia. Progressive fluent aphasia with temporal lobe atrophy. *Brain: A Journal of Neurology, 115*(Pt 6), 1783–1806.

Holland, A. L., McBurney, D. H., Moossy, J., & Reinmuth, O. M. (1985). The dissolution of language in Pick's disease with neurofibrillary tangles: A case study. *Brain and Language, 24*(1), 36–58.

Hoppitt, T., Pall, H., Calvert, M., Gill, P., Yao, G., Ramsay, J.,...Sackley, C. (2011). A systematic review of the incidence and prevalence of long-term neurological conditions in the UK. *Neuroepidemiology, 36*(1), 19–28.

Hu, W. T., Mandrekar, J. N., Parisi, J. E., Knopman, D. S., Boeve, B. F., Petersen, R. C.,...Josephs, K. A. (2007). Clinical features of pathologic subtypes of behavioral–variant frontotemporal dementia. *Archives of Neurology, 64*(11), 1611–1616.

Huey, E. D., Putnam, K. T., & Grafman, J. (2006). A systematic review of neurotransmitter deficits and treatments in frontotemporal dementia. *Neurology, 66*(1), 17–22.

Izzo, K. L., DiLorenzo, P., & Roth, A. (1986). Rehabilitation in progressive supranuclear palsy: Case report. *Archives of Physical Medicine and Rehabilitation, 67*(7), 473–476.

Jicha, G. A., & Nelson, P. T. (2011). Management of frontotemporal dementia: Targeting symptom management in such a heterogeneous disease requires a wide range of therapeutic options. *Neurodegenerative Disease Management, 1*(2), 141–156.

Johnson, J. K., Diehl, J., Mendez, M. F., Neuhaus, J., Shapira, J. S., Forman, M.,...Miller, B. L. (2005). Frontotemporal lobar degeneration: Demographic characteristics of 353 patients. *Archives of Neurology, 62*(6), 925–930.

Josephs, K. A., Whitwell, J. L., Weigand, S. D., Senjem, M. L., Boeve, B. F., Knopman, D. S.,... Petersen, R. C. (2011). Predicting functional decline in behavioural variant frontotemporal dementia. *Brain: A Journal of Neurology, 134*(Pt 2), 432–448.

Kertesz, A., Martinez-Lage, P., Davidson, W., & Munoz, D. G. (2000). The corticobasal degeneration syndrome overlaps progressive aphasia and frontotemporal dementia. *Neurology, 55*(9), 1368–1375.

Kertesz, A., & McMonagle, P. (2010). Behavior and cognition in corticobasal degeneration and progressive supranuclear palsy. *Journal of the Neurological Sciences, 289*(1–2), 138–143.

Kertesz, A., McMonagle, P., Blair, M., Davidson, W., & Munoz, D. G. (2005). The evolution and pathology of frontotemporal dementia. *Brain: A Journal of Neurology, 128*(Pt 9), 1996–2005.

Kipps, C. M., Hodges, J. R., & Hornberger, M. (2010). Nonprogressive behavioural frontotemporal dementia: Recent developments and clinical implications of the "bvFTD phenocopy syndrome." *Current Opinion in Neurology, 23*(6), 628–632.

Kirshner, H. S. (2010). Frontotemporal dementia and primary progressive aphasia: An update. *Current Neurology and Neuroscience Reports, 10*(6), 504–511.

Kuniyoshi, S., Riley, D. E., Zee, D. S., Reich, S. G., Whitney, C., & Leigh, R. J. (2002). Distinguishing progressive supranuclear palsy from other forms of Parkinson's disease: Evaluation of new signs. *Annals of the New York Academy of Sciences, 956*, 484–486.

Lepow, L., Van Sweringen, J., Strutt, A. M., Jawaid, A., MacAdam, C., Harati, Y.,...York, M. K. (2010). Frontal and temporal lobe involvement on verbal fluency measures in amyotrophic lateral sclerosis. *Journal of Clinical and Experimental Neuropsychology, 32*(9), 913–922.

Litvan, I. (1997). Progressive supranuclear palsy and corticobasal degeneration. *Baillière's Clinical Neurology, 6*(1), 167–185.

Litvan, I., Bhatia, K. P., Burn, D. J., Goetz, C. G., Lang, A. E., McKeith, I.,...Wenning, G. K.; Movement Disorders Society Scientific Issues Committee. (2003). Movement Disorders Society Scientific Issues Committee report: SIC Task Force appraisal of clinical diagnostic criteria for Parkinsonian disorders. *Movement Disorders, 18*(5), 467–486.

Litvan, I., Campbell, G., Mangone, C. A., Verny, M., McKee, A., Chaudhuri, K. R.,... D'Olhaberriague, L. (1997). Which clinical features differentiate progressive supranuclear palsy (Steele-Richardson-Olszewski syndrome) from related disorders? A clinicopathological study. *Brain: A Journal of Neurology, 120*(Pt 1), 65–74.

Litvan, I., Phipps, M., Pharr, V. L., Hallett, M., Grafman, J., & Salazar, A. (2001). Randomized placebo-controlled trial of donepezil in patients with progressive supranuclear palsy. *Neurology, 57*(3), 467–473.

Lund and Manchester Groups. (1994). Clinical and neuropathological criteria for frontotemporal dementia. *Journal of Neurology, Neurosurgery, and Psychiatry, 57,* 416–418.

Mahapatra, R. K., Edwards, M. J., Schott, J. M., & Bhatia, K. P. (2004). Corticobasal degeneration. *Lancet Neurology, 3*(12), 736–743.

Mantovan, M. C., Baggio, L., Dalla Barba, G., Smith, P., Pegoraro, E., Soraru', G., Bonometto, P., & Angelini, C. (2003). Memory deficits and retrieval processes in ALS. *European Journal of Neurology, 10*(3), 221–227.

Mesulam, M. M. (1982). Slowly progressive aphasia without generalized dementia. *Annals of Neurology, 11*(6), 592–598.

Miller, R. G., Mitchell, J. D., Lyon, M., & Moore, D. H. (2007). Riluzole for amyotrophic lateral sclerosis (ALS)/motor neuron disease (MND). *The Cochrane Database of Systematic Reviews,* (1), CD001447.

Mitsuyama, Y., & Inoue, T. (2009). Clinical entity of frontotemporal dementia with motor neuron disease. *Neuropathology, 29*(6), 649–654.

Moon, S. Y., Lee, B. H., Seo, S. W., Kang, S. J., & Na, D. L. (2008). Slow vertical saccades in the frontotemporal dementia with motor neuron disease. *Journal of Neurology, 255*(9), 1337–1343.

Nath, U., Ben-Shlomo, Y., Thomson, R. G., Lees, A. J., & Burn, D. J. (2003). Clinical features and natural history of progressive supranuclear palsy: A clinical cohort study. *Neurology, 60*(6), 910–916.

Nath, U., Ben-Shlomo, Y., Thomson, R. G., Morris, H. R., Wood, N. W., Lees, A. J., & Burn, D. J. (2001). The prevalence of progressive supranuclear palsy (Steele-Richardson-Olszewski syndrome) in the UK. *Brain: A Journal of Neurology, 124*(Pt 7), 1438–1449.

Neary, D., & Snowden, J. (2013). Frontal lobe dementia, motor neuron disease, and clinical and neuropathological criteria. *Journal of Neurology, Neurosurgery, and Psychiatry, 84*(7), 713–714.

Neary, D., Snowden, J., & Mann, D. (2005). Frontotemporal dementia. *Lancet Neurology, 4*(11), 771–780.

Neary, D., Snowden, J. S., Gustafson, L., Passant, U., Stuss, D., Black, S., … Benson, D. F. (1998). Frontotemporal lobar degeneration: A consensus on clinical diagnostic criteria. *Neurology, 51*(6), 1546–1554.

O'Keeffe, F. M., Murray, B., Coen, R. F., Dockree, P. M., Bellgrove, M. A., Garavan, H., … Robertson, I. H. (2007). Loss of insight in frontotemporal dementia, corticobasal degeneration and progressive supranuclear palsy. *Brain: A Journal of Neurology, 130*(Pt 3), 753–764.

Olney, R. K., Murphy, J., Forshew, D., Garwood, E., Miller, B. L., Langmore, S., … Lomen-Hoerth, C. (2005). The effects of executive and behavioral dysfunction on the course of ALS. *Neurology, 65*(11), 1774–1777.

Onari, K., & Spatz, H. (1926). Anatomische Beiträge zur Lehre von der Pickschen umschriebenen Grosshirnrinden-Atrophie ("Picksche Krankheit"). *Zeitschrift für die Gesamte Neurologie und Psychiatrie, 101,* 470–511.

Peigneux, P., Salmon, E., Garraux, G., Laureys, S., Willems, S., Dujardin, K., … Van der Linden, M. (2001). Neural and cognitive bases of upper limb apraxia in corticobasal degeneration. *Neurology, 57*(7), 1259–1268.

Phukan, J., Pender, N. P., & Hardiman, O. (2007). Cognitive impairment in amyotrophic lateral sclerosis. *Lancet Neurology, 6*(11), 994–1003.

Pick, A. (1892). Über die Beziehungen der senilen Hirnatrophie zur Aphasie. *Pragur Medicinsche Wochenschrift, 17*, 165–167.

Piguet, O., Halliday, G. M., Reid, W. G., Casey, B., Carman, R., Huang, Y.,...Kril, J. J. (2011). Clinical phenotypes in autopsy-confirmed Pick disease. *Neurology, 76*(3), 253–259.

Piguet, O., Hornberger, M., Mioshi, E., & Hodges, J. R. (2011). Behavioural-variant frontotemporal dementia: Diagnosis, clinical staging, and management. *Lancet Neurology, 10*(2), 162–172.

Rabinovici, G. D., & Miller, B. L. (2010). Frontotemporal lobar degeneration: Epidemiology, pathophysiology, diagnosis and management. *CNS Drugs, 24*(5), 375–398.

Rascovsky, K., Hodges, J. R., Kipps, C. M., Johnson, J. K., Seeley, W. W., Mendez, M. F.,...Miller, B. M. (2007). Diagnostic criteria for the behavioral variant of frontotemporal dementia (bvFTD): Current limitations and future directions. *Alzheimer Disease and Associated Disorders, 21*(4), S14–S18.

Rascovsky, K., Salmon, D. P., Hansen, L. A., & Galasko, D. (2008). Distinct cognitive profiles and rates of decline on the Mattis Dementia Rating Scale in autopsy-confirmed frontotemporal dementia and Alzheimer's disease. *Journal of the International Neuropsychological Society, 14*(3), 373–383.

Rebeiz, J. J., Kolodny, E. H., & Richardson, E. P. (1967). Corticodentatonigral degeneration with neuronal achromasia: A progressive disorder of late adult life. *Transactions of the American Neurological Association, 92*, 23–26.

Ringholz, G. M., Appel, S. H., Bradshaw, M., Cooke, N. A., Mosnik, D. M., & Schulz, P. E. (2005). Prevalence and patterns of cognitive impairment in sporadic ALS. *Neurology, 65*(4), 586–590.

Rinne, J. O., Lee, M. S., Thompson, P. D., & Marsden, C. D. (1994). Corticobasal degeneration. A clinical study of 36 cases. *Brain: A Journal of Neurology, 117*(Pt 5), 1183–1196.

Robbins, T. W., James, M., Owen, A. M., Lange, K. W., Lees, A. J., Leigh, P. N.,...Summers, B. A. (1994). Cognitive deficits in progressive supranuclear palsy, Parkinson's disease, and multiple system atrophy in tests sensitive to frontal lobe dysfunction. *Journal of Neurology, Neurosurgery, and Psychiatry, 57*(1), 79–88.

Rosser, A., & Hodges, J. R. (1994). Initial letter and semantic category fluency in Alzheimer's disease, Huntington's disease, and progressive supranuclear palsy. *Journal of Neurology, Neurosurgery, and Psychiatry, 57*(11), 1389–1394.

Rusina, R., Ridzon, P., Kulist'ák, P., Keller, O., Bartos, A., Buncová, M.,...Matej, R. (2010). Relationship between ALS and the degree of cognitive impairment, markers of neurodegeneration and predictors for poor outcome. A prospective study. *European Journal of Neurology, 17*(1), 23–30.

Salmon, E., Garraux, G., Delbeuck, X., Collette, F., Kalbe, E., Zuendorf, G.,...Herholz, K. (2003). Predominant ventromedial frontopolar metabolic impairment in frontotemporal dementia. *NeuroImage, 20*(1), 435–440.

Schmitt, F., Shih, W., & DeKosky, S. (1992). Neuropsychological correlates of single photon emission computed tomography (SPECT) in Alzheimer's disease. *Neuropsychology, 6*(2), 159–171.

Schrag, A., Ben-Shlomo, Y., & Quinn, N. P. (1999). Prevalence of progressive supranuclear palsy and multiple system atrophy: A cross-sectional study. *Lancet, 354*(9192), 1771–1775.

Seeley, W. W., Allman, J. M., Carlin, D. A., Crawford, R. K., Macedo, M. N., Greicius, M. D.,... Miller, B. L. (2007). Divergent social functioning in behavioral variant frontotemporal dementia and Alzheimer disease: Reciprocal networks and neuronal evolution. *Alzheimer Disease and Associated Disorders, 21*(4), S50–S57.

Shoji, M., Matsubara, E., Murakami, T., Manabe, Y., Abe, K., Kanai, M., ... Hirai, S. (2002). Cerebrospinal fluid tau in dementia disorders: A large scale multicenter study by a Japanese study group. *Neurobiology of Aging, 23*(3), 363–370.

Snowden, J. S., Goulding, P. J., & Neary, D. (1989). Semantic dementia: A form of circumscribed cerebral atrophy. *Behavioral Neurology, 2*(3), 167–182.

Snowden, J., Neary, D., & Mann, D. (2007). Frontotemporal lobar degeneration: Clinical and pathological relationships. *Acta Neuropathologica, 114*(1), 31–38.

Soliveri, P., Monza, D., Paridi, D., Carella, F., Genitrini, S., Testa, D., & Girotti, F. (2000). Neuropsychological follow up in patients with Parkinson's disease, striatonigral degeneration-type multisystem atrophy, and progressive supranuclear palsy. *Journal of Neurology, Neurosurgery, and Psychiatry, 69*(3), 313–318.

Stamelou, M., de Silva, R., Arias-Carrión, O., Boura, E., Höllerhage, M., Oertel, W. H.,... Höglinger, G. U. (2010). Rational therapeutic approaches to progressive supranuclear palsy. *Brain: A Journal of Neurology, 133*(Pt 6), 1578–1590.

Steele, J. C., Richardson, J. C., & Olszewski, J. (1964). Progressive supranuclear palsy. A heterogeneous degeneration involving the brain stem, basal ganglia and cerebellum with vertical gaze and pseudobulbar palsy, nuchal dystonia and dementia. *Archives of Neurology, 10*, 333–359.

Takeda, N., Kishimoto, Y., & Yokota, O. (2012). Pick's disease. In S. Ahmad (Ed.), *Neurodegenerative diseases* (pp. 300–316). New York: Springer.

Talbot, P. R., Goulding, P. J., Lloyd, J. J., Snowden, J. S., Neary, D., & Testa, H. J. (1995). Inter-relation between "classic" motor neuron disease and frontotemporal dementia: Neuropsychological and single photon emission computed tomography study. *Journal of Neurology, Neurosurgery, and Psychiatry, 58*(5), 541–547.

Tashiro, K., Ogata, K., Goto, Y., Taniwaki, T., Okayama, A., Kira, J., & Tobimatsu, S. (2006). EEG findings in early-stage corticobasal degeneration and progressive supranuclear palsy: A retrospective study and literature review. *Clinical Neurophysiology, 117*(10), 2236–2242.

Thompson, J. C., Stopford, C. L., Snowden, J. S., & Neary, D. (2005). Qualitative neuropsychological performance characteristics in frontotemporal dementia and Alzheimer's disease. *Journal of Neurology, Neurosurgery, and Psychiatry, 76*(7), 920–927.

Thompson, P. D., Day, B. L., Rothwell, J. C., Brown, P., Britton, T. C., & Marsden, C. D. (1994). The myoclonus in corticobasal degeneration: Evidence for two forms of cortical reflex myoclonus. *Brain, 117*(Pt. 5), 1197–1207.

Watts, R. L., Williams, R. S., Growdon, J. D., Young, R. R., Haley, E. C., Jr., & Beal, M. F. (1985). Cortico-basal ganglionic degeneration. *Neurology, 35*(Suppl. 1), 178.

Weiner, W. J., Minagar, A., & Shulman, L. M. (1999). Pramipexole in progressive supranuclear palsy. *Neurology, 52*(4), 873–874.

Williams, D. R., de Silva, R., Paviour, D. C., Pittman, A., Watt, H. C., Kilford, L.,...Lees, A. J. (2005). Characteristics of two distinct clinical phenotypes in pathologically proven progressive supranuclear palsy: Richardson's syndrome and PSP-parkinsonism. *Brain: A Journal of Neurology, 128*(Pt 6), 1247–1258.

Zampieri, C., & Di Fabio, R. P. (2008). Balance and eye movement training to improve gait in people with progressive supranuclear palsy: Quasi-randomized clinical trial. *Physical Therapy, 88*(12), 1460–1473.

CHAPTER 10

Semantic Dementia

Daniel Rexroth

The prevalence of dementia in the United States is approximately 3.4 million individuals (Plassman et al., 2007). Because dementia is an age-related disorder and the older adult segment of the population is growing rapidly, the prevalence is expected to climb to 8 to 13 million individuals by 2050 (Sloane et al., 2002). Frontotemporal dementia (FTD) is the third leading cause of dementia in large pathological series (Barker et al., 2002) but tends to have an earlier age of onset than Alzheimer's disease (AD) and Lewy body dementia, the most frequent and second most frequent forms of dementia. The majority of FTD cases have onset prior to 65 years of age. The early age of onset combined with the distinctive symptom cluster of FTD spectrum illnesses creates a different and quite challenging set of employment, social, and family management issues for patients, families, and clinicians.

HISTORY

One form of the syndrome now termed FTD was first described by psychiatrist and neurologist Arnold Pick in 1892 when he reported on a man who had threatened his wife with a knife and showed progressive loss of language; severe atrophy of the frontotemporal lobes was discovered at autopsy. However, the term *Pick's disease* was first used by Onari and Spatz in 1926 (Binetti, Locascio, Corkin, Vonsattel, & Growdon, 2000). Over the next several decades, this cluster of symptoms continued to be called Pick's disease although much of the focus was on patients with the behavioral variant of the disease. In 1975, Elizabeth Warrington described the clinical symptoms in three of her patients that had deficits in semantic memory and expressive language (Warrington, 1975). Then in 1998, Neary et al. (Faber, 1999; Neary et al., 1998) developed a consensus diagnosis of frontotemporal lobar degeneration that included three neurobehavioral syndromes: (a) behavioral, (b) progressive nonfluent aphasia (PNFA), and (c) semantic. The behavioral variant of FTD (bvFTD) involves changes in character and social appropriateness, and often includes emotional blunting, decline in interpersonal relationships, lack of insight into one's behavior, and an inability to control one's behavior. Neary et al. also noted other behavior changes that may be present during the course of the illness such as a decline in self-care, mental inflexibility, hyperorality (examines objects by mouth), changes in diet, and perseveration.

The clinical features of PNFA include nonfluent spontaneous speech with some presence of agrammatism, phonemic paraphasias, or anomia (Neary et al., 1998). Other symptoms that may be present include stuttering, difficulties with repetition, alexia, or agraphia. Semantic dementia (SD) includes impairment in the understanding of the meanings of words and difficulty in identifying objects (Neary et al., 1998). This may include fluent, yet empty speech as well as a loss of the meanings of words and the occurrence of semantic paraphasias. More recently, efforts have been made to further classify language disorders (Gorno-Tempini et al., 2004, 2011; Mesulam et al., 2009b) into agrammatic, semantic, and logopenic variants in order to further define the divisions of Neary et al. (1998). Primary PNFA has been further divided into agrammatic and logopenic subtypes. The agrammatic subtype refers to a disorder in which the individual has difficulty with speech production that includes difficulty with word order and preserved single-word comprehension (Mesulam et al., 2009b). In the logopenic subtype, word retrieval and phonemic paraphasias are most evident (Mesulam et al., 2009b). Semantic primary progressive aphasia, also known as SD, includes difficulties with naming and single-word comprehension although grammar and fluency are often spared (Bonner, Ash, & Grossman, 2010). This poor comprehension of single words is often one of the first symptoms observed in the disease. There is often also impaired object knowledge, particularly for lower-frequency items, and difficulty reading words that sound different from how they are spelled; speech production and repetition speech are usually normal (Gorno-Tempini et al., 2011).

EPIDEMIOLOGY

The prevalence of FTD has ranged from 2.7/100,000 (Rosso et al., 2003) in a study of 60- to 69-year-olds in the Netherlands to 15.1/100,000 (Ratnavalli, Brayne, Dawson, & Hodges, 2002) in a study of adults younger than 65 years of age in the United Kingdom. Approximately 10% to 20% of dementia patients have FTD (Hodges & Miller, 2001; Neary et al., 1998; Snowden et al., 2001). Of the FTD subtypes, the behavioral variant is the most common followed by PNFA and SD (Johnson et al., 2005; Kertesz, Blair, McMonagle, & Munoz, 2007; Neary et al., 1998); between 25% and 33% have the SD subtype (Chow et al., 2005).

The age of onset for FTD is typically between 45 and 64 years although there are reports that as many as 20% to 30% of cases occur outside of this range (Hodges et al., 2010; Ikeda, Ishikawa, & Tanabe, 2004; Johnson et al., 2005; Ratnavalli et al., 2002; Weder, Aziz, Wilkins, & Tampi, 2007). SD and bvFTD usually occur at younger ages than PNFA (Kertesz, 2008). The average age of onset for SD symptoms to occur is between 53 and 61.5 years (Hodges, Davies, Xuereb, Kril, & Halliday, 2003; Hodges et al., 2010; Kertesz et al., 2007; Ratnavalli et al., 2002). One study found that the median time between symptom onset and institutionalization for FTD patients was 5 years but only 1 year after diagnosis (Hodges et al., 2003), presumably due to families having difficulty managing the patient's behavioral changes. This differs from a study on AD patients who were institutionalized an average of 2.5 years from evaluation and 5.6 years from onset of symptoms (Severson et al., 1994). The average life expectancy after diagnosis ranges from 3.0 to 7.8 years for all of the types of FTD (Hodges et al., 2003; Kertesz et al., 2007). SD has been shown to have an average of a 4-year span between diagnosis and death (Hodges et al., 2003). Regarding gender, some studies have found that the rates of disease between the genders are equal (Hodges & Patterson, 2007; Kertesz et al., 2007), while others have found that men tend to have higher rates of SD than women (Hodges et al., 2003; Johnson et al., 2005; Roberson et al., 2005). Education level has not been shown to differentiate between diagnostic FTD subgroups (Chow et al., 2005; Johnson et al., 2005; Kertesz et al., 2007). Patients with SD tend to survive 11.9 years from symptom onset (Rabinovici & Miller, 2010), which is longer on average than those with FTD or PNFA (Roberson et al., 2005). SD is usually sporadic and has the least heritability of the FTDs (Rabinovici & Miller, 2010; Rohrer et al., 2009). In a study by Goldman et al. only 1.9% of cases were autosomal dominant and 17% of patients with SD had a positive family history of dementia or amyotrophic lateral sclerosis (Goldman et al., 2005). Among the various subtypes of FTD, SD has the least heritability (Goldman et al., 2005; Rabinovici & Miller, 2010; Rohrer et al., 2009), with one study suggesting a rate between 2% and 7% (Hodges et al., 2010).

CLINICAL FEATURES AND DIAGNOSTIC CRITERIA

SD is a disorder that involves loss of semantic memory, anomia, receptive aphasia, and an actual loss of word meaning. Speech often remains fluent and grammatically intact but there is a loss of ability to remember the names of objects (anomia) or understand the meaning of words and objects (Boxer & Miller, 1997; Neary et al., 1998). Loss of knowledge about the world is often one of the first symptoms. Speech is often described as being a fluent aphasia because rate and production are normal although the words are often devoid of meaning. Early on, there may be semantic paraphasias, which involves substitution of the correct word with a word that, while incorrect, may be related (e.g., saying cat instead of dog). There is also evidence for a loss of subordinate categories while knowledge for superordinate categories remains (Warrington, 1975). Specifically, the patient often loses the ability to distinguish between objects within a group, and later has trouble distinguishing the group itself from other groups, eventually resulting in referring to all objects in the group as "things." An example of this would be a person forgetting the word *frog* while maintaining the larger category of *animal*, before later forgetting the category and referring to all animals as *things*. With regard to word-finding difficulty, the patient may have an idea of the overall category of the term but loses the preciseness of language; circumlocution becomes common. Repetition, prosody, and syntax are often preserved early in the disease. Word comprehension difficulties are also present early on and patients are often unaware of this deficit. Over time, word finding becomes more pronounced and, while the individual is often able to pronounce words correctly, his or her ability to communicate is reduced to a jumble of words or "word salad." Because of this, speech is often empty with semantic paraphasias present. Reading and writing abilities are also likely to decline over time. Phonetic reading (i.e., being able to read words with spelling-to-sounds correspondence) remains normal but the ability to read words that have irregular orthography (e.g., "rough" is read as "rug") is impaired. Writing ability is often similar in that there is preserved ability to spell dictated words that are spelled phonetically but an inability to spell words that have irregular orthography. Although SD patients lose the language abilities necessary to name objects or their category, they are still generally able to utilize familiar objects for activities such as cooking or participating in hobbies (Lauro-Grotto, Piccini, & Shallice, 1997).

EVALUATION AND ASSESSMENT

Several different disciplines may be involved in order to provide a thorough evaluation. The following assessment tools are those conducted by a psychologist or a neuropsychologist. Such an evaluation should include a clinical interview and neuropsychological examination.

Clinical Interview

Given that the patient may have difficulties with communication and possible cognitive deficits, it is ideal to be able to interview the patient along with a family member/caregiver who is very familiar with the patient's current level of functioning. Information that should be gathered includes a history of the present illness, medical history, psychiatric history, family history, social history, and information regarding the patient's current functional status, including mood, occupational status, and activities of daily living. The main symptoms to look for when interviewing a patient and caregiver with possible SD are fluent speech that is grammatically correct, loss of meaning for objects and words along with anomia, difficulty reading and comprehending words that were previously familiar (Hodges, Patterson, Oxbury, & Funnell, 1992), and possible behavior abnormalities similar to those in bvFTD (Deramecourt et al., 2010). However, several of these may also present early in other dementias and language disorders such as AD and PNFA. According to Kertesz, Jesso, Harciarek, Blair, and McMonagle (2010) there are several cardinal diagnostic features that a health professional may look for when meeting with the patient. One of the most striking of these is loss of the meaning of words resulting in the patient asking "What is ____?" when presented with a noun. While some of the other dementias and language disorders present with difficulties with anomia, expressive speech, or receptive speech, none of them has such a loss of meaning of nouns. The interviewer will also want to listen for semantic paraphasias, such as substituting the word *marker* for *pencil,* as these are more frequent in SD than in other dementias; phonological errors in which the person mispronounces the word or says syllables out of sequence are uncommon (Hodges & Patterson, 2007; Kertesz et al., 2010). As compared to AD, SD patients are more likely to have greater deficits in semantic memory but lesser deficits in episodic memory. SD patients are also more likely to be aware of their deficits than those patients with bvFTD (Allison, Schauer, Diehl, Miller, & Rosen, 2006). Changes in behaviors such as a tendency toward social withdrawal, low mood, and changes in eating patterns are areas that should be explored carefully with caregivers (Bozeat, Gregory, Ralph, & Hodges, 2000; Forman et al., 2007).

Cognitive Testing

The cognitive domains most likely to be affected in SD are confrontation naming, word–picture matching, and semantic knowledge (Rascovsky, Growdon, Pardo, Grossman, & Miller, 2009). Diehl et al. (2005) compared patients with bvFTD, SD, and AD on the Consortium to Establish a Registry for Alzheimer's Disease Neuropsychological Assessment Battery and found that SD patients performed worse than AD patients on the Animal Fluency and Boston Naming Test. In AD, low scores on the Boston Naming Test were associated with low scores on the Mini-Mental State Examination (MMSE). However, SD patients who scored poorly on the Boston Naming Test often scored well on the MMSE. Multivariable logistic regression revealed that a combination of Boston Naming Test and the MMSE correctly differentiated 96.3% of SD and AD patients. Lambon Ralph, Graham, Ellis, and Hodges (1998) were able to further define the difficulty that SD patients had with naming and found that object frequency in spoken language and the age at which most people learn the name of the object all played a role in determining whether the word would be remembered (Lambon Ralph et al., 1998). A later study by Woollams, Cooper-Pye, Hodges, and Patterson (2008) discovered that the broad semantic domain to which the object belonged also played a small but significant role in the severity of the anomia (Woollams et al., 2008).

In addition to confrontation naming, category fluency and vocabulary are some of the tests that are most difficult for the patient with SD (Boxer & Miller, 2005). Hodges, Graham, and Patterson (1995) furthered knowledge in this area by discovering that patients tend to lose the details of the items within the categories before losing their knowledge about the categories themselves. Gorno-Tempini et al. (2011) note that the four language abilities that separate SD from other aphasias are impaired single-word comprehension, confrontation naming, object/people knowledge, and reading/spelling. Single-word comprehension is usually worse for low-frequency items (e.g., *kiwi* vs. more familiar *apple*), and this may be the only symptom along with anomia during the earliest stages of SD (Gorno-Tempini et al., 2011). This poor comprehension for single words is one of the most obvious symptoms of a semantic memory deficit that interferes with object/people knowledge. Difficulties with reading and spelling are most often for words with irregular spelling-to-sound associations (e.g., *knee* or *two*), a disorder known as surface dyslexia. They suggest several tests that may be helpful in eliciting these deficits in the patient. For single-word comprehension, it is suggested that a word-to-picture or word-to-definition test be used. To test confrontation naming, they suggest using tests that involve single-word identification of sounds, foods, and pictures. Picture–picture or gesture–object matching can assist with assessing object/people knowledge. Having the patient orally read word lists of regular and irregular words can help assess reading and having them spell similar types of words can help determine surface dyslexia.

Visuospatial deficits such as associative agnosia and prosopagnosia may also occur (Boxer & Miller, 2005). This means that individuals may be able to identify individual features in a drawing or even copy it although they will be unable to identify what the drawing is; they will also have difficulty recognizing what should be familiar faces. Reading may also be difficult, particularly words that are irregular in that they sound differently from how they are spelled (Boxer & Miller, 2005); repetition speech is generally preserved. They have little difficulty repeating words or sentences (Boxer & Miller, 2005). There is some evidence that, compared to nonfluent aphasia patients, SD patients have more difficulty with the oral or written naming of nouns as opposed to verbs (Hillis, Oh, & Ken, 2004; Robinson, Druks, Hodges, & Garrard, 2009) and more difficulty with written as opposed to oral naming (Hillis et al., 2004). SD patients have also been shown to have difficulty with both imageable and abstract concepts (Jefferies, Patterson, Jones, & Lambon Ralph, 2009).

As opposed to AD, episodic memory is relatively well preserved for the SD patient; it is the well-learned semantic knowledge that becomes impaired. This should be tested with verbal and nonverbal tests. Examples of tests that can be used to verbally test semantic knowledge include confrontation naming, category fluency, and a vocabulary test. The Pyramid and Palm Trees Test (Howard, 1992) can assist the practitioner with testing conceptual knowledge without having to rely on language. It helps determine whether the patient is having difficulty remembering semantic information from pictures or from words, or is having difficulty remembering the correct spoken form of the word. An example from the test is that the patient is presented with a picture of a pyramid as well as pictures of a pine tree and a palm tree; she must choose which of the two trees matches with the pyramid.

There is also often a decline in arithmetic skills and calculation performance for the patient with SD (Julien, Thompson, Neary, & Snowden, 2008). Knowledge of tunes and lyrics from music is relatively spared as to other forms of knowledge (Hailstone, Omar, & Warren, 2009; Robinson et al., 2009). There is also evidence that visuospatial skills and concentration skills are preserved given that patients with SD generally maintain excellent skills at completing jigsaw puzzles (Julien et al., 2008).

Behavior rating scales can be helpful in differentiating among FTD subtypes. The Behavior Rating Inventory of Executive Function (BRIEF) is one (Roth, Isquith, & Gioia, 2005) that consists of a self-report form and an informant report form, each of which has 75 questions measuring change in the patient's ability to inhibit, self-monitor, plan/organize, shift, initiate, task monitor, and display emotional control, working memory, and organization of materials. Another measure of executive function is the Frontal Systems Behavioral Scale (FrSBe) by Grace and Malloy (2001). It is a 46-item behavior rating scale that also has patient and informant forms and measures apathy, disinhibition, and executive functions. It has been shown to be helpful in discriminating between bvFTD and AD, due to increased reports of disinhibited behavior on the rating scales (Malloy, Tremont, Grace, & Frakey, 2007). The Frontal Behavioral Inventory (FBI) is also helpful in diagnosing FTD. The FBI helps inventory some of the core features associated with bvFTD such as apathy, personal neglect, and loss of insight more effectively than cognitive testing (Kertesz, Davidson, McCabe, & Munoz, 2003; Malloy & Grace, 2005). It is comprised of 24 questions that are answered by the caregiver that assess for negative and positive behaviors that are rated on a 4-point scale (0–3); the cutoff is 27. One study found that SD patients were second only to bvFTD in obtaining high scores on the FBI and helped differentiate it from PNFA and AD (Kertesz et al., 2010).

IMAGING

For many dementias, including FTD, imaging is usually conducted in clinical practice to rule out other disorders that can produce symptoms that mimic a dementia illness. However, there have been some patterns of atrophy that can be expected with the three variants of FTD. Atrophy is often present in the left inferior frontal and insular areas in PNFA patients (Gorno-Tempini et al., 2004). Both SD and bvFTD often have atrophy in the ventromedial frontal cortex, bilaterally in the insular and orbital frontal regions, and in the left anterior cingulate cortex (Rosen et al., 2002). However, there are some patterns of atrophy that are different between these two variants as well. The bvFTD often has atrophy that affects the frontal lobes bilaterally, with particular atrophy of the right dorsolateral frontal cortex and the left premotor cortex (Rosen et al., 2002). SD often has a pattern that shows bilateral, although asymmetric, atrophy of the anterior temporal lobes; left-sided atrophy is more commonly seen at a ratio of 3:1 (Rabinovici & Miller, 2010), as well as in the anterior hippocampal region bilaterally. There have been several studies that analyzed structural changes through imaging in the SD patient. It had been hypothesized that the cognitive deficits of SD such as anomia would be associated with polar and inferolateral temporal atrophy but that the hippocampus would be spared (Galton et al., 2001). Compared to controls, there is often widespread volume loss in SD patients, with particular loss in the anterior temporal lobes surrounding the perirhinal cortex (Davies, Halliday, Xuereb, Kril, & Hodges, 2009). However, a study by Galton et al. (2001) of 26 patients with AD, 18 with SD, and 21 matched controls revealed that in addition to the expected changes in the temporal pole bilaterally and the left amygdala, parahippocampal gyrus, fusiform gyrus, and the inferior and middle temporal gyri, the hippocampus had more significant atrophy on the left side than that in the AD patients (Galton et al., 2001). A study of SD by Mesulam et al. revealed three characteristics of these patients on MRI: (a) greater atrophy on the left than the right hemisphere, (b) atrophy of the anterior sections of the perisylvian language network, particularly in the superior and middle temporal gyri, and (c) atrophy of the anterior components of the inferior and medial temporal lobes (Mesulam et al., 2009a). Other imaging studies have also confirmed that alterations usually occur more in the left temporal lobe and that the hippocampus is often involved (Gorno-Tempini et al., 2004; Hodges & Patterson, 2007; Lehmann et al., 2010; Mesulam et al., 2009a; Rosen et al., 2002). However, a study by Bright, Moss, Stamatakis, and Tyler (2008) claimed that greater atrophy in the left hemisphere is not how the disease always presents itself and instead argue that there is heterogeneity (Bright et al., 2008). They also argue that the variability in pattern and rate of atrophy over time is important; earlier damage is generally in the ventral temporal cortex (object processing/semantic memory) and that language dysfunction usually occurs later, after the perisylvian language areas become involved (Bright et al., 2008). Sapolsky et al. (2010) noted that left inferior frontal thinning was well correlated with impaired grammar, syntax, and fluency; left temporopolar thinning correlated with poor word comprehension. Interestingly, they discovered that a "combination of left inferior frontal, left temporopolar, and left superior temporal sulcal thickness separated the three primary progressive subtypes from each other with 100% accuracy" (Sapolsky et al., 2010). Peelle et al. (2008) analyzed sentence comprehension and voxel-based morphometry in the three FTD subtypes and found that SD patients' difficulties with sentence comprehension correlated with left inferolateral temporal lobe damage and theorized that this was related to impairment of lexical processing (Peelle et al., 2008). Gorno-Tempini et al. (2004) studied nonfluent, semantic, and logopenic FTD patients on voxel-based morphometry on MRI. SD patients are characterized by loss of volume in the anterior temporal region. In nonfluent aphasia, volume loss occurred in the left posterior frontal and insular regions, while in the logopenic variant, it was in the left temporoparietal region.

Temporal variant FTD and some of the related clinical changes can look somewhat different at the beginning of the disease process depending on whether atrophy begins in the left or right temporal lobe. The loss of semantic knowledge including anomia and word-finding difficulties with some semantic paraphasic errors is usually a sign that the left temporal lobe has been affected, while changes in emotion, sleep, appetite, and sex drive at the beginning of the disease process usually indicated degeneration of the right temporal lobe (Seeley et al., 2005). After an average of 3 years, however, the symptom not present at inception usually emerges and the two variants begin to look similar. After 5 to 7 years, other symptoms are revealed such as compulsions, disinhibition, prosopagnosia (impaired face recognition), and changes in food preference (Seeley et al., 2005).

Diffusion MRI has revealed that SD is linked to damage to the major superior and inferior temporal white-matter connections of the left hemisphere that are involved in lexical and semantic processes (Agosta et al., 2010).

The use of PET and functional MRI (fMRI) has shown that there is a network of areas involved in semantic tasks (Démonet et al., 1992; Friederici, Opitz, & von Cramon, 2000; Mummery, Patterson, Hodges, & Wise, 1996; Wise et al., 1991); in particular, semantic tasks utilize activation of the left pars triangularis of the inferior frontal gyrus and the posterior section of the left middle and superior temporal gyrus (Friederici et al., 2000). There is some evidence that in SD, some deficits are due to damage to the atrophied anterior temporal regions and underactivation of the posterior inferior temporal region (Mummery et al., 1999).

C-labeled Pittsburgh Compound-B (C-PIB) binds to fibrillar amyloid-beta ($A\beta$) that is detected in AD. A study was conducted that hypothesized that PET imaging with C-PIB would correctly identify control subjects, AD patients, and FTD patients (Rabinovici et al., 2007). All of the AD patients had positive C-PIB scans; however, 4 out of 12 FTD patients and 1 out of 8 control subjects also had positive scans. The authors noted that pathological correlation will be necessary to better explain whether the PIB-positive FTD patients were simply false positives, had comorbid AD/FTLD pathology, or were AD patients with comorbid FTD clinical behaviors (Rabinovici et al., 2007).

NEUROPATHOLOGY

Most FTD cases are sporadic, although there is some evidence that as many as 50% of patients have a family history of neurodegenerative disease (Binetti et al., 2003; Bird et al., 2003; Chow, Miller, Hayashi, & Geschwind, 1999). The behavioral variant group of FTD has been shown to be more associated with having a family history, with SD having the smallest proportion (Rohrer et al., 2009). Approximately 10% of cases have an autosomal dominant inheritance (Goldman et al., 2005; Rohrer et al., 2009). The different variants of FTD are at least partially determined by how pathology is disseminated in the brain. A number of genes on chromosomes 3, 9, and 17 have been identified as being contributory to FTD (Sikkink, Rollinson, & Pickering-Brown, 2007). The two genes that are most contributory to FTD are the *microtubule-associated protein tau* (*MAPT*) and the *progranulin* (*PGRN*) genes, both of which occur on chromosome 17q21. The *MAPT* gene codes for the tau protein. Abnormal amounts of tau results in tau-positive inclusions and is implicated in various types of neuropathology such as AD and FTD. There are two phenotypes associated with MAPT. One is more related to dementia and results in changes in behavior such as apathy or disinhibition, obsessive compulsiveness, or memory difficulties (vanSwieten & Spillantini, 2007). The other is more Parkinson-like and results in changes such as gait impairment, rigidity, postural instability, vertical gate palsy, and axial rigidity (vanSwieten & Spillantini, 2007). The PGRN gene codes the protein progranulin, which helps stimulate cell growth and wound healing (Mackenzie et al., 2006a). Alterations to PGRN may result in tau-negative and ubiquitive TAR-DNA-binding protein-43 (TDP-43)-positive inclusions (Mackenzie et al., 2006a). SD has been associated with ubiquitin-positive, TDP-43-positive, tau-negative inclusions (Davies et al., 2005; Mackenzie et al., 2006b); however, although rarer, there have been reported cases of SD related to tau-positive or AD pathologies (Davies et al., 2005; Rabinovici & Miller, 2010). The greatest amount of damage in SD is done to the anteroinferomedial temporal lobe (Davies et al., 2005). A study by Rossor, Revesz, Lantos, and Warrington (2000) found neurites in the frontotemporal cortices and ubiquitin-positive intracytoplasmic inclusions in the granule cells of the dentate fascia in addition to the ubiquitin-positive, tau-negative inclusions.

Interestingly, these inclusions are similar to those often associated with amyotrophic lateral sclerosis, but in these cases, none was found in the spinal cord motor neurons or brain stem.

NEUROLOGICAL FINDINGS

With the exception of language, much of the neurological examination should be normal. This includes a normal examination of the cranial nerves, strength, reflexes, gait, and cerebellar testing. However, all of the subtypes of FTD can co-occur with motor neuron disease, although this happens most frequently with the behavior variant and least commonly with SD (Seelaar, Rohrer, Pijnenburg, Fox, & van Swieten, 2011). Mild parkinsonism including gait disturbance, bradykinesia, and rigidity is more commonly seen in PNFA and progressive logopenic aphasia than in SD. This may be due to the relative absence of tau pathology in SD (Kremen, Mendez, Tsai, & Teng, 2011).

PHARMACOLOGICAL TREATMENT

There are no Food and Drug Administration (FDA)-approved medications for any of the subtypes of frontotemporal lobar degeneration. Because of this, the medications that are used were developed for other conditions (Rabinovici & Miller, 2010); medications that treat AD and psychiatric conditions are often being used (Vossel & Miller, 2008). However, early in the SD process, individuals may have normal recent memory although they may have a loss for memory of autobiographical events, suggesting that there is a different progression of neuronal functional loss than in AD; cholinergic deficits have not been found in FTD patients. Because of this, it is thought that acetylcholinesterase inhibitors are not likely to be helpful in SD (Boxer & Boeve, 2007) and they may actually increase irritability. There can be an overlap of symptoms between frontal variant FTD and SD in that both can exhibit disinhibited and compulsive behaviors. These are often treated with selective serotonin reuptake inhibitors (SSRIs) to help with compulsive behaviors; those with more right temporal lobe involvement may benefit from the addition of an atypical antipsychotic (Boxer & Boeve, 2007). Of course, the possibility of medication-induced parkinsonism should be monitored. It is more common to have sleep difficulties with SD than the other FTD subtypes (Cairns et al., 2007). Once nonmedical educational interventions such as teaching about sleep hygiene are attempted, trazodone may be a good choice for treating both the insomnia and possible behavior symptoms (Vossel & Miller, 2008).

NON-PHARMACOLOGICAL TREATMENT

Perhaps the most important thing for patients and families to do is to become educated about what they will face in dealing with a degenerative disease such as SD. Asking questions to the doctor or other health care professional can be very helpful. Getting a referral to a speech therapist can also be helpful to learn specific techniques for enhancing communication with the patient with SD. Caregivers should seek out support groups either in person or online. Doing so can provide emotional support, ideas for coping with a progressive disease, and a source for new friendships with others who understand and are coping with similar situations. Family members may also learn about behavior changes that sometimes accompany SD, such as lack of empathy or change in personality that can be very difficult for the patient's family to deal with. It is also important for caregivers to learn about mechanisms for coping with diseases that entail loss of cognitive functioning such as maintaining a structured schedule for the patient, learning new methods of communication with a loved one who is losing the meaning of things around him- or herself, and the importance of making sure that they are taking care of themselves as well as the patient throughout the disease process. In talking to family members, it is also important to emphasize that SD is the least heritable form of frontotemporal lobar degeneration; so they can be assured that their risk for getting the disease is low. Potential sources for support are the Association for Frontotemporal Dementia and the Frontotemporal Dementia Caregiver Support Center.

Another potential avenue for treatment is the utilization of errorless learning to help relearn object naming, definition, and use in SD (Robinson et al., 2009). Errorless learning is a method that attempts to prevent errors from occurring during the learning phase in order to prevent the strengthening of synaptic connections for wrong information that occurs with trial-and-error learning; this method always provides the correct information during the learning phase.

FUTURE DIRECTIONS

While much progress in the research of the variants of FTD has been made in the past 20 years, more needs to be done. This should include more research to improve clinical diagnosis, especially in the realms of clinical-pathology studies and MRI-clinical studies. Improving current cognitive tests for these disorders and agreeing on a cognitive and behavioral test battery would also be helpful. Work should also continue toward developing an imaging ligand that marks tau/TDP-43, similar to the way PIB labels amyloid in patients with AD.

More research is also needed in the realm of the molecular components of SD as well as improved treatment options. Obviously, more must also be learned about tau, TDP-43, and the progranulin gene (PRGN). One obvious benefit from this would be that treatments could become more targeted. This should include work toward an agent that will be successful in treating tauopathies. It would also be helpful to have an organized manual-based set of behavioral treatment interventions for families to utilize for dealing with the problematic behaviors associated with the variants of FTD.

FTD is the third leading cause of dementia. AD is the leading cause of dementia and receives more attention, funding, and services. However, FTD is no less debilitating. Increased public awareness about this devastating illness would help increase attention, research, and funding for this disease.

REFERENCES

Agosta, F., Henry, R. G., Migliaccio, R., Neuhaus, J., Miller, B. L., Dronkers, N. F.,...Gorno-Tempini, M. L. (2010). Language networks in semantic dementia. *Brain: A Journal of Neurology, 133*(Pt 1), 286–299.

Allison, S. C., Schauer, G. F., Diehl, J., Miller, B. L., & Rosen, H. J. (2006). Awareness of deficits in two variants of frontotemporal lobar degeneration. *Neurology, 66*(5), A55.

Barker, W. W., Luis, C. A., Kashuba, A., Luis, M., Harwood, D. G., Loewenstein, D.,...Duara, R. (2002). Relative frequencies of Alzheimer disease, Lewy body, vascular and frontotemporal dementia, and hippocampal sclerosis in the State of Florida Brain Bank. *Alzheimer Disease and Associated Disorders, 16*(4), 203–212.

Binetti, G., Locascio, J. J., Corkin, S., Vonsattel, J. P., & Growdon, J. H. (2000). Differences between Pick disease and Alzheimer disease in clinical appearance and rate of cognitive decline. *Archives of Neurology, 57*(2), 225–232.

Binetti, G., Nicosia, F., Benussi, L., Ghidoni, R., Feudatari, E., Barbiero, L.,...Alberici, A. (2003). Prevalence of TAU mutations in an Italian clinical series of familial frontotemporal patients. *Neuroscience Letters, 338*(1), 85–87.

Bird, T., Knopman, D., VanSwieten, J., Rosso, S., Feldman, H., Tanabe, H.,...Hutton, M. (2003). Epidemiology and genetics of frontotemporal dementia/Pick's disease. *Annals of Neurology, 54*(Suppl 5), S29–S31.

Bonner, M. F., Ash, S., & Grossman, M. (2010). The new classification of primary progressive aphasia into semantic, logopenic, or nonfluent/agrammatic variants. *Current Neurology and Neuroscience Reports, 10*(6), 484–490.

Boxer, A. L., & Boeve, B. F. (2007). Frontotemporal dementia treatment: Current symptomatic therapies and implications of recent genetic, biochemical, and neuroimaging studies. *Alzheimer Disease and Associated Disorders, 21*(4), S79–S87.

Boxer, A. L., & Miller, B. L. (2005). Clinical features of frontotemporal dementia. *Alzheimer Disease and Associated Disorders, 19*(Suppl 1), S3–S6.

Bozeat, S., Gregory, C. A., Ralph, M. A., & Hodges, J. R. (2000). Which neuropsychiatric and behavioural features distinguish frontal and temporal variants of frontotemporal dementia from Alzheimer's disease? *Journal of Neurology, Neurosurgery, and Psychiatry, 69*(2), 178–186.

Bright, P., Moss, H. E., Stamatakis, E. A., & Tyler, L. K. (2008). Longitudinal studies of semantic dementia: The relationship between structural and functional changes over time. *Neuropsychologia, 46*(8), 2177–2188.

Cairns, N. J., Bigio, E. H., Mackenzie, I. R., Neumann, M., Lee, V. M., Hatanpaa, K. J.,...Mann, D. M.; Consortium for Frontotemporal Lobar Degeneration. (2007). Neuropathologic diagnostic and nosologic criteria for frontotemporal lobar degeneration: Consensus of the Consortium for Frontotemporal Lobar Degeneration. *Acta Neuropathologica, 114*(1), 5–22.

Chow, T. W., Hodges, J. R., Dawson, K. E., Miller, B. L., Smith, V., Mendez, M. F., & Lipton, A. M.; National Alzheimer's Coordinating Center. (2005). Referral patterns for syndromes associated with frontotemporal lobar degeneration. *Alzheimer Disease and Associated Disorders, 19*(1), 17–19.

Chow, T. W., Miller, B. L., Hayashi, V. N., & Geschwind, D. H. (1999). Inheritance of frontotemporal dementia. *Archives of Neurology, 56*(7), 817–822.

Davies, R. R., Halliday, G. M., Xuereb, J. H., Kril, J. J., & Hodges, J. R. (2009). The neural basis of semantic memory: Evidence from semantic dementia. *Neurobiology of Aging, 30*(12), 2043–2052.

Davies, R. R., Hodges, J. R., Kril, J. J., Patterson, K., Halliday, G. M., & Xuereb, J. H. (2005). The pathological basis of semantic dementia. *Brain: A Journal of Neurology, 128*(Pt 9), 1984–1995.

Démonet, J. F., Chollet, F., Ramsay, S., Cardebat, D., Nespoulous, J. L., Wise, R.,...Frackowiak, R. (1992). The anatomy of phonological and semantic processing in normal subjects. *Brain: A Journal of Neurology, 115*(Pt 6), 1753–1768.

Deramecourt, V., Lebert, F., Debachy, B., Mackowiak-Cordoliani, M. A., Bombois, S., Kerdraon, O.,...Pasquier, F. (2010). Prediction of pathology in primary progressive language and speech disorders. *Neurology, 74*(1), 42–49.

Diehl, J., Monsch, A. U., Aebi, C., Wagenpfeil, S., Krapp, S., Grimmer, T.,...Kurz, A. (2005). Frontotemporal dementia, semantic dementia, and Alzheimer's disease: The contribution of standard neuropsychological tests to differential diagnosis. *Journal of Geriatric Psychiatry and Neurology, 18*(1), 39–44.

Faber, R. (1999). Frontotemporal lobar degeneration: A consensus on clinical diagnostic criteria. *Neurology, 53*(5), 1159.

Forman, M. S., Farmer, J., Johnson, J., Clark, C., Arnold, S., Coslett, H.,...Grossman, M. (2007). Frontotemporal dementia: Clinicopathological correlations. *Neurology, 68*(12), A351.

Friederici, A. D., Opitz, B., & von Cramon, D. Y. (2000). Segregating semantic and syntactic aspects of processing in the human brain: An fMRI investigation of different word types. *Cerebral Cortex, 10*(7), 698–705.

Galton, C. J., Patterson, K., Graham, K., Lambon-Ralph, M. A., Williams, G., Antoun, N.,... Hodges, J. R. (2001). Differing patterns of temporal atrophy in Alzheimer's disease and semantic dementia. *Neurology, 57*(2), 216–225.

Goldman, J. S., Farmer, J. M., Wood, E. M., Johnson, J. K., Boxer, A., Neuhaus, J.,...Miller, B. L. (2005). Comparison of family histories in FTLD subtypes and related tauopathies. *Neurology, 65*(11), 1817–1819.

Gorno-Tempini, M. L., Dronkers, N. F., Rankin, K. P., Ogar, J. M., Phengrasamy, L., Rosen, H. J.,…Miller, B. L. (2004). Cognition and anatomy in three variants of primary progressive aphasia. *Annals of Neurology, 55*(3), 335–346.

Gorno-Tempini, M. L., Hillis, A. E., Weintraub, S., Kertesz, A., Mendez, M., Cappa, S. F.,… Grossman, M. (2011). Classification of primary progressive aphasia and its variants. *Neurology, 76*(11), 1006–1014.

Grace, J., & Malloy, P. (2001). *Frontal Systems Behavior Scale (FrSBe): Professional manual.* Lutz, FL: Psychological Assessment Resources.

Hailstone, J. C., Omar, R., & Warren, J. D. (2009). Relatively preserved knowledge of music in semantic dementia. *Journal of Neurology, Neurosurgery, and Psychiatry, 80*(7), 808–809.

Hillis, A. E., Oh, S., & Ken, L. (2004). Deterioration of naming nouns versus verbs in primary progressive aphasia. *Annals of Neurology, 55*(2), 268–275.

Hodges, J. R., & Miller, B. (2001). The neuropsychology of frontal variant frontotemporal dementia and semantic dementia. Introduction to the special topic papers: Part II. *Neurocase, 7*(2), 113–121.

Hodges, J. R., & Patterson, K. (2007). Semantic dementia: A unique clinicopathological syndrome. *Lancet Neurology, 6*(11), 1004–1014.

Hodges, J. R., Davies, R., Xuereb, J., Kril, J., & Halliday, G. (2003). Survival in frontotemporal dementia. *Neurology, 61*(3), 349–354.

Hodges, J. R., Graham, N., & Patterson, K. (1995). Charting the progression in semantic dementia: Implications for the organisation of semantic memory. *Memory, 3*(3–4), 463–495.

Hodges, J. R., Mitchell, J., Dawson, K., Spillantini, M. G., Xuereb, J. H., McMonagle, P.,… Patterson, K. (2010). Semantic dementia: Demography, familial factors and survival in a consecutive series of 100 cases. *Brain: A Journal of Neurology, 133*(Pt 1), 300–306.

Hodges, J. R., Patterson, K., Oxbury, S., & Funnell, E. (1992). Semantic dementia. Progressive fluent aphasia with temporal lobe atrophy. *Brain: A Journal of Neurology, 115*(Pt 6), 1783–1806.

Howard, D. P. K. (1992). *The pyramids and palm trees test.* San Antonio, TX: Pearson Assessments.

Ikeda, M., Ishikawa, T., & Tanabe, H. (2004). Epidemiology of frontotemporal lobar degeneration. *Dementia and Geriatric Cognitive Disorders, 17*(4), 265–268.

Jefferies, E., Patterson, K., Jones, R. W., & Lambon Ralph, M. A. (2009). Comprehension of concrete and abstract words in semantic dementia. *Neuropsychology, 23*(4), 492–499.

Johnson, J. K., Diehl, J., Mendez, M. F., Neuhaus, J., Shapira, J. S., Forman, M.,…Miller, B. L. (2005). Frontotemporal lobar degeneration: Demographic characteristics of 353 patients. *Archives of Neurology, 62*(6), 925–930.

Julien, C. L., Thompson, J. C., Neary, D., & Snowden, J. S. (2008). Arithmetic knowledge in semantic dementia: Is it invariably preserved? *Neuropsychologia, 46*(11), 2732–2744.

Kertesz, A. (2008). Frontotemporal dementia: A topical review. *Cognitive and Behavioral Neurology, 21*(3), 127–133.

Kertesz, A., Blair, M., McMonagle, P., & Munoz, D. G. (2007). The diagnosis and course of frontotemporal dementia. *Alzheimer Disease and Associated Disorders, 21*(2), 155–163.

Kertesz, A., Davidson, W., McCabe, P., & Munoz, D. (2003). Behavioral quantitation is more sensitive than cognitive testing in frontotemporal dementia. *Alzheimer Disease and Associated Disorders, 17*(4), 223–229.

Kertesz, A., Jesso, S., Harciarek, M., Blair, M., & McMonagle, P. (2010). What is semantic dementia?: A cohort study of diagnostic features and clinical boundaries. *Archives of Neurology, 67*(4), 483–489.

Kremen, S. A., Mendez, M. F., Tsai, P. H., & Teng, E. (2011). Extrapyramidal signs in the primary progressive aphasias. *American Journal of Alzheimer's Disease and Other Dementias, 26*(1), 72–77.

Lambon Ralph, M. A., Graham, K. S., Ellis, A. W., & Hodges, J. R. (1998). Naming in semantic dementia—what matters? *Neuropsychologia, 36*(8), 775–784.

Lauro-Grotto, R., Piccini, C., & Shallice, T. (1997). Modality-specific operations in semantic dementia. *Cortex, 33*(4), 593–622.

Lehmann, M., Douiri, A., Kim, L. G., Modat, M., Chan, D., Ourselin, S.,...Fox, N. C. (2010). Atrophy patterns in Alzheimer's disease and semantic dementia: A comparison of FreeSurfer and manual volumetric measurements. *NeuroImage, 49*(3), 2264–2274.

Mackenzie, I. R., Baborie, A., Pickering-Brown, S., Du Plessis, D., Jaros, E., Perry, R. H.,...Mann, D. M. (2006a). Heterogeneity of ubiquitin pathology in frontotemporal lobar degeneration: Classification and relation to clinical phenotype. *Acta Neuropathologica, 112*(5), 539–549.

Mackenzie, I. R., Baker, M., Pickering-Brown, S., Hsiung, G. Y., Lindholm, C., Dwosh, E.,... Feldman, H. H. (2006b). The neuropathology of frontotemporal lobar degeneration caused by mutations in the progranulin gene. *Brain: A Journal of Neurology, 129*(Pt 11), 3081–3090.

Malloy, P., & Grace, J. (2005). A review of rating scales for measuring behavior change due to frontal systems damage. *Cognitive and Behavioral Neurology, 18*(1), 18–27.

Malloy, P., Tremont, G., Grace, J., & Frakey, L. (2007). The Frontal Systems Behavior Scale discriminates frontotemporal dementia from Alzheimer's disease. *Alzheimer's & Dementia, 3*(3), 200–203.

Mesulam, M., Rogalski, E., Wieneke, C., Cobia, D., Rademaker, A., Thompson, C., & Weintraub, S. (2009a). Neurology of anomia in the semantic variant of primary progressive aphasia. *Brain: A Journal of Neurology, 132*(Pt 9), 2553–2565.

Mesulam, M., Wieneke, C., Rogalski, E., Cobia, D., Thompson, C., & Weintraub, S. (2009b). Quantitative template for subtyping primary progressive aphasia. *Archives of Neurology, 66*(12), 1545–1551.

Mummery, C. J., Patterson, K., Hodges, J. R., & Wise, R. J. (1996). Generating "tiger" as an animal name or a word beginning with T: Differences in brain activation. *Proceedings. Biological Sciences/The Royal Society, 263*(1373), 989–995.

Mummery, C. J., Patterson, K., Wise, R. J., Vandenberghe, R., Vandenbergh, R., Price, C. J., & Hodges, J. R. (1999). Disrupted temporal lobe connections in semantic dementia. *Brain: A Journal of Neurology, 122*(Pt 1), 61–73.

Neary, D., Snowden, J. S., Gustafson, L., Passant, U., Stuss, D., Black, S.,...Benson, D. F. (1998). Frontotemporal lobar degeneration: A consensus on clinical diagnostic criteria. *Neurology, 51*(6), 1546–1554.

Onari, K., & Spatz, H. (1926). Anatomische Beitrage zur Lehre von Pickscnen umschriebenen Grosshirninden-Atrophie ("Picksche Krankheit'). *Zeitschrift fur die Gesamte Neurology und Psychiatrie, 101*, 470–511.

Peelle, J. E., Troiani, V., Gee, J., Moore, P., McMillan, C., Vesely, L., & Grossman, M. (2008). Sentence comprehension and voxel-based morphometry in progressive nonfluent aphasia, semantic dementia, and nonaphasic frontotemporal dementia. *Journal of Neurolinguistics, 21*(5), 418–432.

Pick, A. (1892). Über die Beziehungen der senilen Hirnatrophie zur Aphasie. *Pragur Medicinsche Wochenschrift, 17*, 165–167.

Plassman, B. L., Langa, K. M., Fisher, G. G., Heeringa, S. G., Weir, D. R., Ofstedal, M....Wallace, R. B. (2007). Prevalence of dementia in the United States: The aging, demographics, and memory study. *Neuroepidemiology, 29*(1–2), 125–132.

Rabinovici, G. D., & Miller, B. L. (2010). Frontotemporal lobar degeneration: Epidemiology, pathophysiology, diagnosis and management. *CNS Drugs, 24*(5), 375–398.

Rabinovici, G. D., Furst, A. J., O'Neil, J. P., Racine, C. A., Mormino, E. C., Baker, S. L.,…Jagust, W. J. (2007). 11C-PIB PET imaging in Alzheimer disease and frontotemporal lobar degeneration. *Neurology, 68*(15), 1205–1212.

Rascovsky, K., Growdon, M. E., Pardo, I. R., Grossman, S., & Miller, B. L. (2009). "The quicksand of forgetfulness": Semantic dementia in one hundred years of solitude. *Brain: A Journal of Neurology, 132*(Pt 9), 2609–2616.

Ratnavalli, E., Brayne, C., Dawson, K., & Hodges, J. R. (2002). The prevalence of frontotemporal dementia. *Neurology, 58*(11), 1615–1621.

Roberson, E. D., Hesse, J. H., Rose, K. D., Slama, H., Johnson, J. K., Yaffe, K.,…Miller, B. L. (2005). Frontotemporal dementia progresses to death faster than Alzheimer disease. *Neurology, 65*(5), 719–725.

Robinson, S., Druks, J., Hodges, J., & Garrard, P. (2009). The treatment of object naming, definition, and object use in semantic dementia: The effectiveness of errorless learning. *Aphasiology, 23*(6), 749–775.

Rohrer, J. D., Guerreiro, R., Vandrovcova, J., Uphill, J., Reiman, D., Beck, J.,…Rossor, M. N. (2009). The heritability and genetics of frontotemporal lobar degeneration. *Neurology, 73*(18), 1451–1456.

Rosen, H. J., Gorno-Tempini, M. L., Goldman, W. P., Perry, R. J., Schuff, N., Weiner, M.,…Miller, B. L. (2002). Patterns of brain atrophy in frontotemporal dementia and semantic dementia. *Neurology, 58*(2), 198–208.

Rosso, S. M., Donker Kaat, L., Baks, T., Joosse, M., de Koning, I., Pijnenburg, Y.,…van Swieten, J. C. (2003). Frontotemporal dementia in The Netherlands: Patient characteristics and prevalence estimates from a population-based study. *Brain: A Journal of Neurology, 126*(Pt 9), 2016–2022.

Rossor, M. N., Revesz, T., Lantos, P. L., & Warrington, E. K. (2000). Semantic dementia with ubiquitin-positive tau-negative inclusion bodies. *Brain: A Journal of Neurology, 123*(Pt 2), 267–276.

Roth, R., Isquith, P., & Gioia, G. (2005). *BRIEF-A: Behavior Rating Inventory of Executive Function-Adult Version*. Lutz, FL: Psychological Assessment Resources, Inc.

Sapolsky, D., Bakkour, A., Negreira, A., Nalipinski, P., Weintraub, S., Mesulam, M. M.,…Dickerson, B. C. (2010). Cortical neuroanatomic correlates of symptom severity in primary progressive aphasia. *Neurology, 75*(4), 358–366.

Seelaar, H., Rohrer, J. D., Pijnenburg, Y. A., Fox, N. C., & van Swieten, J. C. (2011). Clinical, genetic and pathological heterogeneity of frontotemporal dementia: A review. *Journal of Neurology, Neurosurgery, and Psychiatry, 82*(5), 476–486.

Seeley, W. W., Bauer, A. M., Miller, B. L., Gorno-Tempini, M. L., Kramer, J. H., Weiner, M., & Rosen, H. J. (2005). The natural history of temporal variant frontotemporal dementia. *Neurology, 64*(8), 1384–1390.

Severson, M. A., Smith, G. E., Tangalos, E. G., Petersen, R. C., Kokmen, E., Ivnik, R. J.,…Kurland, L. T. (1994). Patterns and predictors of institutionalization in community-based dementia patients. *Journal of the American Geriatrics Society, 42*(2), 181–185.

Sikkink, S., Rollinson, S., & Pickering-Brown, S. M. (2007). The genetics of frontotemporal lobar degeneration. *Current Opinion in Neurology, 20*(6), 693–698.

Sloane, P. D., Zimmerman, S., Suchindran, C., Reed, P., Wang, L., Boustani, M., & Sudha, S. (2002). The public health impact of Alzheimer's disease, 2000–2050: Potential implication of treatment advances. *Annual Review of Public Health, 23*, 213–231.

Snowden, J. S., Bathgate, D., Varma, A., Blackshaw, A., Gibbons, Z. C., & Neary, D. (2001). Distinct behavioural profiles in frontotemporal dementia and semantic dementia. *Journal of Neurology, Neurosurgery, and Psychiatry, 70*(3), 323–332.

vanSwieten, J., & Spillantini, M. G. (2007). Hereditary frontotemporal dementia caused by Tau gene mutations. *Brain Pathology, 17*(1), 63–73.

Vossel, K. A., & Miller, B. L. (2008). New approaches to the treatment of frontotemporal lobar degeneration. *Current Opinion in Neurology, 21*(6), 708–716.

Warrington, E. K. (1975). The selective impairment of semantic memory. *The Quarterly Journal of Experimental Psychology, 27*(4), 635–657.

Weder, N. D., Aziz, R., Wilkins, K., & Tampi, R. R. (2007). Frontotemporal dementias: A review. *Annals of General Psychiatry, 6,* 15.

Wise, R., Chollet, F., Hadar, U., Friston, K., Hoffner, E., & Frackowiak, R. (1991). Distribution of cortical neural networks involved in word comprehension and word retrieval. *Brain: A Journal of Neurology, 114*(Pt 4), 1803–1817.

Woollams, A. M., Cooper-Pye, E., Hodges, J. R., & Patterson, K. (2008). Anomia: A doubly typical signature of semantic dementia. *Neuropsychologia, 46*(10), 2503–2514.

CHAPTER 11

Primary Progressive Aphasia

Rhonda Friedman, Sally Long, and R. Scott Turner

Primary progressive aphasia (PPA) is the term applied to a clinical syndrome characterized by insidious progressive language impairment that is initially unaccompanied by other cognitive deficits (Mesulam, 1982, 2001). This presentation contrasts with that of probable Alzheimer's disease (AD), whose primary identifying symptom during the early stages is significant memory impairment. There is general agreement that the diagnosis of PPA requires a progressive language impairment of *at least 2 years'* duration (Gorno-Tempini et al., 2011; Mesulam, 2001, 2003). It must be the *primary* presenting symptom, and the main cause of any dysfunction in the patient's activities of daily living (ADL). Clear and pronounced verbal and visual memory impairment and visuospatial deficits are relatively absent. Behavioral symptoms may be present, but to a lesser degree and are not the primary concern of the patient. There are several variants of PPA, to be described in the following pages, and more than one etiology. As with aphasia consequent to stroke, nearly all individuals with PPA have some degree of anomia (word-finding problem; Mesulam, 2001).

It is important to understand that PPA is a clinical description and not a neuropathological disease. As we will see in this chapter, most (but not all) individuals with PPA have a form of frontotemporal lobar dementia (FTLD); some have the pathology of AD.

HISTORY

Current classification of the PPAs is best understood within the context of its history. In the late 19th century, two papers appeared, one in German (Pick, 1892) and one in French (Serieux, 1893), describing cases of progressive language impairment with atrophy of the frontal and temporal lobes of the left hemisphere. But the focus on progressive impairment limited to language function did not reemerge until 90 years later, with the publication of Marsel Mesulam's landmark article in which he described six patients with "the insidious onset of an aphasia and its gradual progression for many years in the absence of other behavioral abnormalities" (Mesulam, 1982). Mesulam drew attention to the differences between these six individuals with isolated language impairments and "those who develop a progressive aphasia in conjunction with Alzheimer's or Pick's disease." Patients with AD or Pick's, he asserted, show concomitant signs of dementia in intellect, behavior, and personality that are parallel to the intensity of their language deficits; and they tend to be apathetic with regard to their disabilities (see Chapters 4 and 9, in this volume, for current review). In contrast, Mesulam's six patients showed no other cognitive impairments, and were quite distressed about their language difficulties. There was a suggestion, then, that the six patients may have "a special type of progressive degeneration of unknown cause(s)." In an editorial in 1987, Mesulam coined the term *primary progressive aphasia*, the term that is in use today (Mesulam, 1987). The criterion of a 2-year progression in which language impairment is the major source of interference with ADL was added a few years later (Mesulam & Weintraub, 1992; Weintraub & Mesulam, 1993). The 2-year requirement has recently been called into question (Mesulam, Wieneke, Thompson, Rogalski, & Weintraub, 2012), but remains widely followed at this time.

Mesulam's (1982) article focused on distinguishing these progressive aphasias from language impairments typically seen with AD or Pick's disease. Distinctions between nonfluent (reduced output; halting, effortful, often agrammatic speech) and fluent (well-articulated speech, normal grammar and phrase length) profiles were not drawn, although it appears that both types of profiles were present in the original six patients. A later article, describing the longitudinal course of PPA (Weintraub, Rubin, & Mesulam, 1990), focused on nonfluent PPA patients.

At the same time, researchers in England were characterizing another type of PPA, which they termed *semantic dementia* (Hodges, Patterson, Oxbury, & Funnell, 1992; Snowden, Goulding, & Neary, 1989). The phenomenon was actually described by Elizabeth Warrington in 1975, but not termed *semantic dementia*. Warrington's study was focused on investigating the underlying impairment causing agnosia in three patients with deteriorating memory. She found that all three had intact "expressive speech" and impaired comprehension of single words, and that some semantic attributes and associations were impoverished. Warrington concluded that the agnosia seen in these individuals reflected a "specific impairment of semantic memory." Snowden et al. (1989) coined the term *semantic dementia* and contrasted this syndrome with *dementia of frontal lobe type* (DFT) and with slowly progressive aphasia. The focus of that study was on the underlying pathology. Hodges et al. (1992) elaborated the characterization of semantic dementia in a detailed study of five patients presenting with this profile. Contemporary with these studies, Luzzatti and Poeck (1991) called attention to a very early description of this syndrome, published by Rosenfeld in 1909. At that time, it was labeled *verbal amnesia*. Autopsy results presented in that study conformed to current profiles of semantic dementia, that is, left temporal lobe atrophy.

The similarities between semantic dementia and other described forms of progressive aphasia were noted, and semantic dementia was soon considered a subtype of PPA. Patients with semantic dementia were included in Westbury and Bub's 1997 review of PPA; and Grossman and Ash (2004) considered semantic dementia to be one of the two subtypes of PPA. The inclusion of semantic dementia within the umbrella of PPA is not without controversy. Mesulam et al. (2003, 2009) divide semantic dementia into two types: Semantic dementia without agnosia is said to be a form of PPA, as it meets the criteria of presenting with a primary deficit in language; in contrast, semantic dementia with agnosia does not meet the criteria of PPA, they claim, as there is a secondary deficit, in object recognition. On the other hand, Adlam et al. (2006) argue that individuals who meet the criteria for fluent PPA can be shown to have nonverbal as well as verbal conceptual deficits, as long as familiarity and typicality are modulated appropriately. Semantic dementia and fluent PPA, then, are one and the same; more obvious signs of agnosia appear as the disorder progresses. The issue of the relationship of semantic dementia to PPA has yet to be completely resolved.

Logopenic PPA was not named and designated as a variant of PPA until 2004 (Gorno-Tempini et al., 2004; although the term *logopenia* was introduced by Mesulam in 1982). However, two decades earlier Pogacar and Williams (1984) described an individual who may have had this form of the syndrome. The focus of that article was on a patient who presented initially with anomia without memory impairment, and was shown upon autopsy to have AD. Because the authors were primarily concerned with the atypicality of this presentation of AD and not with the specifics of the language profile per se, it is difficult to know what type of PPA the patient had. There is no mention, for example, of word comprehension abilities. His speech was described as fluent, and there were paraphasic and grammatical errors made on "repetitive tests." If by "repetitive" the authors meant repetition tasks, then the profile fits that of logopenic PPA. The specific mention of a lack of any visual agnosia further suggests that this fluent aphasia was more like logopenic PPA than semantic dementia.

VARIANTS AND THEIR DIAGNOSES

In the past decade, the major PPA researchers, recognizing that different terms were being applied to similar or identical syndromes, got together to develop a common terminology for the PPAs in an attempt to improve reliability of research results across study centers. This group of 20 investigators met on three separate occasions between 2006 and 2009, and the results of their deliberations were published in the journal *Neurology* (Gorno-Tempini et al., 2011). Three main variants of PPA were identified, and criteria for their diagnoses were described. Each of the variants has *core* features that must be present and *other* features, a certain number of which must be present. Some of these "other" features are not, in fact, symptoms that are present, but rather reflect findings of spared abilities, that is, the *absence* of certain symptoms. Despite this recent development of consensus criteria for three different variants of PPA, it is important to note that some patients may present with mixed symptoms that overlap across the three subtypes, or only one symptom.

Semantic Variant of PPA; Also Called Semantic Dementia or PPA-S

Following an initial diagnosis of PPA (see previous definition), the subtype is labeled semantic variant of PPA (svPPA) if both impaired naming-to-confrontation and impaired single-word comprehension are demonstrated. There are four additional features associated with svPPA, and at least three of these must be present: impaired object knowledge, intact repetition, intact motor speech and grammar, and surface alexia or agraphia (reading or writing impairment characterized by difficulty with words that have irregular spellings, e.g., *yacht* or *come*).

Nonfluent/Agrammatic Variant of PPA; Also Called PNFA or PPA-G

To make the clinical diagnosis of nonfluent/agrammatic variant of PPA (nfvPPA) at least one of the two core features must be present: (a) agrammatic speech and (b) halting effortful speech with inconsistent speech sound errors. Two of the following features must also be present: impaired comprehension of syntactically complex sentences, intact object knowledge, and intact single-word comprehension.

Logopenic Variant of PPA; Also Called PPA-L

The two core features of logopenic variant of PPA (lvPPA), both of which must be present for the diagnosis, are impaired repetition at the sentence and phrase level and impaired word retrieval in both spontaneous speech and naming. Associated features, at least two of which must be present, are the following: phonologic errors in speech, intact single-word comprehension and object knowledge, intact motor speech, and grammatic speech.

Problems With Diagnosis of Subtypes

Diagnosis of the subtypes of PPA is not always simple or clear-cut. Given the heterogeneity in the PPA syndrome, even clinicians and researchers who have considerable experience with PPA may disagree on diagnosis. The reasons for this are several. One reason is variability in tests and normative datasets used across clinics to assess language. Additionally, some of the symptoms that characterize the primary variants of PPA overlap, which can make it difficult to distinguish one subtype from another. This is particularly true for nfvPPA and lvPPA. Finally, as the underlying disease progresses, a greater number of cognitive impairments become manifest. The addition of problems in attention or short-term memory, for example, can interfere with the accurate assessment of deficits that are specifically linguistic. Thus, the length of time from initial onset of symptoms to when the individual's language is assessed might affect the diagnosis given.

LANGUAGE PROFILE AND ASSESSMENT

Nonfluent/Agrammatic Variant

nfvPPA is primarily characterized by a core deficit in syntactic processing, or the ability to comprehend and construct sentences (Gorno-Tempini et al., 2011). The poor syntactic processing may result in agrammatic speech, recognizable by the use of short, simple phrases that lack grammatical morphemes such as *the*, *of*, or *–ed*, sometimes termed "telegraphic speech."

For these individuals, normally fluent speech becomes quite effortful, halting, and full of errors, and includes distortions such as word deletions, substitutions, insertions, and transposition of speech sounds. During assessment of these individuals, differentiating deficits in syntactic processing from problems with speech production, single-word comprehension, word finding, or working memory can be challenging (Weintraub et al., 2009).

Agrammatism in speech production is often evident early in the course of the syndrome. A variety of methods are used to evaluate sentence production in the assessment of aphasia (Weintraub et al., 2009). One commonly used task is sentence completion, in which the individual is provided with the beginning words of a sentence and is required to complete it, or, provided with a sentence containing some blanks that they must fill in with an appropriate choice of words. Perhaps more commonly, sentence production is evaluated indirectly by examining phrase length or fluency in a person's speech sample while describing a picture scene orally, such as those found in the *Boston Diagnostic Aphasia Examination*, third edition (BDAE-3; Goodglass, Kaplan, & Barresi, 2001) or *Western Aphasia Battery, Revised* (WAB-R; Kertesz, 2006). However, while shorter phrases or reduced fluency can be indicative of agrammatism, they can also be caused by other problems such as dysarthria, or may simply be due to reduced effort. Providing more visual stimuli in an effort to direct the patient's discourse can help increase speech output, as in the Aesop's

Fables subtest of the BDAE-3 (Goodglass et al., 2001), where the person is required to tell a story that corresponds to a set of ordered pictures. Spontaneous speech elicited through conversation with the individual provides another opportunity to evaluate speech output patterns, although procedures for the analysis of syntax in speech samples can be cumbersome and time consuming (Weintraub et al., 2009). Finally, some tests (e.g., Northwestern Anagram Test; Weintraub et al., 2009) assess syntax by requiring patients to arrange word cards in the appropriate order to create meaningful sentences.

Sentence comprehension is complex and requires several different cognitive processes, including grammatical knowledge, working memory, inhibitory control, and processing speed (Grossman, Rhee, & Moore, 2005). Deficits in any of these components can interfere with the ability to comprehend sentences correctly. In individuals with nfvPPA, deficient syntax comprehension is typically evident through impaired sentence comprehension of more grammatically complex sentences, while comprehension of simple sentences and single words remains intact early in the disease course (Gorno-Tempini et al., 2011). One commonly used clinical assessment tool for evaluating sentence processing is a sentence–picture matching task, in which the patient is presented with an aural sentence and is then required to point to the corresponding picture in a visual array (Weintraub et al., 2009). Well-known traditionally used assessment tools of aphasia, such as the BDAE-3 (Goodglass et al., 2001), often include such tasks. An alternative method of assessing sentence comprehension is to present a sentence and ask a series of follow-up questions to assess the patient's understanding of the sentence content and structure (Grossman et al., 1996), provided the patient has sufficient speech production skills to permit adequate responses.

Additional language deficits observed in nfvPPA include disrupted prosody and slowed speech rate, which can be evident during free conversational speech (Gorno-Tempini et al., 2011). Apraxia of speech, an articulation planning deficit, is very common in this variant and can be the first symptom experienced by the patient. Motor speech can be observed during conversation and evaluated more objectively through repetition of syllables and words (Bonner, Ash, & Grossman, 2010). Repetition of single words is typically spared, but repetition of sentences or phrases can be compromised. Both object knowledge and single-word comprehension are generally intact in nfvPPA.

Semantic Variant of PPA

The core deficit in the svPPA is the loss of semantic memory knowledge, rather than degradation of specific language processes such as syntax or phonology, which remain preserved (Gorno-Tempini et al., 2011). The gradual loss of semantic information causes anomia, or severe naming deficits with little improvement when provided phonemic cues. Some researchers have found that patients with svPPA have more difficulty naming verbs than nouns (Bonner et al., 2009). Within the word class of verbs, svPPA patients tend to have the most difficulty naming concrete rather than abstract verbs, which is an unusual finding that researchers hypothesize may be due to an underlying deficit in visual feature integration of concrete objects (Bonner et al., 2009; Weinstein et al., 2011).

Reports of individuals suffering from the profound naming and comprehension deficits characteristic of this syndrome while maintaining preserved musical knowledge and number concepts also provide some support for the hypothesis that different types of information may be dissociated in semantic memory (Weinstein et al.,

2011). Therefore, extended testing of confrontation naming to include concrete and abstract verbs, collections of different semantic categories, different kinds of semantic information, and information presented in different sensory modalities may be useful in characterizing the extent of the naming deficit.

The loss of semantic knowledge characteristic of this PPA variant is also evident in impairment of single-word comprehension. Comprehension deficits are typically observed initially for words that are less commonly used in everyday language and then progress to include higher-frequency items, resulting in a severe loss of expressive and receptive vocabulary over the course of the disease (Mesulam et al., 2009). While objective evidence of comprehension problems can be established with word-to-picture matching tests, loss of word knowledge can be evident in free conversation as well. Kertesz, Jesso, Harciarek, Blair, and McMonagle (2010) noted in a research study of individuals with svPPA, nfvPPA, and AD that 34 of 37 individuals with svPPA asked for the meaning of commonly used words during conversation with the examiners, while none of the individuals in either of the other two patient groups required any clarification of word meaning. The authors suggested that querying of word meaning was so unique to the patients with svPPA that it might be considered a primary diagnostic feature of this group. An example of an objective test of object knowledge that does not require expressive language is the Pyramids and Palm Trees test (Howard & Patterson, 1992), in which pictures of objects must be matched with pictures of related objects.

Surface alexia and surface agraphia, or impairments in the ability to read and write irregular words, are also features of svPPA. These can be detected by asking the individual to read or write irregularly spelled words such as *doubt* that are matched in frequency and length with regularly spelled words. Such a list can be found as part of the Psycholinguistic Assessments of Language Processing in Aphasia (PALPA; Kay, Lesser, & Coltheart, 1992).

Repetition should be tested with short and long words, and with multisyllabic nonwords. Repetition is generally intact in patients with svPPA, in contrast to patients with lvPPA.

Speech output, assessed in conversation and in picture descriptions (such as the Cookie Theft picture of the BDAE; Goodglass et al., 2001) should be fluent and lacking in motor speech impairment. It is typically characterized by intact grammar, although some paragrammatism may be present along with circumlocutions and paraphasic errors. The paraphasic errors made by these patients tend to be semantic substitution errors, with few or no phonologic errors (Kertesz et al., 2010). However, Budd et al. (2010) compared the three subtypes of PPA on errors made during a confrontation naming task and found that the types of errors made did not differentiate the groups. The authors interpreted these findings to suggest that naming errors may result from different types of cognitive processes underlying the naming deficits associated with damage in different brain regions in the three subtypes.

Logopenic Variant PPA

The language profile of the lvPPA, in comparison to the semantic and agrammatic/nonfluent variants, was first characterized by Gorno-Tempini et al. in 2004. The most prominent symptom in the logopenic variant is a deficit in single-word retrieval evident in free speech and confrontation naming tasks, although the impairment is not as severe as that seen in svPPA. *Logopenic* is Greek for "lack of words" (Gorno-Tempini et al., 2004), and the term is applied to this variant of PPA due to the prominent word-finding pauses typical of speech in these patients. Phonological errors are often observed during conversation and naming tasks, although patients typically recognize most of the objects that they cannot name correctly and retain object knowledge in the early course of the syndrome.

In lvPPA, the rate of speech is slowed due to prominent word-finding problems. However, syntactic processing remains intact in these individuals; therefore, they do not exhibit the agrammatism that is evident in the nfvPPA (Gorno-Tempini et al., 2004). Due to the slow speech and word-finding hesitations, examiners may perceive these individuals to have nonfluent speech, although their speech is typically classified as fluent by common aphasia batteries that emphasize grammar and motor speech in assessment of fluency (Gorno-Tempini et al., 2008). Given that the historical use of the construct fluency emphasized articulation and syntax, Gorno-Tempini et al. (2008) suggest reserving the term *nonfluent* for the agrammatic variant of PPA, and engaging the term *logopenic* for the slowed speech with spared grammar and motor speech characteristic of the logopenic variant.

Impaired repetition of sentences and phrases is also characteristic of the logopenic variant, although single-word repetition remains intact. Sentence repetition tests are typically included in standard aphasia batteries. Additionally, these patients show deficits in comprehension of both simple and grammatically complex sentences and phrases, but intact single-word comprehension.

Gorno-Tempini et al. (2008) hypothesize that the speech problems observed in the logopenic variant are due to an underlying deficit in the phonological loop of verbal working memory. In support of this theory, they found that individuals with lvPPA have intact immediate recall of single and pairs of digits but are severely impaired in recall of sequences greater than three digits. The patients also do not exhibit the typical pattern of better short-term memory of phonologically dissimilar letter strings compared to phonologically similar letter strings, which the authors interpret as additional evidence of a disruption of the storage component of the phonological loop system of auditory working memory. This working memory deficit would explain the poor comprehension of sentences and phrases that is independent of grammatical complexity, and the sentence repetition deficits observed in the logopenic variant.

COGNITIVE AND BEHAVIORAL PROFILES OF PPA SUBTYPES

The defining symptom of PPA is the presence of a language impairment for at least 2 years in the absence of any other significant cognitive problem. The history of the time course of symptoms is usually provided by the patient or a family member. The precise beginning of the PPA syndrome may be difficult to establish given the slow and insidious onset. Still, careful inquiry about the history of symptoms is important since it is the preserved abilities in other areas of cognition, such as episodic memory, executive functioning, and visual-spatial skills, that differentiate PPA from other progressive dementia syndromes like probable AD (prAD) or the behavioral variant of frontotemporal dementia (bvFTD).

Assessment of other cognitive domains is challenging because many tests of memory, attention, executive functioning, and visual-spatial skills rely on language processes in some manner. Research studies using cognitive measures that require little or no receptive or expressive language skills provide support for the isolated impairment in language in the early stages of PPA. Wicklund, Johnson, and Weintraub (2004) demonstrated that a group of individuals in the mild-to-moderate stages of PPA combined across different subtypes perform similarly to a healthy control sample on a brief measure of nonverbal reasoning, while groups of patients with prAD and behavioral FTD both performed significantly worse than the control and PPA samples on this task. Further research comparing the different variants of PPA provides evidence of neuropsychological profiles that distinguish the three groups from each other and from other neurodegenerative dementia syndromes (Gorno-Tempini et al., 2004; Kramer et al., 2003; Libon et al., 2007, 2009).

Gorno-Tempini et al. (2004) reported a post hoc analysis of the cognitive profiles of a sample of patients with each of the three types of PPA. Patients with lvPPA demonstrated deficient learning and recall for verbal material, but normal recognition of both verbal and nonverbal material. This suggests that encoding of episodic information is intact but that underlying language or working memory problems interfere with recall of verbal material. Visual-spatial skills were also comparable to those of a healthy control group. Deficient scores were obtained on tests of working memory, which support the authors' hypothesis that a disruption in the phonological loop of the verbal working memory system underlies the observed language problems in lvPPA. This sample of patients also had difficulty performing arithmetic calculations. The reason for this is unclear because the task procedure was not described, but may be explained, at least in part, by deficits in working memory.

Patients with svPPA have a primary deficit in semantic memory. Relatively preserved episodic memory in these individuals is cited as one differentiating factor between svPPA and AD (Kramer et al., 2003; Libon et al., 2007; Perry & Hodges, 2000). However, at least one study (Gorno-Tempini et al., 2004) reported significantly worse scores on verbal learning, recall, and recognition measures relative to a control group, and worse scores on a recognition test of faces, suggesting difficulty with episodic memory. Little information about symptom duration in participants was provided in either of these studies; therefore, it is possible that the samples represent different stages of disease, and that episodic memory remains intact in early stages of the syndrome but declines as the disease progresses over time (Libon et al., 2009). Patients with svPPA have difficulty recalling autobiographical information (Greenberg et al., 2011), while visual-constructional abilities remain intact (Gorno-Tempini et al., 2004). Interestingly, these patients also tend to show behavioral symptoms (Kertesz et al., 2010), especially those related to mood (i.e., anxiety, apathy, and irritability) earlier and disinhibition later in the disease course (Banks & Weintraub, 2008), and these individuals are more likely to develop the bvFTD syndrome secondarily as their symptoms worsen (Kertesz et al., 2010).

Patients with nfvPPA suffer most from a deficit in syntactic processing. Other areas of cognitive functioning remain relatively intact in the early stages of the disease. Gorno-Tempini et al. (2004) found that these individuals demonstrated intact verbal recall and intact recognition of both verbal and nonverbal information. Performance on visuoconstruction tasks was also comparable to a healthy control group. Some studies have shown reduced auditory working memory capacity (Gorno-Tempini et al., 2004; Libon et al., 2007) in nfvPPA. However, auditory working memory is typically assessed with tasks requiring verbal output (i.e., tests of digit or letter span), and scores on these tests might be negatively impacted by the speech and language deficits present in this variant of PPA.

ANATOMY/IMAGING

Research studies using a variety of brain-imaging techniques have provided evidence that individuals with PPA have greater amounts of brain abnormalities in the left hemisphere regions of the language network (Gorno-Tempini et al., 2004;

Mesulam, 1982; Mesulam et al., 2009). Although all three variants of PPA show overlap in regional brain atrophy patterns, these research findings further indicate the presence of unique patterns of peak atrophy that distinguish the three different subtypes. These distinctive brain-imaging patterns are included as supporting criteria in the recently published diagnostic criteria for PPA variants (Gorno-Tempini et al., 2011).

nfvPPA is associated with atrophy predominantly in left posterior frontal regions, including the inferior frontal gyrus (IFG) and insular regions (Das, Avants, Grossman, & Gee, 2009; Gorno-Tempini et al., 2004; Josephs et al., 2006; Mesulam et al., 2009). These findings are not surprising given that the IFG is involved in aspects of grammatical processing such as syntax (Indefrey, Hellwig, Herzog, Seitz, & Hagoort, 2004; Mesulam et al., 2009; Rogalski, Cobia, et al., 2011), a core deficit in this PPA variant. Additional areas of atrophy are reported in the premotor and dorsolateral prefrontal cortex (Mesulam et al., 2009). Additional evidence for this distinguishing pattern of brain abnormality is found using both fluorodeoxyglucose-PET (FDG-PET; Grossman et al., 1996; Nestor et al., 2003) and single-photon emission computed tomography (SPECT; Newberg, Mozley, Sadek, Grossman, & Alavi, 2000) neuroimaging techniques.

svPPA has greater abnormalities relative to the other PPA variants in bilateral (left greater than right) anterior temporal lobe regions, including superior, middle, and inferior temporal gyri and the fusiform gyrus (Das et al., 2009; Gorno-Tempini et al., 2004; Hodges et al., 1992; Mesulam et al., 2009; Mummery et al., 2000). Anterior temporal lobe areas are found to be involved in aspects of word comprehension (Gitelman, Nobre, Sonty, Parrish, & Mesulam, 2005; Rogalski, Cobia, et al., 2011), which is severely compromised in svPPA.

lvPPA is associated with greater abnormalities in the left temporoparietal junction when compared with the other PPA variants, in addition to posterior temporal, supramarginal, and angular gyri (Das et al., 2009; Gorno-Tempini et al., 2004, 2008; Mesulam et al., 2009). The temporoparietal junction in particular is associated with phonological processing (Graves, Grabowski, Mehta, & Gupta, 2008).

Results from FDG-PET activation studies (Rabinovici et al., 2008) are consistent with anatomic localizations found using MRI. Patients with nfvPPA showed frontal hypometabolism, with left greater than right; patients with svPPA showed left anterior temporal lobe hypometabolism; and patients with lvPPA showed predominantly left temporoparietal hypometabolism. Autopsy results (see the following text) provide further evidence of the association between these brain areas and the subtypes of PPA.

GENETICS

Affected individuals and their relatives often inquire about the potential inherited risk of PPA and its underlying clinical diagnosis and molecular or pathological etiologies. Due to the complexity of PPA genetics, referral to a genetic counselor may be indicated—before and after genetic testing—to review all the risks and benefits associated with testing and disclosure of results. Approximately 5% to 10% of individuals with nfvPPA and svPPA have a mutation in *PRGN* (progranulin, associated with TAR DNA-binding protein [TDP-43] inclusions; also known as FTLD TDP-43) and another 5% to 10% of individuals have a mutation in *MAPT* (microtubule-associated protein tau, associated with phospho-tau inclusions, including Pick bodies). Rare individuals and pedigrees with FTLD or amyotrophic lateral sclerosis (ALS) have a mutation in *TDP-43*, and these individuals may present first with signs and symptoms of either ALS or FTLD, which then converge with disease progression. Rare pedigrees with a mutation in *FUS* (fused in sarcoma—another DNA/RNA-binding protein) may also present with FTLD–ALS. Likewise, mutations in *VCP* (valosin-containing protein) or *CHMP2B* (a trafficking protein) are rare causes of FTLD. To date, mutations in *TDP-43*, *FUS*, *VCP*, or *CHMP2B* have not been specifically linked to PPA. Individuals with *GRN* mutations may present with varied clinical syndromes including PPA and corticobasal syndrome, although bvFTD is the most common clinical diagnosis. The H1 haplotype of *MAPT* and heterozygosity of codon 129 in *PrP* (prion protein) may increase the risk of sporadic PPA. Although apolipoprotein e4 (Apo E-e4)-positive individuals have a fourfold increased risk of developing AD (compared to Apo E-e4-negative individuals), the Apo E-e4 genotype does not influence the risk of FTLD or PPA (Rogalski, Rademaker, et al., 2011). Rare individuals and pedigrees with autosomal-dominant AD carry mutations in either *APP* (*amyloid precursor protein*), *PS1* (*presenilin-1*), or *PS2* (*presenilin-2*), but their clinical presentation with PPA or one of its variants has not been specifically reported. A positive family history of PPA, FTLD, or AD increases the likelihood of identifying a genetic mutation. An autosomal-dominant pattern is suggested in about 10% of FTLD pedigrees, and in less than 1% of AD pedigrees. However, the great majority of PPA, FTLD (and AD) cases remain sporadic, and it is likely that several genetic and environmental factors contribute to their development. A major recent discovery identified *C9ORF72* (chromosome 9 open reading frame 72) as the most common genetic abnormality in familial bvFTD (about 11% of cases) and ALS (about 23% of cases). This mutation is an expansion of the noncoding hexanucleotide repeat GGGGCC on chromosome 9P (Dejesus-Hernandez et al., 2011; Dobson-Stone et al., 2012; Renton et al., 2011; Sha et al., 2012). Molecular mechanisms leading to neurodegeneration remain obscure; hypotheses include haploinsufficiency as well as toxic gain of function. From anatomic localization and pathology, it is anticipated that *C9ORF72* mutations may more likely associate with semantic or nonfluent than logopenic aphasia, but more data are needed.

TREATMENT AND MANAGEMENT

Nonpharmacological interventions begin with providing the most accurate diagnosis and prognosis possible, with continuing education provided to the patient, caregiver, and family with regard to their particular PPA variant and its potential for certain clinical and pathological etiologies. Speech therapy is indicated for further evaluation and possible rehabilitation of language dysfunction (see the following text), as well as for evaluation and dietary management of possible dysphagia. While in the earlier stages of PPA or dementia, training may be initiated with alternate means of communication such as point-boards, tablets, and other computer-assisted devices as directed by a speech therapist. Occupational or physical therapy may also be indicated for motor disturbances, including evaluation of gait and balance with fall-prevention training if indicated. Clinical evaluation at follow-up visits should monitor disease progression and the possible onset of parkinsonism, motor neuron disease, or dysphagia. Functional issues should be reviewed, including impaired ADL, home safety, driving, living situation, and supervision of daily medications and household finances. Identification and nonpharmacological management of triggers for episodic behavioral disturbances may be addressed. Advance directives regarding medical, legal, and financial affairs should be discussed, with subsequent legal referral. Finally, caregivers and patients should be referred to appropriate support groups and community resources.

Cognitive Treatment for Language Dysfunction

To date, there have been very few studies of cognitive treatments for the progressive deficits of PPA, or indeed for any progressive decline in cognitive function. The few studies that do exist are case studies or case series of at most three individuals with PPA.

The majority of such studies focus on word retrieval, the symptom seen in most patients with PPA. Some studies focus on boosting semantic representations (Henry, Beeson, & Rapcsak, 2008), while others focus on training self-cueing strategies (Henry et al., 2013). Some compare types of treatment. For example, a semantically based treatment produced better results for one patient with semantic dementia (SD) than an alphabetically based treatment did for another patient with SD (Graham, Patterson, Pratt, & Hodges, 1999, 2001) although maintenance of learning was poor for both cases.

Snowden and Neary (2002) used a cueing hierarchy treatment with their svPPA patients, and demonstrated some improvement but poor maintenance. They noted that personal "meaningfulness" was positively correlated with maintenance. A cued hierarchy paradigm was also used in a treatment study of nfvPPA patients (Jokel, Cupit, Rochon, & Leonard, 2009). Both patients improved and maintenance was demonstrated at 1-month post-treatment but not at 6 months. Another treatment study that used a standard cueing hierarchy method included a patient with lvPPA and a patient with svPPA (Newhart et al., 2009). Both patients improved on trained items; only the lvPPA patient showed generalization to untrained items. Maintenance testing was not reported.

A recent computer-based treatment study of an SD patient included items the patient was unable to name as well as items he could still name (Jokel, Rochon, & Anderson, 2010). Treatment effects were obtained for all trained items, and maintenance at 3 months post-treatment was demonstrated. Another treatment study that attempted to strengthen items that could still be named (prophylaxis of naming) involved a bilingual patient with lvPPA. The patient practiced naming a set of pictures using a multimodal treatment paradigm. The treatment was performed only in English. The result was better retention of the trained versus untrained items in the untrained language (Norwegian), suggesting a crosslinguistic effect of treatment (Friedman et al., 2010).

One recent treatment study targeted motor speech errors in a patient with nfvPPA. The treatment, which relied on oral text reading, resulted in improved speech output that was maintained for several months post-treatment.

It is encouraging to see that the virtual taboo has been broken, and studies of cognitive treatment for anomia in patients with *progressive* language impairments are beginning to emerge (indeed, an entire issue of *Aphasiology* was devoted to this topic; Jokel et al. [2009]). New treatment approaches for PPA are beginning to appear, such as transcranial magnetic stimulation (Trebbastoni, Raccah, de Lena, Zangen, & Inghilleri, 2013) and transcranial direct current stimulation (Wang, Wu, Chen, Yuan, & Zhang, 2013). Group studies are also beginning to emerge. A recent study found that both a reading/writing treatment and a repetition treatment had a prophylactic effect for treated words in nine participants with PPA, and were effective in remediating anomia in six participants with PPA (Meyer et al., 2013).

Pharmacological Treatment

There are few published drug trials for individuals diagnosed with FTLD, and even fewer for PPA or one of its variants. The literature on this topic consists primarily of case reports and inadequately powered, open-label studies. Reliable and reproducible quantitative outcome measures of behavioral dysfunction, as well as cognitive and functional decline, remain a work in progress, and provide another source of impediments to successful clinical trials. Therefore, the quality of evidence remains poor at best with regard to specific drug recommendations for individuals with PPA or FTLD. There are no drug therapies proven to arrest progression of signs and symptoms of PPA due to FTLD or AD pathologies. Because there is no significant central nervous system (CNS) cholinergic deficit found in FTLD, there is no rationale for prescribing cholinesterase inhibitors. Published studies of these drugs tested for PPA or FTLD report either worsening agitation and disinhibition or mixed results, with worsening in some cognitive, functional, or behavioral domains (and outcome measures) and simultaneous improvement in others (Rabinovici & Miller, 2010).

As the logopenic variant in particular may represent an atypical focal onset of AD, drugs with proven benefits for individuals with AD may be prescribed. The cholinesterase inhibitors donepezil, galantamine, and rivastigmine arrest the progression of cognitive and functional decline for individuals with mild-to-moderate dementia due to AD—for up to 1 to 2 years on average, when cognitive and functional declines resume. Memantine may be beneficial for individuals with moderate to severe (but not mild) dementia due to AD, and is frequently prescribed in addition to one of the three cholinesterase inhibitors (Holtzman, Morris, & Goate, 2011). These medications provide symptomatic benefits either by supporting cholinergic neurotransmission (cholinesterase inhibitors) or by blocking excitotoxic (NMDA-receptor mediated) neuronal morbidity and mortality (memantine). These drugs may also have some benefits for the manifold behavioral manifestations of dementia due to AD. Because a small fraction of individuals with the nonfluent and semantic PPA variants may have an atypical focal onset of AD (instead of one of the expected FTLD pathologies), these individuals may also benefit from drugs approved for AD. In support of this notion, Kertesz et al. (2008) report a benefit of galantamine in some individuals with progressive nonfluent aphasia. As NMDA-mediated neuronal toxicity may also play a role in the neuronal loss associated with FTLD, memantine is now under active investigation in a randomized, placebo-controlled clinical trial. In summary, there is currently inadequate evidence to support the clinical use of cholinesterase inhibitors or memantine in individuals with PPA or FTLD, and such use is considered off-label. Perhaps in the near future, drugs typically prescribed for individuals with AD may have overall benefit for the subset of individuals with PPA *and a positive AD biomarker* (amyloid PET imaging or high Abeta42 or low tau in the cerebrospinal fluid; McKhann et al., 2011). Multicenter, randomized, placebo-controlled studies are now warranted to address this hypothesis.

Individuals with PPA may have significant depression, anxiety, and other behavioral abnormalities that may benefit from one of the antidepressant medications (selective serotonin reuptake inhibitors [SSRIs] or serotonin–norepinephrine reuptake inhibitors [SNRIs]). The SSRIs or SNRIs may also benefit other behavioral manifestations such as disinhibition and repetitive or obsessive/compulsive behaviors. In fact, symptomatic therapy with escitalopram, citalopram, sertraline, bupropion (with parkinsonism), or venlafaxine (with prominent apathy) is often a first-line therapy for individuals with FTLD (Rabinovici & Miller, 2010). Trazodone, a low-affinity serotonin reuptake inhibitor, may also significantly improve behavioral disturbances associated with FTLD (Kaye, Petrovic-Poljak, Verhoeff, & Freedman, 2010). Behavioral difficulties such as agitation, pacing, wandering, delusions, paranoia, and hallucinations that are refractory to SSRIs may be treated with atypical antipsychotics despite little evidence of efficacy and the potential for adverse effects. There are few published studies with olanzapine, risperidone, aripiprazole, and the drug of choice quetiapine, due to its lower risk of extrapyramidal adverse effects (especially in the elderly). Use of atypical antipsychotics also warrants extreme caution due to the increased risk of mortality when prescribed to individuals with dementia (prompting the U.S. Food and Drug Administration [FDA] to issue a black box warning on their use in this patient population). The risks and benefits of these drugs should be reviewed with the patient and his or her family/caregiver, and their continued use reassessed in the face of advancing disease.

CLINICAL COURSE

The sine qua non clinical criterion for PPA remains a prominent and isolated language deficit as the predominant presenting sign and symptom (Gorno-Tempini et al., 2011). The onset of PPA is insidious and its progression is gradual—typically 9 to 11 years, on average, in duration, although some patients can progress more rapidly. A recent study that followed 11 patients with svPPA and 13 patients with lvPPA for 3 years found a more rapid cognitive decline in the lvPPA cohort (Leyton, Hsieh, Mioshi, & Hodges, 2013). Aphasia due to an ischemic stroke or mass lesion is readily ruled out by a thorough history, physical and neurological examination, and neuroimaging study (MRI or CT of the brain), thus leaving primarily neurodegenerative etiologies for PPA. By definition, individuals with PPA have little difficulty with complex ADL (with the exception of those requiring language functions, such as using a telephone) until later in the disease course (arbitrarily, more than 2 years later; Mesulam, 2001). Other cognitive domains (memory, praxis, gnosis, visuospatial skills, executive functions) are mostly spared at first, but become progressively involved as the disease worsens and spreads to include other brain regions. Thus, individuals typically evolve from a PPA variant to a frank dementing illness—becoming increasingly dependent with regard to complex and then basic ADL. Complex ADLs include handling one's own daily medications and household finances, and driving and shopping independently; basic ADLs include dressing, bathing, grooming, walking, toileting, transfers, and eating. Marked weight loss or repeated hospitalizations may signal end-stage disease and serve as a trigger for hospice management and terminal care.

Due to convergence of cognitive and functional deficits over time, individuals with PPA may be most accurately classified by examination early in the disease course and by following their evolution with serial evaluations. Some individuals will present with an isolated sign or with mixed signs, and a clearer picture allowing a more accurate categorization to emerge over time. Although some individuals with PPA are difficult to classify, most will fall into one of the three major variants: nonfluent, semantic, or logopenic. Even speech and language experts, however, do not always agree on categorization of examined or videotaped individuals. Behavioral disturbances are more common in the nonfluent and semantic variants. Mild limb apraxia may be apparent in all variants, particularly with fine motor tasks, but evidence of extrapyramidal signs or parkinsonism (including rigidity, bradykinesia, and tremor) suggests alternative diagnoses. By definition, PPA is restricted to individuals without significant parkinsonism or other major disabling motor syndromes.

nfvPPA is marked by effortful, nonfluent speech with agrammatism that gradually progresses to complete mutism. With disease progression, deficits in memory and executive function add to the presenting deficits in language fluency and comprehension of grammatically complex sentences. Apathy, abulia, and disorders of social function may become more disabling over time. Some individuals with the nonfluent variant progress to include motor problems consistent with a diagnosis of corticobasal degeneration (CBD, marked by asymmetric rigidity with apraxia and myoclonus) or progressive supranuclear palsy (PSP, marked by axial rigidity, poor balance with falls, and a supranuclear vertical gaze palsy).

CBD and PSP are now classified under the umbrella term FTLD and are known to be tauopathies (by genetic and molecular classification). nfvPPA and svPPA are two of the three presentations of FTLD, along with the behavioral variant—the most common of the three. Individuals with PPA may evolve to FTLD either with or without subsequent ALS, which includes atrophy, fasciculations, and weakness of denervated bulbar and limb muscles (often asymmetric, affecting the right side of the body).

svPPA will typically progress to include a social disorder with concomitant marked lack of insight. Signs and symptoms may include personality changes, disinhibition, socially inappropriate behaviors, lack of empathy, rigidity, compulsions, eating disorders, hyperorality, and hypersexuality (components of the Kluver–Bucy syndrome), particularly as disease spreads bilaterally to also involve the right anterior temporal pole. The logopenic variant may evolve to include the language deficits of a more typical AD presentation—including anomia, word-finding difficulties, circumlocutions, impaired repetition, and impaired comprehension and fluency. lvPPA will progressively worsen and impact other cognitive domains (memory, visuospatial, and executive skills). In general, individuals with tauopathies (most often associated with nonfluent aphasia) are often significantly more impaired in executive skills compared to individuals with TDP-43 or AD pathologies. Likewise, episodic memory is more impaired in individuals with AD pathologies (most often associated with the logopenic variant). In summary, a syndromic diagnosis of PPA will ultimately evolve into FTLD (FTLD-ALS, PSP, CBD), AD, or rarely, Lewy body dementia (or have mixed diagnoses/pathologies at autopsy) with a severe dementia associated with eventual mutism, a vegetative state, decubitus ulcers, and weight loss/inanition. A bacterial infection with sepsis (from a urinary tract infection, decubitus ulcer, or aspiration pneumonia) is often the proximate cause of death after many years of progressive neurological disabilities.

PATHOLOGY

On gross examination of the autopsied brain, individuals with nfvPPA and svPPA may present with striking frontal and anterior temporal atrophy ("knife-edge" gyri). The disease is often bilateral, but typically worse on the left, or language-dominant, brain hemisphere. Imaging and neuropathological studies demonstrate particular involvement of the left posterior fronto-insular cortex in the nonfluent variant, and of the anterior temporal lobes with the semantic variant. Individuals with logopenic AD have more widespread cortical atrophy at autopsy, especially of the left perisylvian and parietal cortex—perhaps consistent with the hypothesis that short-term memory deficits underlie the language deficits in this variant. The logopenic variant is also linked to biomarkers consistent with a diagnosis of AD, such as a positive amyloid PET scan and decreased Abeta42 or increased tau levels in the cerebrospinal fluid (McKhann et al., 2011).

Similar to distinct clinical and neuroimaging features, pathological analysis of brain sections also divide PPA into three major categories: nonfluent, agrammatic aphasia is most often linked to FTLD tau pathology (and less often to FTLD TDP-43), whereas semantic dementia is often linked to FTLD TDP-43, and logopenic aphasia is often linked to other or AD pathologies (amyloid plaques composed primarily of Abeta and neurofibrillary tangles composed primarily of phospho-tau). (FTLD with

Pick bodies [a tauopathy] on microscopic examination of brain sections is also called Pick's disease.) Neuronal loss is common to all forms of FTLD, and corresponds to atrophy in gross pathology and the degree of atrophy and hypometabolism on neuroimaging studies. In general, proteinaceous inclusions within CNS neurons and dystrophic neurites are abnormal and marked by ubiquitin-positive immunostaining, which remains useful in defining the degree and extent of microscopic inclusions in brain sections. Additional immunostaining, however, with antibodies to tau, TDP-43, or alpha-synuclein (staining Lewy bodies and Lewy neurites), is useful to further characterize these ubiquitin-positive aggregates. Interestingly, the TDP-43 pathology of semantic dementia is localized only to dystrophic neurites, while nonfluent PPA may also reveal neuronal cytoplasmic or nuclear TDP-43 inclusions. Similar to findings with progranulin (*PGN*) mutations, the newly reported *C9ORF72* mutation is associated with deposits of TDP-43 (Whitwell et al., 2012). Literature older than 2006 reports FTLD with tau-negative ubiquitin-positive neuronal inclusions or dystrophic neurites (FTLD-U), or perhaps as dementia lacking distinctive histopathology (DLDH)—examined today, many or most of these cases would likely be classified or reclassified as FTLD TDP-43. A recent review by Grossman (2010) reports the underlying molecular pathology of 145 autopsied cases of PPA; FTLD-tau is most commonly associated with the nonfluent variant, FTLD-U is most commonly associated with semantic dementia, and other or AD pathology is most commonly associated with the logopenic variant.

Although pathology at autopsy is considered the gold standard of diagnosis in neurological diseases, the pathology of PPA may evolve during its protracted course. Coincident findings at autopsy may include one or more lacunar infarcts and a few amyloid plaques, neurofibrillary tangles, or Lewy bodies. These may be insufficient in density or distribution to meet diagnostic criteria, and irrelevant to the PPA etiology at clinical presentation. Autopsy evaluation is valuable in identifying the predominant pathological and molecular basis of PPA, and its gross and microscopic localization in the brain. Typically, the regions most severely affected at autopsy are those affected first—at clinical presentation.

SUMMARY

It should be clear that differing clinical and pathological definitions, nosologies, and genetic and molecular identifications of PPA, FTLD, and AD, and their continual flux over time, all contribute to the controversies and lack of consensus in the medical literature. Even our current criteria represent a work in progress, because much remains unknown.

Thus, the association of a particular variant of PPA to a particular underlying clinical and pathological diagnosis is currently an overgeneralization, with published exceptions to every rule, and some individuals having mixed pathologies at autopsy (with an unclear primary pathology many years before—at clinical presentation). Further longitudinal assessments with autopsy confirmation of diagnosis are required, particularly for the logopenic variant. Because this variant represents a relatively new clinical concept, the least is known regarding its natural history and molecular etiology and pathology. Incorporation of new biomarkers, including amyloid and other PET neuroimaging and proteomics of blood and cerebrospinal fluid, will likely clarify nosology and etiology to improve diagnostic accuracy in the future. For now, the consensus criteria for PPA variants do not accurately predict the clinical course and underlying pathology in an individual presenting with the symptoms of PPA. Diagnostic clarity, however, is an essential and critical first step to successful novel *disease-specific* treatment strategies. As FTLD is the cause of approximately

15% of all neurodegenerative dementias, this large and growing patient population is clearly under-researched and thus underserved by the medical community.

Nevertheless, the growth in interest in PPA, particularly over the last decade, bodes well for future research. Indeed, individuals with PPA are participating in large-scale studies in several major universities and research sites. In addition to getting involved in studies focused on clinical aspects of PPA, the participation of these individuals is also aiding researchers in their quest to better understand the functional architecture of language in the brain.

REFERENCES

Adlam, A. L., Patterson, K., Rogers, T. T., Nestor, P. J., Salmond, C. H., Acosta-Cabronero, J., & Hodges, J. R. (2006). Semantic dementia and fluent primary progressive aphasia: Two sides of the same coin? *Brain: A Journal of Neurology, 129*(Pt 11), 3066–3080.

Banks, S. J., & Weintraub, S. (2008). Neuropsychiatric symptoms in behavioral variant frontotemporal dementia and primary progressive aphasia. *Journal of Geriatric Psychiatry and Neurology, 21*(2), 133–141.

Bonner, M. F., Ash, S., & Grossman, M. (2010). The new classification of primary progressive aphasia into semantic, logopenic, or nonfluent/agrammatic variants. *Current Neurology and Neuroscience Reports, 10*(6), 484–490.

Bonner, M. F., Vesely, L., Price, C., Anderson, C., Richmond, L., Farag, C.,...Grossman, M. (2009). Reversal of the concreteness effect in semantic dementia. *Cognitive Neuropsychology, 26*(6), 568–579.

Budd, M. A., Kortte, K., Cloutman, L., Newhart, M., Gottesman, R. F., Davis, C.,...Hillis, A. E. (2010). The nature of naming errors in primary progressive aphasia versus acute post-stroke aphasia. *Neuropsychology, 24*(5), 581–589.

Das, S. R., Avants, B. B., Grossman, M., & Gee, J. C. (2009). Registration based cortical thickness measurement. *NeuroImage, 45*(3), 867–879.

DeJesus-Hernandez, M., Mackenzie, I. R., Boeve, B. F., Boxer, A. L., Baker, M., Rutherford, N. J.,...Rademakers, R. (2011). Expanded GGGGCC hexanucleotide repeat in noncoding region of C9ORF72 causes chromosome 9p-linked FTD and ALS. *Neuron, 72*(2), 245–256.

Dobson-Stone, C., Hallupp, M., Bartley, L., Shepherd, C. E., Halliday, G. M., Schofield, P. R.,... Kwok, J. B. (2012). C9ORF72 repeat expansion in clinical and neuropathologic frontotemporal dementia cohorts. *Neurology, 79*(10), 995–1001.

Friedman, R., Carney, A., Lott, S. N., Snider, S., Ullrich, L., & Eckmann, C. (2010). Longitudinal decline of language in a bilingual patient with logopenic variant primary progressive aphasia. *Procedia Social and Behavioral Sciences, 6*, 215–216.

Gitelman, D. R., Nobre, A. C., Sonty, S., Parrish, T. B., & Mesulam, M. M. (2005). Language network specializations: An analysis with parallel task designs and functional magnetic resonance imaging. *NeuroImage, 26*(4), 975–985.

Goodglass, H., Kaplan, E., & Barresi, B. (2001). *Boston diagnostic aphasia examination*. Baltimore, MD: Lippincott Williams & Wilkins.

Gorno-Tempini, M. L., Brambati, S. M., Ginex, V., Ogar, J., Dronkers, N. F., Marcone, A.,... Miller, B. L. (2008). The logopenic/phonological variant of primary progressive aphasia. *Neurology, 71*(16), 1227–1234.

Gorno-Tempini, M. L., Dronkers, N. F., Rankin, K. P., Ogar, J. M., Phengrasamy, L., Rosen, H. J.,... Miller, B. L. (2004). Cognition and anatomy in three variants of primary progressive aphasia. *Annals of Neurology, 55*(3), 335–346.

Gorno-Tempini, M. L., Hillis, A. E., Weintraub, S., Kertesz, A., Mendez, M., Cappa, S. F.,... Grossman, M. (2011). Classification of primary progressive aphasia and its variants. *Neurology, 76*(11), 1006–1014.

Graham, K. S., Patterson, K., Pratt, K. H., & Hodges, J. R. (2001). Can repeated exposure to "forgotten" vocabulary help alleviate word-finding difficulties in semantic dementia? An illustrative case study. *Neuropsychological Rehabilitation, 11*(3/4), 429–454.

Graham, K. S., Patterson, K., Pratt, K. H., & Hodges, J. R. (1999). Relearning and subsequent forgetting of semantic category exemplars in a case of semantic dementia. *Neuropsychology, 13*(3), 359–380.

Graves, W. W., Grabowski, T. J., Mehta, S., & Gupta, P. (2008). The left posterior superior temporal gyrus participates specifically in accessing lexical phonology. *Journal of Cognitive Neuroscience, 20*(9), 1698–1710.

Greenberg, D. L., Ogar, J. M., Viskontas, I. V., Gorno Tempini, M. L., Miller, B., & Knowlton, B. J. (2011). Multimodal cuing of autobiographical memory in semantic dementia. *Neuropsychology, 25*(1), 98–104.

Grossman, M. (2010). Primary progressive aphasia: Clinicopathological correlations. *Nature Reviews. Neurology, 6*(2), 88–97.

Grossman, M., & Ash, S. (2004). Primary progressive aphasia: A review. *Neurocase, 10*(1), 3–18.

Grossman, M., Mickanin, J., Onishi, K., Hughes, E., D'Esposito, M., Ding, X. S.,... Reivich, M. (1996). Progressive nonfluent aphasia: Language, cognitive, and PET measures contrasted with probable Alzheimer's disease. *Journal of Cognitive Neuroscience, 8*(2), 135–154.

Grossman, M., Rhee, J., & Moore, P. (2005). Sentence processing in frontotemporal dementia. *Cortex, 41*(6), 764–777.

Henry, M. L., Beeson, P. M., & Rapcsak, S. Z. (2008). Treatment for lexical retrieval in progressive aphasia. *Aphasiology, 22*(7–8), 826–838.

Henry, M. L., Rising, K., DeMarco, A. T., Miller, B. L., Gorno-Tempini, M. L., & Beeson, P. M. (2013). Examining the value of lexical retrieval treatment in primary progressive aphasia: Two positive cases. *Brain and Language, 127*(2), 145–156.

Hodges, J. R., Patterson, K., Oxbury, S., & Funnell, E. (1992). Semantic dementia. Progressive fluent aphasia with temporal lobe atrophy. *Brain: A Journal of Neurology, 115*(Pt 6), 1783–1806.

Holtzman, D. M., Morris, J. C., & Goate, A. M. (2011). Alzheimer's disease: The challenge of the second century. *Science Translational Medicine, 3*(77), 77sr1.

Howard, D., & Patterson K. (1992). *Pyramids and palm trees: A test of semantic access from pictures and words*. Bury St Edmunds, UK: Thames Valley Publishing.

Indefrey, P., Hellwig, F., Herzog, H., Seitz, R. J., & Hagoort, P. (2004). Neural responses to the production and comprehension of syntax in identical utterances. *Brain and Language, 89*(2), 312–319.

Jokel, R., Cupit, J., Rochon, E., & Leonard, C. (2009). Relearning lost vocabulary in nonfluent progressive aphasia with MossTalk words. *Aphasiology, 23*(2), 175–191.

Jokel, R., Rochon, E., & Anderson, N. D. (2010). Errorless learning of computer-generated words in a patient with semantic dementia. *Neuropsychological Rehabilitation, 20*(1), 16–41.

Josephs, K. A., Duffy, J. R., Strand, E. A., Whitwell, J. L., Layton, K. F., Parisi, J. E.,... Petersen, R. C. (2006). Clinicopathological and imaging correlates of progressive aphasia and apraxia of speech. *Brain: A Journal of Neurology, 129*(Pt 6), 1385–1398.

Kay, J., Lesser, R., & Coltheart, M. (1992). *PALPA: Psycholinguistic Assessments of Language Processing in Aphasia*. London: Lawrence Erlbaum Associates.

Kaye, E. D., Petrovic-Poljak, A., Verhoeff, N. P., & Freedman, M. (2010). Frontotemporal dementia and pharmacologic interventions. *The Journal of Neuropsychiatry and Clinical Neurosciences, 22*(1), 19–29.

Kertesz, A. (2006). *Western aphasia battery—Revised (WABOR)*. Austin, TX: Pro-Ed.

Kertesz, A., Jesso, S., Harciarek, M., Blair, M., & McMonagle, P. (2010). What is semantic dementia?: A cohort study of diagnostic features and clinical boundaries. *Archives of Neurology, 67*(4), 483–489.

Kertesz, A., Morlog, D., Light, M., Blair, M., Davidson, W., Jesso, S., & Brashear, R. (2008). Galantamine in frontotemporal dementia and primary progressive aphasia. *Dementia and Geriatric Cognitive Disorders, 25*(2), 178–185.

Kramer, J. H., Jurik, J., Sha, S. J., Rankin, K. P., Rosen, H. J., Johnson, J. K., & Miller, B. L. (2003). Distinctive neuropsychological patterns in frontotemporal dementia, semantic dementia, and Alzheimer disease. *Cognitive and Behavioral Neurology, 16*(4), 211–218.

Leyton, C. E., Hsieh, S., Mioshi, E., & Hodges, J. R. (2013). Cognitive decline in logopenic aphasia: More than losing words. *Neurology, 80*(10), 897–903.

Libon, D. J., Xie, S. X., Moore, P., Farmer, J., Antani, S., McCawley, G., . . . Grossman, M. (2007). Patterns of neuropsychological impairment in frontotemporal dementia. *Neurology, 68*(5), 369–375.

Libon, D. J., Xie, S. X., Wang, X., Massimo, L., Moore, P., Vesely, L., . . . Grossman, M. (2009). Neuropsychological decline in frontotemporal lobar degeneration: A longitudinal analysis. *Neuropsychology, 23*(3), 337–346.

Luzzatti, C., & Poeck, K. (1991). An early description of slowly progressive aphasia. *Archives of Neurology, 48*(2), 228–229.

McKhann, G. M., Knopman, D. S., Chertkow, H., Hyman, B. T., Jack, C. R. Jr., Kawas, C. H., . . . Phelps, C. H. (2011). The diagnosis of dementia due to Alzheimer's disease: Recommendations from the National Institute on Aging-Alzheimer's Association workgroups on diagnostic guidelines for Alzheimer's disease. *Alzheimer's and Dementia, 7*(3), 263–269.

Mesulam, M., Rogalski, E., Wieneke, C., Cobia, D., Rademaker, A., Thompson, C., & Weintraub, S. (2009). Neurology of anomia in the semantic variant of primary progressive aphasia. *Brain: A Journal of Neurology, 132*(Pt 9), 2553–2565.

Mesulam, M. M. (1982). Slowly progressive aphasia without generalized dementia. *Annals of Neurology, 11*(6), 592–598.

Mesulam, M. M. (1987). Primary progressive aphasia–differentiation from Alzheimer's disease. *Annals of Neurology, 22*(4), 533–534.

Mesulam, M. M. (2001). Primary progressive aphasia. *Annals of Neurology, 49*(4), 425–432.

Mesulam, M. M. (2003). Primary progressive aphasia—a language-based dementia. *The New England Journal of Medicine, 349*(16), 1535–1542.

Mesulam, M. M., & Weintraub, S. (1992). Spectrum of primary progressive aphasia. In M. N. Rossor (Ed.), *Unusual dementias* (pp. 583–609). London: Baillière Tindall.

Mesulam, M. M., Wieneke, C., Thompson, C., Rogalski, E., & Weintraub, S. (2012). Quantitative classification of primary progressive aphasia at early and mild impairment stages. *Brain: A Journal of Neurology, 135*(Pt 5), 1537–1553.

Meyer, A., Getz, H., Snider, S., Sullivan, K., Long, S., Turner, R., & Friedman, R. (2013). Remediation and prophylaxis of anomia in primary progressive aphasia. *Procedia—Social and Behavioral Sciences, 94*, 275–276.

Mummery, C. J., Patterson, K., Price, C. J., Ashburner, J., Frackowiak, R. S., & Hodges, J. R. (2000). A voxel-based morphometry study of semantic dementia: Relationship between temporal lobe atrophy and semantic memory. *Annals of Neurology, 47*(1), 36–45.

Nestor, P. J., Graham, N. L., Fryer, T. D., Williams, G. B., Patterson, K., & Hodges, J. R. (2003). Progressive non-fluent aphasia is associated with hypometabolism centred on the left anterior insula. *Brain: A Journal of Neurology, 126*(Pt 11), 2406–2418.

Newberg, A. B., Mozley, P. D., Sadek, A. H., Grossman, M., & Alavi, A. (2000). Regional cerebral distribution of [Tc-99m] hexylmethylpropylene amineoxine in patients with progressive aphasia. *Journal of Neuroimaging, 10*(3), 162–168.

Newhart, M., Davis, C., Kannan, V., Heidler-Gary, J., Cloutman, L., & Hillis, A. E. (2009). Therapy for naming deficits in two variants of primary progressive aphasia. *Aphasiology, 23*(7–8), 823–834.

Perry, R. J., & Hodges, J. R. (2000). Differentiating frontal and temporal variant frontotemporal dementia from Alzheimer's disease. *Neurology, 54*(12), 2277–2284.

Pick, A. (1892). On the relationship between senile cerebral atrophy and aphasia. *Prager Medicinische Wochenschrift, xvii*(17), 165–167. As translated by D. M. Girling and G. E. Berrios. (1994). *History of Psychiatry, 5*, 542–547.

Pogacar, S., & Williams, R. S. (1984). Alzheimer's disease presenting as slowly progressive aphasia. *Rhode Island Medical Journal, 67*(4), 181–185.

Rabinovici, G. D., & Miller, B. L. (2010). Frontotemporal lobar degeneration: Epidemiology, pathophysiology, diagnosis and management. *CNS Drugs, 24*(5), 375–398.

Rabinovici, G. D., Jagust, W. J., Furst, A. J., Ogar, J. M., Racine, C. A., Mormino, E. C.,…Gorno-Tempini, M. L. (2008). Abeta amyloid and glucose metabolism in three variants of primary progressive aphasia. *Annals of Neurology, 64*(4), 388–401.

Renton, A. E., Majounie, E., Waite, A., Simón-Sánchez, J., Rollinson, S., Gibbs, J. R.,…Traynor, B. J.; ITALSGEN Consortium. (2011). A hexanucleotide repeat expansion in C9ORF72 is the cause of chromosome 9p21-linked ALS-FTD. *Neuron, 72*(2), 257–268.

Rogalski, E., Cobia, D., Harrison, T. M., Wieneke, C., Thompson, C. K., Weintraub, S., & Mesulam, M. M. (2011). Anatomy of language impairments in primary progressive aphasia. *The Journal of Neuroscience, 31*(9), 3344–3350.

Rogalski, E. J., Rademaker, A., Harrison, T. M., Helenowski, I., Johnson, N., Bigio, E.,…Mesulam, M. M. (2011). ApoE e4 is a susceptibility factor in amnestic but not aphasic dementias. *Alzheimer Disease and Associated Disorders, 25*(2), 159–163.

Rosenfeld, M. (1909). Die partielle Grosshirnatrophie. *Journal für Psychologie und Neurologie, 14*, 115–130.

Serieux, P. (1893). Sur un cas de surdite verbal pure. *Revue Medicale, 13*, 733–750.

Sha, S. J., Takada, L. T., Rankin, K. P., Yokoyama, J. S., Rutherford, N. J., Fong, J. C.,…Boxer, A. L. (2012). Frontotemporal dementia due to C9ORF72 mutations: Clinical and imaging features. *Neurology, 79*(10), 1002–1011.

Snowden, J. S., Goulding, P. J., & Neary, D. (1989). Semantic dementia: A form of circumscribed cerebral atrophy. *Behavioural Neurology, 2*(3), 167–182.

Snowden, J. S., & Neary, D. (2002). Relearning of verbal labels in semantic dementia. *Neuropsychologia, 40*(10), 1715–1728.

Trebbastoni, A., Raccah, R., de Lena, C., Zangen, A., & Inghilleri, M. (2013). Repetitive deep transcranial magnetic stimulation improves verbal fluency and written language in a patient with primary progressive aphasia-logopenic variant (LPPA). *Brain Stimulation, 6*(4), 545–553.

Wang, J., Wu, D., Chen, Y., Yuan, Y., & Zhang, M. (2013). Effects of transcranial direct current stimulation on language improvement and cortical activation in nonfluent variant primary progressive aphasia. *Neuroscience Letters, 549*, 29–33.

Warrington, E. K. (1975). The selective impairment of semantic memory. *The Quarterly Journal of Experimental Psychology, 27*(4), 635–657.

Weinstein, J., Koenig, P., Gunawardena, D., McMillan, C., Bonner, M., & Grossman, M. (2011). Preserved musical semantic memory in semantic dementia. *Archives of Neurology, 68*(2), 248–250.

Weintraub, S., & Mesulam, M. M. (1993). Four neuropsychological profiles in dementia. In F. Boller and J. Grafman (Eds.), *Handbook of neuropsychology* (pp. 99–114). Amsterdam: Elsevier Science Publishers B.V. *4*, 253–281.

Weintraub, S., Mesulam, M. M., Wieneke, C., Rademaker, A., Rogalski, E. J., & Thompson, C. K. (2009). The Northwestern Anagram Test: Measuring sentence production in primary progressive aphasia. *American Journal of Alzheimer's Disease and Other Dementias, 24*(5), 408–416.

Weintraub, S., Rubin, N. P., & Mesulam, M. M. (1990). Primary progressive aphasia. Longitudinal course, neuropsychological profile, and language features. *Archives of Neurology, 47*(12), 1329–1335.

Westbury, C., & Bub, D. (1997). Primary progressive aphasia: A review of 112 cases. *Brain and Language, 60*(3), 381–406.

Whitwell, J. L., Weigand, S. D., Boeve, B. F., Senjem, M. L., Gunter, J. L., DeJesus-Hernandez, M., ... Josephs, K. A. (2012). Neuroimaging signatures of frontotemporal dementia genetics: C9ORF72, tau, progranulin and sporadics. *Brain: A Journal of Neurology, 135*(Pt 3), 794–806.

Wicklund, A. H., Johnson, N., & Weintraub, S. (2004). Preservation of reasoning in primary progressive aphasia: Further differentiation from Alzheimer's disease and the behavioral presentation of frontotemporal dementia. *Journal of Clinical and Experimental Neuropsychology, 26*(3), 347–355.

CHAPTER 12

Prion Diseases

Brian S. Appleby

Transmissible spongiform encephalopathies (TSEs) are a group of illnesses characterized by a pathological form of the native prion protein that is widely believed to be transmissible without the aid of nucleic acids. In general, TSEs (a.k.a. prion disease) are rapidly progressive neurodegenerative illnesses that affect sheep (scrapie), mink (transmissible mink encephalopathy), cows (bovine spongiform encephalopathy [BSE]), cervids (chronic wasting disease), and humans (Creutzfeldt–Jakob disease [CJD]; they also are responsible for Gerstmann–Sträussler–Scheinker [GSS] syndrome and fatal familial insomnia [FFI]), and they have been produced experimentally in several other animals. CJD is the most common TSE in humans.

Human prion diseases have three etiologies: (a) sporadic, (b) genetic, and (c) acquired. Similar to other protein misfolding disorders (e.g., Alzheimer's disease [AD], Parkinson's disease, and frontotemporal dementia), prion diseases can originate from a spontaneous posttranslational modification of the native prion protein (PrP^c), resulting in a pathological isoform (PrP^{Sc}). Another common feature that is shared among the protein misfolding disorders is genetic occurrences caused by a mutation in the gene encoding the affected protein. However, prion diseases can also be transmitted interspecies and intraspecies via the ingestion of contaminated food (variant CJD [vCJD]) and through certain medical procedures (iatrogenic CJD [iCJD]).

Human prion diseases are important to understand because of their underlying pathophysiology, public health implications, and clinical features that often result in misdiagnosis. This chapter reviews the historical discovery of prion diseases and the formulation of the prion hypothesis. Both historical discovery and the prion hypothesis have demonstrated a large socioeconomic impact on several major countries, resulting in important epidemiological studies and active surveillance programs. The prion hypothesis and the neuropathogenesis of prion diseases are also explored in greater detail. Finally, the chapter ends with a description of the diagnosis, prognosis, and experimental treatment of human prion diseases.

DISCOVERY OF PRION DISEASES

Scrapie

Scrapie was the first recognized prion disease. The disease affects sheep and goats, and people have known about it since at least the 18th century, during which a discussion within the British House of Commons centered on its economic cost (Brown & Bradley, 1998). Characterized by encephalopathy and pruritus that resulted in sheep "scraping" against objects, scrapie was later found to be infectious. Experimental transmission studies performed by Cuillé and Chelle in 1936 demonstrated transmission of scrapie to normal sheep following inoculation of central nervous system (CNS) tissue from affected sheep (Cuillé & Chelle, 1936). Incubation periods varied and were affected by the route of inoculation, with the shortest incubation periods occurring when brains were inoculated and the longest periods occurring with peripheral routes of inoculation. The infectious agent remained elusive for several decades, and the search for it was later aided by the discovery of similar diseases in humans.

Creutzfeldt–Jakob Disease

The first human prion disease was described in the early 1920s by two neuropsychiatrists, Hans Creutzfeldt and Alfons Jakob. Creutzfeldt first described a case in 1920 (Creutzfeldt, 1920) that was later included in a case series of Jakob's own patients that he classified as having "spastic pseudosclerosis" (Jakob, 1921). Jakob chose this terminology because, "... from a pathophysiological and clinical point of view, this disease occupies a place between the spastic system diseases...and the disease processes primarily localized to the striatum.... From the standpoint of symptoms it comes closest perhaps to multiple sclerosis, from which it differs sharply on the basis of the histologic substrate" (Jakob, 1921). There was early speculation regarding the pertinence of Creutzfeldt's case to Jakob's newly described disease entity because of his patient's young age at disease onset (teenage years), family history of early-life neuropsychiatric illness, and a several-month period of clinical improvement (Kirschbaum, 1968). Thus, some have changed the name of the syndrome to CJD to emphasize Jakob's role in its discovery. However, later neuropathological review of Jakob's cases revealed that only two of his originally described five cases would currently be consistent with a diagnosis of CJD (Masters & Gajdusek, 1982).

The first complete description of what is now considered CJD was detailed by Nevin, McMenemey, Behrman, & Jones in their 1960 characterization of "subacute spongiform encephalopathy" (Nevin et al., 1960). The authors detailed the neuropathological characteristics of status spongiosus and neuronal loss, especially in the cerebral cortex, which is observed in the condition. Patients were affected in mid-to-late life and experienced an insidious onset of disease with rapid neurocognitive deterioration leading to death in weeks to months. Clinical manifestations of the disease often included dementia, myoclonus, motor impairment, language impairment, cerebellar dysfunction, visual disturbances, and neuropsychiatric symptoms. They also observed that affected patients frequently exhibited periodic generalized sharp wave complexes during EEG testing.

Kuru

A dramatic increase in our understanding of human prion diseases occurred following the discovery of kuru. Restricted to the Eastern Highlands of Papua New Guinea, a fatal, rapidly progressive neurodegenerative illness affected the Fore tribe who termed the illness *kuru,* meaning "to be afraid" or "to shiver" (Gajdusek & Zigas, 1957). The disease primarily affected children and adult females and was responsible for more than half of the deaths that occurred over the prior 5 years in some communities. Kuru usually commenced with symptoms of gait ataxia that progressed to further cerebellar disturbances of incoordination, dysarthria, and diffuse tremors. Patients exhibited affective symptoms such as apathy and pseudobulbar palsy, and became immobile and mute, eventually dying of starvation or opportunistic infections within 3 to 6 months of disease onset. The authors were puzzled over the etiology of kuru, raising the possibility of genetic and infectious causes.

The large vacuoles observed in the brains of those affected by kuru were soon compared to those seen in animals affected by scrapie. In 1959, Hadlow compared the similarities between these two diseases, including endemic outbreaks in confined populations; rapid neurodegeneration over several months that was mostly fatal; neurological symptoms of ataxia, tremors, and behavioral changes; and neuropathological characteristics of neuronal degeneration, astrocytic gliosis, and large vacuoles (Hadlow, 1959). Hadlow also noted that scrapie could be induced in unaffected sheep via intracerebral or subcutaneous inoculation of brain tissue from scrapie-affected sheep following a prolonged incubation period (Gordon, 1946). He proposed a similar experiment in primates using tissue from kuru patients.

Hadlow's suspicions that kuru may be transmissible was confirmed several years later in a report by Gajdusek, Gibbs, and Alpers. Gajdusek's laboratory had inoculated many primates with brain tissue from humans affected by a wide array of neurodegenerative diseases, including amyotrophic lateral sclerosis, parkinsonism diseases, myasthenia gravis, multiple sclerosis, and others (Gajdusek, Gibbs, & Alpers, 1966). None of the primates developed these diseases except for three chimpanzees that had been intracerebrally inoculated with brain tissue from kuru patients. The affected chimpanzees developed a rapid neurodegenerative illness that shared a similar clinical phenotype to that seen in kuru patients following an 18- to 21-month incubation period. Neuropathological changes were also similar to those observed in kuru patients (Beck, Daniel, Alpers, Gajdusek, & Gibbs, 1966). Once an infectious etiology was established, researchers and laypeople alike assumed that kuru was transmitted via the endocannibal mourning rituals of the Eastern Highlands people (Gajdusek, 1979). The initial transmission likely occurred during a ritual of an individual with CJD, and the connection between the rituals and the development of kuru was likely not made within the tribal community due to its slow incubation period.

The similar clinical and neuropathological characteristics seen in kuru and CJD raised the question whether CJD was also transmissible. Gajdusek's kuru transmission study was soon followed by another report from his laboratory that described the experimental transmission of a rapid neurodegenerative illness in a chimpanzee that was intracerebrally inoculated with brain tissue from a CJD patient (Gibbs et al., 1968). Thirteen months following inoculation, the chimpanzee developed a rapidly progressive illness that was clinically similar to CJD. Neuropathological characteristics also included those frequently observed in CJD patients: status spongiosis, loss of cortical neurons, astrocyte proliferation, and hypertrophy. These results led the researchers to conclude that CJD was caused by a similar transmissible agent.

THE PRION HYPOTHESIS

Although transmissibility of spongiform encephalopathies had been demonstrated in multiple species, the etiologic agent remained to be identified. Various theories abounded within the field, and TSEs were largely regarded to be caused by atypical or "slow viruses." However, several data argued against a viral agent as demonstrated by its resistance to inactivation via formalin, heat treatments, and high doses of ultraviolet light, suggesting that the agent did not employ the use of nucleic acids to propagate (Alper, Haig, & Clarke, 1966; Gordon, 1946).

TSE infectivity, primarily scrapie, was widely thought to be caused by protein without nucleic acid, although there had been no natural precedent for this type of biological mechanism. In 1967, a mathematician by the name of J. S. Griffith proposed three theoretical mechanisms by which proteins could self-replicate (Griffith, 1967). The further development of a "protein-only" hypothesis of TSEs was proposed by Stanley Prusiner in a 1982 manuscript for which he later won the Nobel Prize (Prusiner, 1982). In this manuscript, he reviewed evidence that largely argued against the use of nucleic acids in TSEs, but for the necessity of certain purified proteins.

Many studies have strengthened the evidence for the prion hypothesis of TSEs, which is widely believed to be the underlying mechanism in these "prion diseases" (see Table 12.1 for evidence supporting the prion hypothesis). The prion protein is a native protein found throughout the human body and primarily in the brain. The exact physiological role of the native prion protein (PrP^c) is unknown. Several researchers have demonstrated its role in binding copper (Brown, Clive, & Haswell, 2001) and normal synaptic functioning (Collinge et al., 1994). PrP^c is also believed to have neuroprotective functions (Rambold et al., 2008; Roucou, Gains, & LeBlanc, 2004). A thorough overview of the physiology of PrP^c can be found in a review by Linden et al. (2008). When the gene that encodes PrP^c (*PRNP*) is knocked out in mice, the mice appear to undergo normal development and do not demonstrate any gross behavioral abnormalities (Büeler et al., 1993).

Prion diseases are caused by a pathological isoform of PrP^c, termed PrP^{Sc}. Prion diseases are unique in that PrP^{Sc} can interact with PrP^c and cause PrP^c to transform into PrP^{Sc} (see Figure 12.1). The interaction of the two proteins is all that is required for the propagation of the disease. No nucleic acids or cofactors have been demonstrated to be essential in this conversion reaction. However, PrP^{Sc} requires PrP^c as a substrate for the conversion process, and mice that do not express PrP^c are resistant to prion

TABLE 12.1 Evidence Supporting the Prion Hypothesis

EVIDENCE	STUDY
Agents that destroy nucleic acids do not affect prion infectivity	Alper, Cramp, Haig, & Clarke, 1967
Purified pathological prion proteins are infectious	Prusiner, Groth, Bolton, Kent, & Hood, 1984
Infectivity is proportional to the concentration of pathological prion proteins	Gabizon, McKinley, Groth, & Prusiner, 1988
Inactivation of the pathological prion protein markedly reduces or eliminates infectivity	Prusiner, Groth, Serban, Stahl, & Gabizon, 1993
Mice devoid of normal prion proteins are resistant to prion disease	Büeler et al., 1993
All genetic forms of prion disease are linked to the prion protein gene (*PRNP*)	Kong, 2004
Pathological prion proteins transform normal prion proteins via an autocatalytic mechanism	Kocisko et al., 1994; Saborio, Permanne, & Soto, 2001
Prion infectivity occurs in the absence of cofactors	Kim et al., 2010

Source: Soto, Estrada, and Castilla (2006).

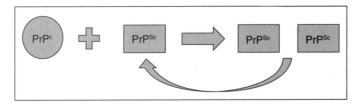

FIGURE 12.1 Prion conversion process.

PrP^c, native prion protein; PrP^{Sc}, pathological isoform of the prion protein.

diseases (Büeler et al., 1993). Because of the necessity of PrP^c in the conversion process, one potential treatment approach would be to block its expression. However, this approach is viewed with caution as science has not entirely established the function of PrP^c, especially its possible role in higher-level thinking and behavior.

HUMAN PRION DISEASES

Human prion diseases, collectively referred to as CJD in the medical field, are rapidly progressive neurodegenerative illnesses. Besides their pathogenic mechanisms, prion diseases are also unique in that they can occur via three separate etiologies: sporadic, genetic, or acquired. The following section explores each etiology in detail.

Sporadic CJD

Sporadic CJD (sCJD) represents the vast majority of human prion diseases, accounting for approximately 85% of all cases. Although the true cause of sCJD is unknown, it is widely believed to be caused by a posttranslational protein modification that results in the conversion of PrP^{Sc} from the native prion protein (Barria, Mukherjee, Gonzalez-Romero, Morales, & Soto, 2009). However, some researchers argue that a proportion of sporadic cases is actually acquired through currently unrecognized methods of transmission such as non-neurological surgeries (Collins et al., 1999; Koperek et al., 2002; Mahillo-Fernandez et al., 2008) and other invasive procedures (Davanipour, Alter, Sobel, Asher, & Gajdusek, 1985). In general, results of risk analysis studies have been varied and inconclusive.

Epidemiology

The worldwide incidence of sCJD is one per million people per year (World Health Organization, 2003a). Epidemiological studies have been completed in many different countries, all with similar incidence rates. Because most surveillance studies have been performed in North America or Europe, little is known about ethnic differences in incidence rates. In a study performed in the United States, the age-adjusted incidence was 2.7 times higher for Whites compared to Blacks (Holman et al., 2010). These results should be viewed with caution given the possibility of ascertainment bias between races that is typically observed in research studies within the United States. Studies have also demonstrated that sCJD affects men and women equally.

The age of onset of sCJD is highly variable. In a meta-analysis, the average age of onset of sCJD was the early 60s (Appleby, Appleby, & Rabins, 2007). However, sCJD has occurred in early, mid, and late life, and should not be discounted based on age of onset alone. sCJD should always be considered in the differential diagnosis of those with young-onset dementia (younger than 65 years). In appropriate clinical settings, it should also be considered in those who are 65 years of age or older, as the average annual incidence in this population was higher at 4.8 per million in one study conducted in the United States (Holman et al., 2010).

Clinical Presentation and Course

Prion diseases have a wide range of clinical presentations. Clinical presentation can range from cognitive to noncognitive symptoms or a combination of the two. Most cases present with some element of cognitive and/or functional impairment (Appleby et al., 2009). Distinctive presentations have also been described in the literature. The Oppenheimer–Brownell variants primarily present with symptoms of ataxia, usually in the absence of cognitive impairment (Brownell & Oppenheimer, 1965). The Heidenhain variant of sCJD presents with profound visual symptoms including cortical blindness, visuospatial impairment, and visual hallucinations (Heidenhain, 1929). Other phenotypes, such as those solely presenting with cognitive or mood symptoms, have also been described (Appleby et al., 2009). Correlations among clinical presentation, diagnostic test results, and survival time have been reported in the literature (Appleby et al., 2009), and neuropathological and molecular determinants have also been described (Parchi et al., 1996, 1999).

Although any neurocognitive symptom is possible in sCJD, some symptoms are observed more than others (Appleby et al., 2007). The most common symptoms observed in sCJD include cerebellar impairment, such as gait ataxia and dysmetria, in addition to cognitive impairment and dementia. Nystagmus and the aforementioned visual symptoms are also frequently observed. Myoclonus, particularly a hyperstartle response, has become popularly associated with sCJD although it is not pathognomonic of the disease. Motor weakness and movement disorders, including extrapyramidal symptoms, are common. As the disease progresses, voluntary movement and speech decrease until the patient reaches a state of akinetic mutism in the terminal stages of the illness. Likewise, ideomotor and swallowing apraxia develop as the disease progresses. The combination of immobility and an inadequately protected airway results in many patients dying from opportunistic infections, including urinary tract infections, infected pressure sores, and pneumonia.

Prion disease is invariably fatal, and it is characterized by a rapid progression. Although the survival time is variable in sCJD, illness duration is typically measured in months as opposed to years. The majority of cases have illness durations of approximately 6 months, and approximately 20% survive a year from illness onset (Pocchiari et al., 2004). On rare occasions, illness durations can last 2 years or more.

Diagnosis

The only way to definitively diagnose prion disease is through neuropathological examination. sCJD is characterized by the presence of spongiform changes, astrogliosis, and neuronal loss (Figure 12.2). Immunohistochemistry and Western blotting are used to further detect the abnormal isoform of the prion protein, which is characteristically resistant to proteinase K digestion. Tissue is usually obtained at postmortem analysis, although brain biopsies are occasionally performed to assist antemortem diagnosis.

A clinical diagnosis of sCJD is made on the basis of symptoms, physical examination findings, and three diagnostic tests. Current diagnostic criteria have been recently updated (Zerr et al., 2009) and are listed in Table 12.2. Any patient suspected of having prion disease should undergo a lumbar puncture (LP), EEG, and brain MRI to assist in diagnosis.

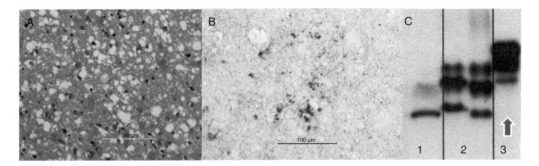

FIGURE 12.2 (*See color insert.*) Definite diagnosis of prion disease requires neuropathological examination. (A) Hematoxylin and eosin stain of the temporal lobe of a patient with prion disease. (B) Immunohistochemistry using 3F4 antibody of the hippocampus of a patient with prion disease. (C) Western blot of a brain homogenate subjected to proteinase K; lanes 1 and 2 display a PrP[27-30] band seen in prion disease compared to lane 3 from a normal control (arrow).

TABLE 12.2 Diagnostic Criteria for Sporadic Creutzfeldt–Jakob Disease

CLINICAL FINDINGS
1. Dementia 2. Cerebellar or visual impairment 3. Pyramidal or extrapyramidal symptoms 4. Akinetic mutism
DIAGNOSTIC TEST RESULTS
1. *EEG*: presence of periodic sharp wave complexes 2. *Cerebrospinal fluid*: presence of 14-3-3 protein *and* illness duration less than 2 years 3. *Brain MRI*: high signal abnormalities in the basal ganglia and/or at least two cortical areas (temporal, parietal, or occipital) on diffusion weighted imaging and/or fluid attenuated inversion recovery sequences
DIAGNOSTIC CRITERIA
Probable sCJD: at least two clinical findings and one diagnostic test result *Possible sCJD*: at least two clinical findings and an illness duration less than 2 years

sCJD, sporadic Creutzfeldt–Jakob disease.

Source: Zerr et al. (2009).

Cerebrospinal Fluid. Any patient with a rapidly progressive dementia should undergo a LP in order to rule out treatable etiologies (Appleby & Lyketsos, 2011). There are several markers that can assist in diagnosing prion disease. The 14–3-3 protein is found in all eukaryotic cells and is present in increased quantities within the cerebrospinal fluid (CSF) of patients with prion disease. Because of the ubiquitous nature of the protein, any pathological process that results in diffuse and rapid death of cells within the nervous system will result in increased 14–3-3 levels in the CSF. Although fairly sensitive, the 14-3-3 test lacks specificity, as several other CNS insults are capable of causing a false-positive test, including traumatic brain injury, seizures, and transverse myelitis. Although less common, false negatives can also occur and may be related to the stage of illness in which the test is performed (Geschwind et al., 2003). More centers are also starting to measure the CSF levels of total-tau protein (t-tau) to assist with the diagnosis of prion disease. Total tau levels are increased in sCJD and less so in AD (Bahl et al., 2009) and may be the most accurate current diagnostic test for sCJD, especially when combined with brain MRI (Satoh et al., 2007).

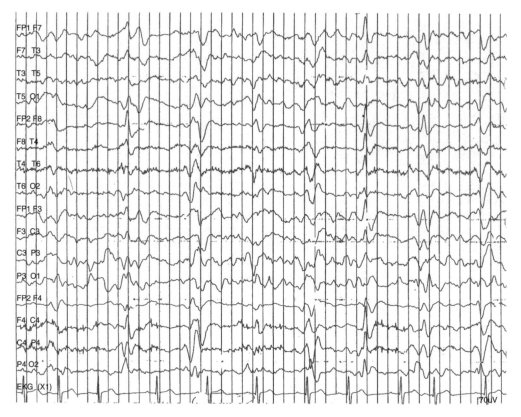

FIGURE 12.3 The "classic" EEG pattern observed in sporadic Creutzfeldt–Jakob disease: periodic sharp wave complexes.

Electroencephalogram. The use of the EEG in the diagnosis of sCJD was popularized following a manuscript published by Jones and Nevin in 1954 (Jones & Nevin, 1954). The "classic" EEG pattern of sCJD is periodic sharp wave complexes (PSWC) that recur every 0.5 to 2 seconds (Figure 12.3; Wieser, Schindler, & Zumsteg, 2006). The finding of PSWC on EEG is highly accurate and reliable (Steinhoff et al., 1996, 2004) but limited by the disease stage in which they are observed. Serial EEGs are often necessary to capture PSWCs. Over the duration of the illness, frontal intermittent rhythmic delta activity (FIRDA) is frequently seen early in the disease course, which later gives rise to PSWCs toward the later stages of the illness (Wieser et al., 2004).

Brain MRI. Readily available and noninvasive, the brain MRI has become one of the most important diagnostic tests to perform in patients with suspected prion disease. The most recent diagnostic criteria for sCJD were published in 2009 and included brain MRI findings for the first time (Zerr et al., 2009). Inclusion of brain MRI findings increased the diagnostic criteria sensitivity from 92.2% to 98% and retained a similar specificity of 70.8%. Brain MRI findings included high signal abnormalities in the caudate and/or putamen on diffusion weighted imaging (DWI) or fluid attenuated inversion recovery (FLAIR) sequences (Figure 12.4). High signal abnormalities within the cortical ribbon of at least two cortical regions (temporal, parietal, or occipital) were also highly suggestive of sCJD. Other cortical regions were not included in

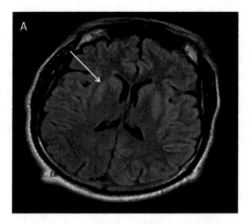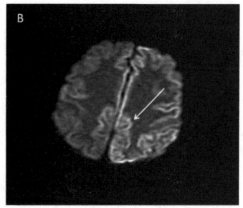

FIGURE 12.4 Brain MRI of a patient with CJD. (A) High signal abnormality in bilateral basal ganglia (arrow) on FLAIR. (B) High signal abnormality throughout the cortical ribbon (arrow) on DWI.

CJD, Creutzfeldt–Jakob disease; DWI, diffusion weighted imaging; FLAIR, fluid attenuated inversion recovery.

the criteria due to low specificity and low inter-rater agreement. False-positive brain MRIs were usually a result of infectious or inflammatory disorders, which would ideally be further characterized via CSF analyses.

Genetic Prion Diseases

The second largest group of human prion diseases is of genetic etiology, comprising 10% to 15% of all prion diseases. More than 40 mutations of the prion protein gene (*PRNP*) have been described to date (Kong, 2004) that include point, insertion, and deletion mutations. Genetic forms of prion disease generally occur in midlife and generally have longer illness durations. The majority of genetic prion diseases are of autosomal dominant inheritance with nearly complete penetrance. Age of disease onset, clinical presentation, disease course, and duration are often affected by the mutation site, which results in specific clinical phenotypes. Those mutations that resemble a classical CJD phenotype are termed genetic or familial CJD. Two other genetic prion disease phenotypes are acknowledged: GSS disease and FFI.

Genetic CJD

Genetic CJD (gCJD) is caused by several mutations of the *PRNP* gene that result in a clinical phenotype resembling that of classical CJD. The clinical phenotype is affected by the mutation type as well as the codon 129 polymorphism of the affected and sometimes unaffected allele. Subsequently, gCJD mutations are often expressed as haplotypes, listing the mutation and the codon 129 polymorphism of the affected allele (e.g., E200K-129M). Despite displaying similar phenotypes, there is a fair amount of clinical heterogeneity among cases with identical mutations. Diagnostic test results also differ among mutation types and are not as reliable as they are in detecting sCJD. Specific information pertaining to individual mutations and haplotypes can be found elsewhere (Gambetti, Parchi, & Chen, 2003; Kong, 2004).

GSS Disease

GSS is another genetic prion disease that displays a unique clinical and neuropathological phenotype. Several mutations of *PRNP* are known to cause GSS, the P102L mutation being the most common (Kong, 2004). The clinical phenotype is determined by mutation type, but most cases of GSS occur in middle age and present with cerebellar impairment that progresses to dementia in the advanced stages of the illness. GSS is also remarkable because of its prolonged survival time of 5 years on average and the presence of PrP-amyloid deposits that are most frequently located within the cerebellum.

Fatal Familial Insomnia

FFI is an autosomal dominant genetic prion disease caused by the D178N, 129M haplotype (Lugaresi et al., 1986). FFI shares the D178N *PRNP* mutation with gCJD, but it differs in the associated codon 129 polymorphism of the affected allele (Goldfarb et al., 1992). Hence, the D178N, 129M haplotype is believed to result in the unique clinical and neuropathological phenotype observed in FFI. Disease onset usually occurs in midlife, and disease duration ranges from months to several years (Kong, 2004). FFI is clinically recognized by intractable insomnia and dysautonomia early in the course of disease and dementia in advanced stages. EEG tracings demonstrate a lack of normal sleep architecture that is likely related to the preferential thalamic involvement of the disease. FDG-PET scans can detect thalamic hypometabolism in FFI mutation carriers prior to disease onset (Cortelli et al., 2006). Spongiform changes, prion protein deposition, neuronal loss, and astrogliosis likewise predominantly affect the thalamus with relative sparing of the neocortex (Parchi et al., 1995).

Acquired Prion Diseases

Acquired prion diseases occur when prion-infected tissue is introduced into an individual and subsequently causes prion disease. All forms of prion disease are potentially transmissible in specific circumstances. Kuru was the first acquired prion disease to be recognized and is covered earlier in this chapter. Other acquired prion diseases include iCJD and vCJD.

Iatrogenic CJD

iCJD is acquired prion disease from a medical intervention. Several routes of transmission have been described (see Table 12.3). All forms of iCJD, with the exception of secondarily transmitted vCJD, have been transmitted through CNS-related tissue contamination. No definitive transmission has been demonstrated through the peripheral nervous system or other organs.

There are several factors that are known to affect the transmission of iCJD. As previously noted, the route of administration has a large effect on transmissibility and incubation period. In general, central areas of contamination are more likely to result in transmission and have shorter incubation periods. For example, the mean incubation period of human growth hormone (hGH) and human pituitary-derived gonadotropins (15 and 13 years, respectively) are much longer than those observed in neurosurgery-related iCJD (Brown, Brandel, Preece, Preese, & Sato, 2006). In the cases of hGH and human pituitary-derived gonadotropin-associated iCJD cases,

TABLE 12.3 Recognized Causes of Iatrogenic Creutzfeldt–Jakob Disease

SURGICAL
1. Dura mater grafts
2. Neurosurgical instruments
3. EEG needles (depth electrodes)
4. Corneal transplants
ENDOCRINE
1. Human growth hormone (hGH)
2. Human pituitary-derived gonadotropins
HEMATOGENOUS[a]
1. Packed red blood cells
2. Plasma products[b]

[a]Hematogenous prion infectivity has only been observed in variant Creutzfeldt–Jakob disease.
[b]One case of asymptomatic infection (Peden et al., 2010).

Source: Brown et al. (2006).

incubation periods correlate with the infective dose amount (Brown et al., 2000). The affected individuals' genotype also influences the likelihood of transmission and incubation period. *PRNP* codon 129 homozygotes (Met-Met or Val-Val) are more predisposed to prion disease transmission, and they experience shorter incubation periods compared to heterozygotes (Met-Val; Brown et al., 1994, 2000).

The argument for prion "strains" is somewhat supported by the clinical presentation of iCJD cases, which most likely share the same contamination source with respect to their route of transmission. Cases of iCJD that were acquired via the same route share clinical similarities. For example, hGH-related cases of iCJD in the United Kingdom all demonstrated profound cerebellar impairment on initial presentation (Markus et al., 1992). Diagnostic test results are also similar to those observed in sCJD. This finding suggests that the initial sources of contamination for most cases of iCJD were index cases of sCJD. The notable exceptions to this are iCJD cases caused by blood transfusions from individuals who later developed vCJD. These blood transfusion recipients displayed initial psychiatric symptoms that are usually observed in cases of vCJD (Brown et al., 2006).

The incidence of iCJD has markedly declined over the years, and newly diagnosed cases have been the result of long incubation periods from previously recognized exposures. The scientific and medical understanding of prion diseases has likely contributed to increasing public health safety in this regard. Human-derived CNS tissue grafts and hormones have largely been replaced by synthetic alternatives, and decontamination practices in operating and mortuary suites have substantially reduced the likelihood of prion disease transmission (World Health Organization, 2003b, 2005). However, knowledge that vCJD can be transmitted between humans via novel routes raises new concerns regarding iCJD.

Variant CJD

vCJD, sometimes referred to as new vCJD, is the most recently recognized acquired prion disease in humans and also the only known zoonotic source of human prion disease. BSE is a prion disease found in cows that grew to epidemic proportions during the 1980s in the United Kingdom. In response, the United Kingdom reestablished a CJD surveillance center to monitor any changes that might occur in the frequency and/or characteristics of human prion disease. Through the surveillance center, Will and Ironside detected a cluster of unusual cases of prion disease (Will et al., 1996). Beginning in 1994, they started seeing cases with a much earlier age of onset (teens to early 30s) and prolonged illness durations of a year or more. These cases also presented with psychiatric symptoms (Zeidler, Johnstone et al., 1997). This new "variant" of CJD that was only observed in the United Kingdom at that time was of concern given the large exposure to BSE that the U.K. population had experienced a decade ago. Molecular analyses of the prion proteins implicated in the two diseases later confirmed that BSE was the likely source of vCJD (Collinge, Sidle, Meads, Ironside, & Hill, 1996).

Epidemiology

As of March 2011, there have been 220 documented cases of vCJD worldwide (www .cjd.ed.ac.uk/vcjdworld.htm). The majority of affected individuals are from the United Kingdom or believed to have acquired the disease while staying in the United Kingdom. The geographic distribution of vCJD cases corresponds to the exposure to BSE throughout the European countries. The incidence of vCJD has followed a bell-shaped curve, with the peak number of reported cases being around 2,000. The typical age of onset is characteristically younger than that for sCJD, with the majority of cases occurring at ages 20 to 35 years (Will, 2003). Similar to iCJD, *PRNP* codon 129 polymorphism affects an individual's predisposition to vCJD. Until recently, all cases were homozygous for methionine at codon 129 (Zeidler, Stewart, Cousens, Estibeiro, & Will, 1997). However, the report of a probable case of vCJD that was heterozygous at codon 129 raises concerns about further cases of vCJD in heterozygotes because of longer incubation periods as found in iCJD (Kaski et al., 2009; Valleron, Boelle, Chatignoux, & Cesbron, 2006).

Although the incidence of vCJD is declining, there is some concern about secondary transmission of the illness. Unlike other forms of prion disease, vCJD is transmissible between humans via blood transfusion. Four secondary transmissions of vCJD have been reported to date (www.cjd.ed.ac.uk/TMER/TMER.htm). Three were symptomatic cases of vCJD that were homozygous for methionine at codon 129. Incubation periods varied from 5 to 8 years. The fourth transmission occurred in an individual who was heterozygous at codon 129 and found to be asymptomatically harboring vCJD on postmortem analysis after dying from an unrelated condition. Several epidemiological studies examining lymphoreticular tissue in the United Kingdom have also raised concerns that a proportion of the population may be asymptomatically infected with vCJD (Clewley et al., 2009; Hilton et al., 2004).

Clinical Presentation and Course

Several clinical characteristics distinguish vCJD from other prion diseases. In addition to its young age of onset, the vast majority of vCJD presents with psychiatric symptoms (Will et al., 1996). Depression, anxiety, and apathy are very common in vCJD, and psychotic symptoms and insomnia are also frequently observed (Zeidler, Johnstone et al., 1997). Sensory symptoms are often described early in the disease course and include dysesthesia and painful sensations (Will et al., 1996). Dementia usually occurs late in the illness. The average disease duration in vCJD is 13 months, approximately twice as long as sCJD (Will, 2003).

Diagnosis

Definitive diagnosis of vCJD is made via pathological examination. vCJD is charac-terized by multiple "florid plaques" that occur in the cerebral and cerebellar cortex and distinct pericellular prion protein deposits (Ironside, 1998). Because vCJD accu-mulates in lymphoreticular tissue, tonsil biopsies can also be performed to achieve a pathological diagnosis.

Diagnostic test results in vCJD differ markedly from those expected in sCJD. None of the initially described cases of vCJD would have met diagnostic criteria for CJD (Will et al., 1996). EEG tracings do not display the typical PSWC pattern observed in classical CJD. CSF 14–3-3 detection lacks the sensitivity (50%) seen in sCJD but maintains equal specificity (Green, 2002). Thus, the positive predictive value of 14-3-3 is high in vCJD (86%), but a negative result does not exclude the diagnosis of vCJD. Brain MRI is the most useful test in vCJD, but the findings differ from those seen in classical CJD. vCJD is characterized by signal abnormalities in the pulvinar nucleus of the thalamus, frequently referred to as the "pulvinar sign" (Zeidler et al., 2000). The pulvinar sign is 78% sensitive and approaches 100% specificity, although this finding has also been described in sCJD (Petzold et al., 2004) and iCJD (Wakisaka et al., 2006).

Treatment

Prion disease is a rapidly progressive and ultimately fatal illness with no currently known treatment. Consequently, symptom management and family and caregiver support and education are crucial as they can help reduce disease burden and maxi-mize quality of life.

Several experimental treatments have been attempted without success. Quinacrine has been the most widely studied treatment for prion disease and was ineffective in three separate trials. Pentosan polysulfate has been used in several case series and case studies with mixed results, but it appears to have possibly slowed the progression of some specific cases. Because it does not cross the blood–brain bar-rier, pentosan polysulfate must be given intraventricularly, which has limited its use and investigation as a possible treatment for prion disease. Finally, doxycycline is currently being investigated as a potential treatment in an international prospective double-blind study. Preliminary results suggest that doxycycline may slow disease progression and its effectiveness may be affected by codon 129 polymorphisms. Further information on investigational treatments of prion disease can be found in multiple reviews on the subject (Appleby & Lyketsos, 2011; Brown, 2009; Riemer et al., 2008; Trevitt & Collinge, 2006; Zerr, 2009).

SUMMARY

The TSEs form a group of illnesses, characterized by a pathological form of the native prion protein, which results in a rapidly progressive neurodegenerative illness. Variations have been noted across many species, including humans. Three forms of TSEs present in humans—CJD, GSS syndrome, and FFI—with CJD representing the most common of the three. The human prion diseases have three etiologies: (a) spo-radic, (b) genetic, and (c) acquired. Variations of human prion diseases exist based on their biological origins. Across all the human prion diseases, diagnosis can only be confirmed on pathology. The human prion diseases are fatal, being resistant to treat-ment. While therapies are not available to treat the disease, symptom management and family support can reduce the burden.

REFERENCES

Alper, T., Cramp, W. A., Haig, D. A., & Clarke, M. C. (1967). Does the agent of scrapie replicate without nucleic acid? *Nature, 214*(5090), 764–766.

Alper, T., Haig, D. A., & Clarke, M. C. (1966). The exceptionally small size of the scrapie agent. *Biochemical and Biophysical Research Communications, 22*(3), 278–284.

Appleby, B. S., Appleby, K. K., Crain, B. J., Onyike, C. U., Wallin, M. T., & Rabins, P. V. (2009). Characteristics of established and proposed sporadic Creutzfeldt-Jakob disease variants. *Archives of Neurology, 66*(2), 208–215.

Appleby, B. S., Appleby, K. K., & Rabins, P. V. (2007). Does the presentation of Creutzfeldt-Jakob disease vary by age or presumed etiology? A meta-analysis of the past 10 years. *The Journal of Neuropsychiatry and Clinical Neurosciences, 19*(4), 428–435.

Appleby, B. S., & Lyketsos, C. G. (2011). Rapidly progressive dementias and the treatment of human prion diseases. *Expert Opinion on Pharmacotherapy, 12*(1), 1–12.

Bahl, J. M., Heegaard, N. H., Falkenhorst, G., Laursen, H., Høgenhaven, H., Mølbak, K.,... Christiansen, M. (2009). The diagnostic efficiency of biomarkers in sporadic Creutzfeldt-Jakob disease compared to Alzheimer's disease. *Neurobiology of Aging, 30*(11), 1834–1841.

Barria, M. A., Mukherjee, A., Gonzalez-Romero, D., Morales, R., & Soto, C. (2009). De novo generation of infectious prions in vitro produces a new disease phenotype. *PLoS Pathogens, 5*(5), e1000421.

Beck, E., Daniel, P. M., Alpers, M., Gajdusek, D. C., & Gibbs, C. J. (1966). Experimental "kuru" in chimpanzees. A pathological report. *Lancet, 2*(7472), 1056–1059.

Brown, D. R., Clive, C., & Haswell, S. J. (2001). Antioxidant activity related to copper binding of native prion protein. *Journal of Neurochemistry, 76*(1), 69–76.

Brown, P. (2009). A historical perspective on efforts to treat transmissible spongiform encephalopathy. *CNS & Neurological Disorders Drug Targets, 8*(5), 316–322.

Brown, P., & Bradley, R. (1998). 1755 and all that: A historical primer of transmissible spongiform encephalopathy. *BMJ, 317*(7174), 1688–1692.

Brown, P., Brandel, J. P., Preece, M., Preese, M., & Sato, T. (2006). Iatrogenic Creutzfeldt-Jakob disease: The waning of an era. *Neurology, 67*(3), 389–393.

Brown, P., Gibbs, C. J., Rodgers-Johnson, P., Asher, D. M., Sulima, M. P., Bacote, A.,...Gajdusek, D. C. (1994). Human spongiform encephalopathy: The National Institutes of Health series of 300 cases of experimentally transmitted disease. *Annals of Neurology, 35*(5), 513–529.

Brown, P., Preece, M., Brandel, J. P., Sato, T., McShane, L., Zerr, I.,...Collins, S. J. (2000). Iatrogenic Creutzfeldt-Jakob disease at the millennium. *Neurology, 55*(8), 1075–1081.

Brownell, B., & Oppenheimer, D. R. (1965). An ataxic form of subacute presenile polioencephalopathy (Creutzfeldt-Jakob disease). *Journal of Neurology, Neurosurgery, and Psychiatry, 28*, 350–361.

Büeler, H., Aguzzi, A., Sailer, A., Greiner, R. A., Autenried, P., Aguet, M., & Weissmann, C. (1993). Mice devoid of PrP are resistant to scrapie. *Cell, 73*(7), 1339–1347.

Clewley, J. P., Kelly, C. M., Andrews, N., Vogliqi, K., Mallinson, G., Kaisar, M.,...Gill, O. N. (2009). Prevalence of disease related prion protein in anonymous tonsil specimens in Britain: Cross sectional opportunistic survey. *BMJ, 338*, b1442.

Collinge, J., Sidle, K. C., Meads, J., Ironside, J., & Hill, A. F. (1996). Molecular analysis of prion strain variation and the aetiology of "new variant" CJD. *Nature, 383*(6602), 685–690.

Collinge, J., Whittington, M. A., Sidle, K. C., Smith, C. J., Palmer, M. S., Clarke, A. R., & Jefferys, J. G. (1994). Prion protein is necessary for normal synaptic function. *Nature, 370*(6487), 295–297.

Collins, S., Law, M. G., Fletcher, A., Boyd, A., Kaldor, J., & Masters, C. L. (1999). Surgical treatment and risk of sporadic Creutzfeldt-Jakob disease: A case-control study. *Lancet, 353*(9154), 693–697.

Cortelli, P., Perani, D., Montagna, P., Gallassi, R., Tinuper, P., Provini, F.,...Gambetti, P. (2006). Pre-symptomatic diagnosis in fatal familial insomnia: Serial neurophysiological and 18FDG-PET studies. *Brain, 129*(Pt 3), 668–675.

Creutzfeldt, H. G. (1920). Über eine eigenartige herdförmige Erkrankung des Zentralnervensystems (vorläufige Mitteilung). *Zeitschrift für die gesamte Neurologie und Psychiatrie, 57,* 1–18.

Cuillé, J., & Chelle, P. (1936). La maladie dite "tremblante" du moutons; est-elle inoculable? *Comptes Rendus à l'Académie des Sciences, 203,* 1552.

Davanipour, Z., Alter, M., Sobel, E., Asher, D., & Gajdusek, D. C. (1985). Creutzfeldt-Jakob disease: Possible medical risk factors. *Neurology, 35*(10), 1483–1486.

Gabizon, R., McKinley, M. P., Groth, D., & Prusiner, S. B. (1988). Immunoaffinity purification and neutralization of scrapie prion infectivity. *Proceedings of the National Academy of Sciences of the United States of America, 85*(18), 6617–6621.

Gajdusek, D. (1979). *Observations on the early history of kuru investigation. Slow transmissible diseases of the nervous system* (Vols. 1–2, Vol. 1, pp. 7–35). London: Academic Press, Inc.

Gajdusek, D. C., Gibbs, C. J., & Alpers, M. (1966). Experimental transmission of a Kuru-like syndrome to chimpanzees. *Nature, 209*(5025), 794–796.

Gajdusek, D. C., & Zigas, V. (1957). Degenerative disease of the central nervous system in New Guinea; the endemic occurrence of kuru in the native population. *The New England Journal of Medicine, 257*(20), 974–978.

Gambetti, P., Parchi, P., & Chen, S. G. (2003). Hereditary Creutzfeldt-Jakob disease and fatal familial insomnia. *Clinics in Laboratory Medicine, 23*(1), 43–64.

Geschwind, M. D., Martindale, J., Miller, D., DeArmond, S. J., Uyehara-Lock, J., Gaskin, D.,... Miller, B. L. (2003). Challenging the clinical utility of the 14-3-3 protein for the diagnosis of sporadic Creutzfeldt-Jakob disease. *Archives of Neurology, 60*(6), 813–816.

Gibbs, C. J., Gajdusek, D. C., Asher, D. M., Alpers, M. P., Beck, E., Daniel, P. M., & Matthews, W. B. (1968). Creutzfeldt-Jakob disease (spongiform encephalopathy): Transmission to the chimpanzee. *Science, 161*(3839), 388–389.

Goldfarb, L. G., Petersen, R. B., Tabaton, M., Brown, P., LeBlanc, A. C., Montagna, P.,... Pendelbury, W. W. (1992). Fatal familial insomnia and familial Creutzfeldt-Jakob disease: Disease phenotype determined by a DNA polymorphism. *Science, 258*(5083), 806–808.

Gordon, W. S. (1946). Advances in veterinary research. *The Veterinary Record, 58*(47), 516–525.

Green, A. J. (2002). Use of 14-3-3 in the diagnosis of Creutzfeldt-Jakob disease. *Biochemical Society Transactions, 30*(4), 382–386.

Griffith, J. S. (1967). Self-replication and scrapie. *Nature, 215*(5105), 1043–1044.

Hadlow, W. J. (1959). Scrapie and kuru. *The Lancet, 274*(7097), 289–290.

Heidenhain, A. (1929). Klinische und anatomische Untersuchungen uber eine eigenartige organische Erkrankung des Zentralnervensystems im Praesenium. *Zeitschrift für die gesamte Neurologie und Psychiatrie, 118,* 49–114.

Hilton, D. A., Ghani, A. C., Conyers, L., Edwards, P., McCardle, L., Ritchie, D.,...Ironside, J. W. (2004). Prevalence of lymphoreticular prion protein accumulation in UK tissue samples. *The Journal of Pathology, 203*(3), 733–739.

Holman, R. C., Belay, E. D., Christensen, K. Y., Maddox, R. A., Minino, A. M., Folkema, A. M.,...Schonberger, L. B. (2010). Human prion diseases in the United States. *PloS One, 5*(1), e8521.

Ironside, J. W. (1998). Neuropathological findings in new variant CJD and experimental transmission of BSE. *FEMS Immunology and Medical Microbiology, 21*(2), 91–95.

Jakob, A. (1921). Uber eine der multiplen Sklerose klinisch nahestehende Erkrankung des Zentralnervensystems (spastische Pseudosklerose) mit bemerkenswertem anatomischem Befunde. Mitteilung eines vierten Falles. *Medizinische Klinik, 17,* 372–376.

Jones, D. P., & Nevin, S. (1954). Rapidly progressive cerebral degeneration (subacute vascular encephalopathy) with mental disorder, focal disturbances, and myoclonic epilepsy. *Journal of Neurology, Neurosurgery, and Psychiatry, 17*(2), 148–159.

Kaski, D., Mead, S., Hyare, H., Cooper, S., Jampana, R., Overell, J.,...Rudge, P. (2009). Variant CJD in an individual heterozygous for PRNP codon 129. *Lancet, 374*(9707), 2128.

Kim, J. I., Cali, I., Surewicz, K., Kong, Q., Raymond, G. J., Atarashi, R.,...Surewicz, W. K. (2010). Mammalian prions generated from bacterially expressed prion protein in the absence of any mammalian cofactors. *The Journal of Biological Chemistry, 285*(19), 14083–14087.

Kirschbaum, W. R. (1968). *Jakob-Creutzfeldt disease: (Spastic pseudosclerosis, A. Jakob; Heidenhain syndrome; subacute spongiform encephalopathy).* New York: American Elsevier Pub. Co.

Kocisko, D. A., Come, J. H., Priola, S. A., Chesebro, B., Raymond, G. J., Lansbury, P. T., & Caughey, B. (1994). Cell-free formation of protease-resistant prion protein. *Nature, 370*(6489), 471–474.

Kong, Q. (2004). *Inherited prion diseases. Prion biology and disease* (2nd ed., pp. 673–775). Cold Spring Harbor, NY: Cold Spring Harbor Laboratory Press.

Koperek, O., Kovács, G. G., Ritchie, D., Ironside, J. W., Budka, H., & Wick, G. (2002). Disease-associated prion protein in vessel walls. *The American Journal of Pathology, 161*(6), 1979–1984.

Linden, R., Martins, V. R., Prado, M. A., Cammarota, M., Izquierdo, I., & Brentani, R. R. (2008). Physiology of the prion protein. *Physiological Reviews, 88*(2), 673–728.

Lugaresi, E., Medori, R., Montagna, P., Baruzzi, A., Cortelli, P., Lugaresi, A.,...Gambetti, P. (1986). Fatal familial insomnia and dysautonomia with selective degeneration of thalamic nuclei. *The New England Journal of Medicine, 315*(16), 997–1003.

Mahillo-Fernandez, I., de Pedro-Cuesta, J., Bleda, M. J., Cruz, M., Mølbak, K., Laursen, H.,... Siden, A.; EUROSURGYCJD Research Group. (2008). Surgery and risk of sporadic Creutzfeldt-Jakob disease in Denmark and Sweden: Registry-based case-control studies. *Neuroepidemiology, 31*(4), 229–240.

Markus, H. S., Duchen, L. W., Parkin, E. M., Kurtz, A. B., Jacobs, H. S., Costa, D. C., & Harrison, M. J. (1992). Creutzfeldt-Jakob disease in recipients of human growth hormone in the United Kingdom: A clinical and radiographic study. *The Quarterly Journal of Medicine, 82*(297), 43–51.

Masters, C., & Gajdusek, D. (1982). *The spectrum of Creutzfeldt-Jakob disease and the virus-induced subacute spongiform encephalopathies. Recent advances in neuropathology* (pp. 139–163). Edinburgh, Scotland: Churchill Livingstone.

Nevin, S., McMenemey, W. H., Behrman, S., & Jones, D. P. (1960). Subacute spongiform encephalopathy—a subacute form of encephalopathy attributable to vascular dysfunction (spongiform cerebral atrophy). *Brain: A Journal of Neurology, 83,* 519–564.

Parchi, P., Castellani, R., Capellari, S., Ghetti, B., Young, K., Chen, S. G.,...Gambetti, P. (1996). Molecular basis of phenotypic variability in sporadic Creutzfeldt-Jakob disease. *Annals of Neurology, 39*(6), 767–778.

Parchi, P., Castellani, R., Cortelli, P., Montagna, P., Chen, S. G., Petersen, R. B.,...Sheller, J. R. (1995). Regional distribution of protease-resistant prion protein in fatal familial insomnia. *Annals of Neurology, 38*(1), 21–29.

Parchi, P., Giese, A., Capellari, S., Brown, P., Schulz-Schaeffer, W., Windl, O.,...Kretzschmar, H. (1999). Classification of sporadic Creutzfeldt-Jakob disease based on molecular and phenotypic analysis of 300 subjects. *Annals of Neurology, 46*(2), 224–233.

Peden, A., McCardle, L., Head, M. W., Love, S., Ward, H. J., Cousens, S. N.,...Ironside, J. W. (2010). Variant CJD infection in the spleen of a neurologically asymptomatic UK adult patient with haemophilia. *Haemophilia, 16*(2), 296–304.

Petzold, G. C., Westner, I., Bohner, G., Einhäupl, K. M., Kretzschmar, H. A., & Valdueza, J. M. (2004). False-positive pulvinar sign on MRI in sporadic Creutzfeldt-Jakob disease. *Neurology, 62*(7), 1235–1236.

Pocchiari, M., Puopolo, M., Croes, E. A., Budka, H., Gelpi, E., Collins, S.,...Will, R. G. (2004). Predictors of survival in sporadic Creutzfeldt-Jakob disease and other human transmissible spongiform encephalopathies. *Brain: A Journal of Neurology, 127*(Pt 10), 2348–2359.

Prusiner, S. B. (1982). Novel proteinaceous infectious particles cause scrapie. *Science, 216*(4542), 136–144.

Prusiner, S. B., Groth, D. F., Bolton, D. C., Kent, S. B., & Hood, L. E. (1984). Purification and structural studies of a major scrapie prion protein. *Cell, 38*(1), 127–134.

Prusiner, S. B., Groth, D., Serban, A., Stahl, N., & Gabizon, R. (1993). Attempts to restore scrapie prion infectivity after exposure to protein denaturants. *Proceedings of the National Academy of Sciences of the United States of America, 90*(7), 2793–2797.

Rambold, A. S., Müller, V., Ron, U., Ben-Tal, N., Winklhofer, K. F., & Tatzelt, J. (2008). Stress-protective signalling of prion protein is corrupted by scrapie prions. *The EMBO Journal, 27*(14), 1974–1984.

Riemer, C., Burwinkel, M., Schwarz, A., Gültner, S., Mok, S. W., Heise, I.,...Baier, M. (2008). Evaluation of drugs for treatment of prion infections of the central nervous system. *The Journal of General Virology, 89*(Pt 2), 594–597.

Roucou, X., Gains, M., & LeBlanc, A. C. (2004). Neuroprotective functions of prion protein. *Journal of Neuroscience Research, 75*(2), 153–161.

Saborio, G. P., Permanne, B., & Soto, C. (2001). Sensitive detection of pathological prion protein by cyclic amplification of protein misfolding. *Nature, 411*(6839), 810–813.

Satoh, K., Shirabe, S., Tsujino, A., Eguchi, H., Motomura, M., Honda, H.,...Eguchi, K. (2007). Total tau protein in cerebrospinal fluid and diffusion-weighted MRI as an early diagnostic marker for Creutzfeldt-Jakob disease. *Dementia and Geriatric Cognitive Disorders, 24*(3), 207–212.

Soto, C., Estrada, L., & Castilla, J. (2006). Amyloids, prions and the inherent infectious nature of misfolded protein aggregates. *Trends in Biochemical Sciences, 31*(3), 150–155.

Steinhoff, B. J., Räcker, S., Herrendorf, G., Poser, S., Grosche, S., Zerr, I.,...Weber, T. (1996). Accuracy and reliability of periodic sharp wave complexes in Creutzfeldt-Jakob disease. *Archives of Neurology, 53*(2), 162–166.

Steinhoff, B. J., Zerr, I., Glatting, M., Schulz-Schaeffer, W., Poser, S., & Kretzschmar, H. A. (2004). Diagnostic value of periodic complexes in Creutzfeldt-Jakob disease. *Annals of Neurology, 56*(5), 702–708.

Trevitt, C. R., & Collinge, J. (2006). A systematic review of prion therapeutics in experimental models. *Brain: A Journal of Neurology, 129*(Pt 9), 2241–2265.

Valleron, A. J., Boelle, P. Y., Chatignoux, E., & Cesbron, J. Y. (2006). Can a second wave of new variant of the CJD be discarded in absence of observation of clinical non Met-Met cases? *Revue d'épidémiologie et de Santé Publique, 54*(2), 111–115.

Wakisaka, Y., Santa, N., Doh-ura, K., Kitamoto, T., Ibayashi, S., Iida, M., & Iwaki, T. (2006). Increased asymmetric pulvinar magnetic resonance imaging signals in Creutzfeldt-Jakob disease with florid plaques following a cadaveric dura mater graft. *Neuropathology, 26*(1), 82–88.

Wieser, H. G., Schindler, K., & Zumsteg, D. (2006). EEG in Creutzfeldt-Jakob disease. *Clinical Neurophysiology, 117*(5), 935–951.

Wieser, H. G., Schwarz, U., Blättler, T., Bernoulli, C., Sitzler, M., Stoeck, K., & Glatzel, M. (2004). Serial EEG findings in sporadic and iatrogenic Creutzfeldt-Jakob disease. *Clinical Neurophysiology, 115*(11), 2467–2478.

Will, R. G. (2003). Acquired prion disease: Iatrogenic CJD, variant CJD, kuru. *British Medical Bulletin, 66*, 255–265.

Will, R. G., Ironside, J. W., Zeidler, M., Cousens, S. N., Estibeiro, K., Alperovitch, A., ... Smith, P. G. (1996). A new variant of Creutzfeldt-Jakob disease in the UK. *Lancet, 347*(9006), 921–925.

World Health Organization. (2003a). *WHO manual for surveillance of human transmissible spongiform encephalopathies including variant Creutzfeldt-Jakob disease.* Geneva, Switzerland: World Health Organization.

World Health Organization. (2003b). *WHO consultation on transmissible spongiform encephalopathies (TSE) in relation to biological and pharmaceutical products.* Geneva, Switzerland: World Health Organization.

World Health Organization. (2005). *WHO guidelines on tissue infectivity distribution in transmissible spongiform encephalopathies.* Geneva, Switzerland: World Health Organization.

Zeidler, M., Johnstone, E. C., Bamber, R. W., Dickens, C. M., Fisher, C. J., Francis, A. F., ... Will, R. G. (1997). New variant Creutzfeldt-Jakob disease: Psychiatric features. *Lancet, 350*(9082), 908–910.

Zeidler, M., Sellar, R. J., Collie, D. A., Knight, R., Stewart, G., Macleod, M. A., ... Colchester, A. F. (2000). The pulvinar sign on magnetic resonance imaging in variant Creutzfeldt-Jakob disease. *Lancet, 355*(9213), 1412–1418.

Zeidler, M., Stewart, G., Cousens, S. N., Estibeiro, K., & Will, R. G. (1997). Codon 129 genotype and new variant CJD. *Lancet, 350*(9078), 668.

Zerr, I. (2009). Therapeutic trials in human transmissible spongiform encephalopathies: Recent advances and problems to address. *Infectious Disorders Drug Targets, 9*(1), 92–99.

Zerr, I., Kallenberg, K., Summers, D. M., Romero, C., Taratuto, A., Heinemann, U., ... Sanchez-Juan, P. (2009). Updated clinical diagnostic criteria for sporadic Creutzfeldt-Jakob disease. *Brain: A Journal of Neurology, 132*(Pt 10), 2659–2668.

CHAPTER 13

Dementia Pugilistica and Chronic Traumatic Encephalopathy

Dominic A. Carone and Shane S. Bush

Dementia pugilistica (DP) is a form of chronic traumatic encephalopathy (CTE) that involves gross impairment of cognitive and motor functioning due to repetitive blows to the head from boxing. The word *pugilistica* is Latin for *boxer*. The term *dementia pugilistica* was coined by Millspaugh (1937) in an effort to develop more specific, nonderisive diagnostic terminology. Until that time, boxers with the condition were commonly referred to as *punch drunk*, a term that originated with the title of Martland's (1928) classic article, the first formal scientific description of the physical effects of repetitive boxing-induced traumatic brain injuries. In that article, Martland described a cluster of characteristic signs and symptoms (e.g., confusion, bradykinesia, tremors, gait disturbance) in boxers that had previously been observed by laymen.

DP symptoms typically emerge between 7 and 35 years after the beginning of a boxer's career, and the symptoms usually are not experienced until after a boxer's career ends (Clausen, McCrory, & Anderson, 2005; Roberts, 1969). DP was initially observed in 17% of retired professional boxers. However, the nature of the sport has changed over the years, with a corresponding change in DP prevalence. The mean number of years a boxer competes dropped from 19 years in 1931 to 5 years in 2002, and the mean number of fights declined from 336 to 13. These changes in competitive boxing over the years represent a considerable decrease in exposure to head injury for contemporary boxers.

Chances of developing DP increase proportionately to boxing exposure (Jordan, et al., 1997; Roberts, 1969). Risk factors include retiring after age 28 years, boxing more than 10 years, participating in more than 150 bouts, and greater sparring exposure. Additionally, the risk of developing DP increases for boxers who have a history of technical knockout (TKO) or knockout (KO; Jordan et al., 1997), those who are "sluggers" rather than "scientific boxers" (Critchley, 1957), and those with the apolipoprotein epsilon 4 allele (ApoE4; Jordan et al., 1997). The risk of DP in amateur boxers is substantially lower (Loosemore, Knowles, & Whyte, 2007).

There are essentially two general types of blows to the head that occur in contact sports: rotational blows and translational blows. A rotational blow is one that is not directed at the center of gravity. As a result of the rotational acceleration, the force of the blow is amplified by the angular momentum, which adds to the acceleration. For this reason, rotational blows are more likely to cause brain injury than translational blows in which the impact is directed to the center of gravity of a freely movable mass (Friedman, 1989). When a blow strikes the head, there is increased pressure in the part of the brain closest to the injury and a relative decrease in the contrecoup region, with pressure waves initially moving back and forth inside the skull.

MIXED MARTIAL ARTS

Rapidly increasing in popularity among fight fans and fighters is mixed martial arts (MMA). With increasing acceptance of MMA, manifested by more than a dozen events held annually, the popularity of the major promotion (Ultimate Fighting Championship) has reached enormous levels since it began in the early 1990s, generating more than $222,766,000 in pay-per-view revenue in 2006, which is a record for pay-per-view events (Colella, 2007). In MMA, the potential for neurological injury exists from striking (using upper and lower extremities), choking, or throwing an opponent. Martial arts that involve striking the opponent (e.g., boxing, kickboxing, karate, and taekwondo) have higher incidences of injury than nonstriking combat arts (e.g., wrestling; Bledsoe, Hsu, Grabowski, Brill, & Li, 2006).

To date, there has been extremely little scientific study of the neurological effects of MMA. Buse (2006) determined that, of 642 bouts reviewed, approximately 28% were stopped because of head impact, 17% because of musculoskeletal stress, 13% because of a neck choke, and approximately 27% because of miscellaneous trauma, which included fighter submission due to head strikes. When including asphyxiation due to neck choke, more than 40% of bouts were stopped because of conditions that potentially affected the brain. These injury rates do not take into account concussive or hypoxic brain injuries that were sustained but did not result in the bouts ending.

A similar observational study of 175 MMA bouts found that the most common ending to a fight was a TKO (26.1%) followed by decisions (24.5%; Bush & Myers, 2008). Overall, 13% of fights ended in a knockout. The TKO/KO rate suggests that many fighters are susceptible to incurring at least mild traumatic brain injuries (MTBIs). Additionally, different weight class fighters are at different risks for sustaining brain trauma (defined by KO or TKO), with heavyweight fighters showing the greatest risk (Bush & Myers, 2009). Furthermore, heavyweight fights were least likely to end in a decision, suggesting that they are at greater risk of overall injury. These findings may have implications for differences in return to fight status, as a function of weight class. Although similarities between boxing and MMA may be expected, much more research is needed before statements about the neurological and neuropsychological effects of MMA can be made with confidence.

TERMINOLOGY

The title of Martland's paper *Punch Drunk* (and the associated term *punch drunk syndrome*) became a colloquial synonym for DP, as did the term *slap happy* (Lacava, 1963). In fact, these terms are still used occasionally in a colloquial sense. Over time, DP has been referred to by many other names, such as *boxer's encephalopathy* (Bogdanoff & Natter, 1989; Lacava, 1963; Wegner, 1963); *boxer's dementia* (Naccache, Slachevsky, Deweer, Habert, & Dubois, 1999); *chronic traumatic brain injury associated with (or in) boxing* (CTBI-B; Jordan, 2000; Jordan et al., 1997); and more recently, *chronic traumatic encephalopathy* (Cantu, 2007; McCrory, Zazryn, & Cameron, 2007; McKee et al., 2009). Although DP and CTE are sometimes used interchangeably, the former is typically used to refer to repetitive brain injuries from boxing, whereas the latter is generally considered a broader term used to refer to repetitive, often subclinical (e.g., asymptomatic), injury to the brain from a variety of contact sports and other causes.

In the area of sport-related concussion, there are two other frequently used terms that are necessary to distinguish from DP and CTE: *postconcussion syndrome* (PCS) and *second impact syndrome* (SIS). PCS is a term used to refer to patients who continue to report persistent nonspecific symptoms after a concussion, typically for 3 or more months. In current scientific nomenclature, a concussion is also known as MTBI. However, in the early to mid-1900s it was common for moderate and severe TBIs to also be referred to as concussions (McCown, 1959), although this is no longer the case. Although TBIs in professional boxing may encompass a mixture of mild, moderate, and severe TBIs, those that occur in football and other noncombat sports are typically of the mild variety. As a result, the chronic effects of multiple TBIs at various severity levels would be expected to exceed the effects of chronic MTBIs. This provides a theoretical rationale for why DP and CTE should be considered as potentially distinct clinical entities rather than synonymous.

Unlike DP, PCS does not involve dementia or localizing neurological signs. In the vast majority of cases, the etiology of PCS is presumed to be related to factors other than the direct neurological effects of concussion. Such factors include psychiatric disorders, psychosomatization, unrelated medical conditions, medication side effects, substance abuse, malingering/exaggeration, psychosocial distress, iatrogenesis, and misperceptions (Iverson, Zasler, & Lange, 2006; McCrea, 2008).

SIS is a controversial term that refers to an exceedingly rare, sudden, and catastrophic (often fatal) neurological condition in youth, during which the athlete rapidly undergoes neurological decompensation (i.e., impaired autoregulation of cerebral vasculature leading to diffused cerebral swelling and brain herniation) after a second concussive injury before complete recovery from the first injury (Bey & Ostick, 2009; Saunders & Harbaugh, 1984). However, some professionals view the term as misleading and question whether SIS exists at all once objective and evidence-based criteria are applied to anecdotally reported cases in the literature (McCrory, 2001).

SIGNS AND SYMPTOMS

The classical clinical signs and symptoms of DP include combinations of dysarthria, incoordination, gait disturbance, pyramidal and extrapyramidal dysfunction, and cognitive impairment (Martland, 1928). Martland's first reported case of DP was a 38-year-old man who boxed from age 16 years to 23 years, quitting due to a tremor in his left hand and unsteadiness in his legs. The man was known to have been knocked out twice, once as long as an hour. He had a staggering and propulsive gait, masked facial expression, stammering and hesitant speech, and fine tremors of the hands and tongue. Martland specifically stated that he believed that his patient suffered from a parkinsonian syndrome. His intelligence was described as "normal" although no formal test results were provided.

Critchley (1957) reported that the neuropsychological deficits of DP are insidious in onset and include emotional lability, progressively slower speech and thought, and significant memory decline. Mendez (1995) reported deficits in processing speed, complex attention, sequencing, memory, executive functions, and finger tapping speed. Motor symptoms include pyramidal, extrapyramidal, and/or cerebellar signs (Jordan, 2000), although some case reports failed to identify the classic motor dysfunction of DP (Rochon, 1994). Motor abnormalities, when present, may progress to ataxia, spasticity, impaired coordination, and parkinsonism.

Very few studies have examined the neuropsychological functioning of professional boxers. One study of professional boxers found that neurocognitive tests measuring planning, attention, concentration, and memory were the most sensitive to brain dysfunction (McLatchie et al., 1987). Another study of professional boxers found neurocognitive test scores 1 month after their bouts to be *better* than their baseline scores, possibly because pre-bout factors such as sparring, cutting weight, and anxiety may have interfered with true baseline abilities (Ravdin, Barr, Jordan, Lathan, & Relkin, 2003).

Neuropsychological investigation of amateur boxers revealed very few neurocognitive deficits (Moriarity et al., 2004; Porter, 2003; Porter & Fricker, 1996; Stewart et al., 1994; Timm, Wallach, Stone, & Ryan, 1993). One study examined amateur boxers participating in multiple bouts during a 7-day tournament and found no evidence of cognitive dysfunction in the immediate post-bout period, except for boxers whose bouts were stopped by the referee (Moriarity et al., 2004). Another study that monitored 20 amateur boxers over a 9-year period found no evidence of decreased neurocognitive test performance; rather, the boxers evidenced significantly better performance over time compared to age-matched controls (Porter, 2003). Similarly, Porter and Fricker (1995) did not find neuropsychological impairment in amateur boxers compared with controls, and found no association between neuropsychological performance and boxing exposure. Timm et al. (1993), having studied boxing safety, determined that serious injuries occur very rarely and that amateur boxing is generally a safe sport.

When neurocognitive deficits were detected in amateur boxers, they occurred primarily in attention, concentration, memory, and motor speed (Brooks, Kupshik, Wilson, Galbraith, & Ward, 1987). Ring experience was associated with greater neuropsychological deficits, but the magnitude of the deficits was considered mild, relative to normative control groups. Neuropsychological tests were found to be more sensitive than other examination procedures (e.g., neurological examination, CT scan, EEG) in the detection of neurological problems in amateur boxers (Ross, Cole, Thompson, & Kim, 1983). Based on these findings, Butler, Forsythe, Beverly, and Adams (1993) concluded that amateur boxing within carefully controlled durations appears to be neuropsychologically safe.

Because of the latency of symptom onset in DP and the symptom overlap with other dementias (e.g., Alzheimer's disease [AD], Parkinson's disease), a primary diagnostic question involves determining whether the neurological dysfunction is best attributed to boxing (Bush & Myers, 2012). To help address diagnostic challenges, Jordan (1993) proposed a symptom-based classification system of the likelihood (probable, possible, or improbable) of neurological dysfunction being caused by boxing. Jordan et al. (1997) also developed a 10-point CTBI rating scale to classify the severity of neurological injury in boxing, based on cognitive, motor, and behavioral symptoms.

NEUROPATHOLOGY AND INJURY MECHANISMS

Based on behavioral observations, neuropathological studies, and autopsy findings of patients with traumatic cerebral hemorrhages, Martland (1928) hypothesized that repeat concussions in boxing caused hemorrhages in the deeper portions of the cerebrum (i.e., caudate, putamen, globus pallidus) due to a displacement of cerebrospinal fluid (CSF) by the effects of contrecoup injury into the perivascular spaces traversing along the vessels supplying these structures (Cassasa, 1924; Osnato & Giliberti, 1927). He also hypothesized that the hemorrhages would be replaced by gliosis or degeneration of these areas, which explained why the late stages of the disease mimicked parkinsonism, and he believed that hemorrhages would almost never be seen in the cerebral cortex or cerebellum. Martland noted that some colleagues doubted the existence of the condition, and he raised concerns that some boxers may try to malinger the condition for undue compensation.

Less than a decade later, Martland's hypothesis began to receive confirmation from other scientists (Carroll, 1936; Critchley, 1937; Jokl & Guttman, 1933; Millspaugh, 1937; Parker, 1934; Winterstein, 1937). Case reports of DP continued to emerge mid-century, such as a German study of a 51-year-old boxer with an 18-year career who developed signs of dementia, parkinsonism, and pathological changes (e.g., cerebral atrophy and an unusually large number of senile plaques, especially in the hippocampus) reminiscent of AD (Brandenburg & Hallervorden, 1954). This boxer was the first known case of DP to undergo autopsy, and the findings were interpreted as a special form of posttraumatic dementia with parkinsonism. Some criticized the findings as a chance association and conceptually criticized the delay between boxing cessation and symptom onset (as reported by Neubuerger, Sinton, & Denst, 1959). However, further neuropathological support came via additional case studies (Courville, 1962; Grahmann & Ule, 1957; Neubuerger et al., 1959; Payne, 1968) followed by a report on the Medical Aspects of Boxing of the Royal College of Physicians of London in 1969 by A.H. Roberts (as cited in Corsellis, Bruton, & Freeman-Browne, 1973). With these studies came the proposition that delayed symptom onset can indeed be a feature of DP due to a slowly progressive disease course.

Although these initial studies laid an important foundation for the conceptualization of DP, it was not until the classic neuropathological study of 15 retired boxers by Corsellis, Bruton, and Freeman-Browne (1973) that the defining neuropathological features of DP were described. Those features are as follows: (a) abnormalities (cavum, fenestrations) of the septum pellucidum (a thin membrane separating the lateral ventricles); (b) scarring on the inferior surface of the lateral cerebellar lobes (mostly in the tonsillar region), with loss of Purkinje cells in these areas; (c) degeneration of the substantia nigra with loss of pigmentation, neurofibrillary changes, and the absence of Lewy bodies; and (d) diffuse neurofibrillary tangles in the cerebral cortex (mostly medial temporal) and brain stem, with very few, if any, senile plaques. Thus, Martland's original hypotheses of basal ganglia damage was confirmed, and advances in microscopic pathological analyses led to a refining of his theory.

Additionally, studies revealed a consistent pattern of ventriculomegaly of the third and lateral ventricles, cerebral atrophy, abnormalities of the septum pellucidum, scarring of the cerebellum, depigmentation of the substantia nigra with neuronal loss, and diffuse neurofibrillary tangles with variable amounts of amyloid plaques depending on the study technique (Casson et al., 1984; Corsellis et al., 1973; Martland, 1928; Morrison, 1986; Payne, 1968; Roberts, 1969; Ross et al., 1983).

METHODS AND MEDIA

Some media reports about concussion and the potential link between repetitive concussions and long-term problems include eye-catching and emotionally provocative titles. However, sensationalistic media reports are often loosely linked to scientific evidence.

Professional Boxing

There is no case that brought the possible neurological dangers of chronic brain damage from professional boxing more into the public consciousness than that of Muhammad Ali. Ali was a world-famous three-time heavyweight champion who fought professionally for 21 years (1960–1981). He became a cultural icon not only for his lightning-fast reflexes but also for his quick-witted rhyming insults of opponents communicated through the media. Some of his fights involved him suffering considerable physical punishment from the likes of Joe Frazier, George Foreman, Larry Holmes, and others. Boxing historians consider his progressive physical decline in boxing to date back to 1975 (Encyclopedia Britannica, 2009). Three years after his last fight (a loss), Ali was diagnosed with Parkinson's disease. The man who once claimed to "float like a butterfly and sting like a bee" was no longer capable of walking without assistance due to severe bradykinesia, tremors, and shuffling gait. His verbal diatribes ended, replaced by masked facial expressions, slurred speech, hypophonia, and markedly restricted verbal output.

In July 1981, Ali was evaluated at the Mayo Clinic because of worsening symptoms. Interestingly, he was cleared to fight by the physicians who evaluated him at the time. The examining physicians stated that his speech was soft and mumbling but nonpathological and that his EEG and brain CT scan were negative. While a brain CT scan at New York University (NYU) Medical Center in July 1981 was read as negative, and a team of 30 physicians at NYU, Mayo Clinic, and the University of California Los Angeles stated there was no evidence of brain damage (attributing his speech problems to a psychosocial response), Dr. Ira Casson (an outside neurologist) firmly disagreed. He stated that the brain CT showed clear evidence of a cavum septum pellucidum and enlarged ventricles for Ali's age (Boyle & Ames, 1983). Around the same time, while being interviewed on British Broadcasting Corporation (BBC) radio, most of his words were so incomprehensible that the interview was cancelled for rebroadcast (Boyle & Ames, 1983).

The public statements to the media about Ali's condition were very different from what was actually written in the famous Mayo Report, which for years had never been formally released despite numerous requests. However, Ali finally decided to allow a biographer to obtain a copy of the report. As it turns out, the actual brain CT report was consistent with Dr. Casson's interpretation of a cavum septum pellucidum (Hauser, 1998). It was also noted that Ali was not hopping with expected agility and was slightly dysmetric on finger to nose testing.

Some professionals have argued that Ali does not have DP due to an absence of cognitive deficits. However, we are unaware of any formal neuropsychological test results that would confirm or refute this assumption. In fact, it is not clear that such testing was ever performed, but it is known that such tests were not performed at NYU (Boyle & Ames, 1983). On one of his neurological examinations, he was reportedly diagnosed with organic mental syndrome, which suggests that he performed poorly on some type of cognitive testing (Boyle & Ames, 1983). The Mayo Report states that he had difficulty with his speech and memory (Hauser, 1998), but it is unclear if such abilities were formally tested. It is difficult to form definitive conclusions about his mental status based on his public appearances because he rarely speaks. Although Parkinson-like changes are a characteristic of DP (likely due to substantia nigra damage), some skeptics have challenged whether boxing had anything to do with his condition and whether he would have developed Parkinson's disease regardless of his profession.

Professional Football

Although the first medical advisory board for boxing dates back to one appointed by New York Governor Thomas Dewey in 1948 (McCown, 1959), the concern regarding repeat concussions on the health of professional football players did not formally begin until the early 1990s. Specifically, in 1992 and 1994, two National Football League (NFL) players (Al Toon and Merrill Hoge, respectively) retired from symptoms reported to be the direct result of repeat concussions. Then NFL Commissioner Paul Tagliabue (2003) created a committee on MTBI and appointed former New York Jets team physician Elliot Pellman (2003) as the committee chair.

Although the NFL's MTBI Committee produced a series of articles in the journal *Neurosurgery* that covered areas such as helmet impacts and impact velocity (Pellman, Powell, et al., 2004; Pellman, Lovell, Viano, & Casson, 2006; Pellman, Viano, Tucker, & Casson, 2003; Viano, Pellman, Withnall, & Shewchenko, 2006); biomechanics (Viano, Casson, & Pellman, 2007; Viano & Pellman, 2005; Viano et al., 2005); brain trauma simulation (Viano et al., 2005); epidemiology and characteristics of single and repeat concussive injuries (Pellman, Powell, et al., 2004; Pellman, Viano, Casson, Tucker, Waekerle, Powell, & Feuer, 2004; Pellman, Viano, Casson, Arfken, & Feuer, 2005; Pellman, Viano, Casson, Arfken, & Powell, 2004); and the neuropsychological effects of concussion (Pellman et al., 2006; Pellman, Lovell, Viano, Casson, & Tucker, 2004), none of the studies were autopsy studies of deceased NFL players thought to be neurologically compromised from repeat concussions.

The main criticisms of the existence of CTE in professional football players have come from former NFL MTBI Committee members Drs. Ira Casson, Eliott Pellman, and David Viano (Casson, 2010; Casson, Pellman, & Viano, 2006a, 2006b, 2009). The MTBI Committee members have continuously stressed that the evidence for CTE in professional football players is limited because the data is based on isolated case reports and survey data with significant methodological limitations. However, the number of reported cases continues to grow, with the Boston research group reporting 68 cases of CTE out of 81 patients studied who were former athletes ($n = 64$; football, boxing, or hockey); military veterans ($n = 21$); and a patient with self-inflicted head injuries ($n = 1$; McKee et al., 2013). In addition, the first Major League Baseball player (Ryan Freel) to be diagnosed with CTE had a career that reportedly involved a very high number of concussive injuries and head traumas (Smith & Moriarty, 2013). In a smaller sample of six retired professional football players from Canada, researchers outside of the Boston research group found CTE in half of the cases (Hazrati et al., 2013). The authors pointed to the need for prospective research designs to better understand the relationship between multiple concussions and CTE, and the risk factors that may mediate the relationship between the two, because they did not believe that a definitive link between multiple concussions and CTE could be established at the time.

Neuropathologically, the former NFL MTBI Committee members listed previously pointed out that the autopsy findings in many CTE cases are not consistent with those of boxers in the classic study by Corsellis et al. (1973). Indeed, CTE appears to be unique based on the location of neuropathology (in the grey matter and perivascular space at the depth of the sulci) and the different distribution of tau-immunoreactive astrocytes with a relative scarcity of beta-amyloid plaques (Gardner, Iverson, & McCrory, 2014; McCrory, Meeuwisse, Kutcher, Jordan, & Gardner, 2013). Autopsy studies have revealed inconsistent neuropathological findings, with the cases being complicated by comorbid cardiovascular disease, psychiatric disorders, brain injuries of varying severities, epilepsy, and developmental delays (Geddes, Vowles, Nicoll, & Révész, 1999; Geddes, Vowles, Robinson, & Sutcliffe, 1996; Omalu et al., 2005, 2006; see Tables 13.1 and 13.2). Many

TABLE 13.1 Summary of Details From the First 11 Professional Sports Players Tested for CTE Whose Results Were Released to the Media

NAME (INITIALS)	AGE	RACE	YEARS PLAYED PROFESSIONALLY	FOOTBALL POSITION OR SPORT	COMPLICATING FACTORS	TESTING FOR CTE
M.W.	50	W	16	C	Anabolic steroid use; history of marked physical abuse; depression; repeatedly stunned himself into unconsciousness with a Taser gun to fall asleep; would not eat for days at a time; chronic use of Ritalin, Dexedrine, Paxil, Prozac, Ultram, Darvocet, Vicodin, Lorcet, and Eldepryl; extensive liver and kidney damage, and heart ailments (coronary atherosclerotic disease with stenting); never treated for a concussion or complained of concussive symptoms during playing career; financial ruin; legal troubles (Garber, 2005a, 2005b, 2005c, 2005d; Omalu et al., 2005)	Positive
T.L.	45	AA	7	OL	Suicide by drinking antifreeze; prior suicide attempt with rat poison; anabolic steroid use; psychiatric disorder characterized by severe major depression, paranoia, agitation, and mood fluctuations; multiple psychiatric hospitalizations; hyperthyroidism with thyroidectomy; business failings; automobile accident during playing career; under federal indictment at time of death (Associated Press [AP], 2006; Omalu et al., 2006)	Positive
A.W.	44	AA	9	DB	Died of gunshot wound to the head; depression, particularly about low-level college coaching jobs and inability to become NFL coach; only small fragments of brain analyzed (Scheiber, 2006; Schwarz, 2007a)	Positive
J.S.	36	W	9	OL	Died of brain injury from MVA; history of anabolic steroid use; chronic marijuana use; often excessive alcohol use; no known prior concussion history; depression; possible undiagnosed bipolar disorder/psychosis; extensive psychosocial stressors (Schwarz, 2007b; Shapiro, 2004)	Positive
J.G.	45	W	9	LB	None known but only one medically documented concussion (Daniloff, 2009)	Positive
T.M.	45	W	8	OG	Overdose of oxycodone and cocaine as well as alcohol combined with Xanax; polysubstance abuse including alcohol; depression (Astleford, 2008; Schwarz, 2009; ScienceDaily, 2009)	Positive

G.S.	52	AA	8	CB	Very little information available although found dead while intoxicated (Laskas, 2009).	Positive
C.W.	39	W	5	C	History of crystal methamphetamine and alcohol abuse (Associated Press [AP], 2008)	Positive
D.N.	24	AA	1	RB	None known; believed to have died of cardiogenic cause; no drugs or alcohol found in his system (Klis, 2007)	Negative
M.B.	42	W	0	WR	Died of alcohol, cocaine, and oxycontin overdose; history of alcohol abuse, pain killer abuse, and other drug abuse (Robertson, 2009)	Positive
C.B.	40	W	22	PW	Died via hanging; Xanax, hydrocodone; high levels of synthetic testosterone in blood upon death; history of anabolic steroid use and alcohol abuse (O'Connor, 2007)	Positive

AA, African American; C, center; CB, cornerback; CTE, chronic traumatic encephalopathy; DB, defensive back; LB, linebacker; MVA, motor vehicle accident; OG, offensive guard; OL, offensive lineman; NFL, National Football League; PW, professional wrestling; RB, running back; W, White; WR, wide receiver.

TABLE 13.2 Common and Contrasting Features of Two Reported Cases of Chronic Traumatic Encephalopathy in Two Retired National Football League Players

CHARACTERISTICS	PATIENT 1	PATIENT 2
Age at death	50 years	45 years
Approximate age when decedent was drafted into the NFL	22 years	25 years
Duration of professional play in the NFL	17 years	8 years
Approximate duration of play of football in high school, college, and/or in the military	5 years	6 years
Interval between retirement from the NFL and death	12 years	12 years
History and diagnosis of major depressive disorder after retirement from the NFL	Present	Present
Gross atrophy of the brain and hydrocephalus ex vacuo	Absent	Absent
Fenestrations of the septum pellucidum	Absent	Absent
Cavum septi pellucidi	Absent	Present
Presence of diffuse amyloid plaques	Present	Absent
Presence of NFTs and NTs	Present	Present
ApoE genotype	E3/E3	E3/E4
Postmortem diagnosis of coronory atherosclerotic disease	Present	Present
Premortem history of steroid use	Present	Present

ApoE, apolipoprotein E; NFL, National Football League; NFTs, neurofibrillary tangles; NTs, neuropil threads.

This table, originally presented in Omalu et al. (2006), is reproduced with permission from Wolters Kluwer.

of the patients who were considered to have CTE based on autopsy were those who died of a neurological cause (e.g., hanging, gunshot wound, drug overdose, severe traumatic brain injury) or who had other potential neurological comorbidities such as polysubstance abuse and anabolic steroid use. Casson (2010) noted that retired football players are not immune to the multiple risk factors and diseases that are associated with dementia in the general population. Some cases were only presented through media press releases and press conferences as opposed to scientific peer-reviewed journal articles (e.g., Hohler, 2009).

Numerous recent critiques have been published on CTE outside of the NFL's former MTBI Committee members. For details, see Gardner et al. (2014); Iverson (2014); Karantzoulis and Randolph (2013); McCrory et al. (2013); Rapp (2013); Wortzel, Brenner, and Arciniegas (2013); and Wortzel, Shura, and Brenner (2013). These critiques make the following points based on systematic reviews of the literature:

1. Pathological studies of CTE are all derived from case studies that are samples of convenience, and some were only presented via media press releases.
2. There is still no published epidemiological prospective or cross-sectional studies on CTE.
3. There is insufficient evidence to conclude that there is a strong causal relationship between CTE and suicide (e.g., basic criteria regarding consistency, temporality, strength, specificity, and coherence of the association has not been met) and current claims of an association between the two involve circular and overly reductionistic reasoning.

4. Most published CTE cases did not die from a neurodegenerative cause but from another cause (unlike in most neurodegenerative diseases).
5. There are numerous other factors or mediating factors that can lead to suicide in patients with a history of repetitive brain/head trauma.
6. There is a significant number of published CTE cases (37%) with pathological comorbidity.
7. Clinical features alone cannot be used to diagnose CTE (as 20%–50% of cases with clinical features suspected of CTE have revealed no neuropathology on autopsy).
8. That the clinical phenotype of CTE is unclear and extremely diverse, overlapping with numerous psychiatric and other neuropathological conditions.
9. The degree to which the underlying neuropathology contributes to the clinical presentation is uncertain.
10. Characterization of CTE in the literature has not adequately considered plausible differential diagnoses and other moderating variables that can explain the presentation.
11. Recent neuropsychological research (Hart et al., 2013; Randolph, Karantzoulis, & Guskiewicz, 2013) comparing retired NFL players showed highly similar neuropsychological profiles to nonathletes diagnosed with mild cognitive impairment (MCI; suggesting that non-CTE factors such as decreased cognitive reserve were responsible) and that none fit the reported profile for CTE.
12. It is unknown if similar or identical neuropathological findings will be found in patients that do not have CTE but share clinical characteristics with CTE, as there are many conditions in which tau aggregation is observed.
13. Causal assumptions between concussions and "subconcussive" impacts and the development of CTE are premature and scientifically unproven and
14. A possible genetic contribution to the neuropathology has not been determined.

Proponents of CTE maintain that while much still needs to be learned about it, it is a genuine and unique neurological condition caused by repetitive MTBIs, and that comorbid neuropathology may be caused by repetitive brain/head trauma (McKee et al., 2013). In fact, McKee et al. (2009) reported that the evidence that repetitive subtle brain trauma causes CTE is "overwhelming" and that the condition often develops before clinical symptoms manifest. Clinical symptoms of CTE are said to involve memory disturbance, parkinsonism, speech abnormalities, gait abnormalities, and changes in behavior and personality. The classic neuropathological features are said to involve cerebral and medial temporal lobe atrophy, ventriculomegaly, enlarged cavum septum pellucidum, and extensive tau-immunoreactive pathology throughout the neocortex, temporal lobe, diencephalon, brain stem, and spinal cord. However, McKee et al. (2009) acknowledged that the plaques and neurofibrillary tangles in reported CTE cases are immunocytochemically identical to those in AD. For a detailed four-stage description of evolving histopathological classifications of CTE compared with dementia pugilistica, see Karantzoulis and Randolph, (2013). In a recent research development, in response to calls (e.g., Casson, 2010) for an in vivo means of diagnosing abnormal brain tau levels in living and retired athletes, Small et al. (2013) reported that a special PET technique identified higher brain tau levels in living retired NFL members compared to controls. However, because the study only involved five players and lacked autopsy confirmation of CTE, the results are considered preliminary at this time. See Tables 13.1 and 13.2 for more detailed information about the complexity of identified cases.

Studies that found neuropsychological symptoms or neuropsychological deficits often suffered from methodological problems, including retrospective report of injury characteristics by the athlete or others, failure to control for confounding variables, attribution of cognitive deficits to isolated low test scores, and failure to consider base rates of neuropsychological symptoms in healthy and general medical populations. Recent studies have shown that normal test performance is easily overpathologized (Brooks, Iverson, Holdnack, & Feldman, 2008; Brooks, Iverson, & White, 2007; Schretlen, Munro, Anthony, & Pearlson, 2003; Schretlen, Testa, Winicki, Pearlson, & Gordon, 2008). In addition, poor effort on neuropsychological testing will lead to invalid and unreliable data (Bush et al., 2005; Green, 2007; Heilbronner, Sweet, Morgan, Larrabee, & Millis, 2009), and very few studies of athletes have included formal measures of symptom validity.

Sometimes, case reports on CTE have been used to draw other pathological inferences that have been quite controversial. A relatively recent example was the autopsy study of two former professional football players and one boxer in which an association was reported between repetitive concussions and the development of CTE and motor neuron disease (McKee et al., 2010). The study suggested that these athletes did not actually have amyotrophic lateral sclerosis (ALS, also known as Lou Gehrig's disease) but instead had a similar motor neuron disease caused by repeated concussions. While Lou Gehrig is not discussed in the actual study, in a *New York Times* article (Schwarz, 2010) about the study, the lead author of the study was quoted as saying, "Here he is, the face of his disease, and he may have had a different disease as a result of his athletic experience" (multiple concussions).

The aforementioned comment led several ALS specialists to publish a joint critique stating that such an inference is a vast overgeneralization of the data and caused anxiety and confusion among patients and families struggling with the disease who expressed concern that they may have been misdiagnosed (Armon & Miller, 2011; Bedlack et al., 2011; Rowland, Mitsumoto, & Hays, 2010; Scelsa, 2010). In a reply to Drs. Armon, Miller, Bedlack, and colleagues, the original study authors apologized for any anguish caused by the comment in the media, but reported an opposite experience of families expressing encouragement, relief, and support of their research.

Historical Parallels

The historical parallels between the current CTE controversy and prior controversies regarding DP are striking. The most well-known article in this regard was by McCown (1959) who was director of the New York State Athletic Commission. McCown criticized the media for unduly publicizing boxing deaths because it only served to "confuse and prejudice the thinking of fair-minded observers and officials" (p. 510), furthering an agenda of those who traditionally opposed boxing in any form. In making this point, McCown was distinguishing between advocacy and science. He believed that the term *punch drunk* had become a slick medical cliché for those who wished to label any boxer whose behavior and performance in or out of the ring was abnormal or not satisfactory. Essentially, he believed the term was being overused and overgeneralized.

Based on his review study of 11,173 boxers, McCown (1959) stated that he did not find a single case of punch drunk syndrome. Although he did not deny that boxing can injure the brain, he denied the existence of a *distinct* neurological syn-drome peculiar to former boxers. He stated that EEG patterns of boxers were prob-ably more due to factors inherent in the person rather than occupational pursuit. Similarly, after examining more than 1,000 professional boxers, Kaplan and Browder (1954) did not find any neurological abnormalities at ringside or during a detailed examination after the bout, including cases where there was a KO. Wright (1965) questioned that boxing caused punch drunk syndrome due to the delayed onset of symptoms and because he stated that identical symptoms could be caused by alco-holism and venereal diseases, two conditions that were common in boxers at the time. However, Corsellis et al. (1973) later countered that the neuropathology of deceased boxers is not observed as the result of other diseases in the brains of non-boxers. In another parallel to the current NFL concussion controversy (see next section), the Medical Advisory Committee of the German Amateur Boxing Association repeat-edly announced that the dangers of boxing are no greater than that of soccer or track and field (as reported by Unterharnscheidt, 1995). In contrast, those holding views that denied the existence of DP were referred to as blind partisans and ostriches who refused to notice the facts and who belittled findings opposed to their own ideas (Unterharnscheidt, 1995).

DEMENTIA RISK FROM NON-SPORTS TBI

As with sports concussion studies, research regarding a possible link between demen-tia and MTBI in the non-sports literature is beset by methodological problems. A primary problem involves the use of retrospective research designs. Additionally, a tendency to generalize the results from studies of persons who sustained moderate-to-severe TBIs to those who sustained mild injuries is problematic. The findings from MTBI and moderate-to-severe TBI studies are not interchangeable (McCrea, 2008). Although a study by Plassman et al. (2000) has been used as evidence to support the notion that TBI is associated with increased risk of dementia, the study showed an increased risk of AD among patients with moderate TBI (hazard ratio [HR] = 2.32) and severe TBI (HR = 4.51), but found that MTBI did not pose a significant risk for AD or dementia compared to a non-head-injured control group.

Fleminger, Oliver, Lovestone, Rabe-Hesketh, and Giora (2003) performed a sys-tematic review of the literature and reported an association between previous his-tory of excess head injury and AD. The findings were specific to a group of males who had sustained moderately severe TBI (odds ratio [OD] = 2.29); it specifically excluded patients with "lesser head injuries" who had not lost consciousness. Wilson (2003) noted that each of the 15 case-controlled studies reviewed by Fleminger suf-fered from significant weaknesses in that they relied on the report of an informant to determine the existence and severity of a head injury with loss of consciousness in the person's lifetime. A *severe* TBI may be a risk factor for AD, especially in those lack-ing the ApoE4 allele (Jellinger, Paulus, Wrocklage, & Litvan, 2001a, 2001b). Overall, despite common assumptions, research has yet to establish an association between MTBI in nonathletes and the development of AD. The importance of clearly differen-tiating TBI severity levels in such studies cannot be overemphasized.

DEMENTIA RISK FROM AGING

Aging boxers, like the general population, experience increased risk of neuropsy-chological problems with increased age. The most common type of dementia, AD, is characterized by neuronal degeneration and an accumulation of neurofibrillary plaques and tangles that begins in the temporal-parietal regions and advances anteriorly (Braak & Braak, 1991). The disease progression clinically coincides with a slowly progressive decline in memory, other cognitive functions (i.e., executive functioning, visual-spatial skills), physical functioning (e.g., motor functions), and personality (Cummings, 2004). Both men and women with the e4 allele of the *ApoE* gene on chromosome 19 are more likely to develop AD (Farrer et al., 1997; Green et al., 2002). Attempting to determine the cause of neuropsychological problems in aging former boxers must take into account the multiple risk factors for neuropsychological problems in older adults.

NEUROPSYCHOLOGICAL ASSESSMENT AND CONSULTATION

Protocols for the assessment and management of sports-related MTBIs have been proposed for a variety of sports, although boxing has received relatively little attention from neuropsychology (for reviews, see Echemendia, 2006; Slobounov & Sebastianelli, 2006). Such programs emphasize the importance of closely monitoring the signs and symptoms of MTBI, including the use of standardized neurocognitive tests, by appropriately trained health care professionals. Although some clinicians advocate for widespread baseline neuropsychological testing of athletes preseason or before competition, followed by serial postconcussion reevaluations and symptom-free waiting periods, comprehensive literature reviews have found that the need for such rigid protocols is not scientifically supported (McCrea et al., 2009; Randolph & Kirkwood, 2009; Randolph, McCrea, & Barr, 2005). Randolph and Kirkwood (2009) concluded that "serious short-term consequences of sport-related concussion are extremely rare and unlikely to be significantly modified *via* management strategies that rely on baseline testing. Other less serious short-term adverse outcomes are also quite rare, transient, and not likely to be altered by specific management guidelines" (p. 512).

Moser et al. (2007) stated, "Neuropsychologists are uniquely qualified to assess the neurocognitive and psychological effects of concussion. The National Academy of Neuropsychology recommends neuropsychological evaluation for the diagnosis, treatment, and management of sports-related concussion at all levels of play" (p. 909). The use of traditional clinical neuropsychological measures to assess the cognitive and emotional functioning of the rare athlete with persisting postconcussive symptoms appears to be a sound approach. Individual clinical decision making appears to be indicated in the neuropsychological assessment and management of boxers.

SAFETY PRECAUTIONS AND TREATMENT

It has been suggested that there is a "critical period" for optimal recovery from MTBI (Prins, Lee, Cheng, Becker, & Hovda, 1996), and returning to training and contact prior to the completion of that recovery period may place fighters at greater risk of subsequent, and possibly more significant, neurological injury (Cantu, 1992). Although the vast majority of sports-related MTBIs seem to resolve completely within days or weeks of the injury, approximately 3% to 5% of athletes appear to have physical, emotional, and/or neurocognitive symptoms that persist beyond 1 month (see McCrea, 2008, for a review). Although waiting periods, such as those mandated by state athletic commissions, for return to competition following MTBI may be beneficial for injured fighters, such guidelines or requirements should be empirically based, maximizing fighter safety without being overly restrictive.

DP symptoms may be treated with the pharmacological agents that are used to treat similar symptoms of other neurological disorders. For example, patients with parkinsonian symptoms may benefit from antiparkinsonism medications (Jordan, 2000). Cholinergic agents and psychotropic medications have yet to be studied for treatment of DP. Because of the lack of empirical support in treating DP, prevention is of primary importance and should include close monitoring of fighters who have risk factors for neurological signs and the use of additional protective equipment such as is used in amateur boxing (Bush & Meyers, 2012).

ETHICAL CONSIDERATIONS

Numerous ethical issues emerge at the intersection of sports, including boxing, and clinical neuropsychology. Bush and Iverson (2010) identified the following ethical issues to be of particular relevance in sports concussion practice: (a) Conflicts of interest in research and program development; (b) competence; (c) bases for scientific and professional judgments; (d) relationship and roles; (e) test selection, use, and interpretation; (f) privacy, confidentiality, and informed consent; and (g) avoidance of false or deceptive statements. Perhaps most importantly, clinicians must consider that the practice of clinical neuropsychology with athletes may have outpaced the supporting science.

Although the safety of athletes is of primary concern, the careers of clinicians should not be built on the promotion of scientifically unsupportable fears or rigid evaluation and management protocols. Athletes have the right to receive information about what is scientifically known and unknown about safety risks and evaluation and treatment options so that they can make informed decisions about their participation in the sport. Neuropsychologists have an obligation to provide that information as accurately and objectively as possible.

FUTURE DIRECTIONS

Continued research is essential for better understanding the neuropsychological effects of, and contributions for, boxing. Such research must address the methodological limitations of many of the previous studies. Prospective research designs and control of potentially confounding factors (including anabolic steroid abuse) are particularly important. The National Academy of Neuropsychology (Heilbronner et al., 2009) recommended the following:

> Although empirical data to answer many questions is still lacking, the available evidence provides some useful information to design methods (e.g., reduced number of rounds and bouts, rule changes) and equipment (e.g., head gear) to improve professional boxing safety. It is recommended that researchers examine high-risk variables such as the number of bouts and sparring matches, previous concussions, age of the fighter, genetic profile, frequency of head blows, and velocity of punches, and identify whether there is a critical number of fights, KOs, or punches that result in cerebral and neurocognitive compromise. (p. 17)

Although a number of medical associations have called for boxing to be banned (e.g., American Academy of Neurology, American Medical Association, British Medical Association, World Medical Association; Hagell, 2000), public interest and athlete participation continue to demonstrate the long-standing relevance of the sport. Calls to ban boxing discount the essential human right to freedom of choice and self-determination for competent adults.

SUMMARY

DP is a neurological condition involving a cluster of characteristic motor, neuropsychiatric, neurocognitive, and neuropathological findings due to chronic brain damage from boxing. Whereas no serious scientific debate currently exists regarding the existence of DP, primarily due to classical studies by Corsellis et al. (1973) and Casson et al. (1984), such debate remains about the precise etiology of a similarly proposed condition—CTE in professional football players, professional wrestlers, and other professional athletes exposed to repeat concussions and head trauma.

Controversy also exists about the association, if any, between concussions and dementia. The debate is largely due to numerous methodological limitations such as retrospective study designs, incomplete case histories, confounding factors that require future study (e.g., the neuropathological effects of anabolic steroid abuse and/or interactions with concussions), and an overreliance on self-report data. Unlike the era when DP was initially studied, we now live in an age where the media sometimes serves as the initial and primary means to disseminate scientific findings. In cases of reported CTE, this is sometimes accompanied by advocacy commentary that has the potential to stifle competing scientific inquiries, criticism, and/or skepticism, such as by suggesting that those who raise such issues are participating in a conspiracy with the NFL. At the same time, one needs to be careful not to deny outright the possibility that CTE is a legitimate clinical entity. While CTE may indeed exist, we believe that the available evidence to date suggests a multifactorial etiology rather than a single etiology (e.g., repetitive head/brain trauma).

Controversies aside, it is clear that professional and nonprofessional athletes are exposed to a risk of concussive head trauma, particularly in contact sports, and that efforts should be made to reduce repeated concussive injuries. Advances in helmet technology and other protective equipment, rule changes, and the use of pre- and postinjury neuropsychological testing are all methods that are currently being utilized to decrease concussive and repeat concussive risk. However, the only way to completely eliminate concussive risk in sports is to ban the sport itself, an extreme measure that we do not believe is practical.

In closing, this chapter has provided an overview of the many complex issues surrounding the effects of repeat concussive trauma, particularly in sports. This is a continuously evolving area that has received intense interest from scientists, the media, and laypersons. We strongly support efforts to improve the protective headgear technology and the reliability, validity, and the psychometric soundness of neuropsychological assessment measures in sports concussion management. We do not recommend that case study findings be released to the media before they have undergone scientific peer review. Although scientific peer review can be a timely process and is not without its flaws, it is the best current method to ensure that our knowledge base increases through the scientific method. In closing, we agree with researchers who have called for large, prospective, longitudinal, clinico-pathological studies to gain a better understanding of CTE followed by blinded neuropathological studies of athletes and controls (Gardner et al., 2014; Karantzoulis & Randolph, 2013; McCrory et al., 2013; Wortzel, Brenner, & Arciniegas, 2013).

REFERENCES

Armon, C., & Miller, R. G. (2011). Correspondence regarding: TDP-43 proteinopathy and motor neuron disease in chronic traumatic encephalopathy. J Neuropathol Exp Neurol 2010:69; 918–929. *Journal of Neuropathology and Experimental Neurology, 70*(1), 97–98; author reply 98.

Associated Press (AP). (2006). *Ex-steeler Long drank antifreeze to commit suicide*. Retrieved March 12, 2009, from http://sports.espn.go.com/nfl/news/story?id=2307003

Associated Press (AP). (2008). *Former NFL center Curtis Whitley dead at 39*. Retrieved May 12, 2008, from www.bostonherald.com/sports/football/other_nfl/view .bg?articleid=1094041&srvc=rss

Astleford, A. (2008). *Seeking relief, McHale's life took a fatal turn*. Retrieved September 9, 2008, from www.washingtonpost.com/wp-dyn/content/story/2008/11/08/ST2008110802509 .html

Bedlack, R. S., Genge, A., Amato, A. A., Shaibani, A., Jackson, C. E., Kissel, J. T., ... Mozaffar, T. (2011). Correspondence regarding: TDP-43 proteinopathy and motor neuron disease in chronic traumatic encephalopathy. J Neuropathol Exp Neurol 2010:69;918–929. *Journal of Neuropathology and Experimental Neurology, 70*(1), 96–97; author reply 98.

Bey, T., & Ostick, B. (2009). Second impact syndrome. *The Western Journal of Emergency Medicine, 10*(1), 6–10.

Bledsoe, G. H., Hsu, E. B., Grabowski, J. G., Brill, J. D., & Li, G. (2006). Incidence of injury in professional mixed martial arts competitions. *Journal of Sports Science & Medicine, 5*(CSSI), 136–142.

Bogdanoff, B., & Natter, H. M. (1989). Incidence of cavum septum pellucidum in adults: A sign of boxer's encephalopathy. *Neurology, 39*(7), 991–992.

Boyle, R. H., & Ames, W. (1983). *Too many punches, too little concern*. Retrieved February 18, 2010, from http://sportsillustrated.cnn.com/vault/article/magazine/MAG1120728/4/ index.htm

Braak, H., & Braak, E. (1991). Neuropathological stageing of Alzheimer-related changes. *Acta Neuropathologica, 82*(4), 239–259.

Brandenburg, W., & Hallervorden, J. (1954). [Dementia pugilistica with anatomical findings]. *Virchows Archiv, 325*(6), 680–709.

Brooks, B. L., Iverson, G. L., Holdnack, J. A., & Feldman, H. H. (2008). Potential for misclassification of mild cognitive impairment: A study of memory scores on the Wechsler Memory Scale-III in healthy older adults. *Journal of the International Neuropsychological Society, 14*(3), 463–478.

Brooks, B. L., Iverson, G. L., & White, T. (2007). Substantial risk of "Accidental MCI" in healthy older adults: Base rates of low memory scores in neuropsychological assessment. *Journal of the International Neuropsychological Society, 13*(3), 490–500.

Brooks, N., Kupshik, G., Wilson, L., Galbraith, S., & Ward, R. (1987). A neuropsychological study of active amateur boxers. *Journal of Neurology, Neurosurgery, and Psychiatry, 50*(8), 997–1000.

Buse, G. J. (2006). No holds barred sport fighting: A 10 year review of mixed martial arts competition. *British Journal of Sports Medicine, 40*(2), 169–172.

Bush, S. S., & Iverson, G. L. (2010). Ethical issues and practical considerations in sports neuropsychology. In F. M. Webbe (Ed.), *Handbook of sport neuropsychology* (pp. 35–52). New York, NY: Spring Publishing Company.

Bush, S. S., & Myers, T. (2008). Disruption of neurocognitive functioning in mixed martial arts: Incidence, assessment, and management. *The Clinical Neuropsychologist, 22*, 390.

Bush, S. S., & Myers, T. (2009). Concussive brain injury in mixed martial arts: Fighter characteristics and bout outcomes. *Applied Neuropsychology, 16*, 289.

Bush, S. S., & Myers, T. (2012). Dementia pugilistica. In C. A. Noggle, R. S. Dean, & A. M. Horton, Jr. (Eds.), *The encyclopedia of neuropsychological disorders* (pp. 258–260). New York, NY: Springer Publishing Co.

Bush, S. S., Ruff, R. M., Tröster, A. I., Barth, J. T., Koffler, S. P., Pliskin, N. H.,...Silver, C. H. (2005). Symptom validity assessment: Practice issues and medical necessity NAN policy & planning committee. *Archives of Clinical Neuropsychology, 20*(4), 419–426.

Butler, R. J., Forsythe, W. I., Beverly, D. W., & Adams, L. M. (1993). A prospective controlled investigation of the cognitive effects of amateur boxing. *Journal of Neurology, Neurosurgery, and Psychiatry, 56*, 1055–1061.

Cantu, R. C. (1992). Cerebral concussion in sport. *Sports Medicine, 14*, 64–74.

Cantu, R. C. (2007). Chronic traumatic encephalopathy in the National Football League. *Neurosurgery, 61*(2), 223–225.

Carroll, E. J. (1936). Punch drunk. *American Journal of the Medical Sciences, 191*, 706–711.

Cassasa, C. B. (1924). Multiple traumatic cerebral hemorrhages. *Proceedings of the New York Pathological Society, 24*, 101–106.

Casson, I. R. (2010). Do the "facts" really support an association between NFL players' concussions, dementia and depression? *Neurology Today, June 3*, 6–7.

Casson, I. R., Pellman, E. J., & Viano, D. C. (2006a). Chronic traumatic encephalopathy in a National Football League player. *Neurosurgery, 58*(5), E1003; author reply E1003; discussion E1003.

Casson, I. R., Pellman, E. J., & Viano, D. C. (2006b). Chronic traumatic encephalopathy in a National Football League player. *Neurosurgery, 59*(5), E1152.

Casson, I. R., Pellman, E. J., & Viano, D. C. (2009). Concussion in the National Football League: An overview for neurologists. *Physical Medicine and Rehabilitation Clinics of North America, 20*(1), 195–214, x.

Casson, I. R., Siegel, O., Sham, R., Campbell, E. A., Tarlau, M., & DiDomenico, A. (1984). Brain damage in modern boxers. *Journal of the American Medical Association, 251*(20), 2663–2667.

Clausen, H., McCrory, P., & Anderson, V. (2005). The risk of chronic traumatic brain injury in professional boxing: Change in exposure variables over the past century. *British Journal of Sports Medicine, 39*(9), 661–664; discussion 664.

Colella, M. (2007). Sports headlines changing the multiplatform game. Ratings from Beckham, brawling, and basketball. *The Bridge, 30*, 1–10.

Corsellis, J. A., Bruton, C. J., & Freeman-Browne, D. (1973). The aftermath of boxing. *Psychological Medicine, 3*(3), 270–303.

Courville, C. B. (1962). Punch drunk. Its pathogenesis and pathology on the basis of a verified case. *Bulletin of the Los Angeles Neurological Society, 27*, 160–168.

Critchley, E. (1937). Nervous disorders in boxers. *Medical Annual*, 318–320.

Critchley, M. (1957). Medical aspects of boxing, particularly from a neurological standpoint. *British Medical Journal, 1*(5015), 357–362.

Cummings, J. L. (2004). Alzheimer's disease. *The New England Journal of Medicine, 351*(1), 56–67.

Daniloff, C. (2009). *The hardest hit*. Retrieved December 4, 2009, from www.bu.edu/bostonia/winter09/concussions/

Echemendia, R. J. (2006). *Sports neuropsychology: Assessment and management of traumatic brain injury*. New York, NY: Guilford Press.

Encyclopedia Britannica. (2009). *Muhammad Ali*. Retrieved December 12, 2009, from www.britannica.com/EBchecked/topic/15252/Muhammad-Ali

Farrer, L. A., Cupples, L. A., Haines, J. L., Hyman, B., Kukull, W. A., Mayeux, R.,...van Duijn, C. M. (1997). Effects of age, sex, and ethnicity on the association between apolipoprotein E genotype and Alzheimer disease. A meta-analysis. APOE and Alzheimer Disease Meta Analysis Consortium. *The Journal of the American Medical Association, 278*(16), 1349–1356.

Fleminger, S., Oliver, D. L., Lovestone, S., Rabe-Hesketh, S., & Giora, A. (2003). Head injury as a risk factor for Alzheimer's disease: The evidence 10 years on; a partial replication. *Journal of Neurology, Neurosurgery, and Psychiatry, 74*(7), 857–862.

Friedman, J. H. (1989). Progressive parkinsonism in boxers. *Southern Medical Journal, 82*(5), 543–546.

Garber, G. (2005a). *Blood and guts*. Retrieved March 12, 2009, from http://sports.espn.go.com /nfl/news/story?id=1972286

Garber, G. (2005b). *Sifting through the ashes*. Retrieved March 12, 2009, from http://sports .espn.go.com/nfl/news/story?id=1972289

Garber, G. (2005c). *A tormented soul*. Retrieved March 12, 2009, from http://sports.espn .go.com/nfl/news/story?id=1972285

Garber, G. (2005d). *Wandering through the fog*. Retrieved March 12, 2009, from http://sports .espn.go.com/nfl/news/story?id=1972288

Gardner, A., Iverson, G. L., & McCrory, P. (2014). Chronic traumatic encephalopathy in sport: A systematic review. *British Journal of Sports Medicine, 48*(2), 84–90.

Geddes, J. F., Vowles, G. H., Nicoll, J. A., & Révész, T. (1999). Neuronal cytoskeletal changes are an early consequence of repetitive head injury. *Acta Neuropathologica, 98*(2), 171–178.

Geddes, J. F., Vowles, G. H., Robinson, S. F., & Sutcliffe, J. C. (1996). Neurofibrillary tangles, but not Alzheimer-type pathology, in a young boxer. *Neuropathology and Applied Neurobiology, 22*(1), 12–16.

Grahmann, H., & Ule, G. (1957). [Diagnosis of chronic cerebral symptoms in boxers (dementia pugilistica & traumatic encephalopathy of boxers)]. *Psychiatria et Neurologia, 134*(3–4), 261–283.

Green, P. (2007). The pervasive influence of effort on neuropsychological tests. *Physical Medicine and Rehabilitation Clinics of North America, 18*(1), 43–68, vi.

Green, R. C., Cupples, L. A., Go, R., Benke, K. S., Edeki, T., Griffith, P. A.,...Farrer, L. A.; MIRAGE Study Group. (2002). Risk of dementia among white and African American relatives of patients with Alzheimer disease. *The Journal of the American Medical Association, 287*(3), 329–336.

Hagell, P. (2000). Should boxing be banned? *The Journal of Neuroscience Nursing, 32*(2), 126–128.

Hart, J., Kraut, M. A., Womack, K. B., Strain, J., Didehbani, N., Bartz, E.,...Cullum, C. M. (2013). Neuroimaging of cognitive dysfunction and depression in aging retired National Football League players: A cross-sectional study. *The Journal of the American Medical Association Neurology, 70*(3), 326–335.

Hauser, T. (1998). *Muhammad Ali and company: Inside the world of professional boxing*. Norwalk: CT: Hastings House.

Hazrati, L. N., Tartaglia, M. C., Diamandis, P., Davis, K. D., Green, R. E., Wennberg, R.,... Tator, C. H. (2013). Absence of chronic traumatic encephalopathy in retired football players with multiple concussions and neurological symptomatology. *Frontiers in Human Neuroscience, 7*, 222.

Heilbronner, R. L., Bush, S. S., Ravdin, L. D., Barth, J. T., Iverson, G. L., Ruff, R. M.,... Broshek, D. K. (2009). Neuropsychological consequences of boxing and recommendations to improve safety: A National Academy of Neuropsychology education paper. *Archives of Clinical Neuropsychology, 24*(1), 11–19.

Heilbronner, R. L., Sweet, J. J., Morgan, J. E., Larrabee, G. J., & Millis, S. R.; Conference Participants. (2009). American Academy of Clinical Neuropsychology Consensus Conference Statement on the neuropsychological assessment of effort, response bias, and malingering. *The Clinical Neuropsychologist, 23*(7), 1093–1129.

Hohler, B. (2009). *Major breakthrough in concussion crisis: Researchers find signs of degenerative brain disease in an 18-year-old high school football player.* Retrieved January 21, 2010, from www.boston.com/sports/other_sports/articles/2009/01/27/major_breakthrough_in_concussion_crisis/

Iverson, G. L. (2014). Chronic traumatic encephalopathy and risk of suicide in former athletes. *British Journal of Sports Medicine, 48*(2), 162–165.

Iverson, G. L., Zasler, N. D., & Lange, R. T. (2006). Post-concussive disorder. In N. D. Zasler, D. I. Katz, & R. D. Zafonte (Eds.), *Brain injury medicine: Principles and practice* (pp. 374–385). New York, NY: Demos Medical Publishing.

Jellinger, K. A., Paulus, W., Wrocklage, C., & Litvan, I. (2001a). Effects of closed traumatic brain injury and genetic factors on the development of Alzheimer's disease. *European Journal of Neurology, 8*(6), 707–710.

Jellinger, K. A., Paulus, W., Wrocklage, C., & Litvan, I. (2001b). Traumatic brain injury as a risk factor for Alzheimer disease. Comparison of two retrospective autopsy cohorts with evaluation of ApoE genotype. *BMC Neurology, 1*, 3.

Jokl, E., & Guttman, E. (1933). Neurologisch-psychiatrische Untersuchung an Boxern. *Munch Med Woch, 1*, 560.

Jordan, B. D. (1993). Chronic neurologic injuries in boxing. In B. D. Jordan (Ed.), *Medical aspects of boxing* (pp. 177–185). Boca Raton, FL: CRC Press.

Jordan, B. D. (2000). Chronic traumatic brain injury associated with boxing. *Seminars in Neurology, 20*(2), 179–185.

Jordan, B. D., Relkin, N. R., Ravdin, L. D., Jacobs, A. R., Bennett, A., & Gandy, S. (1997). Apolipoprotein E epsilon4 associated with chronic traumatic brain injury in boxing. *The Journal of the American Medical Association, 278*(2), 136–140.

Kaplan, H. A., & Browder, J. (1954). Observations on the clinical and brain wave patterns of professional boxers. *Journal of the American Medical Association, 156*(12), 1138–1144.

Karantzoulis, S., & Randolph, C. (2013). Modern chronic traumatic encephalopathy in retired athletes: What is the evidence? *Neuropsychology Review, 23*(4), 350–360.

Klis, M. (2007). *Nash death cause not determined.* Retrieved December 5, 2009, from www.denverpost.com/sports/ci_5849665

Lacava, G. (1963). Boxer's encephalopathy. *Journal of Sports Medicine and Physical Fitness, 168*, 87–92.

Laskas, J. (2009). *Game brain.* Retrieved December 5, 2009, from www.gq.com/sports/profiles/200909/nfl-players-brain-dementia-study-memory-concussions?currentPage=all

Loosemore, M., Knowles, C. H., & Whyte, G. P. (2007). Amateur boxing and risk of chronic traumatic brain injury: Systematic review of observational studies. *British Medical Journal, 335*(7624), 809.

Martland, H. S. (1928). Punch drunk. *The Journal of the American Medical Association, 91*, 1103–1107.

McCown, I. A. (1959). Boxing injuries. *American Journal of Surgery, 98*, 509–516.

McCrea, M. (2008). *Mild traumatic brain injury and postconcussion syndrome: The new evidence base for diagnosis and treatment.* New York, NY: Oxford University Press.

McCrea, M., Guskiewicz, K., Randolph, C., Barr, W. B., Hammeke, T. A., Marshall, S. W., & Kelly, J. P. (2009). Effects of a symptom-free waiting period on clinical outcome and risk of reinjury after sport-related concussion. *Neurosurgery, 65*(5), 876–882; discussion 882.

McCrory, P. (2001). Does second impact syndrome exist? *Clinical Journal of Sport Medicine, 11*(3), 144–149.

McCrory, P., Meeuwisse, W. H., Kutcher, J. S., Jordan, B. D., & Gardner, A. (2013). What is the evidence for chronic concussion-related changes in retired athletes: Behavioural, pathological and clinical outcomes? *British Journal of Sports Medicine, 47*(5), 327–330.

McCrory, P., Zazryn, T., & Cameron, P. (2007). The evidence for chronic traumatic encephalopathy in boxing. *Sports Medicine, 37*(6), 467–476.

McKee, A. C., Cantu, R. C., Nowinski, C. J., Hedley-Whyte, E. T., Gavett, B. E., Budson, A. E.,... Stern, R. A. (2009). Chronic traumatic encephalopathy in athletes: Progressive tauopathy after repetitive head injury. *Journal of Neuropathology and Experimental Neurology, 68*(7), 709–735.

McKee, A. C., Gavett, B. E., Stern, R. A., Nowinski, C. J., Cantu, R. C., Kowall, N. W.,... Budson, A. E. (2010). TDP-43 proteinopathy and motor neuron disease in chronic traumatic encephalopathy. *Journal of Neuropathology and Experimental Neurology, 69*(9), 918–929.

McKee, A. C., Stern, R. A., Nowinski, C. J., Stein, T. D., Alvarez, V. E., Daneshvar, D. H.,... Cantu, R. C. (2013). The spectrum of disease in chronic traumatic encephalopathy. *Brain: A Journal of Neurology, 136*(Pt 1), 43–64.

McLatchie, G., Brooks, N., Galbraith, S., Hutchison, J. S., Wilson, L., Melville, I., & Teasdale, E. (1987). Clinical neurological examination, neuropsychology, electroencephalography and computed tomographic head scanning in active amateur boxers. *Journal of Neurology, Neurosurgery, and Psychiatry, 50*(1), 96–99.

Mendez, M. F. (1995). The neuropsychiatric aspects of boxing. *International Journal of Psychiatry in Medicine, 25*(3), 249–262.

Millspaugh, J. A. (1937). Dementia pugilistica. *US Naval Medical Bulletin, 35,* 297–303.

Moriarity, J., Collie, A., Olson, D., Buchanan, J., Leary, P., McStephen, M., & McCrory, P. (2004). A prospective controlled study of cognitive function during an amateur boxing tournament. *Neurology, 62*(9), 1497–1502.

Morrison, R. G. (1986). Medical and public health aspects of boxing. *The Journal of the American Medical Association, 255*(18), 2475–2480.

Moser, R. S., Iverson, G. L., Echemendia, R. J., Lovell, M. R., Schatz, P., Webbe, F. M.,... Barth, J. T.; NAN Policy and Planning Committee; Donna K. Broshek, Shane S. Bush, Sandra P. Koffler, Cecil R. Reynolds, Cheryl H. Silver. (2007). Neuropsychological evaluation in the diagnosis and management of sports-related concussion. *Archives of Clinical Neuropsychology, 22*(8), 909–916.

Naccache, L., Slachevsky, A., Deweer, B., Habert, M. O., & Dubois, B. (1999). ["Boxer's dementia" without motor signs]. *Presse Médicale, 28*(25), 1352–1354.

Neubuerger, K. T., Sinton, D. W., & Denst, J. (1959). Cerebral atrophy associated with boxing. *American Medical Association Archives of Neurology and Psychiatry, 81*(4), 403–408.

O'Connor, A. (2007). *Wrestler found to have taken testosterone.* Retrieved December 5, 2009, from www.nytimes.com/2007/07/18/us/18wrestler.html

Omalu, B. I., DeKosky, S. T., Hamilton, R. L., Minster, R. L., Kamboh, M. I., Shakir, A. M., & Wecht, C. H. (2006). Chronic traumatic encephalopathy in a national football league player: Part II. *Neurosurgery, 59*(5), 1086–1092; discussion 1092.

Omalu, B. I., DeKosky, S. T., Minster, R. L., Kamboh, M. I., Hamilton, R. L., & Wecht, C. H. (2005). Chronic traumatic encephalopathy in a National Football League player. *Neurosurgery, 57*(1), 128–34; discussion 128.

Osnato, M., & Giliberti, V. (1927). Posttraumatic neurosis–traumatic encephalitis. *Archives of Neurology and Psychiatry, 18,* 181–214.

Parker, H. L. (1934). Traumatic encephalopathy ("Punch Drunk") of professional pugilists. *The Journal of Neurology and Psychopathology, 15*(57), 20–28.

Payne, E. E. (1968). Brains of boxers. *Neurochirurgia, 11*(5), 173–188.

Pellman, E. J. (2003). Background on the National Football League's research on concussion in professional football. *Neurosurgery, 53*(4), 797–798.

Pellman, E. J., Lovell, M. R., Viano, D. C., & Casson, I. R. (2006). Concussion in professional football: Recovery of NFL and high school athletes assessed by computerized neuropsychological testing–Part 12. *Neurosurgery, 58*(2), 263–274; discussion 263.

Pellman, E. J., Lovell, M. R., Viano, D. C., Casson, I. R., & Tucker, A. M. (2004). Concussion in professional football: Neuropsychological testing–part 6. *Neurosurgery, 55*(6), 1290–1303; discussion 1303.

Pellman, E. J., Powell, J. W., Viano, D. C., Casson, I. R., Tucker, A. M., Feuer, H.,...Robertson, D. W. (2004). Concussion in professional football: Epidemiological features of game injuries and review of the literature–part 3. *Neurosurgery, 54*(1), 81–94; discussion 94.

Pellman, E. J., Viano, D. C., Casson, I. R., Arfken, C., & Feuer, H. (2005). Concussion in professional football: Players returning to the same game–part 7. *Neurosurgery, 56*(1), 79–90; discussion 90.

Pellman, E. J., Viano, D. C., Casson, I. R., Arfken, C., & Powell, J. (2004). Concussion in professional football: Injuries involving 7 or more days out–Part 5. *Neurosurgery, 55*(5), 1100–1119.

Pellman, E. J., Viano, D. C., Casson, I. R., Tucker, A. M., Waeckerle, J. F., Powell, J. W., & Feuer, H. (2004). Concussion in professional football: repeat injuries–part 4. *Neurosurgery, 55*(4), 860–873; discussion 873–876.

Pellman, E. J., Viano, D. C., Tucker, A. M., & Casson, I. R.; Committee on Mild Traumatic Brain Injury, National Football League. (2003). Concussion in professional football: Location and direction of helmet impacts–Part 2. *Neurosurgery, 53*(6), 1328–1340; discussion 1340.

Pellman, E. J., Viano, D. C., Withnall, C., Shewchenko, N., Bir, C. A., & Halstead, P. D. (2006). Concussion in professional football: Helmet testing to assess impact performance–part 11. *Neurosurgery, 58*(1), 78–96; discussion 78.

Plassman, B. L., Havlik, R. J., Steffens, D. C., Helms, M. J., Newman, T. N., Drosdick, D.,...Breitner, J. C. (2000). Documented head injury in early adulthood and risk of Alzheimer's disease and other dementias. *Neurology, 55*(8), 1158–1166.

Porter, M. D. (2003). A 9-year controlled prospective neuropsychologic assessment of amateur boxing. *Clinical Journal of Sport Medicine, 13*(6), 339–352.

Porter, M. D., & Fricker, P. A. (1996). Controlled prospective neuropsychological assessment of active experienced amateur boxers. *Clinical Journal of Sport Medicine, 6*(2), 90–96.

Prins, M. L., Lee, S. M., Cheng, C. L., Becker, D. P., & Hovda, D. A. (1996). Fluid percussion brain injury in the developing and adult rat: A comparative study of mortality, morphology, intracranial pressure and mean arterial blood pressure. *Brain Research. Developmental Brain Research, 95*(2), 272–282.

Randolph, C., Karantzoulis, S., & Guskiewicz, K. (2013). Prevalence and characterization of mild cognitive impairment in retired national football league players. *Journal of the International Neuropsychological Society, 19*(8), 873–880.

Randolph, C., & Kirkwood, M. W. (2009). What are the real risks of sport-related concussion, and are they modifiable? *Journal of the International Neuropsychological Society, 15*(4), 512–520.

Randolph, C., McCrea, M., & Barr, W. B. (2005). Is neuropsychological testing useful in the management of sport-related concussion? *Journal of Athletic Training, 40*(3), 139–152.

Rapp, G. C. (2013). *Suicide, concussions, and the NFL*. Retrieved from http://ssrn.com/abstract=2233383

Ravdin, L. D., Barr, W. B., Jordan, B., Lathan, W. E., & Relkin, N. R. (2003). Assessment of cognitive recovery following sports related head trauma in boxers. *Clinical Journal of Sport Medicine, 13*(1), 21–27.

Roberts, A. H. (1969). *Brain damage in boxers—A study of the prevalence of traumatic encephalopathy among ex-professional boxers.* London: Pitman.

Robertson, L. (2009). *Borich case shows the damage hits can cause.* Retrieved December 5, 2009, from www.miamiherald.com/sports/columnists/linda-robertson/story/1297607.html

Rochon, M. (1994). [Presentation of a case: Encephalopathy of boxers]. *Canadian Journal of Psychiatry, 39*(4), 211–214.

Ross, R. J., Cole, M., Thompson, J. S., & Kim, K. H. (1983). Boxers–computed tomography, EEG, and neurological evaluation. *The Journal of the American Medical Association, 249*(2), 211–213.

Rowland, L. P., Mitsumoto, H., & Hays, A. (2010). Did Lou Gehrig have Lou Gehrig's disease? *Neurology Today, 10*, 6.

Saunders, R. L., & Harbaugh, R. E. (1984). The second impact in catastrophic contact-sports head trauma. *The Journal of the American Medical Association, 252*(4), 538–539.

Scelsa, S. (2010). The Mayo Clinic got it right: Lou Gehrig had ALS. *Neurology News, 18*, 20.

Scheiber, D. (2006). *The mysterious death of Andre Waters.* Retrieved from www.sptimes.com/2006/12/11/Sports/The_mysterious_death_.shtml

Schretlen, D. J., Munro, C. A., Anthony, J. C., & Pearlson, G. D. (2003). Examining the range of normal intraindividual variability in neuropsychological test performance. *Journal of the International Neuropsychological Society, 9*(6), 864–870.

Schretlen, D. J., Testa, S. M., Winicki, J. M., Pearlson, G. D., & Gordon, B. (2008). Frequency and bases of abnormal performance by healthy adults on neuropsychological testing. *Journal of the International Neuropsychological Society, 14*(3), 436–445.

Schwarz, A. (2007a). *Expert ties ex-player's suicide to brain damage.* Retrieved April 12, 2009, from www.nytimes.com/2007/01/18/sports/football/18waters.html?pagewanted=1&_r=2&ref=sports

Schwarz, A. (2007b). *Lineman, dead at 36, exposes brain injuries.* Retrieved April 12, 2009, from www.nytimes.com/2007/06/15/sports/football/15brain.html?_r=2

Schwarz, A. (2009). *New sign of brain damage in N.F.L.* Retrieved May 12, 2009, from www.nytimes.com/2009/01/28/sports/football/28brain.html?_r=2&hp

Schwarz, A. (2010). *Study says brain trauma can mimic A.L.S.* Retrieved 19 December, 2013, from http://www.nytimes.com/2010/08/18/sports/18gehrig.html?pagewanted=all&_r=0

ScienceDaily. (2009). *First former college football player diagnosed with chronic traumatic encephalopathy.* Retrieved December 5, 2009, from www.sciencedaily.com/releases/2009/10/091022101657.htm

Shapiro, L. (2004). *After football, a tragic free fall.* Retrieved April 12, 2009, from www.washingtonpost.com/wp-dyn/articles/A8578–2004Nov23.html

Slobounov, S., & Sebastianelli, W. (2006). *Foundations of sport-related brain injuries.* New York, NY: Springer Press.

Small, G. W., Kepe, V., Siddarth, P., Ercoli, L. M., Merrill, D. A., Donoghue, N.,... Barrio, J. R. (2013). PET scanning of brain tau in retired national football league players: preliminary findings. *The American Journal of Geriatric Psychiatry, 21*(2), 138–144.

Smith, S., & Moriarty, D. (2013). *First major league baseball player diagnosed with CTE.* Retrieved December 18, 2009, from http://edition.cnn.com/2013/12/15/health/baseball-ryan-freel-cte-suicide/index.html?hpt=hp_t1

Stewart, W. F., Gordon, B., Selnes, O., Bandeen-Roche, K., Zeger, S., Tusa, R. J.,... Hall, C. (1994). Prospective study of central nervous system function in amateur boxers in the United States. *American Journal of Epidemiology, 139*(6), 573–588.

Tagliabue, P. (2003). Tackling concussions in sports. *Neurosurgery, 53*(4), 796.

Timm, K. E., Wallach, J. M., Stone, J. A., & Ryan, E. J. (1993). Fifteen years of amateur boxing injuries/illnesses at the United States olympic training center. *Journal of Athletic Training, 28*(4), 330–334.

Unterharnscheidt, F. (1995). A neurologist's reflections on boxing. V. Conclude remarks. *Revista de Neurologia, 23*(123), 1027–1032.

Viano, D. C., & Pellman, E. J. (2005). Concussion in professional football: Biomechanics of the striking player–part 8. *Neurosurgery, 56*(2), 266–280; discussion 266.

Viano, D. C., Casson, I. R., & Pellman, E. J. (2007). Concussion in professional football: Biomechanics of the struck player–part 14. *Neurosurgery, 61*(2), 313–327; discussion 327.

Viano, D. C., Casson, I. R., Pellman, E. J., Zhang, L., King, A. I., & Yang, K. H. (2005). Concussion in professional football: Brain responses by finite element analysis: Part 9. *Neurosurgery, 57*(5), 891–916; discussion 891.

Viano, D. C., Pellman, E. J., Withnall, C., & Shewchenko, N. (2006). Concussion in professional football: Performance of newer helmets in reconstructed game impacts–Part 13. *Neurosurgery, 59*(3), 591–606; discussion 591.

Wegner, W. (1963). Boxer's encephalopathy. *The Journal of Sports Medicine and Physical Fitness, 3*, 170–173.

Wilson, J. T. (2003). Head injury and Alzheimer's disease. *Journal of Neurology, Neurosurgery, and Psychiatry, 74*(7), 841.

Winterstein, C. E. (1937). Head injuries attributable to boxing. *The Lancet, 2*, 719–720.

Wortzel, H. S., Brenner, L. A., & Arciniegas, D. B. (2013). Traumatic brain injury and chronic traumatic encephalopathy: A forensic neuropsychiatric perspective. *Behavioral Sciences and the Law, 31*(6), 721–738.

Wortzel, H. S., Shura, R. D., & Brenner, L. A. (2013). Chronic traumatic encephalopathy and suicide: A systematic review. *Biomed Research International, 2013*, 424280.

Wright, A. D. (1965). Head injuries. In A. L. Bass, J. L. Blonstein, R. D. James, & J. P. Williams (Eds.), *Medical aspects of boxing* (pp. 61–61). London: Pergamon Press.

CHAPTER 14

Mild Cognitive Impairment: Many Questions, Some Answers

Kevin Duff

Mr. N is a 76-year-old, married, White male who presented to the Memory Disorders Clinic with a 1- to 2-year history of gradually worsening problems with his memory, including trouble recalling names, misplacing common objects, poor recall of details of conversations, and mild word-finding difficulties. He denied any other cognitive problems. Despite the memory problems, he denied any significant functional limitations at the time of this study (e.g., continues to drive, manages his finances and medications, prepares meals, and participates in household chores and hobbies). He also denied any symptoms associated with depression, although he did report some worry about his memory problems. Mrs. N largely corroborated her husband's report of his cognition, daily functioning, and mood. His medical history is notable for hypertension, diabetes, and arthritis. No psychiatric history was reported. The patient denied use of tobacco and illegal drugs, but did report minimal use of alcohol (currently and in the past). Family medical and psychiatric history is unremarkable. Mr. N completed 16 years of school, and he denied any early academic difficulties. He retired from his position as a manager of a retail store approximately 10 years ago. He lives with his wife. He was pleasant and cooperative with the evaluation, although he did tend to make self-deprecating comments during the memory tests. He was alert and oriented to person, place, and time. Premorbid intellect was estimated to be in the average range. Overall cognition was intact (Mini-Mental State Examination [MMSE] = 29/30) and current intellect was average. Most other cognitive abilities (e.g., attention, perception and construction, executive functioning) also met expectations. Performance on language measures (e.g., naming, verbal fluency) was borderline to below average. Learning and memory, however, were well below expectations, with most scores falling in the moderately to severely impaired range.

Diagnostically, how would you describe Mr. N's condition? Is this normal aging? Probably not, as his performance on measure of learning and memory falls well below expectations, both for himself and his peer group. Is this dementia? According to the *Diagnostic and Statistical Manual of Mental Disorders, Fourth Edition, Text Revision* (American Psychiatric Association [APA], 2000) and many other diagnostic criteria, dementia typically requires evidence of both impairment in multiple cognitive domains and functional decline (e.g., occupationally, socially). As Mr. and Mrs. N denied any functional impairment in the patient at the time of this study, dementia seems to be an inappropriate diagnosis. Although there are other diagnostic entities to consider (e.g., amnestic disorder, cognitive disorder not otherwise specified), Mr. N may be better labeled as having mild cognitive impairment (MCI).

WHAT IS MCI?

Most broadly, MCI can be conceptualized as "not normal, but not demented." Theoretically, MCI represents a transitional phase between normal aging and dementia. From this theoretical standpoint, the concept of MCI makes a lot of sense in that individuals are typically not "normal" one day and "demented" the next. In theory, especially for progressive neurodegenerative conditions (e.g., Alzheimer's disease [AD], frontotemporal dementia [FTD]), the development of dementia may take months or years. During that transitional period from normal to pathological, the concept of MCI allows us to identify and study these individuals. MCI allows us the opportunity to learn more about both ends of that transitional spectrum. For example, comparisons between normal aging and MCI can give insights into the earliest indicators of disease (vs. "normal" variability). Comparisons of MCI and full-blown dementia could be useful in understanding how a disease progresses from its mild to more severe stages.

Operationally, there have been many definitions of MCI. However, a general rubric to differentiate MCI from normal aging and dementia is presented in Table 14.1. In this model, the two key variables are cognition and daily functioning (e.g., driving, managing medication, preparing meals, keeping track of finances). The "normal" or "intact" individual will be able to perform adequately on both of these key variables. The demented individual will suffer impairment on both cognition and daily functioning. As expected, the individual with MCI will fall between the other two, with impairment in cognition but relatively intact daily functioning. Although this schematic is an oversimplification, it can serve as an introduction into this evolving diagnostic concept.

IS MCI A NEW CONCEPT?

Admittedly, MCI is not an entirely new concept. Prior literature has touched on similar topics. Early distinctions between "benign" and "malignant" forgetfulness were made, with the former appearing to reflect normal aging and the latter reflecting pathological decline (Kral, 1962). Others (Crook et al., 1986) followed up on benign senescent forgetfulness as they described age-associated memory impairment (i.e., objective memory deficits in older adults compared to younger adults). However, these earlier concepts viewed the memory impairment as relatively "normal for age" and not necessarily as a cause of concern. In a report for a working group associated

TABLE 14.1 Overview of the Differences Among Normal Aging, Mild Cognitive Impairment, and Dementia

	NORMAL AGING	MCI	DEMENTIA
Cognition	Intact	Impaired	Impaired
Daily functioning	Intact	Intact	Impaired

MCI, mild cognitive impairment.

with the World Health Organization (WHO), diagnostic criteria for aging-associated cognitive decline were presented (Levy, 1994). These criteria include: (a) complaint of cognitive decline by patient or informant; (b) gradual decline over at least 6 months; (c) cognitive decline occurring in one of several specific domains (e.g., memory, language, attention, executive functions); (d) scores on cognitive tests fall at least 1 standard deviation (SD) below age- and education-corrected normative data; and (e) exclusion criteria (e.g., dementia, depression, delirium, substance abuse), which are not met. The criteria described by Levy appeared to be a significant advance toward the current concept of MCI, as these criteria no longer reflected normal aging. These criteria provided a more objective cutoff for impairment (i.e., greater than 1 SD below peers), allowed for individual difference variables (e.g., age- and education-corrected normative data), and allowed for impairment to occur in memory or non-memory domains. For readers already familiar with MCI, Levy's criteria are quite similar to those used by Petersen et al. in their descriptions of MCI (Petersen et al., 1999, 2009). Others have also touched on the concept of MCI, before there was MCI (e.g., cognitive impairment—no dementia [Graham et al., 1997], mild cognitive disorder [Christensen et al., 1995]).

HOW DID THE CONCEPT OF MCI DEVELOP?

In 1999, Ronald Petersen et al. from the Mayo Clinic published one of their first articles on MCI (Petersen et al., 1999). In this influential six-page article, they present data on 76 older patients at the "mild end of the cognitive spectrum." More formally, they classified individuals with MCI as having: (a) memory complaint, (b) normal activities of daily living (ADL), (c) normal general cognitive functioning, (d) abnormal memory for age, and (e) not demented. In comparison to a cohort of cognitively healthy peers and patients with AD, individuals with MCI tended to fall between the other two groups on most relevant measures. For example, on global rating scales of dementia, cognitive screening scales (e.g., MMSE), and formal neuropsychological instruments (including IQ, memory, naming, and phonemic fluency), controls performed the best, AD patients performed the worst, and MCI patients fell in the middle. These patients were also followed across time, and annual rates of change on dementia rating scales and cognitive screening measures showed that again MCI fell between the other two groups (i.e., controls with the least decline and AD with the most decline). In 4-year follow-up data, 12% of the MCI cases converted to AD per year (compared with 1%–2% per year in healthy controls). It is this last finding that suggested that MCI may be a particularly important group to study to learn more about AD.

HOW HAS THIS CONCEPT CONTINUED TO EVOLVE?

Following this 1999 article on the clinical characterization and outcome in MCI, research in this area exploded. As can be seen in Figure 14.1, there were 30 articles listed on PubMed that mentioned the term *mild cognitive impairment* in 1999. In 2003, there were 176 articles using this term. By 2007 and 2010, 457 and 738 articles referred to MCI, respectively. And in 2013, that number had jumped to over 1,300! Admittedly, not all of these articles directly focus on MCI, but they do demonstrate that there is continually growing interest in this and related topics.

As this evidence has accumulated over time, the concept of MCI and its operational definition has changed. For example, in its 2001 article, the Mayo group (Petersen et al., 2001) had already refined its own diagnostic criteria for MCI to

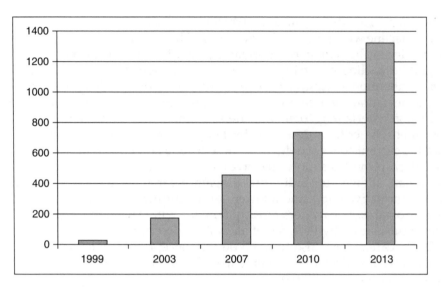

FIGURE 14.1 Number of publications citing "mild cognitive impairment."

include subjective complaints *corroborated by an informant* (vs. only the patient), *age- and education-corrections* for memory impairment, and *preserved* (vs. "normal") general cognitive function. Additionally, they acknowledged that MCI could affect domains *other than memory*. And these different subtypes of MCI could be prodromal periods of different dementing illnesses. For example, the purely memory-impaired MCI (i.e., amnestic subtype) would likely lead to AD. MCI-like impairment in memory and other cognitive domains (i.e., multidomain subtype) could lead to AD or vascular dementia (VaD). Impairment in domains other than memory (i.e., non-amnestic subtype) could lead to FTD (perhaps with primarily executive dysfunction), dementia with Lewy bodies (perhaps with primarily attention deficits), or primary progressive aphasia (perhaps with primarily language disturbances). At the time, the idea that different MCI subtypes would lead to different dementias was purely theoretical, but it provided a broader framework for the concept of MCI. Although MCI continues to be most commonly referred to as a prodrome of AD, recent studies have identified MCI-like states in VaD (Hachinski et al., 2006), Parkinson's disease (Caviness et al., 2007), Huntington's disease (Duff, Paulsen, et al., 2010), multiple sclerosis (Calabrese et al., 2010), and other neurological and psychiatric conditions (Gualtieri & Morgan, 2008).

Another major modification of the MCI criteria occurred in 2004. Following the First Key Symposium on MCI, an international consensus group (including Dr. Petersen) provided general recommendations for MCI (Winblad et al., 2004). These criteria, which are presented in Table 14.2, had some similarities to the original criteria, but also some departures. Consistent with the original criteria, evidence of subjective and objective cognitive decline was needed. The absence of dementia and the preservation of most functional abilities were also consistent with the initial MCI criteria. However, for the first time, the criteria specifically use the phrase "not normal, not demented." Although this phrase had been implied by the original criteria, it allows for a much broader application of the criteria. Similarly, the types of cognitive impairment are much wider with the new definition. There is no mention of memory or any other specific cognitive domain, which indicates that any/all cognitive domains could be affected. Again, although this was implied, especially following

TABLE 14.2 Criteria for MCI Based on Winblad et al. (2004)

1. Not normal, not demented
2. Cognitive decline • Self and/or informant report and impairment on objective test, and/or • Evidence of decline over time on objective tests
3. Activities of daily living • Basic activities are preserved, and • Complex activities can only be minimally impaired

MCI, mild cognitive impairment.

the Petersen et al. (2001) article, it has not been formally stated. No mention is made about corrections for individual difference variables, neither age nor education, when determining impairment. Based on several studies that have demonstrated that mild functional difficulties can occur in MCI (Farias et al., 2006; Griffith et al., 2003; Wadley et al., 2009), these new criteria allow for some "minimal impairment" in complex daily functions. Lastly, and perhaps the greatest departure from the original criteria, is that cognitive decline criterion in MCI can be documented by actual decline on cognitive tests over time. This provides a stronger rationale for including neuropsychological evaluations in the diagnosis of MCI.

Most recently, a working group from National Institute on Aging and the Alzheimer's Association issued a new set of diagnostic criteria for MCI (Albert et al., 2011). In setting these criteria, they were hoping to focus on MCI due to AD, rather than other etiologies. Their clinical core criteria do not stray too far from previous descriptors of MCI, including: (a) concern about change in cognition (from the patient, an informant, or a clinician), (b) objective evidence of impairment in one or more cognitive domains (but no cutoff point identified), (c) independence of daily functioning, with minimal aids or assistance, and (d) not demented. The clinical syndrome of MCI due to AD can be identified via a neuropsychological evaluation or less-sensitive cognitive screening measures. These authors note that it is important to rule out other etiologies (e.g., vascular, psychiatric, medical comorbidities). In addition to the clinical core criteria, research criteria are also put forth based on the presence of biomarkers of AD that can be used to support the suspected etiology and to determine the likelihood of progression. These biomarkers include beta-amyloid deposition (e.g., via cerebrospinal fluid [CSF] or PET imaging); neuronal injury (e.g., via tau, hippocampal atrophy, or cerebral hypometabolism); and biochemical change (e.g., via inflammatory markers or oxidative stress). The clinical and research criteria can be used in concert. For example, an individual who meets the clinical core criteria and has evidence of increased beta-amyloid deposition and neuronal injury via fluro-2-deoxy-D-glucose (FDG)-PET hypometabolism may be identified as having "MCI due to AD—High likelihood," whereas another individual meeting the clinical core criteria but having "normal" beta-amyloid and cerebral metabolism may be identified as having "MCI—Unlikely due to AD."

Despite the evolution of the diagnostic criteria for MCI over the years, there remains an uncomfortable amount of ambiguity in them. For example, what constitutes "impairment" on objective cognitive tests? Will the unofficial cutoff of 1.5 SD be retained? Similarly, and perhaps more complexly, what constitutes evidence of decline on cognitive tests over time? Currently, neuropsychologists use a variety of methods (e.g., Reliable Change Index with and without corrections for practice, Standardized Based Regression formulas) and cutoffs (e.g., ±1.645 or ±1.96) to determine if a change is reliable and meaningful (Chelune, Naugle, Luders, Sedlak, & Awad, 1993; Duff, Beglinger, Moser, & Paulsen, 2010a; McSweeny, Naugle, Chelune, & Luders, 1993). Which method will be adopted for MCI? Lastly, it remains quite unclear how independent one has to be on daily activities to still meet criteria for MCI. If a patient continues to handle day-to-day and monthly financial transactions (e.g., purchasing items at a store, paying monthly bills) but has turned over a major financial undertaking (e.g., selling some real-estate holdings) to his adult child, would this meet the criterion for MCI? It is expected that the concept and diagnostic criteria of MCI will continue to evolve in the future.

Much of what we are learning about MCI, and therefore refining its diagnostic criteria, is coming from two large-scale studies of cognition and aging: Alzheimer's Disease Neuroimaging Initiative (ADNI) and Australian Imaging, Biomarkers and Lifestyle (AIBL). ADNI is an ongoing, longitudinal, multicenter study designed to develop clinical, imaging, genetic, and biochemical biomarkers for the early detection and tracking of AD. ADNI's enrollment targeted those with MCI and early AD, as well as healthy controls. Funding for ADNI has been provided by both the public and private sectors, including the National Institutes on Aging, pharmaceutical companies, and foundations. AIBL is an ongoing, longitudinal, multicenter investigation to determine which biomarkers, cognitive characteristics, and health and lifestyle factors determine subsequent development of symptomatic AD. Like ADNI, AIBL has recruited healthy elderly individuals, as well as those with MCI and early AD. Support for AIBL comes from the Australian Commonwealth Scientific Industrial and Research Organization, universities, and foundations. Although both of these studies are ongoing, the initial cohorts of MCI in ADNI ($N = 398$; see Petersen et al., 2010) and AIBL ($N = 133$; see Ellis et al., 2009) are providing vast amounts of information about MCI and its progression.

IS MCI REALLY JUST DEMENTIA?

Despite the growing popularity of MCI, it does have its detractors. The most notable group that refutes the concept of MCI is from Washington University. In their opinion, cases of MCI are really just very early or mild cases of dementia. To support their view, they followed a large cohort of "MCI" subjects (i.e., rated as 0.5 on the Clinical Dementia Rating [CDR] scale) over 9.5 years (Morris et al., 2001). Of these "MCI" cases with very mild impairment in memory and other functional domains, 100% progressed to a more severe dementia on follow-up. Given this single outcome for these subjects, the authors conclude that they must all have had very mild AD from the baseline visit. In their more recent articles on the development of dementia (Morris et al., 2009), the Washington University group refers to the progression from cognitively intact (CDR = 0) to very mild dementia (CDR = 0.5), entirely omitting an MCI category. Although the actual differences between this group's CDR = 0.5 and Petersen's MCI might come down to semantics, it continues to be a topic of debate in the study of AD.

HOW FREQUENT IS MCI?

The prevalence and incidence of MCI appear to depend on several factors, including the diagnostic criteria (e.g., Petersen criteria vs. modified versions); methods to implement those criteria (e.g., screening measures vs. comprehensive evaluations); recruitment sites and procedures (e.g., specialty memory disorder clinics vs. community-based settings); and demographic characteristics of the sample (e.g., age, education, ethnicity). Despite these caveats, some general information can be garnered from the existing literature. In a systematic review of nine relevant studies, Luck, Luppa, Briel, and Riedel-Heller (2010) found incident rates of MCI to range from 1.7% to 22.6%. If any MCI subtype was considered, these studies found an average of approximately 10% of MCI. Single-domain MCI (amnestic or non-amnestic) tended to occur more frequently than multidomain MCI. Studies that required the subjective cognitive complaint criterion tended to have lower rates of MCI than those studies that did not require this criterion.

WHO IS AT RISK OF MCI?

Relatively little research has identified the risk factors associated with the development of MCI. In a review of four relevant studies (Luck et al., 2010), it was observed that higher age tended to be a consistent risk factor for MCI. Similarly, individuals with lower education tended to be at higher risk of MCI. Hypertension also led to increased risk. Gender was not associated with MCI risk. Other factors were inconsistent. For example, ethnicity entered into some models as significantly related to MCI, but not others. One study found apolipoprotein E (ApoE) e4 as a significant risk factor, but another did not.

WHO PROGRESSES FROM MCI TO DEMENTIA?

As noted in the conceptual description of MCI and the Petersen et al. (1999) article, cases of MCI tend to progress to dementia. But just as current rates of MCI are subject to considerable heterogeneity due to methodological factors of the individual studies, rates of progression to dementia are similarly variable. Nonetheless, a recent meta-analysis (Mitchell & Shiri-Feshki, 2009) provides some useful information. In their review of 41 studies with an average 4-year follow-up period, the authors reported annual conversion rates from MCI to dementia to be 6.7%. Conversion to probable AD was 6.5% per year, and conversion to VaD was much lower, at 1.6% per year. In general, conversion rates in specialty clinics tended to be higher than rates in community-based studies (9.6% vs. 4.9%, respectively). Conversion rates were also higher if Petersen criteria were used compared to some modified version of these criteria. Additionally, conversion to dementia was higher in amnestic and multidomain MCI subtypes compared to non-amnestic MCI (11.7%, 12.2%, and 4.1%, respectively).

Manly et al. (2008) provide some insight into the risk factors for progression from MCI to dementia. In their particular study, they were focusing on AD as the only dementia outcome. Having any subtype of MCI put individuals at greater risk of developing AD across their 5-year follow-up (e.g., 10.3% progress from intact to AD vs. 21.8% progress from MCI to AD). Albeit more conservative progression numbers, these findings support the initial observations by Petersen and his Mayo colleagues that MCI status is a risk factor for dementia. Manly et al. also reported that the amnestic and multidomain subtypes of MCI put individuals at greater risk of AD than other subtypes. It was noted that the severity of baseline memory impairment, as well as impairment in language and visuospatial abilities and the presence of memory complaints, also put an individual at greater risk of progression to AD. This latter finding was also observed in ADNI's 398 MCI participants (69 who progressed to dementia and 329 who did not progress) over the first year of that study (Petersen et al., 2010). In addition to cognitive variables, there are other prognostic markers that seem to predict likelihood of progression to dementia, including genetic information and neuroimaging data. For example, a recent meta-analysis (Elias-Sonnenschein, Viechtbauer, Ramakers, Verhey, & Visser, 2011) reported that patients with MCI who also have the ApoE e4 allele are 2.3 times more likely to progress than those without this allele. In a genome-wide association study, Ramanan et al. (2012) identified 27 possible genetic pathways that seem to predict progression. Although these genetic links to dementia progression need further study, they may be some of the best predictors in the future. For more immediate prognostic markers, baseline and yearly change scores on MRI seem to be beneficial. For example, Risacher et al. (2010) reported that MCI participants who converted to dementia in ADNI showed significantly greater hippocampal atrophy across 1 year compared to those with MCI who remained stable. Lastly, given the complexity of this prediction, a combination of biomarkers and cognitive test scores might provide the most sensitive prognostic information. Using ADNI data on 130 individuals with amnestic MCI, Ewers et al. (2012) observed that scores on Trail Making Test part B, right hippocampal volume, phosphorylated tau181/Aβ1–42, and age were the best combination of predictors for progression, yielding a classification accuracy of 76.3%. Using a larger sample of all MCI subjects in ADNI, Liu et al. (2013) noted that subjects with key markers of AD (e.g., poor scores on the Rey Auditory Verbal Learning Test, medial temporal lobe atrophy, CSF markers) converted at a rate of 65%, whereas subjects without these key markers converted at a rate of only 7%.

Although we are learning about how to better predict progression in MCI, an astute reader will notice that MCI converting to dementia is not a foregone conclusion. In one of the early MCI articles by the Mayo group (Petersen et al., 2001), nearly 20% of their sample did not convert to dementia after 6 years of follow-up. Across nearly 5 years, 77% of Manly's sample had not yet converted (Manly et al., 2008). It is possible that longer follow-up periods would have led to 100% conversion in both studies, but other data appear to refute this idea.

Although it has not been widely publicized by the Mayo group, several studies have identified that a sizable minority of cases of MCI "revert" to normal on follow-up. For example, in one study (de Rotrou et al., 2005), 34% of older individuals classified as MCI at baseline had reverted to normal by 6 months. By the 12-month follow-up, 48% of the baseline MCI cases were no longer sufficiently impaired to warrant that diagnosis. These reverting cases have been labeled as "accidental" or "reversible" MCI. In a larger, community-based aging study (Manly et al., 2008), 30.2% of individuals classified as MCI were later classified as normal/intact. A closer look at these cases found that nearly half (48%) no longer met the objective cognitive impairment criterion on follow-up. Smaller numbers of cases failed to meet the subjective complaint criterion (17%) and the functional impairment criterion (12%). Not surprisingly, single-domain MCI (amnestic or non-amnestic) tended to revert more commonly than multidomain MCI. The presence of a sizable number of reverting cases is one of the main controversies in the MCI literature.

BESIDES PROGRESSION TO DEMENTIA, WHAT ARE THE OTHER NEGATIVE OUTCOMES OF MCI?

Although conversion to dementia has been the primary outcome variable examined in longitudinal studies of MCI, other negative effects have been observed for those "not normal, but not demented." Psychiatric symptoms (e.g., depression, apathy, irritability) appear to be relatively common in MCI (Edwards, Spira, Barnes, & Yaffe, 2009; Ellis et al., 2009; Lyketsos et al., 2002; Zahodne et al. 2013). Additionally, the presence of psychiatric symptoms in MCI seems to put the individuals at greater risk of conversion (Palmer et al., 2010). A variety of other neurological events have been associated with MCI, including parkinsonism (Boyle et al., 2005); gait disturbance (Verghese et al., 2008); and cerebrovascular accidents (Mariani et al., 2007). Individuals with MCI were at greater risk of nursing home placement (Fisk, Merry, & Rockwood, 2003; Storandt, Grant, Miller, & Morris, 2006). Lastly, mortality rates appear higher in this group (Wilson et al., 2009).

WHAT ARE THE NEUROPSYCHOLOGICAL FINDINGS IN MCI?

Almost by definition, it should be expected that neuropsychological impairment would be observed in cases of MCI. However, the cognitive domains affected obviously depend on the subtype of MCI examined. For example, if a purely amnestic subtype is studied, then primarily deficits of learning and memory should be observed. If multidomain MCI is the focus, then a number of domains could be impaired.

In their initial description of amnestic MCI, Petersen et al. (1999) provided a fair amount of cognitive data to demonstrate the circumscribed memory deficits in their patients. For example, the mean MMSE score in the MCI patients was 26.0, which is above the traditional cutoff for dementia. Additionally, IQ scores were all around 100. Compared to Mayo's Older Americans Normative Studies (MOANS) normative data, scores on measures of language functioning were also average (e.g., Boston Naming Test = 25th percentile, Controlled Oral Word Association Test = 37th percentile). However, performance on measures of learning and memory was more noticeably below expectations (Wechsler Memory Scale—Revised: Logical Memory I = 9th percentile, Logical Memory II = 5th percentile, Visual Reproductions I = 16th percentile, Visual Reproductions II = 16th percentile; Auditory Verbal Learning Test Percent Retention = 9th percentile). The other expected finding in these cognitive data was that scores for the MCI group tended to fall between those of the healthy controls and those with AD. This relative rank ordering of subjects (i.e., controls > MCI > AD) meets both the conceptual and operational definition of MCI, and it will be observed across a variety of markers of disease. In ADNI's nearly 400 amnestic MCI participants, learning and memory scores tended to be impaired (e.g., Auditory Verbal Learning Test: Trials 1–5 = 8th percentile, Delayed Recall = 12th percentile) relative to controls (Petersen et al., 2010). Non-memory scores tended to be somewhat comparable to those of the controls in this cohort (e.g., MMSE = 27, Boston Naming Test = 16th percentile, Category Fluency = 24th percentile, Trail Making Test part B = 19th percentile). On all cognitive measures in this trial, the controls outperformed those with MCI, who in turn outperformed those with AD (i.e., controls > MCI > AD). These similar findings were observed in AIBL's MCI cohort (e.g., California Verbal Learning Test [CVLT]-II Long Delay Free Recall $z = -1.6$; Ellis et al., 2009).

Despite the relatively consistent finding that learning and memory measures are mildly impaired in patients with amnestic MCI, there are still areas that need further elucidation. For example, there are growing data to suggest that not all memory measures identify "impairment" in MCI in the same way. Tremont, Miele, Smith, and Westervelt observed that a list-learning task identified significantly more cases of MCI than a story-recall task (Tremont, Miele, Smith, & Westervelt, 2010). Similarly, our group observed that traditional memory tests (e.g., Hopkins Verbal Learning Test—Revised, Brief Visuospatial Memory Test—Revised) identified memory deficits better than brief screening batteries (e.g., Repeatable Battery for the Assessment of Neuropsychological Status) in amnestic MCI (Duff, Hobson, Beglinger, & O'Bryant, 2010). Another area in need of additional investigation is the role of recognition memory in identifying MCI and its progression. Although performance on delayed recall trials has typically been the focus in amnestic MCI studies, recent findings suggest that recognition memory (e.g., number of false positives) may also be useful in MCI trials (Chapman et al., 2011). Lastly, a number of studies report that patients with amnestic MCI have "relative" deficits in other cognitive domains, including attention and working memory (Saunders & Summers, 2010); processing speed (Economou, Papageorgiou, Karageorgiou, & Vassilopoulos, 2007); verbal fluency (Murphy, Rich, & Troyer, 2006; Nutter-Upham et al., 2008); executive functioning (Brandt et al., 2009); and olfaction (Devanand et al., 2010; Westervelt, Bruce, Coon, & Tremont, 2008). The heterogeneity of findings with amnestic MCI (e.g., prevalence, course, cognitive deficits) may be partially explained by some of these yet-to-be clarified diagnostic issues.

Because most of the existing literature has focused on the amnestic subtype of MCI, less is known about the neuropsychological profiles in the non-amnestic and multidomain subtypes. However, it can also be surmised that mild deficits would appear across a range of cognitive domains in these other subtypes. For example, in a study of MCI subtypes (Libon et al., 2010), a cluster analysis identified three subtypes: amnestic, dysexecutive, and mixed. Not surprisingly, these three different subtypes performed differently on cognitive tests. The dysexecutive subtype performed poorly on measures of executive functioning (e.g., mental control and phonemic fluency = 3rd percentile), but adequately on measures of memory (e.g., delayed free recall of a list of words = 37th percentile). Conversely, the amnestic subtype performed poorly on the memory measures (2nd percentile), but adequately on the executive functioning measures (40th percentile). The mixed subtype performed mildly below expectations on both the memory and executive functioning measures (16th and 20th percentiles, respectively). Similarly, in another study of MCI subtypes (Delano-Wood et al., 2009), three neuropsychologically separate subgroups were identified: pure memory (e.g., Consortium to Establish a Registry in Alzheimer's Disease [CERAD] Word List Free Recall = 11th percentile); memory and language (e.g., CERAD Word List Free Recall = 8th percentile, Category Fluency = 9th percentile); and executive and processing speed (e.g., Trail Making Test Part B = 1st percentile, Stroop Color Word Test = 4th percentile). These studies highlight the differential cognitive profiles expected to be seen in various MCI subtypes.

Neuropsychological studies have also examined the cognitive changes observed across time in these cases. In general, individuals diagnosed with MCI tend to demonstrate greater cognitive decline than healthy controls, but lesser decline than patients with AD (i.e., decline across a year: AD > MCI > controls). In the original clinical characterization article on MCI (Petersen et al., 1999), yearly declines on two cognitive screening measures were reported. On the MMSE, controls showed no change across 1 year, patients with MCI declined by 1 point, and patients with AD declined by 2 to 3 points. On the total score of the Mattis Dementia Rating Scale, again controls showed no change, but patients with MCI declined by 2 points and patients with AD declined by 7 points. More than 10 years later, the initial results of the ADNI trial showed a similar annual cognitive decline pattern: AD > MCI > controls (Petersen et al., 2010). Two additional interesting findings come from examining these cognitive change scores in this large trial. First, although these patients were almost exclusively suffering from amnestic MCI, they demonstrated changes across nearly all cognitive tasks (e.g., Auditory Verbal Learning Test Delayed Recall = −0.4 words, Trail Making Test Part B = +9.0 seconds, Category Fluency = −0.7 words, Boston Naming Test = −0.2 correct). This finding seems to suggest a spreading of the cognitive impairment beyond memory, which could be an indicator of the development of full-blown dementia. A second interesting finding is that both the MCI and AD groups declined on nearly all measures across time, but the controls tended to improve on measures across time. The improvement in cognitive test scores across time by controls is likely due to practice effects (McCaffrey, Duff, & Westervelt, 2000); however, this provides an avenue for additional research.

While others have previously identified that practice effects can be absent in MCI and dementia (Cooper et al., 2001; Cooper, Lacritz, Weiner, Rosenberg, & Cullum, 2004; Darby, Maruff, Collie, & McStephen, 2002), we have identified that practice effects may have diagnostic, prognostic, and treatment implications in MCI. In a group of 62 older adults classified with MCI (both pure amnestic and amnestic plus other deficits; Duff et al., 2008), nearly all subjects demonstrated some practice effects when reevaluated after 1 week. However, 49% of the MCI subjects improved so significantly that they could no longer be classified as having MCI. For example, in the "low practice effects" group, performance on the Brief Visuospatial Memory Test—Revised improved from the 1st percentile at baseline to the 6th percentile after 1 week. In the "high practice effects" group, performance on this same measure across this same interval improved from the 5th percentile to the 61st percentile (see Figure 14.2). If some patients with MCI dramatically improve with retesting across 1 week, then these findings have some practical clinical implications. First, short-term practice effects might be useful in diagnosing MCI. The individuals who failed to benefit from repeated exposure to test materials clearly seem to have amnestic MCI, and this is consistent with prior work (Darby et al., 2002). However, what should be said about those that do significantly benefit from practice? These individuals did have memory impairment on the baseline testing that would qualify for MCI, but they normalized on retesting. It is possible that these individuals reflect a "pre-MCI" phase (Saykin et al., 2006) or "accidental MCI" (Brooks, Iverson, & White, 2007). A second implication of these practice effect findings relates to treatment recommendations. If these patients, who are mildly to severely memory impaired, can benefit from practice, then should additional efforts be made at cognitive rehabilitation? Even the "low practice effects" group improved on short-term retesting, despite averaging at the 1st percentile on a visual memory measure. Clinicians might rethink the treatment

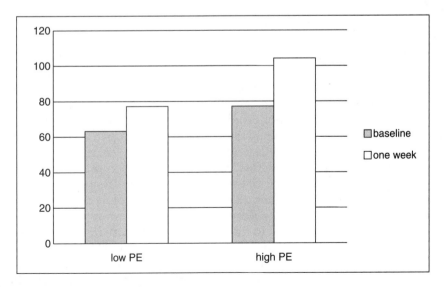

FIGURE 14.2 One-week practice effects in two groups of individuals with amnestic MCI.

MCI, mild cognitive impairment; PE, practice effects.

Note: Y-axis is age-corrected standard score on Brief Visuospatial Memory Test—Revised.

possibilities for these individuals, or at least use some measure of learning (e.g., practice effects) to make decisions about treatment recommendations (Duff, Beglinger, Moser, Schultz, & Paulsen, 2010c). A final implication of these findings is that practice effects appear to have some prognostic value as well, as individuals with lower practice effects tended to demonstrate more decline across time compared to those with higher practice effects (Duff et al., 2007, 2010b). We have also observed that MCI patients who do not show the expected short-term practice effects are more likely to have amyloid deposition than those who do show the expected practice effects (Duff et al., 2014). Although these findings need to be replicated, practice effects appear to have some value to clinicians who evaluate these mildly impaired patients.

WHAT CUTOFF SHOULD BE USED FOR DETERMINING IMPAIRMENT IN MCI?

Although many clinicians and researchers working in MCI tend to use 1.5 SD below the mean as a cutoff for "impairment," others have used different cutoffs (e.g., –1.0 SD, –2.0 SD). Interestingly, for neuropsychologists, the original article on the clinical characterization of MCI (Petersen et al., 1999) did not provide a strict cutoff for determining memory impairment. Similarly, it did not provide any guidance on what constituted normal general cognitive functioning. Only in their Comment section did the authors mention anything that appears to be a more formal operational definition for cognitive scores in MCI. They noted that the objective cognitive tests would corroborate the subjective complaint, and that an impaired memory score was "generally 1.5 SD below age- and education-matched control subjects" and normal scores on other cognitive tasks were "within 0.5 SD of appropriate controls." Nonetheless, this has been popularly interpreted to mean that 1.5 SD below normative data is the only appropriate cutoff for the diagnosis of MCI. In subsequent writings, Petersen has tried to clarify this point. For example, he indicated that the original MCI cohort had a *mean* performance of 1.5 SD below the controls, which indicates that approximately half of the sample had scores above this "cutoff" (Petersen, 2004). He also noted that individual difference variables (e.g., premorbidly high or low functioning abilities) may alter what reflects impairment for different patients. Others have similarly argued against a strict application of these criteria (Duff, Hobson et al., 2010).

On a related point, should an absolute cutoff for impairment be used, or a relative one? An absolute cutoff would use exactly the same cutoff for all individuals, regardless of age, education, or premorbid intellect. In this scenario, an absolute cutoff of 1.5 SD below the mean (e.g., standard score of 78 [7th percentile]) would be used for individuals who are premorbidly average (e.g., standard score of 100 [50th percentile]); high average (e.g., standard score of 112 [80th percentile]); or low average (e.g., standard score of 87 [20th percentile]). However, if an individual needs to decline past the cutoff to be classified as having MCI, then the amount of decline in these three individuals will be dramatically different. The person with average premorbid abilities should decline by 22 standard score points to break the cutoff of MCI. In the high-average person, a decline of 34 standard score points should occur to break the same absolute cutoff. In the low-average person, he or she must decline by only 9 standard score points before being identified with the cognitive impairment associated with MCI. A relative cutoff would use a dynamic or floating cutoff that accounts for the individual difference variables of interest (e.g., premorbid intellect). In this scenario, the cutoff could still be 1.5 SD below the mean, but the relative decline would be tied to the person's premorbid level. That is, all individuals would need to decline by the same 1.5 SD to be classified as having MCI. The premorbidly average person would still need to decline by 22 standard score points. However, with this relative cutoff, the high-average and low-average persons also must decline by the same number of relative units (i.e., 22 standard score points). The high-average person needs to drop to a standard score of 90 or lower (i.e., 112 − 22 = 90), and the low-average person must drop to a standard score of 65 or lower (i.e., 87 − 22 = 65). Although premorbid intellect was used in the current example, relative cutoffs could be applied to other individual difference variables. Neuropsychologists already use some type of relative cutoff in their clinical practice, but it may be useful to lobby for including this approach into the diagnostic criteria for MCI and dementia.

WHAT ARE THE NEUROPATHOLOGICAL FEATURES ASSOCIATED WITH MCI?

If MCI is a precursor to dementia, then it is expected that these individuals will display a milder profile of neuropathological features than that seen in dementia. According to the most recent research diagnostic criteria for MCI due to AD (Albert et al., 2011), evidence of beta-amyloid deposition, neuronal injury, and/or other biochemical changes needs to be seen to increase confidence of the etiology of MCI. In studies examining these biomarkers, they are consistent with many of the other abnormalities in MCI; that is, they fall between healthy elders and patients with dementia.

In a meta-analysis of 14 structural imaging studies in MCI, significant bilateral hippocampal atrophy was found in individuals with MCI (Shi, Liu, Zhou, Yu, & Jiang, 2009). Compared to controls, the average volume reduction of the hippocampi was 12.5% in MCI and 23.6% in AD. More recent results from the ADNI (Leung et al., 2010) and AIBL (Villemagne et al., 2013) trials were comparable, with decreasing hippocampal volumes from controls to MCI to AD. Overall, hippocampal atrophy can be used as evidence of neuronal injury in the research criteria for MCI. However, these authors also provided information about subgroups of MCI based on their follow-up status. MCI patients who went on to convert to dementia had significantly smaller hippocampi than those who remained stable on follow-up. MCI "reverters" (i.e., classified as intact/normal on follow-up) had the largest hippocampi of any of the MCI subgroups. Also using the ADNI sample, the value of serial MRI studies can be seen (Vemuri et al., 2010). Annual decreases in ventricular volume linearly increased from controls (1.4 cm^3) to amnestic MCI (2.9 cm^3) to AD (4.4 cm^3) patients, and these annual changes in ventricular volumes were related to changes on cognitive and functional measures (MMSE and CDR). Using diffuse tensor imaging (DTI), patients with MCI have been found to have a profile similar to those with AD, including decreased fractional anisotropy, a measure of white matter connectivity (Sexton, Kalu, Filippini, Mackay, & Ebmeier, 2011). Despite the strength of these structural imaging modalities in MCI, another meta-analysis found that memory testing had a larger effect size than MRI-measured medial temporal lobe volumes (Schmand, Huizenga, & van Gool, 2010).

Another biomarker of neuronal injury in suspected AD has been FDG-PET hypometabolism. In the ADNI trial, their FDG-PET outcome variable was regional cerebral metabolic rate for glucose (CMRgl). Consistent with the MRI data from this same trial, MCI and AD patients had significantly lower CMRgl bilaterally compared to controls, and the regions primarily affected were in posterior cingulate, precuneus, and parietotemporal and frontal cortices (Langbaum et al., 2009). In an examination of the 1-year follow-up FDG-PET data (Chen et al., 2010), the MCI and AD groups each had significant declines in CMRgl compared to controls, and these declines were most noticeable in the cingulate, parietal, temporal, frontal, and occipital cortices. The declines in FDG-PET metabolism were also correlated with clinical measures of decline.

Amyloid imaging via PET has also been used to examine the pathology associated with MCI due to AD. In ADNI trials using F18-AV-45, participants with "early" MCI had significantly greater levels of cortical amyloid deposition compared to healthy controls (Wu et al., 2012). In this same study, individuals identified as "late" MCI tended to have comparable amyloid levels as those already diagnosed with AD. Using a different amyloid imaging compound (C11-PIB), 67% of AIBL's MCI subjects were found to have elevated amyloid levels at baseline, whereas 26% of their healthy controls and 95% of the AD participants had elevated amyloid levels at baseline (Villemagne et al., 2013).

Other biomarkers that have frequently been examined in AD (e.g., ApoE e4, beta-amyloid, tau) have also been studied in the case of MCI. Although a systematic review and meta-analysis (Diniz, Pinto Júnior, & Forlenza, 2008) found that individuals with MCI had lower amyloid beta, higher total tau, and higher phosphorylated tau in their CSF compared to controls, these measures appear to be far from diagnostics for MCI (or dementia) at this point. ADNI and AIBL observed similar findings in their cohorts (Ellis et al., 2009; Petersen et al., 2010). Studies combine biomarkers (e.g., MRI volumes, beta-amyloid, cognitive test scores) to best diagnose and predict the course in MCI (Bouwman et al., 2007).

WHAT TREATMENT OPTIONS ARE AVAILABLE FOR MCI?

Cholinesterase inhibitors remain the primary pharmacological treatment for AD. Similarly, they appear to be the first-line choice in MCI. However, the empirical evidence to support this choice is limited. In a meta-analysis of four randomized clinical trials of cholinesterase inhibitors in MCI (Diniz et al., 2009), approximately 15% of patients converted to dementia while on the drug compared to 20% taking placebo. Although this difference was statistically significant, it might be countered by the additional information that dropout rates were higher in the medication group compared to those in the placebo. In the largest treatment trial of MCI to date, donepezil (another cholinesterase inhibitor) was associated with less progression to AD in the first year of the study, but no differences in progression rates between donepezil and placebo were observed after 3 years (Petersen et al., 2005).

There have been multiple meta-analyses and systematic reviews of cognitive rehabilitation-like programs for MCI. For example, Li et al. (2011) found benefits of these programs on objective and subjective outcome measures. Significant post-intervention improvements occurred on 44% of objective measures of memory and 12% of objective measures of other cognition domains (Jean, Bergeron, Thivierge, & Simard, 2010). Improvements were also observed in nearly half of the subjective measures of memory, quality of life, or mood. Although most of these studies appeared far less rigorously controlled than the pharmacological studies, they do offer promise for nonmedical treatment options in MCI.

WHAT TO CONCLUDE ABOUT MCI?

Believe in it or not, like it or not, MCI, as a diagnostic category, appears to be here to stay for the foreseeable future. Although the concept has evolved considerably over the past 15 years, there are many areas where it still needs development. More formal criteria for defining the cognitive and functional impairment in MCI are needed. These criteria would allow us to better estimate its prevalence, morbidity, and outcomes. These criteria would allow us to design and conduct better treatment trials. These criteria would allow us to learn more about individuals who are "not normal" but "not demented."

REFERENCES

Albert, M. S., DeKosky, S. T., Dickson, D., Dubois, B., Feldman, H. H., Fox, N. C.,…Phelps, C. H. (2011). The diagnosis of mild cognitive impairment due to Alzheimer's disease: Recommendations from the National Institute on Aging-Alzheimer's Association workgroups on diagnostic guidelines for Alzheimer's disease. *Alzheimer's & Dementia, 7*(3), 270–279.

American Psychiatric Association (APA). (2000). *Diagnostic and statistical manual of mental disorders* (4th ed., text rev.). Washington, DC: Author.

Bouwman, F. H., Schoonenboom, S. N., van der Flier, W. M., van Elk, E. J., Kok, A., Barkhof, F.,…Scheltens, P. (2007). CSF biomarkers and medial temporal lobe atrophy predict dementia in mild cognitive impairment. *Neurobiology of Aging, 28*(7), 1070–1074.

Boyle, P. A., Wilson, R. S., Aggarwal, N. T., Arvanitakis, Z., Kelly, J., Bienias, J. L., & Bennett, D. A. (2005). Parkinsonian signs in subjects with mild cognitive impairment. *Neurology, 65*(12), 1901–1906.

Brandt, J., Aretouli, E., Neijstrom, E., Samek, J., Manning, K., Albert, M. S., & Bandeen-Roche, K. (2009). Selectivity of executive function deficits in mild cognitive impairment. *Neuropsychology, 23*(5), 607–618.

Brooks, B. L., Iverson, G. L., & White, T. (2007). Substantial risk of "Accidental MCI" in healthy older adults: Base rates of low memory scores in neuropsychological assessment. *Journal of the International Neuropsychological Society, 13*(3), 490–500.

Calabrese, M., Rinaldi, F., Mattisi, I., Grossi, P., Favaretto, A., Atzori, M.,…Gallo, P. (2010). Widespread cortical thinning characterizes patients with MS with mild cognitive impairment. *Neurology, 74*(4), 321–328.

Caviness, J. N., Driver-Dunckley, E., Connor, D. J., Sabbagh, M. N., Hentz, J. G., Noble, B.,… Adler, C. H. (2007). Defining mild cognitive impairment in Parkinson's disease. *Movement Disorders, 22*(9), 1272–1277.

Chapman, R. M., Mapstone, M., McCrary, J. W., Gardner, M. N., Porsteinsson, A., Sandoval, T. C.,…Reilly, L. A. (2011). Predicting conversion from mild cognitive impairment to Alzheimer's disease using neuropsychological tests and multivariate methods. *Journal of Clinical and Experimental Neuropsychology, 33*(2), 187–199.

Chelune, G. J., Naugle, R. I., Luders, H., Sedlak, J., & Awad, I. A. (1993). Individual change after epilepsy surgery: Practice effects and base-rate information. *Neuropsychology, 7*(1), 41–52.

Chen, K., Langbaum, J. B., Fleisher, A. S., Ayutyanont, N., Reschke, C., Lee, W.,… Reiman, E. M.; Alzheimer's Disease Neuroimaging Initiative. (2010). Twelve-month metabolic declines in probable Alzheimer's disease and amnestic mild cognitive impairment assessed using an empirically pre-defined statistical region-of-interest: Findings from the Alzheimer's Disease Neuroimaging Initiative. *NeuroImage, 51*(2), 654–664.

Christensen, H., Henderson, A. S., Jorm, A. F., Mackinnon, A. J., Scott, R., & Korten, A. E. (1995). ICD-10 mild cognitive disorder: Epidemiological evidence on its validity. *Psychological Medicine, 25*(1), 105–120.

Cooper, D. B., Epker, M., Lacritz, L., Weine, M., Rosenberg, R. N., Honig, L., & Cullum, C. M. (2001). Effects of practice on category fluency in Alzheimer's disease. *The Clinical Neuropsychologist, 15*(1), 125–128.

Cooper, D. B., Lacritz, L. H., Weiner, M. F., Rosenberg, R. N., & Cullum, C. M. (2004). Category fluency in mild cognitive impairment: Reduced effect of practice in test-retest conditions. *Alzheimer Disease and Associated Disorders, 18*(3), 120–122.

Crook, T., Bartus, R. T., Ferris, S. H., Whitehouse, P., Cohen, G. D., & Gershon, S. (1986). Age-associated memory impairment: Proposed diagnostic criteria and measures of clinical change. Report of a National Institute of Mental Health Work Group. *Developmental Neuropsychology, 2*, 261–276.

Darby, D., Maruff, P., Collie, A., & McStephen, M. (2002). Mild cognitive impairment can be detected by multiple assessments in a single day. *Neurology, 59*(7), 1042–1046.

de Rotrou, J., Wenisch, E., Chausson, C., Dray, F., Faucounau, V., & Rigaud, A. S. (2005). Accidental MCI in healthy subjects: A prospective longitudinal study. *European Journal of Neurology, 12*(11), 879–885.

Delano-Wood, L., Bondi, M. W., Sacco, J., Abeles, N., Jak, A. J., Libon, D. J., & Bozoki, A. (2009). Heterogeneity in mild cognitive impairment: Differences in neuropsychological profile and associated white matter lesion pathology. *Journal of the International Neuropsychological Society, 15*(6), 906–914.

Devanand, D. P., Tabert, M. H., Cuasay, K., Manly, J. J., Schupf, N., Brickman, A. M., . . . Mayeux, R. (2010). Olfactory identification deficits and MCI in a multi-ethnic elderly community sample. *Neurobiology of Aging, 31*(9), 1593–1600.

Diniz, B. S., Pinto Júnior, J. A., & Forlenza, O. V. (2008). Do CSF total tau, phosphorylated tau, and beta-amyloid 42 help to predict progression of mild cognitive impairment to Alzheimer's disease? A systematic review and meta-analysis of the literature. *The World Journal of Biological Psychiatry, 9*(3), 172–182.

Diniz, B. S., Pinto, J. A., Gonzaga, M. L., Guimarães, F. M., Gattaz, W. F., & Forlenza, O. V. (2009). To treat or not to treat? A meta-analysis of the use of cholinesterase inhibitors in mild cognitive impairment for delaying progression to Alzheimer's disease. *European Archives of Psychiatry and Clinical Neuroscience, 259*(4), 248–256.

Duff, K., Beglinger, L. J., Schultz, S. K., Moser, D. J., McCaffrey, R. J., Haase, R. F., . . . Paulsen, J. S.; Huntington's Study Group. (2007). Practice effects in the prediction of long-term cognitive outcome in three patient samples: A novel prognostic index. *Archives of Clinical Neuropsychology, 22*(1), 15–24.

Duff, K., Beglinger, L. J., Moser, D. J., & Paulsen, J. S. (2010a). Predicting cognitive change within domains. *The Clinical Neuropsychologist, 24*(5), 779–792.

Duff, K., Beglinger, L. J., Moser, D. J., Paulsen, J. S., Schultz, S. K., & Arndt, S. (2010b). Predicting cognitive change in older adults: The relative contribution of practice effects. *Archives of Clinical Neuropsychology, 25*(2), 81–88.

Duff, K., Beglinger, L. J., Moser, D. J., Schultz, S. K., & Paulsen, J. S. (2010c). Practice effects and outcome of cognitive training: Preliminary evidence from a memory training course. *The American Journal of Geriatric Psychiatry, 18*(1), 91.

Duff, K., Beglinger, L. J., Van Der Heiden, S., Moser, D. J., Arndt, S., Schultz, S. K., & Paulsen, J. S. (2008). Short-term practice effects in amnestic mild cognitive impairment: Implications for diagnosis and treatment. *International Psychogeriatrics/IPA, 20*(5), 986–999.

Duff, K., Foster, N. L., & Hoffman, J. M. (2014). Practice effects and amyloid deposition: Preliminary data on a method for enriching samples in clinical trials. *Alzheimer Disease and Associated Disorders, 28*(3), 247–252.

Duff, K., Hobson, V. L., Beglinger, L. J., & O'Bryant, S. E. (2010). Diagnostic accuracy of the RBANS in mild cognitive impairment: Limitations on assessing milder impairments. *Archives of Clinical Neuropsychology, 25*(5), 429–441.

Duff, K., Paulsen, J., Mills, J., Beglinger, L. J., Moser, D. J., Smith, M. M.,…Harrington, D. L.; PREDICT-HD Investigators and Coordinators of the Huntington Study Group. (2010). Mild cognitive impairment in prediagnosed Huntington disease. *Neurology, 75*(6), 500–507.

Economou, A., Papageorgiou, S. G., Karageorgiou, C., & Vassilopoulos, D. (2007). Nonepisodic memory deficits in amnestic MCI. *Cognitive and Behavioral Neurology, 20*(2), 99–106.

Edwards, E. R., Spira, A. P., Barnes, D. E., & Yaffe, K. (2009). Neuropsychiatric symptoms in mild cognitive impairment: Differences by subtype and progression to dementia. *International Journal of Geriatric Psychiatry, 24*(7), 716–722.

Elias-Sonnenschein, L. S., Viechtbauer, W., Ramakers, I. H., Verhey, F. R., & Visser, P. J. (2011). Predictive value of APOE-e4 allele for progression from MCI to AD-type dementia: A meta-analysis. *Journal of Neurology, Neurosurgery, and Psychiatry, 82*(10), 1149–1156.

Ellis, K. A., Bush, A. I., Darby, D., De Fazio, D., Foster, J., Hudson, P.,…Ames, D.; AIBL Research Group. (2009). The Australian Imaging, Biomarkers and Lifestyle (AIBL) study of aging: Methodology and baseline characteristics of 1112 individuals recruited for a longitudinal study of Alzheimer's disease. *International Psychogeriatrics/IPA, 21*(4), 672–687.

Ewers, M., Walsh, C., Trojanowski, J. Q., Shaw, L. M., Petersen, R. C., Jack, C. R.,…Hampel, H.; North American Alzheimer's Disease Neuroimaging Initiative (ADNI). (2012). Prediction of conversion from mild cognitive impairment to Alzheimer's disease dementia based upon biomarkers and neuropsychological test performance. *Neurobiology of Aging, 33*(7), 1203–1214.

Farias, S. T., Mungas, D., Reed, B. R., Harvey, D., Cahn-Weiner, D., & Decarli, C. (2006). MCI is associated with deficits in everyday functioning. *Alzheimer Disease and Associated Disorders, 20*(4), 217–223.

Fisk, J. D., Merry, H. R., & Rockwood, K. (2003). Variations in case definition affect prevalence but not outcomes of mild cognitive impairment. *Neurology, 61*(9), 1179–1184.

Graham, J. E., Rockwood, K., Beattie, B. L., Eastwood, R., Gauthier, S., Tuokko, H., & McDowell, I. (1997). Prevalence and severity of cognitive impairment with and without dementia in an elderly population. *Lancet, 349*(9068), 1793–1796.

Griffith, H. R., Belue, K., Sicola, A., Krzywanski, S., Zamrini, E., Harrell, L., & Marson, D. C. (2003). Impaired financial abilities in mild cognitive impairment: A direct assessment approach. *Neurology, 60*(3), 449–457.

Gualtieri, C. T., & Morgan, D. W. (2008). The frequency of cognitive impairment in patients with anxiety, depression, and bipolar disorder: An unaccounted source of variance in clinical trials. *The Journal of Clinical Psychiatry, 69*(7), 1122–1130.

Hachinski, V., Iadecola, C., Petersen, R. C., Breteler, M. M., Nyenhuis, D. L., Black, S. E.,… Leblanc, G. G. (2006). National Institute of Neurological Disorders and Stroke-Canadian Stroke Network vascular cognitive impairment harmonization standards. *Stroke, 37*(9), 2220–2241.

Jean, L., Bergeron, M. E., Thivierge, S., & Simard, M. (2010). Cognitive intervention programs for individuals with mild cognitive impairment: Systematic review of the literature. *The American Journal of Geriatric Psychiatry, 18*(4), 281–296.

Kral, V. A. (1962). Senescent forgetfulness: Benign and malignant. *Canadian Medical Association Journal, 86*, 257–260.

Langbaum, J. B., Chen, K., Lee, W., Reschke, C., Bandy, D., Fleisher, A. S.,…Reiman, E. M.; Alzheimer's Disease Neuroimaging Initiative. (2009). Categorical and correlational analyses of baseline fluorodeoxyglucose positron emission tomography images from the Alzheimer's Disease Neuroimaging Initiative (ADNI). *NeuroImage, 45*(4), 1107–1116.

Leung, K. K., Barnes, J., Ridgway, G. R., Bartlett, J. W., Clarkson, M. J., Macdonald, K.,... Ourselin, S.; Alzheimer's Disease Neuroimaging Initiative. (2010). Automated cross-sectional and longitudinal hippocampal volume measurement in mild cognitive impairment and Alzheimer's disease. *NeuroImage, 51*(4), 1345–1359.

Levy, R. (1994). Aging-associated cognitive decline. Working Party of the International Psychogeriatric Association in collaboration with the World Health Organization. *International Psychogeriatrics/IPA, 6*(1), 63–68.

Li, H., Li, J., Li, N., Li, B., Wang, P., & Zhou, T. (2011). Cognitive intervention for persons with mild cognitive impairment: A meta-analysis. *Ageing Research Reviews, 10*(2), 285–296.

Libon, D. J., Xie, S. X., Eppig, J., Wicas, G., Lamar, M., Lippa, C.,... Wambach, D. M. (2010). The heterogeneity of mild cognitive impairment: A neuropsychological analysis. *Journal of the International Neuropsychological Society, 16*(1), 84–93.

Liu, Y., Mattila, J., Ruiz, M. Á., Paajanen, T., Koikkalainen, J., van Gils, M.,... Soininen, H.; The Alzheimer's Disease Neuroimaging Initiative. (2013). Predicting AD conversion: Comparison between prodromal AD guidelines and computer assisted PredictAD tool. *PLoS One, 8*(2), e55246. doi: 10.1371/journal.pone.0055246

Luck, T., Luppa, M., Briel, S., & Riedel-Heller, S. G. (2010). Incidence of mild cognitive impairment: A systematic review. *Dementia and Geriatric Cognitive Disorders, 29*(2), 164–175.

Lyketsos, C. G., Lopez, O., Jones, B., Fitzpatrick, A. L., Breitner, J., & DeKosky, S. (2002). Prevalence of neuropsychiatric symptoms in dementia and mild cognitive impairment: Results from the cardiovascular health study. *JAMA, 288*(12), 1475–1483.

Manly, J. J., Tang, M. X., Schupf, N., Stern, Y., Vonsattel, J. P., & Mayeux, R. (2008). Frequency and course of mild cognitive impairment in a multiethnic community. *Annals of Neurology, 63*(4), 494–506.

Mariani, E., Monastero, R., Ercolani, S., Mangialasche, F., Caputo, M., Feliziani, F. T.,... Mecocci, P.; ReGAl Study Group. (2007). Vascular risk factors in mild cognitive impairment subtypes. Findings from the ReGAl project. *Dementia and Geriatric Cognitive Disorders, 24*(6), 448–456.

McCaffrey, R. J., Duff, K., & Westervelt, H. J. (2000). *Practitioner's guide to evaluating change with neuropsychological assessment instruments.* New York, NY: Plenum/Kluwer.

McSweeny, A. J., Naugle, R. I., Chelune, G. J., & Luders, H. (1993). T scores for change: An illustration of a regression approach to depicting change in clinical neuropsychology. *The Clinical Neuropsychologist, 7,* 300–312.

Mitchell, A. J., & Shiri-Feshki, M. (2009). Rate of progression of mild cognitive impairment to dementia—meta-analysis of 41 robust inception cohort studies. *Acta Psychiatrica Scandinavica, 119*(4), 252–265.

Morris, J. C., Roe, C. M., Grant, E. A., Head, D., Storandt, M., Goate, A. M.,... Mintun, M. A. (2009). Pittsburgh compound B imaging and prediction of progression from cognitive normality to symptomatic Alzheimer disease. *Archives of Neurology, 66*(12), 1469–1475.

Morris, J. C., Storandt, M., Miller, J. P., McKeel, D. W., Price, J. L., Rubin, E. H., & Berg, L. (2001). Mild cognitive impairment represents early-stage Alzheimer disease. *Archives of Neurology, 58*(3), 397–405.

Murphy, K. J., Rich, J. B., & Troyer, A. K. (2006). Verbal fluency patterns in amnestic mild cognitive impairment are characteristic of Alzheimer's type dementia. *Journal of the International Neuropsychological Society, 12*(4), 570–574.

Nutter-Upham, K. E., Saykin, A. J., Rabin, L. A., Roth, R. M., Wishart, H. A., Pare, N., & Flashman, L. A. (2008). Verbal fluency performance in amnestic MCI and older adults with cognitive complaints. *Archives of Clinical Neuropsychology, 23*(3), 229–241.

Palmer, K., Di Iulio, F., Varsi, A. E., Gianni, W., Sancesario, G., Caltagirone, C., & Spalletta, G. (2010). Neuropsychiatric predictors of progression from amnestic-mild cognitive impairment to Alzheimer's disease: The role of depression and apathy. *Journal of Alzheimer's Disease, 20*(1), 175–183.

Petersen, R. C. (2004). Mild cognitive impairment as a diagnostic entity. *Journal of Internal Medicine, 256*(3), 183–194.

Petersen, R. C., Aisen, P. S., Beckett, L. A., Donohue, M. C., Gamst, A. C., Harvey, D. J.,… Weiner, M. W. (2010). Alzheimer's Disease Neuroimaging Initiative (ADNI): Clinical characterization. *Neurology, 74*(3), 201–209.

Petersen, R. C., Doody, R., Kurz, A., Mohs, R. C., Morris, J. C., Rabins, P. V.,…Winblad, B. (2001). Current concepts in mild cognitive impairment. *Archives of Neurology, 58*(12), 1985–1992.

Petersen, R. C., Roberts, R. O., Knopman, D. S., Boeve, B. F., Geda, Y. E., Ivnik, R. J.,…Jack, C. R. (2009). Mild cognitive impairment: Ten years later. *Archives of Neurology, 66*(12), 1447–1455.

Petersen, R. C., Smith, G. E., Waring, S. C., Ivnik, R. J., Tangalos, E. G., & Kokmen, E. (1999). Mild cognitive impairment: Clinical characterization and outcome. *Archives of Neurology, 56*(3), 303–308.

Petersen, R. C., Thomas, R. G., Grundman, M., Bennett, D., Doody, R., Ferris, S.,…Thal, L. J.; Alzheimer's Disease Cooperative Study Group. (2005). Vitamin E and donepezil for the treatment of mild cognitive impairment. *The New England Journal of Medicine, 352*(23), 2379–2388.

Ramanan, V. K., Kim, S., Holohan, K., Shen, L., Nho, K., Risacher, S. L.,…Saykin, A. J.; Alzheimer's Disease Neuroimaging Initiative (ADNI). (2012). Genome-wide pathway analysis of memory impairment in the Alzheimer's Disease Neuroimaging Initiative (ADNI) cohort implicates gene candidates, canonical pathways, and networks. *Brain Imaging and Behavior, 6*(4), 634–648.

Risacher, S. L., Shen, L., West, J. D., Kim, S., McDonald, B. C., Beckett, L. A.,…Saykin, A. J.; Alzheimer's Disease Neuroimaging Initiative (ADNI). (2010). Longitudinal MRI atrophy biomarkers: Relationship to conversion in the ADNI cohort. *Neurobiology of Aging, 31*(8), 1401–1418.

Saunders, N. L., & Summers, M. J. (2010). Attention and working memory deficits in mild cognitive impairment. *Journal of Clinical and Experimental Neuropsychology, 32*(4), 350–357.

Saykin, A. J., Wishart, H. A., Rabin, L. A., Santulli, R. B., Flashman, L. A., West, J. D.,… Mamourian, A. C. (2006). Older adults with cognitive complaints show brain atrophy similar to that of amnestic MCI. *Neurology, 67*(5), 834–842.

Schmand, B., Huizenga, H. M., & van Gool, W. A. (2010). Meta-analysis of CSF and MRI biomarkers for detecting preclinical Alzheimer's disease. *Psychological Medicine, 40*(1), 135–145.

Sexton, C. E., Kalu, U. G., Filippini, N., Mackay, C. E., & Ebmeier, K. P. (2011). A meta-analysis of diffusion tensor imaging in mild cognitive impairment and Alzheimer's disease. *Neurobiology of Aging, 32*(12), 2322.e5–2322.18.

Shi, F., Liu, B., Zhou, Y., Yu, C., & Jiang, T. (2009). Hippocampal volume and asymmetry in mild cognitive impairment and Alzheimer's disease: Meta-analyses of MRI studies. *Hippocampus, 19*(11), 1055–1064.

Storandt, M., Grant, E. A., Miller, J. P., & Morris, J. C. (2006). Longitudinal course and neuropathologic outcomes in original vs revised MCI and in pre-MCI. *Neurology, 67*(3), 467–473.

Tremont, G., Miele, A., Smith, M. M., & Westervelt, H. J. (2010). Comparison of verbal memory impairment rates in mild cognitive impairment. *Journal of Clinical and Experimental Neuropsychology, 32*(6), 630–636.

Vemuri, P., Wiste, H. J., Weigand, S. D., Knopman, D. S., Trojanowski, J. Q., Shaw, L. M.,... Jack, C. R.; Alzheimer's Disease Neuroimaging Initiative. (2010). Serial MRI and CSF biomarkers in normal aging, MCI, and AD. *Neurology, 75*(2), 143–151.

Verghese, J., Robbins, M., Holtzer, R., Zimmerman, M., Wang, C., Xue, X., & Lipton, R. B. (2008). Gait dysfunction in mild cognitive impairment syndromes. *Journal of the American Geriatrics Society, 56*(7), 1244–1251.

Villemagne, V. L., Burnham, S., Bourgeat, P., Brown, B., Ellis, K. A., Salvado, O.,... Masters, C. L.; Australian Imaging Biomarkers and Lifestyle (AIBL) Research Group. (2013). Amyloid ß deposition, neurodegeneration, and cognitive decline in sporadic Alzheimer's disease: A prospective cohort study. *Lancet Neurology, 12*(4), 357–367.

Wadley, V. G., Okonkwo, O., Crowe, M., Vance, D. E., Elgin, J. M., Ball, K. K., & Owsley, C. (2009). Mild cognitive impairment and everyday function: An investigation of driving performance. *Journal of Geriatric Psychiatry and Neurology, 22*(2), 87–94.

Westervelt, H. J., Bruce, J. M., Coon, W. G., & Tremont, G. (2008). Odor identification in mild cognitive impairment subtypes. *Journal of Clinical and Experimental Neuropsychology, 30*(2), 151–156.

Wilson, R. S., Aggarwal, N. T., Barnes, L. L., Bienias, J. L., Mendes de Leon, C. F., & Evans, D. A. (2009). Biracial population study of mortality in mild cognitive impairment and Alzheimer disease. *Archives of Neurology, 66*(6), 767–772.

Winblad, B., Palmer, K., Kivipelto, M., Jelic, V., Fratiglioni, L., Wahlund, L. O.,... Petersen, R. C. (2004). Mild cognitive impairment—beyond controversies, towards a consensus: Report of the International Working Group on Mild Cognitive Impairment. *Journal of Internal Medicine, 256*(3), 240–246.

Wu, L., Rowley, J., Mohades, S., Leuzy, A., Dauar, M. T., Shin, M.,... Rosa-Neto, P.; Alzheimer's Disease Neuroimaging Initiative. (2012). Dissociation between brain amyloid deposition and metabolism in early mild cognitive impairment. *PLoS One, 7*(10), e47905. doi: 10.1371/journal.pone.0047905

Zahodne, L. B., Gongvatana, A., Cohen, R. A., Ott, B. R., & Tremont, G.; Alzheimer's Disease Neuroimaging Initiative. (2013). Are apathy and depression independently associated with longitudinal trajectories of cortical atrophy in mild cognitive impairment? *The American Journal of Geriatric Psychiatry, 21*(11), 1098–1106.

CHAPTER 15

Delirium: From Pathology to Treatment

Melanie Rylander and Chad A. Noggle

Delirium, also known as acute confusional state, organic brain syndrome, brain failure, and encephalopathy, is a common occurrence among medical and surgical patients and causes extensive morbidity and mortality. Conceptually, delirium represents a crucial interface among internal medicine, neurology, and psychiatry. Historically, clinicians have focused most of their attention on the underlining disorder that accompanies delirium. However, the grave prognostic implications of delirium have sparked interest in conceptualizing this disorder as a separate entity apart from the underlining illness. Though it is commonly discussed in relation to dementia, as noted by Khan, Kahn, and Bourgeois (2009), delirium remains badly neglected in terms of fundamental research attention within the clinical neurosciences, as well as poorly understood and managed in terms of routine clinical care.

Watt, Budding, and Koziol (2012) recently offered an excellent review and reconceptualization of delirium. As stated by these authors "Delirium is consistently underdiagnosed, all too frequently blamed on a 'dementia' (instead of appreciating its superposition and reversible etiologies), and too often iatrogenically created by a number of medical interventions and untoward events (frequent and less-than-optimally circumspect use of benzodiazepines, opiates, and anticholinergics in elderly patients; surgeries; severe sleep deprivation in most ICUs; and hospital-based infections)." Watt et al. (2012) reiterated Hufschmidt, Shabarin, and Zimmer (2009), noting that while distinction is typically drawn between chronic confusional states (in later stages of Alzheimer's disease [AD]) and more acute deliriums, they are symptomatically and behaviorally indistinguishable.

In this chapter, we provide an updated review of delirium, including pathophysiological correlates, clinical features, diagnostic considerations, and contemporary treatment options.

EPIDEMIOLOGY

Delirium is a common occurrence among medical and surgical patients and causes extensive morbidity and mortality. The *Diagnostic and Statistical Manual of Mental Disorders, Fourth Edition, Text Revision* (*DSM-IV-TR*; American Psychiatric Association

TABLE 15.1 *DSM-IV-TR* and *DSM-5* Components of Delirium

DSM-IV-TR
1. Disturbance of consciousness with reduced ability to focus, shift attention, or sustain attention.
2. A change in cognition or development of a perceptual disturbance that is not better accounted for by a preexisting, established, or evolving dementia.
3. The disturbance develops over a short period of time (hours to days) and tends to fluctuate during the course of the day.
4. There is evidence from the history, physical examination, or laboratory findings that the disturbance is caused by the direct physiological consequences of a general medical condition.

DSM-5
1. Attention and awareness are significantly disrupted.
2. Delirium develops over a short period of time, typically hours to days. There is a change in baseline attention and awareness. It fluctuates throughout the day.
3. There is also another disturbance in cognition, such as in memory, orientation, language, and perception.
4. The disturbances in (1) and (3) are not better explained by another preexisting, established, or evolving neurocognitive disorder. (Having a neurocognitive disorder, however, increases the risk of the development of delirium.)
5. There must also be evidence that the delirium is due to a direct physiological consequence of another medical condition, substance intoxication or withdrawal, or exposure to a toxin, or is due to multiple etiologies.

[APA], 2000) suggested that delirium consisted of four components, which was slightly modified during the release of the fifth edition. These components are summarized in Table 15.1.

The defining features of delirium include an acute change in mental status characterized by altered consciousness, cognition, and fluctuations. Delirium frequently occurs in the setting of an acute medical illness or substance intoxication or withdrawal. The incidence of delirium varies depending on the setting. Among patients undergoing elective noncardiac surgery, the incidence has been estimated to be 11% (Franco, Litaker, Locala, & Bronson, 2001). Among general medical inpatients, the incidence is estimated to range from 11% to 42% with high-risk groups having rates close to 60% (Inouye & Charpentier, 1996; Siddiqi, House, & Holmes, 2006). Patients with advanced cancer are estimated to have rates more than 70% (Lawlor et al., 2000). The reported incidence of delirium in ICU patients ranges from 16% to 87%, with higher rates reported in patients with mechanical ventilation (Dubois, Bergeron, Dumont, Dial, & Skrobik, 2001; Ely et al., 2001; Kishi, Iwasaki, Takezawa, Kurosawa, & Endo, 1995; Milbrandt et al., 2004; Thomason et al., 2005).

Delirium has been associated with increased length of stay, institutionalization, and mortality (Franco et al., 2001; Milbrandt et al., 2004; Siddiqi et al., 2006; Thomason et al., 2005). Even after adjusting for confounding factors, it has been estimated that delirium increases hospital costs by at least 30% (Milbrandt et al., 2004). ICU delirium alone has been estimated to cost between 6.5 and 20.4 billion dollars a year (Milbrandt et al., 2004).

RISK FACTORS

The risk factors for delirium have been well studied. These can be divided into two categories: predisposing factors and precipitating factors. Predisposing factors are those that are non-modifiable and specific to the individual patient while precipitating causes are related to the acute illness. Predisposing factors include age more than 70 years; sensory impairment; previous stroke; depression; history of substance abuse; baseline polypharmacy, particularly opioids, anticholinergics, antihistamines, and benzodiazepines; severity of comorbidities (Michaud et al., 2007); smoking history; history of hypertension (Dubois et al., 2001); and poor physical conditioning (van der Mast, van den Broek, Fekkes, Pepplinkhuizen, & Habbema, 2000). Additionally, baseline cognitive impairment is a significant risk factor. McNicoll et al. (2003) did a prospective study of 118 consecutively admitted ICU patients aged 65 years and older. Overall, 70% of patients had delirium at some point during their hospitalization. Patients with baseline dementia were 40% more likely to develop delirium even after controlling for comorbidity, baseline functional status, illness severity, and invasive procedures.

Precipitating causes include respiratory illness, respiratory failure, heart failure, infection, fever, anemia, hypotension, renal failure, hepatic failure, metabolic acidosis, acute stroke, central nervous system (CNS) disease, electrolyte and endocrine disturbances, drug intoxication/withdrawal, polypharmacy with special emphasis on narcotics, anticholinergics, antihistamines and benzodiazepines, physical restraints, number of room changes, absence of a clock, absence of glasses, number of windows in the room, mechanical ventilation, indwelling lines and catheters, and ICU admission (Aldemir, Ozen, Kara, Sir, & Baç, 2001; Michaud et al., 2007).

PATHOPHYSIOLOGY

The mechanism underlining delirium is not understood. Evidence suggests that delirium involves a complex interplay among a series of factors with a common final pathway toward global cerebral dysfunction. Separate factors identified in the literature as having causative roles include inflammatory markers, neurotransmitters, and hormones.

The observation that drugs effecting neurotransmission seem to precipitate and ameliorate delirium leads to the hypothesis that delirium was the result of altered neurotransmission. Anticholingeric drugs have repeatedly been identified as a risk factor for delirium. Therefore, the cognitive dysfunction in delirium may be related to cholinergic deficits (Gunther, Morandi, & Ely, 2008). Serum anticholingeric activity (SAA) is a surrogate marker used in some studies to evaluate the relationship between anticholinergic processes and delirium. Thomas et al. (2008) reported that SAA was higher in delirious ICU patients than in those without delirium. Mach et al. (1995) reported elevated SAA levels in 11 delirious medical patients compared to controls. They found that levels fell with improvement of symptoms. Flacker et al. (1998) observed that SAA levels were independently associated with delirium in elderly medical patients. Although the previous findings support an association between delirium and cholinergic deficits, a cause-and-effect relationship cannot be established.

Imbalances in the synthesis, release, and degradation in gamma-aminobutyric acid (GABA), glutamate, acetylcholine, and the monoamines have also been hypothesized to have roles in delirium. GABA is the primary inhibitory neurotransmitter in the CNS and medications such as benzodiazepines and propofol have known actions at GABA receptors and have been associated with delirium. It has been speculated that decreased CNS arousal caused by increased GABA-ergic activity results in the global cognitive impairment that characterizes delirium (Gunther et al., 2008).

Given widespread projections of the monoamines and their role in other psychiatric conditions, a possible role in the pathogenesis of delirium is intuitive.

Perturbations in dopamine transmission have been linked with parkinsonism on one end and psychosis on the other. Additionally, dopamine antagonists are commonly used to control behavior symptoms in delirious patients. Norepinephrine plays established roles in arousal and attention, both of which are abnormal in delirium. However, studies have failed to elicit the role of monoamines in delirium (Gunther et al., 2008).

van der Mast, van den Broek, Fekkes, Pepplinkhuizen, and Habbema (2000) observed increased levels of phenylalanine and decreased levels of tryptophan to be associated with delirium in 296 patients undergoing elective cardiac surgery. They speculated that alterations in these precursor amino acids could lead to aberrations in the synthesis of monoamines, as well as serotonin and melatonin, respectively. Robinson, Raeburn, Angles, and Moss (2008) found low levels of tryptophan on postoperative day 2, predicting future development of delirium in 50 patients undergoing elective surgery with anticipated postoperative ICU admission.

The frequent association of delirium with sepsis has led many to speculate about the role of inflammatory markers. Sepsis is characterized by a systemic inflammatory response. Sepsis-related delirium is hypothesized to result in altered permeability of the blood–brain barrier (BBB) and vasogenic edema leading to impaired neurotransmission. Aberrations in capillary permeability and blood flow limit oxygen and nutrient delivery to cells resulting in cellular hypoxia and possible cell death. Inflammatory markers such as tumor necrosis factor-alpha, interleukin-1, nitric oxide, and other cytokines and chemokines result in endothelial activation, hypercoagulability, and disseminated intravascular coagulation, resulting in further ischemia (Gunther et al., 2008; Sharshar, Hopkinson, Orlikowski, & Annane, 2005). van Gool, van de Beek, and Eikelenboom (2010) hypothesized that cognitive changes characterizing delirium were the result of unabated activation by microglial cells. Altered permeability of the BBB allows increased amounts of systemic inflammatory markers to enter the CNS and activate microglia. Normally regulated by acetylcholine, the authors stated that the cholinergic deficit observed in delirium or premorbid cholinergic deficits in those with existing dementia lead to unchecked activation and a dysregulated CNS immune response. Activated microglia release cytotoxic substances including chemokines and cytokines that can lead to neuronal death with long-term exposure.

Alterations in vasopressin and cortisol have also been observed in cases of delirium, particularly those associated with sepsis (Sharshar et al., 2005). How these alterations lead to cerebral dysfunction has not been determined. The observation that sleep dysregulation is associated with delirium and improved sleep cycle regulation associated with improvement has led some investigators to speculate about the role of melatonin. Balan et al. (2003) observed variations in 6-sulfatoxymelatonin (6-SMT), the chief metabolite of melatonin, which resolved with symptom resolution in seven patients with hyperactive delirium and ten patients with hypoactive delirium. They did not observe any differences in 6-SMT levels during and after delirium resolution in 14 mixed patients. The high prevalence of delirium in ICU patients further supports a role for melatonin given the high prevalence of sleep disturbances in this population (Figueroa-Ramos, Arroyo-Novoa, Lee, Padilla, & Puntillo, 2009; Mistraletti et al., 2008).

Although several radiographic studies have been performed to elicit information about the mechanism of delirium, the varying methodologies and patient variability have limited the findings. Koponen et al. (1989) found significant differences in ventricular dilation, cortical atrophy, as well as correlations between Mini-Mental State Examination (MMSE) scores and sylvian fissure width in

69 elder delirious patients compared with 31 controls similar in gender and age. It is speculated that these structural changes were present prior to onset of delirium and highlight the importance of baseline structural brain changes as the predisposing factor for delirium. Piazza, Cotena, De Robertis, Caranci, and Tufano (2009) found evidence of vasogenic edema in cerebral MRI in a series of four patients with sepsis-associated delirium. These findings were further substantiated by Sharshar et al. (2007) who analyzed MRI scans in nine patients with sepsis and delirium. Two patients had normal scans, two had evidence of multiple ischemic strokes, and the remaining showed white matter lesions characteristic of ischemia. MRI findings were associated with poor outcomes. The mechanism of this is unclear but may relate to alterations in the BBB stemming from inflammatory mediators involved in sepsis and hyperthermia resulting in chronic ischemia, cellular hypoxia, and ultimately brain dysfunction.

Functional brain imaging has yielded additional findings. Several studies have demonstrated reduced cerebral perfusion in the frontal, parietal, and occipital regions. The perfusion abnormalities were reversible when the delirium resolved (Yokota, Ogawa, Kurokawa, & Yamamoto, 2003). These findings underscore the possible role of cerebral hypoperfusion.

CLINICAL PRESENTATION

Delirium presents with alterations in consciousness, a fluctuating course, perceptual disturbances, motor agitation or retardation, and disorganized thinking. Psychotic symptoms are thought to be present in 40% to 67% of patients (Cutting, 1987; Ross, Peyser, Shapiro, & Folstein, 1991; Webster & Holroyd, 2000). Visual hallucinations are the most common type of hallucinations while paranoia is the most common delusional feature. The presence of psychosis is related to a higher number of comorbid medical problems and having multiple versus single etiology of delirium (Webster & Holroyd, 2000).

Three motor subtypes have been identified: hyperactive, hypoactive, and mixed. Hyperactive delirium is characterized by motor agitation, restlessness, and hypervigilance. Hypoactive is characterized by lethargy and motor retardation. Patients with a mixed subtype demonstrate features of both hypoactive and hyperactive delirium. Mixed delirium is the most common clinical presentation (Meagher, O'Hanlon, O'Mahony, Casey, & Trzepacz, 2000; O'Keeffe & Lavan, 1999). The subtypes differ in terms of phenomenology and prognosis. In general, the hyperactive form has been more strongly associated with alcohol or benzodiazepine withdrawal, younger age, earlier recognition, more frequent use of neuroleptics, and decreased mortality relative to the hypoactive subtype (Kiely, Jones, Bergmann, & Marcantonio, 2007; Meagher, O'Hanlon, O'Mahony, Casey, & Trzepacz, 2000; Peterson et al., 2006). The hypoactive subtype is associated with older age, decreased detection, longer length of hospital stay, increased treatment complications, and increased mortality (Kiely, Jones, Bergmann, & Marcantonio, 2007; O'Keeffe & Lavan, 1999; Yang et al., 2009). Although studies have tried to link motor subtypes with specific etiologies of delirium, there is no clear consensus on this topic.

On a cognitive level, delirium is oftentimes erroneously regarded as a disruption of attention, which is a significant oversimplification. In reality, virtually all "global-state" cognitive operations collapse in direct proportion to the severity of any confusional state; given that these processes are foundational for virtually all other cognitive operations, their joint collapse brings down the entire cognitive apparatus (Mesulam, 1990; Mesulam & Geschwind, 1976; Watt et al., 2012).

DIAGNOSIS

The development of delirium has several prognostic implications making prompt and accurate diagnosis essential. Unfortunately, delirium is often overlooked with non-detection rates reported to be as high as 66% (Brown & Boyle, 2002; Inouye, 1994). Barriers to detection include lack of provider awareness of clinical presentation or experience; hypoactive presentation that is often overlooked; and symptom attribution to another disorder like dementia, depression, or psychosis. Another issue, eluded by others (e.g., Watt et al., 2012), is that delirium, when superimposed on a more chronic presentation such as dementia, may suffer from the impact of diagnostic overshadowing. Often moderately to severely demented patients are regarded as untreatable due to their mental decay being associated with an inescapable structural degeneration in the form of generalized (and regional) atrophy. As clinicians adopt this "there is nothing we can do" mindset, patients are abandoned both in regards to treatment and research (Watt et al., 2012), and thus delirium is not appreciated clinically.

Although the gold standard for delirium diagnosis is the criteria outlined in the *DSM-IV-TR* and now the *DSM-5* (APA, 2013), the use of this in clinical settings is limited by the fact that most care providers are nonpsychiatrists. Furthermore, as discussed by Watt et al. (2012), the *DSM-IV-TR* criteria featured "a number of significant and poorly appreciated problems." As noted by these authors, the *DSM-IV* criteria did not appreciate the range of severity that can be seen across cases and the use of the term *confusional* or its variants is highly nonspecific. However, the recently released *DSM-5* did not rectify this issue. Watt et al. (2012) offered additional insight regarding issues with the *DSM-IV-TR* criteria itself in relation to delirium, which holds true for the *DSM-5*. One issue outlined by these authors was that the first criteria of the *DSM-IV-TR*, that remains for the *DSM-5*, is that it does not provide an adequate operational definition for "a disturbance of consciousness or attention" that might be indexed or manifest. Watt et al. (2012) suggested that a more useful criteria would be a "failure to register incoming stimuli into some form of working memory on a consistent basis, with the associated collapse of stable representation of those stimuli in working memory, along with loss of the organized segues within working memory that define a coherent train of thought."

These same authors noted that Criterion #2 in the *DSM-IV-TR*, which is now outlined in Criterion #3 in the *DSM-5*, is in many ways duplicative as "a change in cognition (which may include deficits of memory, language, or orientation) or onset of a perceptual disturbance not better accounted for by a dementia" would be anticipated if attentional registration of stimuli, along with working memory and executive functioning are impaired as they serve as a foundation upon which other cognitive domains are based (Watt et al., 2012). This argument holds true with Lurian theory, which suggests that activities depend on the cooperation of all three units described by Luria in which the first unit regulates activation, muscle tone, and vigilance; the second unit is responsible for registration, analysis, and storage of sensory information; and the third unit regulates complex mental activity, such as planning, abstract thought, and organization. Watt et al. (2012) further criticized Criteria #3 and #4 of the *DSM-IV-TR* stating a "short period," as discussed in Criterion #3 of the *DSM-IV-TR*, now Criterion #2 of the *DSM-5*, can mean weeks or longer in the case of slowly progressive metabolic disorders and that Criterion #4 of the *DSM-IV-TR*, now Criterion #5 of the *DSM-5*, neglects the fact that many etiologies are mixed and multifactorial and that an unequivocal etiology is not always found. The *DSM-5* has offered specifiers regarding possible cause, course, and presentation, as noted in Table 15.2, but these issues remain.

TABLE 15.2 Delirium Specifiers

1. Substance intoxication delirium
2. Substance withdrawal delirium
3. Medication-induced delirium
4. Delirium due to another medical condition
5. Delirium due to multiple etiologies
6. Acute
7. Persistent
8. Hyperactive
9. Hypoactive
10. Mixed level of activity

In response to these issues, Watt et al. (2012) have suggested that delirium may better fit a more comprehensive taxonomy of diseases of consciousness ranging from the most severe to the least severe, which was also suggested by Watt and Pincus (2004). At the most severe end would fall coma followed by persistent vegetative state, stupor/obtunded, akinetic mutism, minimally conscious state, and finally delirium/confusional states. Table 15.3 includes the outline proposed by Watt et al. (2012) detailing a continuum of severity from mildest to most severe, which, as noted by the authors, "contrasts the *DSM*'s current 'one size fits all' assumption, which has encouraged the mistaken belief in the relative uniformity of syndrome manifestation." The authors believe such a continuum would correct the failure to diagnose milder confusional states. Furthermore, they argue that the mildest manifestation of this continuum (i.e., low-grade encephalopathy, "a state probably too mild to be considered part of delirium proper,") is often misdiagnosed on neuropsychological testing as a prodromal or early stage of a frontal system neurodegenerative disorder due to the appearance of working memory and executive function deficits. Watt et al. (2012) note that this "underlines the importance of clinicians making a concerted effort to determine *whether or not a patient undergoing neuropsychological assessment is truly at a representative baseline or not*, as prodromal stages of confusional states (what one might term 'subclinical delirium') still merit a review of potential (generative) etiologies. Readers are strongly encouraged to review the Watt et al. (2012) chapter themselves.

Beyond *DSM-5* criteria, the use of routine screening assessments by providers has been shown to improve detection rates (Devlin et al., 2007). There are several available screening tools designed for bedside use that have been developed including Confusion Assessment Method (CAM and CAM-ICU), Delirium Rating Scale (DRS), NEECHAM Confusion Scale, and Memorial Delirium Assessment Scale (MDS), Cognitive Test for Delirium (CTD), Delirium Detection Score, and Intensive Care Delirium Screening Checklist (ICDS). Although the content of the scales and populations targeted differ, all have been validated in the literature (Bergeron, Dubois, Dumont, Dial, & Skrobik, 2001; Ely et al., 2001; Hart et al., 1996; Immers, Schuurmans, & van de Bijl, 2005; Inouye et al., 1990; Otter et al., 2005). Although all are validated, important differences exist among these scales in their ability to detect hypoactive delirium, specific components of the syndrome they focus on, ability of patients with compromised level of consciousness to participate, and ease of use. A recent systemic review suggests that the CAM may have the strongest evidence base and is featured in Figure 15.1 (Wong, Holroyd-Leduc, Simel, & Straus, 2010).

TABLE 15.3 Stages and Levels of Confusional State

SEVERITY	CLINICAL FEATURES
Mildest possible encephalopathy	Lowered cognitive efficiency and speed of processing, poor working memory, other mild cognitive disruption (especially in short-term memory and executive function) but with preserved orientation to place and situation (basic lucidity). *Patients at this level are probably better diagnosed with reversible mild cognitive impairment rather than delirium proper.* However, as the physiological condition(s) underlying this mildest possible manifestation of encephalopathy worsen (or as additional etiologies are added to the clinical picture), patients begin to segue into the stages of delirium proper. Patients at this stage are frequently misdiagnosed with early stage dementing disorders if they are undergoing neuropsychological testing. Conversely, without such formal cognitive assessment, this stage (essentially a preclinical or prodromal stage of delirium proper) is rarely detected. Mental status examinations may pick up on this condition if they include more challenging probes such as backward serial sevens or Go No Go testing. This stage of the process is often clinically almost invisible, except to the exceptionally sensitive observer who realizes that the patient is cognitively "off" without being more severely impaired. Insightful and introspective patients may also report that they feel "fuzzyheaded," "can't focus," "are not sharp," "not themselves," "feel spacey," or other similar descriptions.
Mild confusional states	Mild confusional states show increasing cognitive disorganization relative to the first stage: There is now more obvious task derailing and basic registration failures of relatively simple stimuli starting to appear within working memory function. Patients are still mostly oriented to situation/place. However, the degree of disorganization is now sufficient to preclude performing any attentionally demanding tasks, and this level of deficit can be detected in many mental status examinations. Patients can no longer successfully complete such relatively simple working memory tasks as months of the year backward or serial arithmetic, and make multiple errors. Simple digit span forward performance can be preserved, but often in concert with remarkably poorer digit span backward (large gap between digits forward and digits backward). Increased anxiety or hypoactivity may be visible.
Mild-to-moderate confusional states	Basic orientation to environment may fluctuate, with the patient occasionally aware of where he or she is but at least intermittently showing disorientation to place, in concert with increasing and now obvious collapse of working memory and task organization. Thinking is more obviously disorganized, with difficulty following any train of thought. In some cases, patients now cannot consistently register questions, and may produce non sequiturs. Even digit span forward performance starts to collapse. Agitation or behavioral slowing may be more obvious.
Moderate confusional states	Orientation to situation/place now consistently impaired, registration of incoming stimuli consistently poor with registration failures becoming endemic/constant, increasing language disorganization, possible hallucinatory phenomena. Patients demonstrate severe behavioral disorganization, with almost no task organization possible. Most attempts at cognitive assessment are now virtually impossible given the patient's poor registration of questions and tasks.
Severe confusional states	Complete failure of registration, lack of orientation to the environment, unintelligible or mute language production, loss of orienting to salient stimuli, approximating a minimally conscious state.

Adapted with permission from Watt et al. (2012).

The diagnosis of delirium requires the presence of (1) and (2) and either (3) or (4):
(1) Acute onset and fluctuating course: Is there an acute change in the mental status from the patient's baseline? Did this behavior fluctuate during the past day?
(2) Inattention: Does the patient have difficulty focusing attention, for example, being easily distractible, or having difficulty keeping track of what was being said?
(3) Disorganized thinking: Is the patient's speech disorganized or incoherent, such as rambling or irrelevant conversation, unclear or illogical flow of ideas, or unpredictable switching from subject to subject?
(4) Altered level of consciousness: Overall, how would you rate this patient's level of consciousness? Alert (normal), Vigilant (hyperalert), Lethargic (drowsy, easily aroused), Stupor (difficult to arouse), Coma (unarousable)

FIGURE 15.1 Confusion Assessment Method (CAM).

TABLE 15.4 Common Precipitating Factors of Delirium

Infection
Iatrogenic (narcotics, anticholinergics, dopamine agonists, antihistamines, benzodiazepines)
Hepatic disease
Pulmonary disease
Renal failure
Sleep deprivation
Metabolic derangement
Intoxication/withdrawal
Cardiac disease
Pain
CNS disease

CNS, central nervous system.

It is important to remember that delirium is the symptom of an underlying problem. Thus, after correctly identifying delirium, the next step becomes identifying and rectifying the precipitating cause. Common precipitators of delirium are listed in Table 15.4. Many of these can be determined by a careful history, review of medications, substance use history, and routine laboratory work. Head imagining can be useful to exclude structural causes including neoplastic processes, intracerebral bleeds, and ischemic strokes. In the setting of delirium, diffuse slowing is found on an EEG, making this a nonspecific tool for diagnosis. However, an EEG can aid in excluding seizure activity although a negative study does not rule this diagnosis out. A 24-hour EEG would be a preferred test if clinical suspicion is high. A lumbar puncture may be necessary to search for CNS infection if the etiology is still not evident after the previous. A summary of the clinical approach to diagnosis is outlined in Figure 15.2.

Delirium can present with similar features to depression, dementia, and psychotic disorders. Often the diagnosis is clear from the history. However, there are several other distinguishing features that can aid in diagnosis (Table 15.5).

TREATMENT

The treatment of delirium is treating the underlining cause. However, antipsychotics are often used to control symptoms of agitation, sleep dysregulation, and psychosis. Traditionally, haloperidol has been the first-line antipsychotic because of its

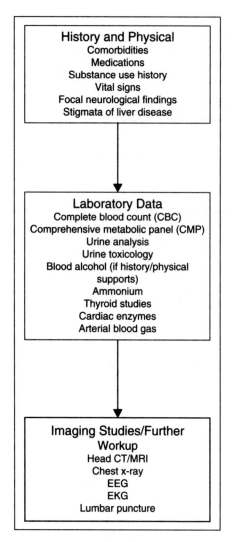

FIGURE 15.2 Diagnostic approach to delirium.

effectiveness in controlling hyperactive symptoms, few active metabolites, minimal risk of sedation, and minimal anticholinergic side effects. However, haloperidol is associated with an increased risk of extrapyramidal side effects, particularly in the elderly and severely ill. The adverse side effects of haloperidol prompted interest in using the newer atypical antipsychotics, which are believed to cause less extrapyramidal symptoms (EPS). Several studies have demonstrated equivalent efficacy in terms of symptom reduction compared to haloperidol and reduced incidence of EPS (Han & Kim, 2004; Liu, Juang, Liang, Lin, & Yeh, 2004; Rea, Battistone, Fong, & Devlin, 2007; Sipahimalani & Masand, 1998; Skrobik, Bergeron, Dumont, & Gottfried, 2004). Despite encouraging results, most of the studies have several limitations including small numbers of patients, questionable equivalents, retrospective nature, and lack of placebo group. However, despite these limitations, atypical antipsychotics appear to be a reasonable alternative to haloperidol.

Further concern about using antipsychotics in this population is the risk of a prolonged QT interval leading to Tosade de Pointes and sudden cardiac death.

TABLE 15.5 Differential Diagnosis of Delirium

FEATURE	DELIRIUM	DEMENTIA	DEPRESSION	PSYCHOTIC DISORDERS
Onset	Acute	Insidious	Slow	Acute or slow
Course	Fluctuating	Chronic, progressive	Single or recurrent	Chronic with exacerbations
Duration	Hours to months	Months to years	Weeks to years	Weeks to years
Consciousness	Impaired	Normal	Normal	Normal
Attention	Impaired	Normal, impaired in late stages	Normal/impaired	Normal/impaired
Orientation	Impaired	Impaired	Normal	Normal
Thought process	Disorganized	Impoverished	Normal	Disorganized
Illusions/ hallucinations	Common	Present in late stages	Not common	Common
Reversibility	Usually	Rarely	Yes	Rarely
EEG findings	Diffuse slowing	Normal or mild diffuse slowing	Normal	Normal

Among the first generation antipsychotics, haloperidol, thioridazine, droperidol, and chlorpromazine have all been associated with prolonged QT and sudden cardiac death. The atypical ziprasidone has caused the most concern about prolonged QT and sudden cardiac death. There have also been case reports of sudden cardiac death with risperdone (Abdelmawla & Mitchell, 2006; Glassman & Bigger, 2001).

In addition to the risk of sudden cardiac death, several studies have implicated the use of antipsychotics with an elevated mortality in elderly demented patients, eventually leading to a Food and Drug Administration (FDA) black box warning (Liperoti et al., 2009; Wang et al., 2005). Additional concerns have arisen in the literature regarding an association between antipsychotic use and cerebral vascular accidents among elderly patients with dementia (Douglas & Smeeth, 2008; van Marum & Jansen, 2005); however, not all studies have confirmed this (Herrmann, Mamdani, & Lanctôt, 2004; Liperoti et al., 2005). Thus, the use of antipsychotics among the elderly is controversial. The risk of stroke and mortality among delirium patients receiving antipsychotics has not been extensively studied. One retrospective study did not find an elevated mortality risk (Elie et al., 2009).

Beyond the use of antipsychotics, other agents have been used to manage delirium. Patients suffering from alcohol or benzodiazepine withdrawal are treated with benzodiazepines. Delirium secondary to pain is often managed with narcotics. Antiepileptics have not been proven effective in the literature. Of growing interest is the novel alpha 2 agonist dexmedetomidine, which has shown to reduce delirium in cardiac surgery patients (Maldonado et al., 2009). Additional interest in the role of melatonin in the treatment of delirium has emerged in light of the frequent sleep cycle disturbances observed in this population. One prospective study suggested that melatonin may have a role in delirium prevention (Al-Aama et al., 2011).

PROGNOSIS

The identification of delirium has important prognostic significance. Several studies have examined the relationship between delirium and mortality. Ely et al. (2004) followed 275 consecutively mechanically ventilated patients admitted to a medical and coronary ICU, looking for mortality, overall length of hospital stay, and length of post-ICU stay. Eighty-one percent of patients developed delirium at some point during their ICU stay. The 6-month mortality of delirious patients was 34% versus 15% in nondelirious patients ($p = .03$), and delirious patients spent an average of 10 days longer in the hospital. After adjustment for age, illness severity, comorbid conditions, coma, and use of sedatives or analgesics, delirium was associated with an increased mortality at 6 months (hazard ratio [HR]: 3.2, confidence interval [CI]: 1.4, 3) and longer post-ICU stay (HR: 1.6, CI: [1.2, 2.3]). McCusker, Cole, Abrahamowicz, Primeau, and Belzile (2002) had similar findings in a prospective study of patients aged 65 years and older admitted to a medical service. The 12-month mortality among delirious patients was 42% versus 14.4% of nondelirious patients. Factors associated with elevated mortality among the delirious cohort included severity of delirium, number of comorbidities, and severity of illness. Rockwood et al. (1999) followed 203 patients admitted to a general medical service for a mean 32.5 months. Only 21% of patients diagnosed with delirium were still alive versus 57% of those without delirium. After adjustment for comorbidities, baseline dementia, demographics, and living arrangements, patients with delirium were 1.7 times more likely to die than those without (CI: [1.02, 2.87]). Curyto et al. (2001) followed 102 elderly residential care patients over the course of 1 year. Patients who were hospitalized and developed delirium were at increased risk of death over the following year (relative risk [RR]: 2.24, CI: [1.02, 4.91]) versus those hospitalized who did not develop delirium. The effect was no longer significant when adjusted for global cognitive performance as measured by prehospital MMSE. Taken together, the literature suggests that delirium is an independent risk factor for mortality.

Delirium also has been demonstrated to have adverse effects on functional status, lead to increased rates of institutionalization, and precipitate cognitive decline. In a study examining the long-term cognitive outcomes of postoperative hip surgery patients, Kat et al. (2008) found that the relative risk of dementia or mild cognitive impairment (MCI) was 1.9 (CI: [1.1, 3.3]) after 30 months of follow-up. The risk of institutionalization was also elevated with a relative risk of 1.8 (CI: [0.9, 3.4]). Levkoff et al. (1992) also found an increased risk of institutionalization. Rockwood et al. (1999) found the incidence of dementia to be 5.6% per year over 3 years in patients admitted to a medical floor without delirium compared to 18.1% per year in those with delirium. The unadjusted odds ratio was 3.23 (CI: [1.86, 5.63]). After adjustment for age, sex, and comorbidities, the odds ratio increased to 5.97 (CI [1.83, 19.54]). In a 3-year prospective study, Bickel, Gradinger, Kochs, and Förstl (2008) found that postoperative delirium highly correlated with cognitive impairment, subjective memory decline, and incident need for long-term care in a group of hip-surgery patients after adjusting for demographics, comorbidities, and preoperative cognitive performance.

Although traditionally believed to resolve when the underlining cause is addressed, recent work has suggested that symptoms of delirium may persist for months after hospital discharge in a large percentage of patients (Siddiqi et al., 2006). McCusker et al. (2002) reported the presence of symptoms of delirium in 41% of patients 12 months after discharge, while Levkoff et al. (1992) reported that only 4% of patients had resolution of all symptoms by hospital discharge and only 17.7% had resolution at 6 months postdischarge.

SUMMARY

Although it is frequently discussed within the clinical neurosciences, and commonly occurs in medical patients, delirium is consistently underdiagnosed. We would argue that delirium has suffered from a consistent oversimplification of the presentation as it is oftentimes chalked up to dementia rather than appreciated as an acute manifestation that would otherwise respond to appropriate treatment. We liken this to the practice of diagnostic overshadowing, whose roads inevitably end with increased morbidity and mortality. As a means of moving forward, it is critical for clinicians to understand the dynamics of delirium, including its pathophysiological correlates and clinical variations. Only through the due diligence of clinicians can the errors commonly made in response to delirium begin to be corrected on a large scale.

REFERENCES

Abdelmawla, N., & Mitchell, A. (2006). Sudden cardiac death and antipsychotics Part 2: Monitoring and prevention. *Advances in Psychiatric Treatment, 12,* 100–109.

Al-Aama, T., Brymer, C., Gutmanis, I., Woolmore-Goodwin, S. M., Esbaugh, J., & Dasgupta, M. (2011). Melatonin decreases delirium in elderly patients: A randomized, placebo-controlled trial. *International Journal of Geriatric Psychiatry, 26*(7), 687–694.

Aldemir, M., Ozen, S., Kara, I. H., Sir, A., & Baç, B. (2001). Predisposing factors for delirium in the surgical intensive care unit. *Critical Care, 5*(5), 265–270.

American Psychiatric Association (APA). (2000). *Diagnostic and statistical manual of mental disorders* (4th ed., text rev.). Washington, DC: Author.

American Psychiatric Association (APA). (2013). *Diagnostic and statistical manual of mental disorders* (5th ed.). Arlington, VA: American Psychiatric Publishing.

Balan, S., Leibovitz, A., Zila, S. O., Ruth, M., Chana, W., Yassica, B.,... Habot, B. (2003). The relation between the clinical subtypes of delirium and the urinary level of 6-SMT. *The Journal of Neuropsychiatry and Clinical Neurosciences, 15*(3), 363–366.

Bergeron, N., Dubois, M. J., Dumont, M., Dial, S., & Skrobik, Y. (2001). Intensive Care Delirium Screening Checklist: Evaluation of a new screening tool. *Intensive Care Medicine, 27*(5), 859–864.

Bickel, H., Gradinger, R., Kochs, E., & Förstl, H. (2008). High risk of cognitive and functional decline after postoperative delirium. A three-year prospective study. *Dementia and Geriatric Cognitive Disorders, 26*(1), 26–31.

Brown, T. M., & Boyle, M. F. (2002). Delirium. *British Medical Journal, 325*(7365), 644–647.

Curyto, K. J., Johnson, J., TenHave, T., Mossey, J., Knott, K., & Katz, I. R. (2001). Survival of hospitalized elderly patients with delirium: A prospective study. *The American Journal of Geriatric Psychiatry, 9*(2), 141–147.

Cutting, J. (1987). The phenomenology of acute organic psychosis. Comparison with acute schizophrenia. *The British Journal of Psychiatry, 151,* 324–332.

Devlin, J. W., Fong, J. J., Schumaker, G., O'Connor, H., Ruthazer, R., & Garpestad, E. (2007). Use of a validated delirium assessment tool improves the ability of physicians to identify delirium in medical intensive care unit patients. *Critical Care Medicine, 35*(12), 2721–2724; quiz 2725.

Douglas, I. J., & Smeeth, L. (2008). Exposure to antipsychotics and risk of stroke: Self controlled case series study. *British Medical Journal, 337,* a1227.

Dubois, M. J., Bergeron, N., Dumont, M., Dial, S., & Skrobik, Y. (2001). Delirium in an intensive care unit: A study of risk factors. *Intensive Care Medicine, 27*(8), 1297–1304.

Elie, M., Boss, K., Cole, M. G., McCusker, J., Belzile, E., & Ciampi, A. (2009). A retrospective, exploratory, secondary analysis of the association between antipsychotic use and mortality in elderly patients with delirium. *International Psychogeriatrics, 21*(3), 588–592.

Ely, E. W., Margolin, R., Francis, J., May, L., Truman, B., Dittus, R.,...Inouye, S. K. (2001). Evaluation of delirium in critically ill patients: Validation of the Confusion Assessment Method for the Intensive Care Unit (CAM-ICU). *Critical Care Medicine, 29*(7), 1370–1379.

Ely, E. W., Shintani, A., Truman, B., Speroff, T., Gordon, S. M., Harrell, F. E.,...Dittus, R. S. (2004). Delirium as a predictor of mortality in mechanically ventilated patients in the intensive care unit. *The Journal of the American Medical Association, 291*(14), 1753–1762.

Figueroa-Ramos, M. I., Arroyo-Novoa, C. M., Lee, K. A., Padilla, G., & Puntillo, K. A. (2009). Sleep and delirium in ICU patients: A review of mechanisms and manifestations. *Intensive Care Medicine, 35*(5), 781–795.

Flacker, J. M., Cummings, V., Mach, J. R., Bettin, K., Kiely, D. K., & Wei, J. (1998). The association of serum anticholinergic activity with delirium in elderly medical patients. *The American Journal of Geriatric Psychiatry, 6*(1), 31–41.

Franco, K., Litaker, D., Locala, J., & Bronson, D. (2001). The cost of delirium in the surgical patient. *Psychosomatics, 42*(1), 68–73.

Glassman, A. H., & Bigger, J. T. (2001). Antipsychotic drugs: Prolonged QTc interval, torsade de pointes, and sudden death. *The American Journal of Psychiatry, 158*(11), 1774–1782.

Gunther, M. L., Morandi, A., & Ely, E. W. (2008). Pathophysiology of delirium in the intensive care unit. *Critical Care Clinics, 24*(1), 45–65, viii.

Han, C. S., & Kim, Y. K. (2004). A double-blind trial of risperidone and haloperidol for the treatment of delirium. *Psychosomatics, 45*(4), 297–301.

Hart, R. P., Levenson, J. L., Sessler, C. N., Best, A. M., Schwartz, S. M., & Rutherford, L. E. (1996). Validation of a cognitive test for delirium in medical ICU patients. *Psychosomatics, 37*(6), 533–546.

Herrmann, N., Mamdani, M., & Lanctôt, K. L. (2004). Atypical antipsychotics and risk of cerebrovascular accidents. *The American Journal of Psychiatry, 161*(6), 1113–1115.

Hufschmidt, A., Shabarin, V., & Zimmer, T. (2009). Drug-induced confusional states: The usual suspects? *Acta Neurologica Scandinavica, 120*(6), 436–438.

Immers, H. E., Schuurmans, M. J., & van de Bijl, L. L. (2005). Recognition of delirium in ICU patients: A diagnostic study of the NEECHAM confusion scale in ICU patients. *BMC Nursing, 13*, 4.

Inouye, S. K. (1994). The dilemma of delirium: Clinical and research controversies regarding diagnosis and evaluation of delirium in hospitalized elderly medical patients. *The American Journal of Medicine, 97*(3), 278–288.

Inouye, S. K., & Charpentier, P. A. (1996). Precipitating factors for delirium in hospitalized elderly persons. Predictive model and interrelationship with baseline vulnerability. *Journal of the Americal Medical Association, 275*(11), 852–857.

Inouye, S. K., van Dyck, C. H., Alessi, C. A., Balkin, S., Siegal, A. P., & Horwitz, R. I. (1990). Clarifying confusion: The confusion assessment method. A new method for detection of delirium. *Annals of Internal Medicine, 113*(12), 941–948.

Kat, M. G., Vreeswijk, R., de Jonghe, J. F., van der Ploeg, T., van Gool, W. A., Eikelenboom, P., & Kalisvaart, K. J. (2008). Long-term cognitive outcome of delirium in elderly hip surgery patients. A prospective matched controlled study over two and a half years. *Dementia and Geriatric Cognitive Disorders, 26*(1), 1–8.

Khan, R. A., Kahn, D., & Bourgeois, J. A. (2009). Delirium: Sifting through the confusion. *Current Psychiatry Reports, 11*(3), 226–234.

Kiely, D. K., Jones, R. N., Bergmann, M. A., & Marcantonio, E. R. (2007). Association between psychomotor activity delirium subtypes and mortality among newly admitted post-acute facility patients. *The Journals of Gerontology, 62*(2), 174–179.

Kishi, Y., Iwasaki, Y., Takezawa, K., Kurosawa, H., & Endo, S. (1995). Delirium in critical care unit patients admitted through an emergency room. *General Hospital Psychiatry, 17*(5), 371–379.

Koponen, H., Hurri, L., Stenbäck, U., Mattila, E., Soininen, H., & Riekkinen, P. J. (1989). Computed tomography findings in delirium. *The Journal of Nervous and Mental Disease, 177*(4), 226–231.

Lawlor, P. G., Gagnon, B., Mancini, I. L., Pereira, J. L., Hanson, J., Suarez-Almazor, M. E., & Bruera, E. D. (2000). Occurrence, causes, and outcome of delirium in patients with advanced cancer: A prospective study. *Archives of Internal Medicine, 160*(6), 786–794.

Levkoff, S. E., Evans, D. A., Liptzin, B., Cleary, P. D., Lipsitz, L. A., Wetle, T. T., … Rowe, J. (1992). Delirium. The occurrence and persistence of symptoms among elderly hospitalized patients. *Archives of Internal Medicine, 152*(2), 334–340.

Liperoti, R., Gambassi, G., Lapane, K. L., Chiang, C., Pedone, C., Mor, V., & Bernabei, R. (2005). Cerebrovascular events among elderly nursing home patients treated with conventional or atypical antipsychotics. *The Journal of Clinical Psychiatry, 66*(9), 1090–1096.

Liperoti, R., Onder, G., Landi, F., Lapane, K. L., Mor, V., Bernabei, R., & Gambassi, G. (2009). All-cause mortality associated with atypical and conventional antipsychotics among nursing home residents with dementia: A retrospective cohort study. *The Journal of Clinical Psychiatry, 70*(10), 1340–1347.

Liu, C. Y., Juang, Y. Y., Liang, H. Y., Lin, N. C., & Yeh, E. K. (2004). Efficacy of risperidone in treating the hyperactive symptoms of delirium. *International Clinical Psychopharmacology, 19*(3), 165–168.

Mach, J. R., Dysken, M. W., Kuskowski, M., Richelson, E., Holden, L., & Jilk, K. M. (1995). Serum anticholinergic activity in hospitalized older persons with delirium: A preliminary study. *Journal of the American Geriatrics Society, 43*(5), 491–495.

Maldonado, J. R., Wysong, A., van der Starre, P. J., Block, T., Miller, C., & Reitz, B. A. (2009). Dexmedetomidine and the reduction of postoperative delirium after cardiac surgery. *Psychosomatics, 50*(3), 206–217.

McCusker, J., Cole, M., Abrahamowicz, M., Primeau, F., & Belzile, E. (2002). Delirium predicts 12-month mortality. *Archives of Internal Medicine, 162*(4), 457–463.

McNicoll, L., Pisani, M. A., Zhang, Y., Ely, E. W., Siegel, M. D., & Inouye, S. K. (2003). Delirium in the intensive care unit: Occurrence and clinical course in older patients. *Journal of the American Geriatrics Society, 51*(5), 591–598.

Meagher, D. J., O'Hanlon, D., O'Mahony, E., Casey, P. R., & Trzepacz, P. T. (2000). Relationship between symptoms and motoric subtype of delirium. *The Journal of Neuropsychiatry and Clinical Neurosciences, 12*(1), 51–56.

Mesulam, M. M. (1990). Large-scale neurocognitive networks and distributed processing for attention, language, and memory. *Annals of Neurology, 28*(5), 597–613.

Mesulam, M. M., & Geschwind, N. (1976). Disordered mental states in the postoperative period. *The Urologic Clinics of North America, 3*(2), 199–215.

Michaud, L., Büla, C., Berney, A., Camus, V., Voellinger, R., Stiefel, F., & Burnand, B.; Delirium Guidelines Development Group. (2007). Delirium: Guidelines for general hospitals. *Journal of Psychosomatic Research, 62*(3), 371–383.

Milbrandt, E. B., Deppen, S., Harrison, P. L., Shintani, A. K., Speroff, T., Stiles, R. A.,...Ely, E. W. (2004). Costs associated with delirium in mechanically ventilated patients. *Critical Care Medicine, 32*(4), 955–962.

Mistraletti, G., Carloni, E., Cigada, M., Zambrelli, E., Taverna, M., Sabbatici, G.,...Iapichino, G. (2008). Sleep and delirium in the intensive care unit. *Minerva Anestesiologica, 74*(6), 329–333.

O'Keeffe, S. T., & Lavan, J. N. (1999). Clinical significance of delirium subtypes in older people. *Age and Ageing, 28*(2), 115–119.

Otter, H., Martin, J., Bäsell, K., von Heymann, C., Hein, O. V., Böllert, P.,...Spies, C. (2005). Validity and reliability of the DDS for severity of delirium in the ICU. *Neurocritical Care, 2*(2), 150–158.

Peterson, J. F., Pun, B. T., Dittus, R. S., Thomason, J. W., Jackson, J. C., Shintani, A. K., & Ely, E. W. (2006). Delirium and its motoric subtypes: A study of 614 critically ill patients. *Journal of the American Geriatrics Society, 54*(3), 479–484.

Piazza, O., Cotena, S., De Robertis, E., Caranci, F., & Tufano, R. (2009). Sepsis associated encephalopathy studied by MRI and cerebral spinal fluid S100B measurement. *Neurochemical research, 34*(7), 1289–1292.

Rea, R. S., Battistone, S., Fong, J. J., & Devlin, J. W. (2007). Atypical antipsychotics versus haloperidol for treatment of delirium in acutely ill patients. *Pharmacotherapy, 27*(4), 588–594.

Robinson, T. N., Raeburn, C. D., Angles, E. M., & Moss, M. (2008). Low tryptophan levels are associated with postoperative delirium in the elderly. *American Journal of Surgery, 196*(5), 670–674.

Rockwood, K., Cosway, S., Carver, D., Jarrett, P., Stadnyk, K., & Fisk, J. (1999). The risk of dementia and death after delirium. *Age and Ageing, 28*(6), 551–556.

Ross, C. A., Peyser, C. E., Shapiro, I., & Folstein, M. F. (1991). Delirium: Phenomenologic and etiologic subtypes. *International Psychogeriatrics, 3*(2), 135–147.

Sharshar, T., Carlier, R., Bernard, F., Guidoux, C., Brouland, J. P., Nardi, O.,...Annane, D. (2007). Brain lesions in septic shock: A magnetic resonance imaging study. *Intensive Care Medicine, 33*(5), 798–806.

Sharshar, T., Hopkinson, N. S., Orlikowski, D., & Annane, D. (2005). The brain in sepsis—culprit and victim. *Critical Care, 9,* 37–44.

Siddiqi, N., House, A. O., & Holmes, J. D. (2006). Occurrence and outcome of delirium in medical in-patients: A systematic literature review. *Age and Ageing, 35*(4), 350–364.

Sipahimalani, A., & Masand, P. S. (1998). Olanzapine in the treatment of delirium. *Psychosomatics, 39*(5), 422–430.

Skrobik, Y. K., Bergeron, N., Dumont, M., & Gottfried, S. B. (2004). Olanzapine vs haloperidol: Treating delirium in a critical care setting. *Intensive Care Medicine, 30*(3), 444–449.

Thomas, C., Hestermann, U., Kopitz, J., Plaschke, K., Oster, P., Driessen, M.,...Weisbrod, M. (2008). Serum anticholinergic activity and cerebral cholinergic dysfunction: An EEG study in frail elderly with and without delirium. *BMC Neuroscience, 9,* 86.

Thomason, J. W., Shintani, A., Peterson, J. F., Pun, B. T., Jackson, J. C., & Ely, E. W. (2005). Intensive care unit delirium is an independent predictor of longer hospital stay: A prospective analysis of 261 non-ventilated patients. *Critical Care, 9*(4), R375–R381.

van der Mast, R. C., van den Broek, W. W., Fekkes, D., Pepplinkhuizen, L., & Habbema, J. D. (2000). Is delirium after cardiac surgery related to plasma amino acids and physical condition? *The Journal of Neuropsychiatry and Clinical Neurosciences, 12*(1), 57–63.

van Gool, W. A., van de Beek, D., & Eikelenboom, P. (2010). Systemic infection and delirium: When cytokines and acetylcholine collide. *Lancet, 375*(9716), 773–775.

van Marum, R. J., & Jansen, P. A. (2005). [Increased risk of stroke during the use of olanzapine or risperidone in patients with dementia]. *Nederlands Tijdschrift Voor Geneeskunde, 149*(4), 165–167.

Wang, P. S., Schneeweiss, S., Avorn, J., Fischer, M. A., Mogun, H., Solomon, D. H., & Brookhart, M. A. (2005). Risk of death in elderly users of conventional vs. atypical antipsychotic medications. *The New England Journal of Medicine, 353*(22), 2335–2341.

Watt, D., Budding, D. E., & Koziol, L. F. (2012). Delirium. In C. A. Noggle & R. S. Dean (Eds.), *The neuropsychology of psychopathology* (pp. 425–440). New York, NY: Springer Publishing Company.

Watt, D. F., & Pincus, D. I. (2004). Neural substrates of consciousness: Implications for clinical psychiatry. In J. Paksepp (Ed.), *Textbook of biological psychiatry* (pp. 75–110). Hoboken, NJ: Wiley.

Webster, R., & Holroyd, S. (2000). Prevalence of psychotic symptoms in delirium. *Psychosomatics, 41*(6), 519–522.

Wong, C. L., Holroyd-Leduc, J., Simel, D. L., & Straus, S. E. (2010). Does this patient have delirium?: Value of bedside instruments. *The Journal of the American Medical Association, 304*(7), 779–786.

Yang, F. M., Marcantonio, E. R., Inouye, S. K., Kiely, D. K., Rudolph, J. L., Fearing, M. A., & Jones, R. N. (2009). Phenomenological subtypes of delirium in older persons: Patterns, prevalence, and prognosis. *Psychosomatics, 50*(3), 248–254.

Yokota, H., Ogawa, S., Kurokawa, A., & Yamamoto, Y. (2003). Regional cerebral blood flow in delirium patients. *Psychiatry and Clinical Neurosciences, 57*(3), 337–339.

Interventions and Other Issues

CHAPTER 16

Pharmacology of Dementing Disorders

Robert H. Howland

More than 25 million people worldwide have dementia (Ferri et al., 2005). In the United States, the prevalence of dementia is approximately 5% to 15% among adults older than 65 years (Plassman et al., 2007). Dementia is a syndrome in which impairment of cortical or subcortical brain function leads to deterioration of cognitive processes or intellectual abilities, including memory, judgment, language, communication, and abstract thinking. In addition to cognitive impairment, other noncognitive behavioral and psychiatric symptoms are very common in patients with dementing disorders. The treatment of dementia can be broadly divided into two domains: those interventions used to improve or preserve cognitive function and those interventions used to control disturbed behavior of individuals with dementia.

CORE FEATURES

Dementing Disorders

The presence of memory impairment plus one or more other cognitive disturbances (i.e., aphasia, apraxia, agnosia, or executive dysfunction) is the hallmark diagnostic characteristic that defines dementia (American Psychiatric Association [APA], 2000). Dementia can result from many conditions, some of which are potentially reversible, but the most common and clinically relevant forms include Alzheimer's disease (AD), vascular dementia (VaD), dementia with Lewy bodies (DLB), Parkinson's disease dementia (PDD), and frontotemporal dementia (FTD).

The most prevalent form of dementia is AD, which is characterized by an insidious onset and gradual progression of cognitive impairment along with associated social and/or vocational functional impairment (Dubois et al., 2010). In AD, the neuropathological findings of amyloid beta (Aβ) plaques, neurofibrillary tau-protein tangles, and cerebral neuronal loss are characteristic. The greatest density of plaques and tangles is found in the frontoparietal cortex, hippocampus, amygdala, locus coeruleus, and dorsal raphe nucleus. A progressive loss of cholinergic neurons of the nucleus basalis, noradrenergic neurons of the locus coeruleus, and serotonergic neurons of the dorsal raphe nucleus also occurs, which is likely to explain the reductions of cortical concentrations of the neurotransmitters acetylcholine (ACh), norepinephrine, and serotonin. The most profound biochemical abnormality found in AD is the reduction of temporoparietal and hippocampal cortical activity of choline acetyl-transferase (CAT). The enzyme CAT is found only in cholinergic neurons, where it catalyzes the synthesis of ACh. Recent work has suggested that a clinical diagnosis of AD can be confirmed by demonstrating the presence of one or more of the following biomarkers: (a) decreased concentrations of Aβ and increased concentrations of tau-protein in the cerebrospinal fluid; (b) identifying specific amyloid-related binding of Pittsburgh compound B (PiB) with the use of PET scanning; (c) medial temporal lobe atrophy with the use of MRI scanning; and/or (d) temporal/parietal hypometabo-lism with the use of PET scanning (Dubois et al., 2010).

The second most common form of dementia is VaD, which is characterized by clinical or laboratory evidence of cerebrovascular disease that is associated with the onset and progression of dementia (Kirshner, 2009). In contrast to AD, VaD often is characterized by an abrupt onset and stepwise deterioration of cognitive impair-ment. Multiple small cortical and/or subcortical infarctions are believed to have a cumulative adverse effect on brain function resulting in dementia. The specific cogni-tive deficits depend on the location of the vascular lesions.

Two related forms of dementia are DLB and PDD (Leroi, Collins, & Marsh, 2006; Miyasaki et al., 2006). DLB has clinical and pathological features that overlap with those of AD and Parkinson's disease. In DLB, the progressive decline in cognitive function is eventually accompanied by the development of parkinsonian symptoms (i.e., bradykinesia, rigidity, resting tremors, and abnormalities of balance, gait, and posture). Two features of DLB are diagnostic: marked day-to-day fluctuations in cog-nitive function and the presence of well-formed visual hallucinations (typically of animals, inanimate objects, or people). Patients are extremely sensitive to the adverse effects of antipsychotic drugs. Neuropathological findings in DLB included extensive Aβ plaques (as seen in AD), but relatively few tangles. Lewy bodies are characteristic and are found extensively throughout the brain. Markers of cholinergic activity are reduced to a magnitude even greater than that found in AD.

While this text is primarily focused on primary dementing disorders, for com-parison, the pharmacological approaches to the treatment of PDD are included. In PDD, patients with Parkinson's disease typically develop dementia later in the course of their illness. Executive cognitive impairment is most common, but progres-sion of the dementia will include other aspects of cognitive function. Although the clinical presentation of DLB and PDD is quite different, there are similar underlying neuropathological abnormalities. Current consensus is that these two disorders exist as part of a spectrum, rather than discrete entities.

In contrast to AD, DLB, and PDD, FTD comprises a group of clinical syn-dromes that share a common pattern of relatively focal degeneration of the frontal and temporal lobes of the brain (Neary, Snowden, & Mann, 2005). In addition to meeting criteria for dementia, the core feature of FTD is an early and prominent decline of social interpersonal conduct, impairment in regulation of personal con-duct, emotional blunting, and loss of insight. The typical neuropathological find-ing is frontal and anterotemporal atrophy. In some cases, Pick's bodies are found. Although these appear to be reactive to neurofibrillary tau-protein, they are distinct from the Aβ plaques and neurofibrillary tau-protein tangles characteristic of AD. Abnormalities in frontotemporal lobes are seen clinically with the use of MRI and/or PET scanning.

Mild cognitive impairment (MCI) is characterized by subjective memory com-plaints, with objective evidence of non-age-related memory impairment from stan-dardized tests, normal mental status, normal activities of daily living (ADL), and no evidence of global dementia (Dubois et al., 2010). Among individuals with MCI, the rate of transition to dementia (typically AD) is about 10% to 15% per year. The early neuropathological findings of early AD can sometimes be detected.

Behavioral and Psychiatric Symptoms Associated With Dementia

Among patients with dementing disorders, noncognitive behavioral and psychiatric symptoms are very common. The most important aspects of behavioral and psychiatric symptoms associated with dementia (BPSAD) are agitation, aggression, and psychosis, and they have serious clinically relevant consequences for patients and caregivers (Jeste et al., 2008). BPSAD occurs in more than 50% of individuals with dementia living in the community and in more than 80% of patients living in nursing homes (Steinberg et al., 2003; Testad, Aasland, & Aarsland, 2007). The lifetime risk of BPSAD approaches 100% (Lyketsos et al., 2000).

Cognitive, Functional, and Behavioral Measures in Dementia Studies

In clinical trials, the effectiveness of drugs for cognitive loss is often measured by the cognitive subscale of the Alzheimer's Disease Assessment Scale (ADAS-Cog) and in severe dementia by the Severe Impairment Battery (SIB). Other tests that assess response to treatment include the Clinical Global Impression of Change (CGIC), the Clinician Interview-Based Impression of Change (CIBIC) or the Clinical Dementia Rating (CDR) for overall clinical benefit, the Neuropsychiatric Inventory (NPI) for behavior, ADL scales for daily function, and the Mini-Mental State Examination (MMSE) for global cognition.

ACETYLCHOLINESTERASE INHIBITOR DRUGS FOR DEMENTIA

The neurotransmitter ACh is important for communication between neurons and muscle at the neuromuscular junction, is the main neurotransmitter in the autonomic parasympathetic nervous system, and is involved in cognitive processing, arousal, and attention (Picciotto, Alreja, & Jentsch, 2002). Cholinergic transmission can occur through muscarinic or nicotinic ACh receptors. Multiple muscarinic and nicotinic receptor subtypes exist throughout the central nervous system (CNS) and the peripheral nervous system (PNS). The effects of ACh on cholinergic transmission are terminated by the action of cholinesterase enzymes that metabolize ACh. Acetylcholinesterase inhibitor (AChI) drugs block the effects of this enzyme, and they are used clinically to boost cholinergic function.

Currently available AChI drugs include tacrine (Cognex); donepezil (Aricept; Aricept ODT); rivastigmine (Exelon; Exelon Transdermal Patch); and galantamine (Reminyl; Razadyne; Razadyne ER). All are approved by the Food and Drug Administration (FDA) for the treatment of cognitive impairment in AD, which is characterized in part by the selective loss of cholinergic neurons in the brain. They also are commonly used in clinical practice for treating other dementing disorders, although there is little to no evidence of their efficacy and safety.

Tacrine

Tacrine was the first AChI drug to be FDA approved for the treatment of mild-to-moderate AD. Tacrine is a centrally active, noncompetitive, and reversible cholinesterase inhibitor (Wagstaff & McTavish, 1994). It also acts as a partial agonist at muscarinic receptors; blocks the reuptake of dopamine, serotonin, and norepinephrine;

inhibits monoamine oxidase activity; and can block sodium and potassium channels. In the placebo-controlled clinical trials, tacrine significantly improved or slowed the decline in various cognitive test scores in a minority of patients, but there was no evidence that its use led to substantial functional improvement. Nausea, vomiting, diarrhea, headache, myalgia, and ataxia are associated with its use, but increased liver enzymes are the most common adverse effects. Because tacrine must be given four times daily and because of concerns about its liver toxicity, it is used much less commonly since the introduction and FDA approval of other AChI drugs.

Donepezil

Donepezil is a centrally active, reversible inhibitor of acetylcholinesterase with little peripheral activity (Seltzer, 2005). The drug has a piperidine structure that distinguishes it from acridine drugs (e.g., tacrine), which are associated with liver toxicity, and from carbamate drugs (e.g., rivastigmine, discussed below). Donepezil is FDA approved for the treatment of mild-to-moderate AD as well as for severe AD.

Among patients with mild-to-moderate AD, donepezil was modestly but statistically and significantly more effective than placebo in improving scores on neuropsychological tests, assessments of behavior and ADL, and a global clinical measure based on the impressions of the physician, the patient, the patient's family, and others. In patients with severe AD living in nursing homes, donepezil was significantly more effective than placebo in ADL, cognition, and global function, but there was no difference in behavior; in another study of outpatients with severe AD, donepezil was more effective than placebo on measures of cognition and global function (Black et al., 2007).

In patients with VaD, some randomized double-blind placebo-controlled trials have shown statistically significant improvements with donepezil on measures of cognition, ADL, and global functioning (Black et al., 2003; Wilkinson et al., 2003). Among patients with DLB and PDD, two small placebo-controlled clinical trials demonstrated modest improvement in cognition, global function, and ADL with donepezil (Ravina et al., 2005; Thomas et al., 2005). In a 3-year randomized double-blind trial comparing donepezil, vitamin E, and placebo in patients with MCI, there was no significant overall difference in the probability of progression from MCI to AD, and in a 48-week placebo-controlled trial in patients with MCI a small but significant effect of donepezil on the primary measure of cognition was found, but with no effect on the primary measure of global function (Doody et al., 2009).

The most common adverse effects of donepezil, resulting from increased cholinergic activity, include nausea, vomiting, and diarrhea. Less common adverse effects include urinary incontinence, vivid dreams, bradycardia, syncope, fatigue, and muscle cramps. Because donepezil is metabolized by cytochrome P450 3A4 (CYP3A4) and CYP2D6 liver enzymes, other drugs that inhibit or induce the activity of these enzymes can lead to increased side effects or decreased efficacy, respectively. A large community-based open-label trial in patients with mild-to-moderate AD taking other drugs (e.g., aspirin, antidepressants, vitamins, antihypertensive drugs, and nonsteroidal anti-inflammatory drugs [NSAIDs]) found that donepezil was not associated with increased adverse effects (Relkin, Reichman, Orazem, & McRae, 2003).

Rivastigmine

Rivastigmine is a carbamate-based, reversible, noncompetitive cholinesterase inhibitor with good penetration into the CNS (Williams, Nazarians, & Gill, 2003). It is FDA approved for the treatment of mild-to-moderate AD and also for mild-to-moderate

PDD. The transdermal patch formulation requires daily applications, but may be a more reliable way to administer the drug to patients with dementia (Wentrup, Oertel, & Dodel, 2009).

Randomized double-blind placebo-controlled trials in mild-to-moderate AD demonstrated that rivastigmine modestly but statistically and significantly slowed the rate of decline in cognitive function, improved ADL, and decreased the severity of dementia symptoms (Birks, Grimley Evans, Iakovidou, Tsolaki, & Holt, 2009). Randomized double-blind placebo-controlled trials also found modest but statistically significant benefits for rivastigmine on measures of behavior in patients with DLB and on measures of attention and cognition in patients with PDD (Wesnes, McKeith, Edgar, Emre, & Lane, 2005). In patients with MCI, a 4-year placebo-controlled trial found no benefit for rivastigmine on reducing the probability of progression from MCI to AD (Feldman et al., 2007).

Similar to other AChI drugs, the most common adverse effects of rivastigmine include nausea, vomiting, and diarrhea, although these are less frequent with the transdermal patch formulation. Less frequent adverse effects include bradycardia and syncope. Rivastigmine is not metabolized by CYP450 liver enzymes and therefore has a low risk of drug interactions.

Galantamine

Galantamine is a reversible, competitive inhibitor of acetylcholinesterase that also acts on nicotinic ACh receptors (Scott & Goa, 2000). It is FDA approved for the treatment of mild-to-moderate AD.

In placebo-controlled clinical trials in patients with mild-to-moderate AD, galantamine had modest but significant benefits on cognitive and clinical global measures. Among patients with VaD, several clinical trials demonstrated significant improvement on measures of cognition, behavior, sleep quality, and ADL with the use of galantamine (Thavichachart et al., 2006). In patients with MCI, two 2-year randomized placebo-controlled trials did not show any benefit of galantamine over placebo on the rate of progression to AD (Winblad et al., 2008).

The most common adverse effects of galantamine are nausea, vomiting, diarrhea, dizziness, anorexia, and weight loss. Less common adverse effects include bradycardia, depression, fatigue, and somnolence. In one study of patients with MCI, more deaths were associated with the use of galantamine than with placebo (Winblad et al., 2008). Because galantamine is metabolized by CYP3A4 and CYP2D6 liver enzymes, inhibitors or inducers of these enzymes can lead to increased side effects or decreased efficacy, respectively.

Comparing the AChI Drugs for Dementia

Donepezil, rivastigmine, and galantamine have relatively similar efficacy and adverse effects. Rivastigmine patches may be better tolerated and easier to administer than the oral formulations. Tacrine is poorly tolerated by many patients and it can cause liver toxicity. Well-controlled comparative trials of the AChI drugs are not available. A meta-analysis of the effectiveness of the five drugs FDA approved for the treatment of dementia (the four AChI drugs plus memantine [Namenda], which is described in the following text) found that they produced statistically significant, but clinically marginal, improvement in cognition and global function (Raina et al., 2008). These drugs do not halt or correct the underlying degenerative process in dementia, but they can slow the progression of memory impairment. They can secondarily diminish the apathy, depression, anxiety, hallucinations, agitation, and other associated psychological and behavioral problems in these patients. Donepezil and rivastigmine each has documented efficacy in VaD, DLB, and PDD. Galantamine has documented efficacy in VaD. There is no clear evidence that the AChI drugs are effective for the treatment of MCI. All of these drugs can potentially exacerbate the motor symptoms of Parkinson's disease. Use of AChI drugs is associated with increased rates of syncope, bradycardia, pacemaker insertion, and hip fracture in older adults with dementia (Gill et al., 2009). Concurrent use of anticholinergic drugs can diminish the clinical benefits of AChI drugs, whereas the use of other cholinergic drugs can increase the occurrence of cholinergic adverse effects.

GLUTAMATE-MODULATING DRUGS FOR DEMENTIA

Glutamate is the major excitatory amino acid neurotransmitter in the brain. Glutamate is important in many normal and abnormal physiological processes, including neurotrophism (neuronal growth and maintenance), cognition (learning and memory), and neurodegeneration (neuronal damage or death; Meldrum, 2000). Glutamate systems have been implicated in various neurodegenerative disorders, including AD (Francis, 2009). Glutamate is released from neurons, binds to receptors, and is removed by reuptake transporters. Glutamate receptor systems are complex and can be segregated into various distinct receptor subtypes according to their molecular and pharmacological properties. One type of glutamate receptor is the N-methyl-D-aspartate (NMDA) receptor, which has multiple subtypes (Kugaya & Sanacora, 2005).

Memantine (Namenda) is an FDA-approved treatment for moderate-to-severe AD, and it has been investigated in other cognitive and neurodegenerative disorders (Robinson & Keating, 2006). Memantine is not an AChI, but it is a weakly binding NMDA-receptor antagonist. The rationale for using memantine in AD is based on the belief that persistent glutamate activation of NMDA receptors contributes to neuronal cell death and the symptoms of dementia. Memantine inhibits the damaging effects of excessive glutamate by blocking the NMDA receptor. It does not affect the inhibitory amino acid gamma-aminobutyric acid (GABA) or other neurotransmitter receptors.

In patients with moderate-to-severe AD, a double-blind placebo-controlled trial demonstrated that memantine had statistically significant benefits on global, functional, and cognitive measures. In one double-blind study of patients with moderate-to-severe AD who were taking donepezil, adding memantine resulted in significantly better outcomes on measures of cognition, behavior, ADL, and global improvement compared to adding placebo. A second double-blind study in patients with mild-to-moderate AD who were taking a cholinesterase inhibitor drug found that adding memantine was not more effective than adding placebo (Porsteinsson, Grossberg, Mintzer, & Olin, 2008). Among patients with mild-to-moderate VaD, two studies found that memantine improved cognition compared to placebo (Orgogozo, Rigaud, Stöffler, Möbius, & Forette, 2002; Wilcock, Möbius, & Stöffler, 2002). In a double-blind placebo-controlled study of patients with DLB or PDD, memantine improved global clinical status and behavioral symptoms in these patients who had mild-to-moderate symptoms (Emre et al., 2010).

Possible adverse effects of memantine include dizziness, headache, constipation, and confusion, but it is not associated with serious adverse neuropsychiatric effects. Memantine does not affect the inhibition of acetylcholinesterase by AChI drugs. Amantadine (Symmetrel), a closely related chemical analog of memantine, is an NMDA receptor antagonist (Blanpied, Boeckman, Aizenman, & Johnson, 1997). It is an FDA-approved treatment for influenza, Parkinson's disease, and drug-induced parkinsonian side effects, and it has been used for many of the same therapeutic purposes as memantine. Amantadine and memantine might have an undesirable additive effect if used together. Memantine does not interact with drugs metabolized by CYP450 liver enzymes.

OTHER DRUG THERAPIES FOR DEMENTIA

Vasodilator Drugs

Many drugs with vasodilator activity were originally tried in dementia when it was hypothesized that the condition was due to cerebrovascular insufficiency. Although these drugs have little evidence of benefit and are rarely used, several are FDA approved for the treatment of dementia. One such drug is the peripheral vasodilator isoxsuprine (Vasodilan), which is classified by the FDA as "possibly effective" for the relief of symptoms associated with senile dementia of the Alzheimer's type and/or multiple infarct dementia (Hussain, Gedye, Naylor, & Brown, 1976). Possible adverse effects of isoxsuprine include rash, dizziness, hypotension, tachyarrhythmia, abdominal discomfort, nausea, and pulmonary edema.

Another such drug is ergoloid mesylates (Hydergine), which acts centrally to decrease vascular tone and slow the heart rate and also acts peripherally to block alpha-adrenergic receptors. Another possible mechanism is the effect of ergoloid mesylates on neuronal cell metabolism, possibly resulting in improved oxygen uptake and improved cerebral metabolism, which in turn may normalize depressed neurotransmitter levels. According to the FDA-approved product label, ergoloid mesylates has been used to treat symptoms of an idiopathic decline in mental capacity (such as cognitive and interpersonal skills, mood, self-care, and apparent motivation) related to aging or to an underlying dementing condition such as primary progressive dementia, Alzheimer's dementia, or senile-onset multi-infarct dementia (Thompson et al., 1990). Possible adverse effects of ergoloid mesylates include flushing, rash, nausea, vomiting, headache, blurred vision, nasal congestion, bradyarrhythmia, and orthostatic hypotension.

Axona for Dementia

Axona (Axona Product Information, 2010) is designated by the FDA as a "medical food." A medical food is defined as "a food which is formulated to be consumed or administered enterally (or orally) under the supervision of a physician and which is intended for the specific dietary management of a disease or condition for which distinctive nutritional requirements, based on recognized scientific principles, are established by medical evaluation." Medical foods are exempt from FDA labeling requirements for health claims and nutrient content, and they are not reviewed or approved by the FDA. They must comply with good manufacturing practice regulations and labeling practices for protection against food allergens.

Axona contains a proprietary formulation of medium-chain triglycerides (mostly caprylic triglyceride). It is currently being marketed for the "clinical dietary management of the metabolic processes associated with mild to moderate AD." The rationale for the use of Axon is based on the finding that cerebral hypometabolism (i.e., impaired glucose metabolism) is an early sign of AD. Medium-chain triglycerides are metabolized in the liver, resulting in the production of the ketone body beta-hydroxybutyrate. Beta-hydroxybutyrate is transported into the brain and provides an alternative fuel source for cerebral metabolism.

A randomized, placebo-controlled, crossover study in 15 patients with AD and 5 patients with MCI found that a single oral dose of Axona produced an increase in serum ketones and an immediate statistically significant improvement in the ADAS-Cog (Reger et al., 2004). More recently, a double-blind, randomized, 90-day, placebo-controlled trial in 152 patients with mild-to-moderate AD found a significant improvement in the ADAS-Cog in patients treated with Axona at 45 days, but not at 90 days (Costantini, Barr, Vogel, & Henderson, 2008).

Medium-chain triglycerides in general and caprylic triglyceride in particular are generally considered safe. In the Axona clinical trials, about 25% of patients developed diarrhea. A few patients showed clinically significant increases in serum triglyceride concentrations. Because Axona contains milk and soy products, it should not be consumed by patients allergic to either. The longer-term efficacy, tolerability, and safety of Axona are unknown.

Nootropic Drugs for Dementia

Nootropic agents refer to a class of drugs that are purported to improve cognitive function. These types of drugs also have been known as "smart drugs," memory enhancers," and "cognitive enhancers." However, the term *nootropic* was first used to describe the cognitive effects of the compound piracetam, which was synthesized in 1964. Nootropic agents most specifically describe the larger class of drugs that are chemically related to piracetam (Malykh & Sadaie, 2010). Piracetam and piracetam-like drugs are cyclic derivatives of GABA. The precise mechanism of action of these drugs is unclear, but they have anticonvulsant and antioxidant properties, may enhance the function of cholinergic receptor systems, and might modulate glutamate receptor systems.

Piracetam is manufactured outside of the United States under various trade names (Nootropil, Nootrop, Nootropyl). In the United States, the drug is designated by the FDA as an orphan drug for the treatment of myoclonus. Orphan drugs are designated as such for the treatment of rare diseases or conditions. Piracetam is not otherwise regulated by the FDA, and it can be obtained in the United States without a prescription.

A meta-analysis of 19 double-blind placebo-controlled studies in a diverse group of patients with age-related dementia or cognitive impairment demonstrated a significant benefit for piracetam (Waegemans et al., 2002). This benefit, however, was based on the outcome measure of CGIC, rather than other standard measures of cognitive function (e.g., ADAS-Cog). The long-term effects of piracetam in these patients are not known.

Possible adverse effects of piracetam include anxiety, insomnia, irritability, headache, agitation, tremor, and nausea. Elevations of liver enzymes have been reported rarely. Because the drug is cleared through the kidneys, patients with impaired renal function have a higher risk of adverse effects. Abrupt discontinuation can be associated with seizures.

There are more than a dozen nootropic agents, but none has been as well studied as piracetam. Levetiracetam (Keppra) currently is the only nootropic agent that is FDA approved. Levetiracetam is the S-enantiomer of the racemate drug etiracetam. Etiracetam is structurally similar to piracetam. Levetiracetam is FDA-approved as adjunctive therapy for partial seizures, generalized seizures, and myoclonic seizures. The drug appears to have fewer adverse cognitive effects compared to other anticonvulsant drugs. It has not been well studied for cognitive impairment or dementia, but an ongoing clinical trial is investigating its use for MCI (www.clinical-trials.gov/show/NCT01044758). Common adverse effects of levetiracetam are dizziness, somnolence, weakness, and irritability. Behavioral changes, hallucinations, and psychosis have also been reported.

Ginkgo Biloba for Dementia

Ginkgo biloba is obtained from the leaves of the *Ginkgo biloba* tree, formerly known as *Salisburia adiantifolia*. It is used alone or is sometimes added as a supplement in various "natural" food products. It has antioxidant, anti-inflammatory, and antiplatelet effects. Because ginkgo produces arterial vasodilation, inhibits arterial spasms, decreases blood viscosity, and increases tissue perfusion and cerebral blood flow, it has been used and studied for peripheral vascular insufficiency, cerebrovascular disease, MCI, dementia, and sexual dysfunction. Early clinical trials for AD, VaD, and MCI found modest, but inconsistent benefits for ginkgo compared to placebo on some cognitive and psychosocial outcome measures (Birks & Grimley Evans, 2004). A recent double-blind, randomized trial found that it was not effective in preventing or treating dementia (DeKosky et al., 2008). A second double-blind, randomized trial found it also was not effective for preventing cognitive decline in older adults (Snitz et al., 2009).

Common side effects are nausea, vomiting, diarrhea, headache, irritability, and dizziness. Bruising and bleeding may occur, with rare reports of serious intracranial bleeding (e.g., subdural hematoma). Seizures have been reported in children who ingested large amounts. Potential drug interactions include anticoagulants and antiplatelet drugs (e.g., aspirin and other nonsteroidal anti-inflammatory medications). Ginkgo may affect liver metabolic enzymes, but this has not been extensively investigated.

Antioxidant and Anti-Inflammatory Drugs

The hypothesis that free radicals may initiate and maintain mechanisms responsible for neurodegeneration in AD has stimulated interest in investigating drugs such as vitamin E (e.g., alpha-tocopherol); ginkgo biloba (discussed previously); and selegiline (Eldepryl; Zelapar) as antioxidant therapies. Some retrospective studies also found an inverse association between the use of anti-inflammatory drugs, such as the NSAIDs, and the risk of developing AD. Similarly, an association between statin drugs, which are used for treating hypercholesterolemia and have anti-inflammatory effects, and a reduced risk of developing dementia has been noted. Evidence reviews conducted by practice guidelines have found no evidence of sufficient efficacy and/ or safety to justify the use of any of these drug therapies for the treatment of dementing disorders, including AD and MCI (O'Brien & Burns, 2011; Rabins et al., 2007). NSAIDs are associated with an increased risk of impaired renal function and bleeding. Vitamin E supplementation has been associated with an increased bleeding risk and an increased mortality risk.

Omega-3 Fatty Acids

Docosahexaenoic acid (DHA) is an omega-3 fatty acid that has been identified as a potential drug treatment for AD. Epidemiological studies have shown that omega-3 fatty acid consumption is associated with a reduced risk of cognitive decline or developing AD. Preclinical animal studies have found that DHA modifies the expression of AD-like neuropathologies. The most abundant fatty acid in the brain is DHA, and it is reduced in the brains of patients with AD. The other major omega-3 fatty acid found in fish, eicosapentaenoic acid (EPA), is virtually absent from the brain. A recent double-blind placebo-controlled trial in patients with mild-to-moderate AD found no benefit for the use of DHA on slowing the rate of cognitive or functional decline in these patients (Quinn et al., 2010).

Hormone Replacement Therapy

Epidemiological studies in humans and preclinical animal studies have suggested that estrogen therapy or combined estrogen and progestagen therapy in post-menopausal women may protect against cognitive decline and dementia. Evidence reviews have found no evidence of sufficient efficacy and/or safety to justify the use of any of these drug therapies for the prevention or treatment of dementing disorders (O'Brien & Burns, 2011; Rabins et al., 2007). Indeed, these studies have suggested that their use is associated with an increased risk of cognitive decline, as well as an increased cancer risk in women.

B Vitamins

Reduced levels of B vitamins (including folate and vitamin B_{12}) have been associated with cognitive impairment and an increased risk of dementia. Evidence reviews have found no evidence of sufficient efficacy to justify their use to prevent or treat dementing disorders (O'Brien & Burns, 2011).

ANTIPSYCHOTIC DRUG THERAPIES FOR BPSAD

Efficacy

The FDA has not approved any drug therapy for the treatment of BPSAD, but antipsychotic drugs are the most commonly used. Consistent with their general clinical popularity, the "atypical" second-generation antipsychotic drugs (SGAs) have been better studied and more often used than "typical" first-generation antipsychotic drugs (FGAs) in elderly patients with BPSAD.

Eight placebo-controlled randomized clinical trials (RCTs) have been conducted with FGAs and 18 trials with SGAs (Ballard & Howard, 2006; Jeste et al., 2008). The studies lasted 6 to 12 weeks; only two lasted for 6 months or longer. Most of the RCTs included the FGA drug haloperidol (Haldol) or the SGA drugs risperidone (Risperdal), olanzapine (Zyprexa), quetiapine (Seroquel), or aripiprazole (Abilify). Approximately half of the clinical trials of antipsychotic drugs in dementia patients recruited individuals primarily with psychosis, whereas the other half selected individuals primarily with agitation or global behavioral disturbances. Because most trials of psychosis did not exclude agitation and most trials of agitation did not exclude psychosis, the vast majority of studies included patients with an admixture of BPSAD. Overall, SGA drugs appear to have modest efficacy at best for treating psychotic symptoms, and some studies did not find a significant advantage of active drug over placebo with respect to psychotic symptoms. Although some analyses suggested a better antipsychotic symptom benefit for risperidone, there was no clear difference in efficacy among the SGA drugs. Some RCTs, but not all, demonstrated modest efficacy for reducing aggression and agitation with antipsychotic drugs. In direct comparisons, only one of four non-placebo-controlled RCTs found significantly greater efficacy with SGAs compared to the FGA haloperidol (Jeste et al., 2008).

Adverse Events

Despite the perceived greater tolerability, lesser risk for parkinsonian side effects, and lower risk for tardive dyskinesia of SGA drugs compared to FGA drugs, other potential side effects of SGA drugs in elderly persons include sedation, postural hypotension, gait disturbances, and falls. In the four comparative studies, haloperidol was associated with more parkinsonian side effects than the SGA drugs. There have been no large-scale published studies of antipsychotic drug-associated obesity, diabetes, and other metabolic disturbances among elderly patients with BPSAD. In recent years, however, two serious adverse events have been associated with the use of antipsychotic drugs in dementia patients: cerebrovascular adverse events (CVAEs; e.g., stroke and transient ischemic attacks) and death.

Concerns about an increased risk of stroke associated with SGAs first arose in Canada in 2002 (Douglas & Smeeth, 2008). Based on RCTs available at that time, Health Canada (a regulatory body in Canada) issued a warning highlighting this risk. The Committee on Safety of Medicines in the United Kingdom recommended avoiding the specific use of the SGAs risperidone and olanzapine in dementia patients in 2004 (Mowat, Fowlie, & MacEwan, 2004).

In the United States, the FDA first issued a warning titled "CVAEs, Including Stroke, in Elderly Patients With Dementia" in 2003. This warning stated that CVAEs, including some deaths, were reported in elderly patients in the risperidone trials for BPSAD. In a combined analysis of data from three published placebo-controlled RCTs, 12 of 744 patients taking risperidone (1.6%) developed serious CVAEs, a rate significantly greater than the 4 of 562 patients taking placebo (0.7%). Four patients on risperidone and two on placebo died. In a second analysis that pooled data from three published and three unpublished placebo-controlled RCTs, the rates of serious CVAEs for risperidone (15 of 1,009 patients; 1.5%) and for placebo (4 of 712 patients; 0.6%) were not significantly different. Risperidone-treated patients, however, had significantly higher rates of nonserious CVAEs (18 of 1,009; 1.8%) than placebo-treated patients (4 of 712; 0.6%; Herrmann & Lanctôt, 2005).

Soon after, the FDA applied a similar warning to olanzapine and aripiprazole. In five olanzapine RCTs, the relative risk of CVAEs was not significantly different than placebo. An analysis combining all 11 studies of risperidone and olanzapine found that 48 of 2,187 drug-treated subjects (2.2%) experienced CVAEs compared with 10 of 1,190 placebo-treated subjects (0.8%), which was significantly different (Herrmann & Lanctôt, 2005). In two other placebo-controlled trials there was an increased incidence of CVAEs, including some deaths, in aripiprazole-treated patients (the specific incident rates were not reported). Analysis of data from two RCTs demonstrated no significant difference in CVAE rates for quetiapine (0.9%) compared to placebo (1.9%). A meta-analysis of all RCTs found that CVAE rates were significantly different for SGA-treated patients (1.9%) compared to placebo-treated patients (0.9%; Schneider et al., 2006).

In April 2005, the FDA issued a new public health advisory warning about an increased risk of death associated with the use of SGAs compared to placebo in elderly patients with BPSAD. Analyses of 17 placebo-controlled RCTs (enrolling 5,377 patients for 10–12 weeks) revealed a risk of death in drug-treated patients (4.5%) that was significantly greater than that seen in placebo-treated patients (2.6%).

According to the FDA, the causes of death varied. Most appeared to be related either to cardiovascular (e.g., heart failure, sudden death) or infectious (e.g., pneumonia) causes. A published meta-analysis of 15 RCTs documented that the risk of mortality associated with SGAs (3.5%) was significantly greater than that associated with placebo (2.3%; Schneider, Dagerman, & Insel, 2005). Based on their analysis, the FDA requested that the manufacturers of all SGA drugs include information about this risk in a *Boxed Warning* and in the *Warnings* section of the drugs' prescribing information.

Most recently, the FDA issued an updated advisory in June 2008 extending its warning about risk of death to include FGA drugs. This warning was based on two published observational epidemiological studies that examined the risk of death in elderly patients who were treated with FGAs. Gill et al. (2007) conducted a retrospective cohort study in Ontario, Canada, of 27,259 elderly adults with a diagnosis of dementia between April 1997 and March 2002. The study compared the risk for death with use of an SGA versus no antipsychotic drug and the risk for death with use of an FGA versus an SGA. The use of SGAs was associated with increased mortality compared to no antipsychotic drug use, beginning as early as 30 days and persisting until the study ended at 180 days. Additionally, FGA use was associated with a marginally higher risk of death compared with SGA use. The causes of death were not reported in this study.

In the second study, Schneeweiss, Setoguchi, Brookhart, Dormuth, and Wang (2007) conducted a retrospective cohort study in British Columbia, Canada, of 37,241 elderly adults who were prescribed FGA or SGA drugs for any reason (not just dementia) between January 1996 and December 2004. The study compared the 180-day all-cause mortality with use of an FGA versus an SGA. The risk of death in FGA-treated patients was comparable to, and possibly greater than, the risk of death in SGA-treated patients. The causes of death with the highest relative risk were cancer and cardiac disease. A more recent analysis of these data demonstrated that patients taking FGA drugs had significantly higher noncancer death rates attributable to cardiovascular, respiratory, nervous system, and other causes (Setoguchi et al., 2008). Despite methodological limitations of epidemiological studies and the characteristics of the patient populations studied, the FDA concluded that the overall weight of evidence, including these and previous studies, indicated that the FGA drugs share the increased risk of death in elderly patients with BPSAD that has been observed for the SGA drugs. The FDA mandated that prescribing information for all antipsychotic drugs include the same risk information in a *Boxed Warning* and in the *Warnings* section.

A clinically useful way of looking at efficacy and safety data from RCTs is through two statistical concepts: "Number Needed to Treat" (NNT) and "Number Needed to Harm" (NNH). NNT is the number of patients that need to receive a therapy to successfully treat one person. An NNT of one is ideal; a value of 10 or less is considered clinically significant. Similarly, NNH is the number of patients that would need to receive a therapy before you would see a harmful outcome (e.g., a serious adverse event or death). In the meta-analysis of RCTs for BPSAD, the NNT for SGA drugs ranged from 5 to 14 depending on the individual studies (Schneider et al., 2006). Hence, treating 5 to 14 patients with an SGA drug would be needed to benefit one patient. By contrast, the mortality NNH for SGAs was about 100 (Schneider et al., 2005). That is, for every 100 patients treated with an SGA, there would be one death due to the SGA. By combining the NNT and NNH calculations, the likelihood of benefit versus serious risk would be modest: for every 9 to 25 individuals helped with SGAs, one death would be expected (Jeste et al., 2008).

NON-ANTIPSYCHOTIC DRUG THERAPIES FOR BPSAD

There are relatively few evidence-based medication alternatives to the use of antipsychotic drugs for BPSAD (Sink, Holden, & Yaffe, 2005). These RCTs have been limited to patients with mild-to-moderate symptoms. Among the FDA-approved treatments for dementia, there is only weak evidence for the use of AChI drugs (e.g., donepezil and rivastigmine) and memantine in the treatment of BPSAD (Figiel & Sadowsky, 2008; Howard et al., 2007; Maidment et al., 2008; Sink et al., 2005). A small number of RCTs of anticonvulsant drugs found some benefit for carbamazepine (Tegretol), but not for valproic acid (Depakene; Depakote; Jeste et al., 2008; Konovalov, Muralee, & Tampi, 2008). Several RCTs of the serotonin reuptake inhibitor (SRI) antidepressant drug citalopram (Celexa) also demonstrated a significant benefit (Pollock et al., 2007), but other antidepressant drug studies have found no benefit (Sink et al., 2005). In patients with FTD, there is some evidence that SRI drugs may help BPSAD, but they do not improve cognitive function (O'Brien & Burns, 2011). Antipsychotic drugs are associated with a greater mortality risk in elderly patients with BPSAD compared to the use of other psychotropic drugs (Kales et al., 2007).

SUMMARY

Many different drug therapies have been developed for the treatment of dementia and cognitive impairment. Currently available FDA-approved drugs for the treatment of AD and other dementing disorders have statistically significant but clinically limited symptomatic improvement (Raina et al., 2008). The AChI drugs donepezil, rivastigmine, galantamine, and the NMDA-receptor antagonist memantine have produced modest and persistent improvements on measures of cognition, ADL, and behavior in patients with disease severity ranging from mild to severe. Among the AChI drugs, the rivastigmine transdermal patch is associated with fewer cholinergic side effects and may be easier to administer in demented patients. In patients with moderate-to-severe dementia, memantine used in combination with an AChI drug may be more effective than an AChI drug alone. None of these agents have been shown to stop or reverse the underlying neurodegenerative process. Most importantly, these drugs do not have significantly demonstrated benefits or safety to justify their use in MCI. For FTD, there is no evidence that AChI drugs or memantine are effective, but there is some evidence that SRI drugs may improve behavioral symptoms. There is no evidence that other drug therapies, including isoxsuprine, ergoloid mesylates, nootropic drugs, ginkgo biloba, Axona, vitamin E, selegiline, NSAIDs, statin drugs, estrogen or combined estrogen plus progestin therapy, or B vitamins, are sufficiently effective and safe to justify their clinical use for the treatment of MCI, AD, or other dementing disorders.

The management of BPSAD should always include nonpharmacological approaches, although their effectiveness has been demonstrated mostly in studies of patients with mild-to-moderate severity (Ayalon, Gum, Feliciano, & Areán, 2006). The overuse or misuse of medications should be avoided. For more severe cases, however, it is not necessarily reasonable to stop prescribing medications completely because of safety concerns. Antipsychotic drugs, especially SGA drugs, have the best supporting evidence, even though their efficacy is modest and their side effects are potentially more serious. For the treatment of BPSAD, antipsychotic drugs should be used judiciously, after a careful assessment of risks and benefits. Weighing small but real risks (e.g., stroke or death) compared with possible benefits (e.g., being able to live in a less restricted environment) is a complex decision involving patients, families, and other caregivers. There are very few alternatives to the use of antipsychotic drugs for BPSAD. Among the FDA-approved treatments for dementia, there is only weak evidence for the effectiveness of AChI drugs and memantine. There also is limited evidence of effectiveness from studies of anticonvulsant drugs and antidepressant drugs.

REFERENCES

American Psychiatric Association (APA). (2000). *Diagnostic and statistical manual of mental disorders* (4th ed., text rev.). Washington, DC: Author.

Axona Product Information. (2010). Retrieved from http://about-axona.com/

Ayalon, L., Gum, A. M., Feliciano, L., & Areán, P. A. (2006). Effectiveness of nonpharmacological interventions for the management of neuropsychiatric symptoms in patients with dementia: A systematic review. *Archives of Internal Medicine, 166*(20), 2182–2188.

Ballard, C., & Howard, R. (2006). Neuroleptic drugs in dementia: Benefits and harm. *Nature Reviews. Neuroscience, 7*(6), 492–500.

Birks, J., & Grimley Evans, J. (2004). Ginkgo biloba for cognitive impairment and dementia. *Cochrane Database of Systematic Reviews, 4.*

Birks, J., Grimley Evans, J., Iakovidou, V., Tsolaki, M., & Holt, F. E. (2009). Rivastigmine for Alzheimer's disease. *The Cochrane Database of Systematic Reviews,* (2), CD001191.

Black, S., Román, G. C., Geldmacher, D. S., Salloway, S., Hecker, J., Burns, A.,... Pratt, R.; Donepezil 307 Vascular Dementia Study Group. (2003). Efficacy and tolerability of donepezil in vascular dementia: Positive results of a 24-week, multicenter, international, randomized, placebo-controlled clinical trial. *Stroke, 34*(10), 2323–2330.

Black, S. E., Doody, R., Li, H., McRae, T., Jambor, K. M., Xu, Y.,... Richardson, S. (2007). Donepezil preserves cognition and global function in patients with severe Alzheimer disease. *Neurology, 69*(5), 459–469.

Blanpied, T. A., Boeckman, F. A., Aizenman, E., & Johnson, J. W. (1997). Trapping channel block of NMDA-activated responses by amantadine and memantine. *Journal of Neurophysiology, 77*(1), 309–323.

Costantini, L. C., Barr, L. J., Vogel, J. L., & Henderson, S. T. (2008). Hypometabolism as a therapeutic target in Alzheimer's disease. *BMC Neuroscience, 9*(Suppl 2), S16.

DeKosky, S. T., Williamson, J. D., Fitzpatrick, A. L., Kronmal, R. A., Ives, D. G., Saxton, J. A.,... Furberg, C. D.; Ginkgo Evaluation of Memory (GEM) Study Investigators. (2008). Ginkgo biloba for prevention of dementia: A randomized controlled trial. *Journal of the American Medical Association, 300*(19), 2253–2262.

Doody, R. S., Ferris, S. H., Salloway, S., Sun, Y., Goldman, R., Watkins, W. E.,... Murthy, A. K. (2009). Donepezil treatment of patients with MCI: A 48-week randomized, placebo-controlled trial. *Neurology, 72*(18), 1555–1561.

Douglas, I. J., & Smeeth, L. (2008). Exposure to antipsychotics and risk of stroke: Self controlled case series study. *British Medical Journal, 337*, a1227.

Dubois, B., Feldman, H. H., Jacova, C., Cummings, J. L., Dekosky, S. T., Barberger-Gateau, P.,... Scheltens, P. (2010). Revising the definition of Alzheimer's disease: A new lexicon. *Lancet Neurology, 9*(11), 1118–1127.

Emre, M., Tsolaki, M., Bonuccelli, U., Destée, A., Tolosa, E., Kutzelnigg, A.,... Jones, R.; 11018 Study Investigators. (2010). Memantine for patients with Parkinson's disease dementia or dementia with Lewy bodies: A randomised, double-blind, placebo-controlled trial. *Lancet Neurology, 9*(10), 969–977.

Feldman, H. H., Ferris, S., Winblad, B., Sfikas, N., Mancione, L., He, Y.,…Lane, R. (2007). Effect of rivastigmine on delay to diagnosis of Alzheimer's disease from mild cognitive impairment: The InDDEx study. *Lancet Neurology, 6*(6), 501–512.

Ferri, C. P., Prince, M., Brayne, C., Brodaty, H., Fratiglioni, L., Ganguli, M.,…Scazufca, M.; Alzheimer's Disease International. (2005). Global prevalence of dementia: A Delphi consensus study. *Lancet, 366*(9503), 2112–2117.

Figiel, G., & Sadowsky, C. (2008). A systematic review of the effectiveness of rivastigmine for the treatment of behavioral disturbances in dementia and other neurological disorders. *Current Medical Research and Opinion, 24*(1), 157–166.

Francis, P. T. (2009). Altered glutamate neurotransmission and behaviour in dementia: Evidence from studies of memantine. *Current Molecular Pharmacology, 2*(1), 77–82.

Gill, S. S., Anderson, G. M., Fischer, H. D., Bell, C. M., Li, P., Normand, S. L., & Rochon, P. A. (2009). Syncope and its consequences in patients with dementia receiving cholinesterase inhibitors: A population-based cohort study. *Archives of Internal Medicine, 169*(9), 867–873.

Gill, S. S., Bronskill, S. E., Normand, S. L., Anderson, G. M., Sykora, K., Lam, K.,… Rochon, P. A. (2007). Antipsychotic drug use and mortality in older adults with dementia. *Annals of Internal Medicine, 146*(11), 775–786.

Herrmann, N., & Lanctôt, K. L. (2005). Do atypical antipsychotics cause stroke? *Central Nervous System Drugs, 19*(2), 91–103.

Howard, R. J., Juszczak, E., Ballard, C. G., Bentham, P., Brown, R. G., Bullock, R.,… Rodger, M.; CALM-AD Trial Group. (2007). Donepezil for the treatment of agitation in Alzheimer's disease. *The New England Journal of Medicine, 357*(14), 1382–1392.

Hussain, S. M., Gedye, J. L., Naylor, R., & Brown, A. L. (1976). The objective measurement of mental performance in cerebrovascular disease. A double-blind controlled study, using a graded-release preparation of isoxsuprine. *The Practitioner, 216*(1292), 222–228.

Jeste, D. V., Blazer, D., Casey, D., Meeks, T., Salzman, C., Schneider, L.,…Yaffe, K. (2008). ACNP white paper: Update on use of antipsychotic drugs in elderly persons with dementia. *Neuropsychopharmacology, 33*(5), 957–970.

Kales, H. C., Valenstein, M., Kim, H. M., McCarthy, J. F., Ganoczy, D., Cunningham, F., & Blow, F. C. (2007). Mortality risk in patients with dementia treated with antipsychotics versus other psychiatric medications. *The American Journal of Psychiatry, 164*(10), 1568–1576; quiz 1623.

Kirshner, H. S. (2009). Vascular dementia: A review of recent evidence for prevention and treatment. *Current Neurology and Neuroscience Reports, 9*(6), 437–442.

Konovalov, S., Muralee, S., & Tampi, R. R. (2008). Anticonvulsants for the treatment of behavioral and psychological symptoms of dementia: A literature review. *International Psychogeriatrics/IPA, 20*(2), 293–308.

Kugaya, A., & Sanacora, G. (2005). Beyond monoamines: Glutamatergic function in mood disorders. *Central Nervous System Spectrums, 10*(10), 808–819.

Leroi, I., Collins, D., & Marsh, L. (2006). Non-dopaminergic treatment of cognitive impairment and dementia in Parkinson's disease: A review. *Journal of the Neurological Sciences, 248*(1–2), 104–114.

Lyketsos, C. G., Steinberg, M., Tschanz, J. T., Norton, M. C., Steffens, D. C., & Breitner, J. C. (2000). Mental and behavioral disturbances in dementia: Findings from the Cache County Study on Memory in Aging. *The American Journal of Psychiatry, 157*(5), 708–714.

Maidment, I. D., Fox, C. G., Boustani, M., Rodriguez, J., Brown, R. C., & Katona, C. L. (2008). Efficacy of memantine on behavioral and psychological symptoms related to dementia: A systematic meta-analysis. *The Annals of Pharmacotherapy, 42*(1), 32–38.

Malykh, A. G., & Sadaie, M. R. (2010). Piracetam and piracetam-like drugs: From basic science to novel clinical applications to CNS disorders. *Drugs, 70*(3), 287–312.

Meldrum, B. S. (2000). Glutamate as a neurotransmitter in the brain: Review of physiology and pathology. *The Journal of Nutrition, 130*(4S Suppl), 1007S–1015S.

Miyasaki, J. M., Shannon, K., Voon, V., Ravina, B., Kleiner-Fisman, G., Anderson, K.,...Weiner, W. J.; Quality Standards Subcommittee of the American Academy of Neurology. (2006). Practice parameter: Evaluation and treatment of depression, psychosis, and dementia in Parkinson disease (an evidence-based review): Report of the Quality Standards Subcommittee of the American Academy of Neurology. *Neurology, 66*(7), 996–1002.

Mowat, D., Fowlie, D., & MacEwan, T. (2004). CSM warning on atypical psychotics and stroke may be detrimental for dementia. *British Medical Journal, 328*(7450), 1262.

Neary, D., Snowden, J., & Mann, D. (2005). Frontotemporal dementia. *Lancet Neurology, 4*(11), 771–780.

O'Brien, J. T., & Burns, A.; BAP Dementia Consensus Group. (2011). Clinical practice with anti-dementia drugs: A revised (second) consensus statement from the British Association for Psychopharmacology. *Journal of Psychopharmacology, 25*(8), 997–1019.

Orgogozo, J. M., Rigaud, A. S., Stöffler, A., Möbius, H. J., & Forette, F. (2002). Efficacy and safety of memantine in patients with mild to moderate vascular dementia: A randomized, placebo-controlled trial (MMM 300). *Stroke, 33*(7), 1834–1839.

Picciotto, M. R., Alreja, M., & Jentsch, J. D. (2002). Acetylcholine. In K. L. Davis, D. Charney, J. T. Coyle, & C. Nemeroff (Eds.), *Neuropsychopharmacology: The fifth generation of progress* (pp. 3–14). Philadelphia, PA: Lippincott Williams & Wilkins.

Plassman, B. L., Langa, K. M., Fisher, G. G., Heeringa, S. G., Weir, D. R., Ofstedal, M. B.,... Wallace, R. B. (2007). Prevalence of dementia in the United States: The aging, demographics, and memory study. *Neuroepidemiology, 29*(1–2), 125–132.

Pollock, B. G., Mulsant, B. H., Rosen, J., Mazumdar, S., Blakesley, R. E., Houck, P. R., & Huber, K. A. (2007). A double-blind comparison of citalopram and risperidone for the treatment of behavioral and psychotic symptoms associated with dementia. *The American Journal of Geriatric Psychiatry, 15*(11), 942–952.

Porsteinsson, A. P., Grossberg, G. T., Mintzer, J., & Olin, J. T.; Memantine MEM-MD-12 Study Group. (2008). Memantine treatment in patients with mild to moderate Alzheimer's disease already receiving a cholinesterase inhibitor: A randomized, double-blind, placebo-controlled trial. *Current Alzheimer Research, 5*(1), 83–89.

Quinn, J. F., Raman, R., Thomas, R. G., Yurko-Mauro, K., Nelson, E. B., Van Dyck, C.,...Aisen, P. S. (2010). Docosahexaenoic acid supplementation and cognitive decline in Alzheimer disease: A randomized trial. *Journal of the Americal Medical Association, 304*(17), 1903–1911.

Rabins, P. V., Blacker, D., Rovner, B. W., Rummans, T., Schneider, L. S., Tariot, P. N.,...Fochtmann, L. J.; APA Work Group on Alzheimer's Disease and Other Dementias. (2007). American Psychiatric Association practice guideline for the treatment of patients with Alzheimer's disease and other dementias. Second edition. *American Journal of Psychiatry, 164*(12 Suppl), 5–56.

Raina, P., Santaguida, P., Ismaila, A., Patterson, C., Cowan, D., Levine, M.,...Oremus, M. (2008). Effectiveness of cholinesterase inhibitors and memantine for treating dementia: Evidence review for a clinical practice guideline. *Annals of Internal Medicine, 148*(5), 379–397.

Ravina, B., Putt, M., Siderowf, A., Farrar, J. T., Gillespie, M., Crawley, A.,...Simuni, T. (2005). Donepezil for dementia in Parkinson's disease: A randomised, double blind, placebo controlled, crossover study. *Journal of Neurology, Neurosurgery, and Psychiatry, 76*(7), 934–939.

Reger, M. A., Henderson, S. T., Hale, C., Cholerton, B., Baker, L. D., Watson, G. S.,…Craft, S. (2004). Effects of beta-hydroxybutyrate on cognition in memory-impaired adults. *Neurobiology of Aging, 25*(3), 311–314.

Relkin, N. R., Reichman, W. E., Orazem, J., & McRae, T. (2003). A large, community-based, open-label trial of donepezil in the treatment of Alzheimer's disease. *Dementia and Geriatric Cognitive Disorders, 16*(1), 15–24.

Robinson, D. M., & Keating, G. M. (2006). Memantine: A review of its use in Alzheimer's disease. *Drugs, 66*(11), 1515–1534.

Schneider, L. S., Dagerman, K. S., & Insel, P. (2005). Risk of death with atypical antipsychotic drug treatment for dementia: Meta-analysis of randomized placebo-controlled trials. *Journal of the American Medical Association, 294*(15), 1934–1943.

Schneider, L. S., Tariot, P. N., Dagerman, K. S., Davis, S. M., Hsiao, J. K., Ismail, M. S.,… Lieberman, J. A.; CATIE-AD Study Group. (2006). Effectiveness of atypical antipsychotic drugs in patients with Alzheimer's disease. *The New England Journal of Medicine, 355*(15), 1525–1538.

Schneeweiss, S., Setoguchi, S., Brookhart, A., Dormuth, C., & Wang, P. S. (2007). Risk of death associated with the use of conventional versus atypical antipsychotic drugs among elderly patients. *Canadian Medical Association Journal, 176*(5), 627–632.

Scott, L. J., & Goa, K. L. (2000). Galantamine: A review of its use in Alzheimer's disease. *Drugs, 60*(5), 1095–1122.

Seltzer, B. (2005). Donepezil: A review. *Expert Opinion on Drug Metabolism & Toxicology, 1*(3), 527–536.

Setoguchi, S., Wang, P. S., Alan Brookhart, M., Canning, C. F., Kaci, L., & Schneeweiss, S. (2008). Potential causes of higher mortality in elderly users of conventional and atypical antipsychotic medications. *Journal of the American Geriatrics Society, 56*(9), 1644–1650.

Sink, K. M., Holden, K. F., & Yaffe, K. (2005). Pharmacological treatment of neuropsychiatric symptoms of dementia: A review of the evidence. *Journal of the American Medical Association, 293*(5), 596–608.

Snitz, B. E., O'Meara, E. S., Carlson, M. C., Arnold, A. M., Ives, D. G., Rapp, S. R.,… DeKosky, S. T.; Ginkgo Evaluation of Memory (GEM) Study Investigators. (2009). Ginkgo biloba for preventing cognitive decline in older adults: A randomized trial. *Journal of the American Medical Association, 302*(24), 2663–2670.

Steinberg, M., Sheppard, J. M., Tschanz, J. T., Norton, M. C., Steffens, D. C., Breitner, J. C., & Lyketsos, C. G. (2003). The incidence of mental and behavioral disturbances in dementia: The cache county study. *The Journal of Neuropsychiatry and Clinical Neurosciences, 15*(3), 340–345.

Testad, I., Aasland, A. M., & Aarsland, D. (2007). Prevalence and correlates of disruptive behavior in patients in Norwegian nursing homes. *International Journal of Geriatric Psychiatry, 22*(9), 916–921.

Thavichachart, N., Phanthumchinda, K., Chankrachang, S., Praditsuwan, R., Nidhinandana, S., Senanarong, V., & Poungvarin, N. (2006). Efficacy study of galantamine in possible Alzheimer's disease with or without cerebrovascular disease and vascular dementia in Thai patients: A slow-titration regimen. *International Journal of Clinical Practice, 60*(5), 533–540.

Thomas, A. J., Burn, D. J., Rowan, E. N., Littlewood, E., Newby, J., Cousins, D.,… McKeith, I. G. (2005). A comparison of the efficacy of donepezil in Parkinson's disease with dementia and dementia with Lewy bodies. *International Journal of Geriatric Psychiatry, 20*(10), 938–944.

Thompson, T. L., Filley, C. M., Mitchell, W. D., Culig, K. M., LoVerde, M., & Byyny, R. L. (1990). Lack of efficacy of hydergine in patients with Alzheimer's disease. *The New England Journal of Medicine, 323*(7), 445–448.

Waegemans, T., Wilsher, C. R., Danniau, A., Ferris, S. H., Kurz, A., & Winblad, B. (2002). Clinical efficacy of piracetam in cognitive impairment: A meta-analysis. *Dementia and Geriatric Cognitive Disorders, 13*(4), 217–224.

Wagstaff, A. J., & McTavish, D. (1994). Tacrine: A review of its pharmacodynamic and pharmacokinetic properties, and therapeutic efficacy in Alzheimer's disease. *Drugs Aging, 4*(6), 510–540.

Wentrup, A., Oertel, W. H., & Dodel, R. (2009). Once-daily transdermal rivastigmine in the treatment of Alzheimer's disease. *Drug Design, Development and Therapy, 2*, 245–254.

Wesnes, K. A., McKeith, I., Edgar, C., Emre, M., & Lane, R. (2005). Benefits of rivastigmine on attention in dementia associated with Parkinson disease. *Neurology, 65*(10), 1654–1656.

Wilcock, G., Möbius, H. J., & Stöffler, A.; MMM 500 group. (2002). A double-blind, placebo-controlled multicentre study of memantine in mild to moderate vascular dementia (MMM500). *International Clinical Psychopharmacology, 17*(6), 297–305.

Wilkinson, D., Doody, R., Helme, R., Taubman, K., Mintzer, J., Kertesz, A., & Pratt, R. D.; Donepezil 308 Study Group. (2003). Donepezil in vascular dementia: A randomized, placebo-controlled study. *Neurology, 61*(4), 479–486.

Williams, B. R., Nazarians, A., & Gill, M. A. (2003). A review of rivastigmine: A reversible cholinesterase inhibitor. *Clinical therapeutics, 25*(6), 1634–1653.

Winblad, B., Gauthier, S., Scinto, L., Feldman, H., Wilcock, G. K., Truyen, L., ... Nye, J. S.; GAL-INT-11/18 Study Group. (2008). Safety and efficacy of galantamine in subjects with mild cognitive impairment. *Neurology, 70*(22), 2024–2035.

CHAPTER 17

Nonpharmacological, Cognitive Interventions in Dementia

Lokesh Shahani and Chad A. Noggle

Dementia is defined as a neurodegenerative condition with progressive impairment of cognitive functioning in the absence of delirium. Dementia is chronic and causes widespread dysfunction in multiple neuropsychological domains. While cognitive symptoms vary across different types of dementia based on their underlying neuropathology, impairments in attention, memory, and comprehension predominate. Furthermore, psychological impairments and problems with mood, behavior, and anxiety are also commonly noted. With these multiple domains being affected, pharmacological interventions are often not effective alone. The current chapter briefly discusses the research on the efficacy of various cognitive and behavioral interventions aimed to improve the neuropsychological symptoms in patients with dementia.

DEMENTIA AND COGNITIVE RESERVE

Patients with dementia vary with regard to their presentation and progression. While there exists a difference related to the severity of neuropathology and the clinical presentation of the patients, it has been hypothesized and demonstrated that patients have a different capacity in coping with their disease. It has been further hypothesized that such differences exist because of the underlying "cerebral reserve" (Stern, 2003). A meta-analysis including more than 29,000 individuals showed that individuals with high cognitive reserve had a 46% reduced risk of developing dementia compared with individuals with low cognitive reserve. Of all the factors that influence cognitive reserve, mentally stimulating activities were shown to have the largest effect on dementia risk. The effect of cognitive reserve was sustained over a median longitudinal follow-up of 7 years (Valenzuela & Sachdev, 2006).

Cognitive reserve has been shown to be influenced by various premorbid factors. Education as a preventive or a risk-reducing factor for dementia is now well known. Various studies have replicated the inverse dose effect relation between the level of education and the risk of developing Alzheimer's dementia. Various studies have replicated the fact that the individuals with a higher level of education have a lower risk of developing the clinical symptoms despite having neuropathological presence of dementia (Letenneur et al., 1999).

Education has been hypothesized to increase the "cerebral reserve" and delay the onset of dementia. It has been shown to increase the synaptic density in the neocortex and offer more resistance to the progressive worsening of the neuronal function (Stern, Alexander, Prohovnik, & Mayeux, 1992). Education further enhances a person's environmental engagement as well as the engagement in mentally stimulating activity leading to an increase in the "cerebral reserve."

As cognitive reserve seems to have such a large effect on the risk of developing dementia, cognitive interventions have been hypothesized to attenuate cognitive decline in healthy elderly individuals and potentially delay the onset of dementia. The SIMA (Maintaining and Supporting Independent Living in Old Age) study demonstrated that a combination of memory and psychomotor training significantly improved cognitive status in healthy elderly people (75–89 years) after 1 year of training. This effect was stable for 5 years, and immediate and long-term transfer effects on nontrained cognitive functions were demonstrated (Oswald, Rupprecht, Gunzelmann, & Tritt, 1996). In addition, the ACTIVE (Advanced Cognitive Training for Independent and vital Elderly) study showed significant improvements in distinct cognitive functions—memory, reasoning, problem solving, and speed of processing—after receiving more than 2 years of cognitive intervention therapy (Ball et al., 2002). Eleven-month follow-up booster training sessions, which were administered to more than 60% of the study participants, successfully improved reasoning and speed of processing abilities. Improvements in these cognitive functions were stable for more than 5 years. In addition, the 5-year follow-up revealed that reasoning training resulted in a reduced decline in everyday functions (Willis et al., 2006). Studies examining the neurobiological basis of training programs indicate that training can alter brain function at the molecular and synaptic levels, as well as at the neural network level (Buonomano & Merzenich, 1998).

There is also considerable neurobiological evidence demonstrating the adaptability of the central nervous system, indicating structural reorganization (neuroplasticity), and certain degrees of functional recovery are possible following damage or pathology. Kleim and Jones (2008) described principles fundamental to experience-dependent neuroplasticity and their implications for rehabilitation following brain damage. These principles are applicable to individuals with dementia, as research on animals with pathology comparable with Alzheimer's disease (AD) has demonstrated that stimulating environments with increased opportunities for learning enhance cellular plasticity (Herring et al., 2009); reduce neuropathological hallmarks delaying memory deficits (Berardi, Braschi, Capsoni, Cattaneo, & Maffei, 2007); and counteract neurovascular dysfunction (Herring et al., 2008).

COGNITIVE TRAINING

Cognitive training refers to nonpharmacological interventions aimed to improve a patient's cognitive function and is specifically designed to improve the patient's functional capacity. Cognitive training generally includes a combination of cognitive stimulation, memory rehabilitation, reality orientation, and neuropsychological rehabilitation (Yu et al., 2009).

- Cognitive stimulation refers to nonregimental involvement in activities that require mental functioning and is less formally programmed than other kinds of cognitive training.

- Memory rehabilitation is based on the hypothesis that memory loss in AD results from defective encoding and storage of information rather than forgetting information.
- Reality orientation relates information such as person, place, and time to individuals with AD and can be done continually or as a classroom technique.
- Neuropsychological rehabilitation in AD aims to optimize functions, minimize excessive disability risk, and prevent the development of negative social psychology.

COGNITIVE STIMULATION

Cognitive stimulation therapies have been designed with a focus on optimizing cognitive function with a socially oriented outcome. These therapies are designed to be enjoyable for the patients and at the same time improve cognitive functioning through increased participation in daily activities, interpersonal relationships, and improving the overall quality of life. Reminiscence therapy, which involves discussion of the past activities or experiences with the use of cornet prompts, is an example of cognitive stimulation. Stimulation could be provided in an active or a passive manner. Active methods could involve discussion of a current event or solving a puzzle. Passive methods of stimulation could include involvement of audio or visual sensations such as listening to music or watching television (Yu et al., 2009).

A recent meta-analysis consisting of 718 subjects (407 receiving cognitive stimulation and 311 in control groups) evaluated the effectiveness of cognitive stimulation in dementia (Aguirre, Woods, Spector, & Orrell, 2013). Results demonstrated a significant benefit in cognitive function following treatment and the benefits appeared to be greater than any medication effects. This remained evident at follow-up up to 3 months after the end of treatment. In secondary analyses, with smaller total sample sizes, significant benefits were also noted for quality of life and well-being, and on staff ratings of communication and social interaction. Furthermore, a randomized clinical trial showed a positive result when cognitive stimulation was combined with pharmacological interventions as compared to pharmacological interventions alone (Chapman, Weiner, Rackley, Hynan, & Zientz, 2004). Compared with the medication-only group, participants in the combination group showed slower decline in Mini-Mental State Examination (MMSE) scores, less irritability, less apathy, and improved quality of life after completion of the training.

MEMORY REHABILITATION

As mentioned earlier, memory rehabilitation focuses on encoding information in areas of the brain that are less affected by the disease. In particular, it focuses on encoding information in areas of the brain that are less affected by AD. Memory rehabilitation training has three characteristics:

1. Specifically targets encoding of memory and recall.
2. Typically examines the effect of one training method per study.
3. Targets the location of active pathology and function of that area.

Some of the common techniques used in memory rehabilitation include explicit learning, errorless learning, errorful learning, implicit learning, and memory aids (Yu et al., 2009). Explicit learning is purposeful and occurs when people use rote memorization and verbally oriented learning in a conscious process to create a memory or learn a skill. Memory recovery training is another type of explicit learning. Patients are given didactic training and, with the help of imagery techniques and problem-solving techniques, they are helped to regain some of their skills for independent living (Liberati, Raffone, & Olivetti Belardinelli, 2012). Implicit memory is nonverbal and observational and may be accomplished during the course of an activity unrelated to what is being learned. It is considered to be automatic and is not performed on a conscious basis.

Errorless learning is a learning approach that avoids, or at least limits, errors during the acquisition phase of learning, thereby reducing the chances of reinforcement of incorrect information. The principle behind errorless learning is that when subjects are allowed to make mistakes during training, it might interfere with learning correct information. Hence, eliminating these mistakes and rehearsing correct information could help facilitate correct learning (Liberati et al., 2012).

Errorful learning, on the other hand, focuses on correcting mistakes made during the acquisition phase of learning. Memory aids include different devices such as an electronic memory aid (EMA), which is a device that uses an alarm system to alert the user to a message regarding an appointment or task to facilitate memory and learning (Yu et al., 2009).

A 2006 meta-analysis of studies evaluating cognitive training for early stage dementia between 1980 and 2004 supports the efficacy of cognitive training. Medium effect sizes were observed for learning, memory, executive functioning, activities of daily living (ADL), general cognitive problems, depression, and self-rated general functioning (Sitzer, Twamley, & Jeste, 2006). Results showed that a combination of cognitive training and medication showed better improvement in cognition in individuals with Alzheimer's dementia. Their MMSE scores increased from an average of 23.50 to 24.33 at the end of the 5-month study, while the medication-only group declined from 21.29 to 19.86 (Bottino et al., 2005).

Only a few neuroimaging studies have investigated the effects of cognitive training or cognitive stimulation in patients with dementia. One of the earliest PET studies of patients with mild AD reported that a combination of cognitive training and drug therapy was associated with increased brain glucose metabolism in temporal–parietal brain areas during a continuous visual recognition task. Furthermore, patients receiving combined cognitive and drug therapies showed increased glucose metabolism and improved cognitive performance compared with control groups receiving either drug or cognitive intervention alone (Heiss, Kessler, Mielke, Szelies, & Herholz, 1994). This study further adds to our knowledge of neuroplasticity, which is enhanced by cognitive training.

SENSORY STIMULATION

It has been hypothesized that the behavioral and psychological symptoms of dementia are related to the disease process; however, the environment also plays a part in further progression of the symptoms. At times patients could have excessive sensory simulation, which could worsen the behavioral problems. Kovach suggested the "sensoristasis" model, which states that older adults with dementia experience intrapsychic discomfort because of imbalances in the pacing of sensory-stimulating or sensory-calming activity. Consequences of this intrapsychic discomfort include agitated behaviors and episodic or premature decline in instrumental and social function. According to this model, interventions in people with dementia must facilitate optimum sensoristasis, that is, to achieve a balance between the sensory-stimulating and the sensory-calming activities (Kovach, 2000).

Agitation, which is defined as inappropriate verbal, vocal, or motor activity, can be caused by psychological, functional, interpersonal relation, and environmental factors. After pooling, the results of three studies ($n = 120$) evaluating the effect of sensory interventions suggested that there were statistically significant differences in agitation between treatment groups and control groups, indicating moderate beneficial effects of sensory interventions on agitation (Kong, Evans, & Guevara, 2009). The study further recommended that sensory interventions might be important practical interventions for agitation in older adults with dementia in terms of significant effect, ease of performance, low cost, and safety.

Multisensory stimulation environment (MSSE) has also been used as nonpharmacological therapy in people with dementia. This concept was developed initially in the Netherlands in 1970s and used effectively for patients with learning difficulties. It was known as "Snoezelen" and took place in a dusky, attractively lit room where soft music was heard; this provided an emphatic appeal to the senses that are stimulated individually (Hulsegge & Verheul, 2005). MSSE aims to stimulate the primary senses through pleasurable sensory experiences without the need for intellectual activity in an atmosphere of trust and relaxation. Stimuli used are nonsequential and unpatterned, experienced moment by moment without relying on short-term memory to link them to previous events (Sánchez, Millán-Calenti, Lorenzo-López, & Maseda, 2013). A review of 18 articles showed that MSSE provides immediate positive effects on the behavior and mood of people with dementia. However, there are no conclusive data about their long-term effectiveness. At the same time, effects on cognition communication, social interaction, and functional state were limited (Sánchez et al., 2013).

Occupational therapy (OT) for patients with dementia has been explored. Meta-analysis was conducted to examine the effects of OT interventions based on sensory stimulation, environmental modification, and functional task activity on the behavioral problems and depression of an individual with dementia. The analysis suggested that OT intervention based on sensory stimulation was an effective intervention to improve behavioral problems (Kim, Yoo, Jung, Park, & Park, 2012).

Music therapy and aromatherapy as forms of sensory stimulation have also been explored. Music therapy is defined by the World Federation of Music Therapy (WFMT, 2013) as "the use of music and/or its musical elements (sound, rhythm, melody and harmony) by a qualified music therapist, with a client or group, in a process designed to facilitate and promote communication, relationships, learning, mobilization, expression, organization and other relevant therapeutic objectives in order to meet physical, emotional, mental, social and cognitive needs." The results of a meta-analysis showed that music therapy influenced behavioral and psychological symptoms in patients with dementia. The effects of music therapy on anxiety symptoms were moderate, while the effects on depression and behavior were small. A long intervention period seemed to be somewhat more effective for anxiety symptoms (Ueda, Suzukamo, Sato, & Izumi, 2013).

Aromatherapy is a form of complementary and alternative medicine. A systemic review of 11 clinical trials showed that aromatherapy had a positive effect on improving cognitive functioning and reducing the frequencies of behavioral and psychological symptoms of dementia (BPSD) in patients with dementia. In addition, improvement in independence in ADL tasks, social functioning, and engagement was reported. Compared with antipsychotic medication, aromatherapy had a better influence on the quality of life of patients with dementia (Fung, Tsang, & Chung, 2012).

It has been recommended that the strongest interventions were multimodal in nature, using at least two different interventions to positively affect multiple outcomes. Community-based programs, as a form of combining interventions, have been proposed to be a possible intervention. They can take many forms, with some programs meeting once per week for approximately 4 to 5 hours and others meeting several days per week over a longer time frame. Health professionals with expertise in care of persons with early-stage dementia often lead such programs, because they have the clinical expertise and dedication to effectively offer continuous programs.

SUMMARY

Cognitive interventions have been shown to improve global cognitive functioning and abilities of daily living, reduce behavioral disturbances, and have positive effects on quality of life in patients with dementia. Neuroimaging results indicate that changes in attention underpin many of the improvements in cognitive performance. Admittedly, more research is needed along these lines, but such interventions are oftentimes not considered when designing treatment plans for patients with dementia. In comparison with the pharmacological treatments currently available for the treatment of Alzheimer's dementia, namely, cholinesterase inhibitors and memantine, nonpharmacological cognitive interventions are safer and associated with lower costs and higher cost-effectiveness; for these reasons, their increased use may be worthwhile.

REFERENCES

Aguirre, E., Woods, R. T., Spector, A., & Orrell, M. (2013). Cognitive stimulation for dementia: A systematic review of the evidence of effectiveness from randomised controlled trials. *Ageing Research Reviews, 12*(1), 253–262.

Ball, K., Berch, D. B., Helmers, K. F., Jobe, J. B., Leveck, M. D., Marsiske, M.,...Willis, S. L.; Advanced Cognitive Training for Independent and Vital Elderly Study Group. (2002). Effects of cognitive training interventions with older adults: A randomized controlled trial. *The Journal of the American Medical Association, 288*(18), 2271–2281.

Berardi, N., Braschi, C., Capsoni, S., Cattaneo, A., & Maffei, L. (2007). Environmental enrichment delays the onset of memory deficits and reduces neuropathological hallmarks in a mouse model of Alzheimer-like neurodegeneration. *Journal of Alzheimer's Disease, 11*(3), 359–370.

Bottino, C. M., Carvalho, I. A., Alvarez, A. M., Avila, R., Zukauskas, P. R., Bustamante, S.E.,... Câmargo, C. H. (2005). Cognitive rehabilitation combined with drug treatment in Alzheimer's disease patients: A pilot study. *Clinical Rehabilitation, 19*(8), 861–869.

Buonomano, D. V., & Merzenich, M. M. (1998). Cortical plasticity: from synapses to maps. *Annual Review of Neuroscience, 21*, 149–186.

Chapman, S. B., Weiner, M. F., Rackley, A., Hynan, L. S., & Zientz, J. (2004). Effects of cognitive-communication stimulation for Alzheimer's disease patients treated with donepezil. *Journal of Speech, Language, and Hearing Research, 47*(5), 1149–1163.

Fung, J. K., Tsang, H. W., & Chung, R. C. (2012). A systematic review of the use of aromatherapy in treatment of behavioral problems in dementia. *Geriatrics & Gerontology International, 12*(3), 372–382.

Heiss, W. D., Kessler, J., Mielke, R., Szelies, B., & Herholz, K. (1994). Long-term effects of phosphatidylserine, pyritinol, and cognitive training in Alzheimer's disease. A neuropsychological, EEG, and PET investigation. *Dementia, 5*(2), 88–98.

Herring, A., Ambrée, O., Tomm, M., Habermann, H., Sachser, N., Paulus, W., & Keyvani, K. (2009). Environmental enrichment enhances cellular plasticity in transgenic mice with Alzheimer-like pathology. *Experimental Neurology, 216*(1), 184–192.

Herring, A., Yasin, H., Ambrée, O., Sachser, N., Paulus, W., & Keyvani, K. (2008). Environmental enrichment counteracts Alzheimer's neurovascular dysfunction in TgCRND8 mice. *Brain Pathology, 18*(1), 32–39.

Hulsegge, J., & Verheul, A. (2005). *Snoezelen: Another world*. Chesterfield, UK: Rompa.

Kim, S. Y., Yoo, E. Y., Jung, M. Y., Park, S. H., & Park, J. H. (2012). A systematic review of the effects of occupational therapy for persons with dementia: A meta-analysis of randomized controlled trials. *NeuroRehabilitation, 31*(2), 107–115.

Kleim, J. A., & Jones, T. A. (2008). Principles of experience-dependent neural plasticity: Implications for rehabilitation after brain damage. *Journal of Speech, Language, and Hearing Research, 51*(1), S225–S239.

Kong, E. H., Evans, L. K., & Guevara, J. P. (2009). Nonpharmacological intervention for agitation in dementia: A systematic review and meta-analysis. *Aging & Mental Health, 13*(4), 512–520.

Kovach, C. R. (2000). Sensoristasis and imbalance in persons with dementia. *Journal of Nursing Scholarship, 32*(4), 379–384.

Letenneur, L., Gilleron, V., Commenges, D., Helmer, C., Orgogozo, J. M., & Dartigues, J. F. (1999). Are sex and educational level independent predictors of dementia and Alzheimer's disease? Incidence data from the PAQUID project. *Journal of Neurology, Neurosurgery, and Psychiatry, 66*(2), 177–183.

Liberati, G., Raffone, A., & Olivetti Belardinelli, M. (2012). Cognitive reserve and its implications for rehabilitation and Alzheimer's disease. *Cognitive Processing, 13*(1), 1–12.

Oswald, W. D., Rupprecht, R., Gunzelmann, T., & Tritt, K. (1996). The SIMA-project: Effects of 1 year cognitive and psychomotor training on cognitive abilities of the elderly. *Behavioural Brain Research, 78*(1), 67–72.

Sánchez, A., Millán-Calenti, J. C., Lorenzo-López, L., & Maseda, A. (2013). Multisensory stimulation for people with dementia: A review of the literature. *American Journal of Alzheimer's Disease and Other Dementias, 28*(1), 7–14.

Sitzer, D. I., Twamley, E. W., & Jeste, D. V. (2006). Cognitive training in Alzheimer's disease: A meta-analysis of the literature. *Acta Psychiatrica Scandinavica, 114*(2), 75–90.

Stern, Y. (2003). The concept of cognitive reserve: A catalyst for research. *Journal of Clinical and Experimental Neuropsychology, 25*(5), 589–593.

Stern, Y., Alexander, G. E., Prohovnik, I., & Mayeux, R. (1992). Inverse relationship between education and parietotemporal perfusion deficit in Alzheimer's disease. *Annals of Neurology, 32*(3), 371–375.

Ueda, T., Suzukamo, Y., Sato, M., & Izumi, S. (2013). Effects of music therapy on behavioral and psychological symptoms of dementia: A systematic review and meta-analysis. *Ageing Research Reviews, 12*(2), 628–641.

Valenzuela, M. J., & Sachdev, P. (2006). Brain reserve and dementia: A systematic review. *Psychological Medicine, 36*(4), 441–454.

Willis, S. L., Tennstedt, S. L., Marsiske, M., Ball, K., Elias, J., Koepke, K. M., . . . Wright, E.; ACTIVE Study Group. (2006). Long-term effects of cognitive training on everyday functional outcomes in older adults. *The Journal of the American Medical Association, 296*(23), 2805–2814.

World Federation of Music Therapy (WFMT). (2013). Retrieved December 2013 from http://www.musictherapyworld.net/WFMT/FAQMusic Therapy.html

Yu, F., Rose, K. M., Burgener, S. C., Cunningham, C., Buettner, L. L., Beattie, E., . . . McKenzie, S. E. (2009). Cognitive training for early-stage Alzheimer's disease and dementia. *Journal of Gerontological Nursing, 35*(3), 23–29.

CHAPTER 18

The Role of Caregivers in the Treatment of Patients With Dementia

Geoffrey Tremont and Jennifer Duncan Davis

Alzheimer's disease (AD) and related cortical dementias are a major health problem. There are currently 5.3 million people with AD in the United States. With the aging of the baby-boomer generation, it is estimated that 7.7 million people will be affected by 2030. Approximately 65% to 75% of dementia patients are cared for at home by family members, including both spouses and adult children (Aneshensel, Pearlin, Mullan, Zarit, & Whitlach, 1995). About 10.9 million Americans provide unpaid care for persons with dementia, totaling 12.5 billion hours of care per year, which is valued at almost $144 million. Over the course of the illness, the individual requires comprehensive care that includes family members, professional caregivers, and interactions with multiple aspects of the health care system. Patients with AD and related dementia have more hospital stays, have more skilled nursing home stays, and utilize more home health care visits compared to older adults without dementia. In fact, nearly half of all individuals older than 65 years admitted to nursing homes have dementia (Alzheimer's Association, 2009). The emotional burden of providing care crosses all of these roles, and can have wide-ranging effects on families and professionals alike.

This chapter will discuss the role of family caregivers and how they interact with in-home assistance, day care, assisted living, and nursing homes in the care of an individual with dementia. Special attention will be given to the family, psychological, and physical/medical effects of dementia caregiving, which can begin with symptom onset and persist into the grieving process following the care recipient's death. We will discuss important transitions in the trajectory of dementia care, including diagnosis, treatment decision making, home and day care issues, long-term care placement, and death. We will highlight the importance of caregiver assessment, education, and intervention as part of the care process.

THEORETICAL MODEL OF CAREGIVER STRESS

Dementia caregiving often serves as the model for studying the effects of chronic stress on an individual's mental and physical health. The most common theoretical model applied to stress experienced by dementia caregivers is Lazarus and Folkman's transactional stress and coping model (see Figure 18.1; Lazarus & Folkman, 1984).

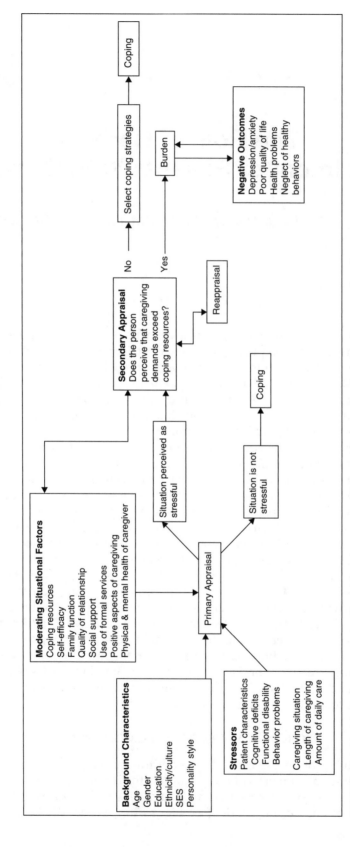

FIGURE 18.1 Model of caregiver stress adapted from Lazarus and Folkman's transactional model of stress and coping.

This model posits that situations or experiences are not inherently stressful but are experienced as stressful after a two-stage appraisal process by the individual. Initial appraisals are influenced by background, past experiences, culture/ethnicity, and personality. Secondary appraisals involve deciding whether an individual is capable of managing the stress and selection of a coping strategy. This secondary process is more situation dependent than the initial appraisal and is generally the target of interventions. Among dementia caregivers, there is evidence that active coping strategies (e.g., seeking education about the disease, seeking family and other social support) lead to lower levels of distress than avoidant coping (e.g., denying the stressor). In a nursing home situation, the model of stressors is very similar except for the addition of nursing home–specific stressors. These could include communication and interaction with the staff and dissatisfaction with placement. The transactional stress and coping framework and related models have been used to study the impact of situational factors, background characteristics, and stressors on negative caregiver outcomes across caregiver transitions.

DIAGNOSIS

AD and related dementias typically begin later in life and involve a long, relentless decline over about 7 to 10 years. Over the course of the illness, there are many transitions that the patient and family member experience. Family caregivers must manage, adjust, and cope with declining cognition and function, changing demands, and unexpected problem behaviors. Although by definition the course of AD and related dementias is gradual, the rate and specific symptoms are often unpredictable.

Typically, family members are the first to notice a change in cognition and memory and often have to prompt the family member to seek medical advice. This can be stressful given the high frequency of anosognosia (i.e., lack of awareness of cognitive decline) and psychological denial in dementia. Up to 80% of individuals with dementia will experience some degree of reduced insight into their cognitive or functional changes (Reed, Jagust, & Coulter, 1993). There also may be a tendency on the part of the patient to minimize, try to normalize, or even cover up his or her problems (Keady, Nolan, & Gilliard, 1995). There may be disagreement among family members about the seriousness of the problem and whether the cognitive change reflects normal aging or some other benign or reversible explanation (e.g., medication effects). Once the individual receives the diagnosis, there may be issues related to accepting the diagnosis and limitations, dealing with stigma, and assuming new responsibilities and role changes (Robinson, Clare, & Evans, 2005). There is evidence, however, that early diagnosis can be beneficial for patients and caregivers to adjust and make sense of their memory loss and to anticipate their future needs (Robinson et al., 2005). Many family members express concern about disclosing the diagnosis to the person with dementia, and there is evidence that individuals who receive the specific diagnosis of AD experience shock and distress (Aminzadeh, Byszewski, Molnar, & Eisner, 2007; Bamford et al., 2004). Interestingly, there is less of a negative emotional reaction to the diagnosis of vascular dementia (VaD), suggesting that the Alzheimer's term is emotionally charged. Interactions among the patient, caregiver, and physician (often referred to as the triad of care) can be stressful, and there are reports of lack of communication and poor understanding about diagnosis, prognosis, treatment decision making, and home care (Beisecker, Chrisman, & Wright, 1997). Caregivers also report a very negative emotional response to receiving a diagnosis of dementia from a physician, whereas physicians tend to believe that diagnostic discussions are well received by family members (Connell, Boise, Stuckey,

Holmes, & Hudson, 2004). Regardless, it is generally accepted that disclosure of the diagnosis to the patient and caregiver is appropriate as long as it is done in a supportive manner.

At the time of diagnosis, it is important that the caregiver has a good understanding of the disease, prognosis, and treatment options. In our current health care model, time with the family is often limited, and care providers must prioritize the information to be discussed. Caregivers consistently express the need for more education about the disease and how to handle the symptoms (Lussignoli et al., 2010). In a survey of memory clinic and community mental health informal caregivers, the most commonly sought information at the time of diagnosis included a definition of dementia, medication treatments available, the common symptoms of dementia, information about services, the course of the illness, and ways to handle crisis situations (Wald, Fahy, Walker, & Livingston, 2003). Education appears to be an important component of the diagnostic process as higher levels of caregiver knowledge about AD are associated with lower levels of depression and greater confidence in their ability to provide care (Graham, Ballard, & Sham, 1997). A good opportunity to provide education and dispel incorrect beliefs about the disease is when meeting with the patient and family to review test results and to present the diagnosis. Table 18.1 presents important topics to be discussed at the time of diagnosis. In addition to being information seeking, caregivers often have misinformation that should be addressed. There also may be important cultural and ethnic differences in caregivers' knowledge and attitudes about AD. For example, Chinese and Hispanic caregivers were more likely than White caregivers to believe that AD is a normal part of aging and can be diagnosed with a blood test (Gray, Jimenez, Cucciare, Tong, & Gallagher-Thompson, 2009).

After receiving the diagnosis, both the patient and caregiver/family members will likely experience feelings of loss. For example, early-stage dementia is associated with a high frequency of depression, which in part may be related to coping with memory loss and other changes (Craig, Mirakhur, Hart, McIlroy, & Passmore, 2005). Caregivers and family can also experience stress and burden even in individuals who may be in the very earliest stages of the illness and diagnosed with mild cognitive impairment (MCI; Bruce, McQuiggan, Williams, Westervelt, & Tremont, 2008). Many of these experiences following a diagnosis of dementia mimic those following death of a loved one. Therefore, family members (especially spouses) may enter a period of grief following the diagnosis. This process may be more complicated than grief associated with death of a loved one given the continued presence of the patient and occasional behaviors that remind the caregiver of his or her former self.

There may be a subset of individuals who take a longer period to receive an accurate diagnosis because of complicating factors. This may be particularly common for the non-Alzheimer's dementias. For example, 50% of Lewy body dementia (LBD) patients saw more than three doctors and more than 10 visits over 1 year to

TABLE 18.1 Key Educational Points for Families at the Time of Diagnosis

• Definition of Alzheimer's disease versus dementia
• Alzheimer's disease and related dementias versus normal aging
• Genetic risk for Alzheimer's disease
• Medications available
• Cognitive and behavioral symptoms of dementia
• Prognosis and staging of the disease
• Support resources
• Effects on caregivers

receive an accurate diagnosis (Galvin et al., 2010). In these situations, the diagnosis may serve as more of a relief than a shock.

TREATMENT DECISIONS

Once an MCI or dementia diagnosis is made, the patient and family members need to make decisions about treatment and management of the condition. Education about the disease and limitations of the current treatment regimen is extremely important, so that patients and their family members can make informed decisions. There is evidence that caregivers lack knowledge about symptoms, treatment, and services, especially spouses and those with low educational levels (Werner, 2001). Caregivers may also play a major role in selecting treatments for their care recipients. Studies suggest that the likelihood that individuals with dementia take and remain on cholinesterase inhibitors is significantly associated with caregivers' willingness to accept greater numbers of side effects (Oremus, Wolfson, Vandal, Bergman, & Xie, 2007). Invariably, patients and family members ask about nonpharmacological strategies such as lifestyle changes, including diet, exercise, and mental stimulation. There is increasing evidence that exercise (Baker et al., 2010); diet (particularly the Mediterranean diet; Scarmeas et al., 2009); and cognitive activity (Wilson et al., 2010) can slow cognitive decline in MCI and AD, but the practitioner must use caution when describing any potential benefits of these strategies so as not to give the impression that these strategies can entirely prevent decline. Rather, the practitioner should encourage lifestyle changes to reduce risk of decline, enhance current functioning, and improve quality of life. Lifestyle changes may also be presented as complementary therapies to traditional treatment with a cholinesterase inhibitor or similar cognitive-enhancing medication (e.g., memantine).

FAMILY CAREGIVER BURDEN

As stated previously, the majority of dementia care is provided at home by family members who are unpaid. As the primary caregivers, family members may experience the greatest levels of distress. In the literature, the emotional experience endured by dementia caregivers is referred to as caregiver burden, which includes both the objective and subjective components of providing care. Examples of the objective aspects of burden involve the time needed for care, physical demands of caregiving aspects of providing care, and financial costs of caregiving, whereas subjective experience of caregiving encompasses the perceptions and emotional reactions to caregiving. The most commonly used measure of dementia caregiver burden is the Zarit Burden Interview (Zarit, Reever, & Bach-Peterson, 1980). The measure contains 22 items that address perceived burden. Factor analysis of the scale demonstrated its multidimensionality, measuring the social and personal aspects of caregiving (e.g., Do you feel that your social life has suffered because you are caring for your relative?); psychological burden (e.g., Do you feel angry when you are around your relative?); and guilt (e.g., Do you feel you should be doing more for your relative?) (Ankri, Andrieu, Beaufils, Grand, & Henrard, 2005). Given that burden is a multifactorial measure of distress, it is not surprising that there are strong correlations between caregiver burden and depression. However, burden and depression do not necessarily represent the same construct (Epstein-Lubow, Davis, Miller, & Tremont, 2008).

Psychological Consequences

Dementia caregivers are at risk of a variety of negative mental health consequences. There is evidence that providing care for an individual with dementia is more stressful than caring for a physically impaired older adult (Ory, Hoffman, Yee, Tennstedt, & Schulz, 1999). It appears that caregivers of non-demented older adults experience similar levels of stress and subjective well-being and physical health as their dementia caregiver counterparts, although they do not report high levels of depression and low self-efficacy seen in dementia caregivers (Pinquart & Sörensen, 2003b). High levels of depression and anxiety are common in dementia caregivers, with about one third of individuals meeting diagnostic criteria for depression (Schulz & Martire, 2004). Correlates of depression and other aspects of distress in caregivers include care recipient behavior problems, severity of cognitive and functional impairment, more hours providing care, greater number of caregiving tasks, and longer duration of caregiving (Davis & Tremont, 2007; Pinquart & Sörensen, 2003a). Greater burden and depression are associated with being a spouse, older, female, and having low levels of social support (Pinquart & Sörensen, 2003b). There continues to be some uncertainty whether long-term caregiving leads to increased risk of problems or some degree of adaptation. Recent findings suggest that persisting high levels of burden are associated with a subsequent increase in depressive symptoms (Epstein-Lubow et al., 2008).

Another important moderating variable for dementia caregiver distress is self-efficacy. Self-efficacy is an individual's belief in his or her ability to perform tasks and to accumulate the necessary motivation, cognitive resources, and course of action required to meet the demands of a difficult situation (Bandura, 1997). Several authors have operationalized the construct into many dimensions. For example, Fortinsky, Kercher, and Burant (2002) identified self-efficacy for symptom management and community support service use, whereas Steffen, McKibbin, Zeiss, Gallagher-Thompson, and Bandura (2002) posited three self-efficacy domains: asking for help, responding to disruptive behaviors, and controlling upsetting thoughts. There are inconsistent findings whether self-efficacy for managing behavior problems serves as a moderator between stress (i.e., patient behavior problems) and emotional distress in caregivers. Interestingly, recent work suggests that high self-efficacy for controlling upsetting thoughts about caregiving may protect caregivers from depression even if they report significant burden (Romero-Moreno et al., 2011).

As evident from the previous discussion, the variables that account for the distress in dementia caregivers are multifactorial and complex. Recent evidence suggests that perceptions of patient suffering are predictive of caregiver depression and antidepressant use, independent of patient characteristics, patient behavior problems, and the amount of time caring for the patient (Schulz et al., 2008). Similarly, there is evidence that noncaregiving family members of persons with dementia experience levels of distress commensurate with their caregiving family members, bringing into question the argument that distress is directly tied to the caregiving experience (Amirkhanyan & Wolf, 2003).

Medical and Physical Effects

In addition to emotional and psychiatric consequences, dementia caregivers are at risk of physical health problems. It is proposed that chronic stress associated with dementia caregiving may negatively impact immunological and hormonal functioning, thereby increasing susceptibility to illness. There are consistent findings showing that dementia caregivers have poor perceived health (Pinquart & Sörensen, 2003b; Vitaliano, Zhang, & Scanlan, 2003). Dementia caregivers also tend to neglect their own health, such as not getting enough sleep and having poor nutrition, which places them at heightened risk of illness (Vitaliano et al., 2003). Meta-analytic studies suggest that behavior problems and cognitive impairment in the care recipient, longer duration of caregiving, low socioeconomic status (SES) and education, receipt of less informal support, older age, not being a spouse, coresidence with the care recipient, and high levels of depression/burden are predictors of poor health among dementia caregivers (Pinquart & Sörensen, 2007). In general, female caregivers and minority caregivers report poorer health than male caregivers and Caucasian caregivers (Pinquart & Sörensen, 2005).

Several studies demonstrate that dementia caregivers are at higher risk of developing chronic medical conditions, such as hypertension, hyperlipidemia, cardiovascular disorders, diabetes, and infectious diseases, compared to noncaregiving controls (Kolanowski, Fick, Waller, & Shea, 2004; Lee, Colditz, Berkman, & Kawachi, 2003; Vitaliano et al., 2002). Dementia caregivers also show evidence of poor immune responses. For example, dementia caregivers failed to show the expected increase in antibody titers compared to noncaregiving controls following influenza vaccination (Kiecolt-Glaser, Glaser, Gravenstein, Malarkey, & Sheridan, 1996). Similarly, spousal caregivers who report more ruminative and intrusive thoughts had smaller antibody response following influenza vaccination compared to caregivers with fewer negative thoughts (Segerstrom, Schipper, & Greenberg, 2008). These studies suggest that chronic stress associated with caregiving can place these individuals at increased risk of developing infectious illnesses. In addition to poor vaccination response, dementia caregivers exhibit high levels of proinflammatory cytokine interleukin-6 (IL-6), which is associated with increased risk of chronic disease (Kiecolt-Glaser et al., 2003). New research reveals that dementia caregivers show evidence of increased cellular aging compared to noncaregiving controls, as measured by telomere length (Damjanovic et al., 2007). Overall, there is convincing evidence that the chronic stress associated with caring for someone with dementia has physiological consequences on the caregiver.

Some of the most interesting findings on the health effects of dementia caregiving come from large, longitudinal epidemiological studies. Schulz and Beach (1999) showed that caregiving was an independent risk factor for mortality, with caregivers experiencing a 63% increase in risk of death over 4 years compared to noncaregivers. Similarly, spousal caregivers of individuals with dementia had a high mortality rate (8.6% for husbands and 5.0% for wives) within 1 year after hospitalization of their spouse, which for husbands was higher than that in any other condition and higher for most conditions for women (Christakis & Allison, 2006). The authors hypothesize that the more that the care recipient's disease interfered with mental or physical abilities, the greater the risk of spousal death. Finally, recent epidemiological data show a sixfold increased risk of dementia in spousal dementia caregivers compared to noncaregivers (Norton et al., 2010). Husbands had a significantly greater risk than wives. Taken together, these findings argue for the importance of attending to family caregivers' needs during the course of care of an individual with dementia.

Family Effects

Serving as a caregiver for someone with dementia can have significant effects on the family system. These effects are not necessarily only negative. There is evidence that family members can feel empathy and respect for caregivers along with the spillover effects of caregiver stress (Szinovacz, 2003). Caregivers with family dysfunction are more likely to be anxious, depressed, have higher levels of caregiver burden, and have been caring for individuals with a longer dementia duration than those caregivers with no family dysfunction (Tremont, Davis, & Bishop, 2006). In addition, better-quality relationships between family caregivers and care recipients are associated with lower patient depression and caregiver burden (Ball et al., 2010). Similarly, unsatisfying predementia relationships are associated with greater reactivity to memory and behavior problems and less burden compared to individuals with satisfying pre-dementia relationships (Steadman, Tremont, & Davis, 2007).

Several studies have addressed the concept of expressed emotion (EE) in dementia caregivers. EE is described as the amount of criticism and emotional over-involvement expressed by the family members toward the patient. Among dementia caregivers, the percentage of caregivers exhibiting high EE ranges from 17% to 58%, depending on the type of caregiver studied (e.g., spouse, adult child) and severity of caregiver depression (Wagner, Logsdon, Pearson, & Teri, 1997). Dementia caregivers who are high in EE have an increased likelihood of a depression diagnosis, report greater burden, and describe fewer positive benefits from caregiving than caregivers low in EE (Wagner et al., 1997). In one study, 53% of dementia caregivers acknowledged some form of abuse of their care recipient (verbal, physical, or neglect) and EE was highly correlated with all forms of abuse (Cooney, Howard, & Lawlor, 2006). Overall, it is important to not only assess the caregiver, but also to attend to the family system. This will be important at each transition of the dementia illness.

Early-Onset AD and Other Cortical Dementias

AD is most common in individuals older than 65 years, and the incidence of the disease increases with advancing age. However, about 10% of AD cases can occur in younger individuals. This can present a unique and challenging situation for patients and their caregivers. For example, these individuals may have young children living in the home or be in the midst of developing their careers. There is evidence that caregivers of early-onset AD patients experience more burden than caregivers of late-onset dementia patients (Freyne, Kidd, Coen, & Lawlor, 1999). There can also be issues in accessing services and resources, which are typically designated for older adults. In addition to early-onset AD, other less common forms of cortical dementia have specific caregiver issues associated with them. Given the strong relationship between care recipient behavior problems and caregiver distress, it is no surprise that caregivers of individuals with frontotemporal dementia (FTD; a condition characterized by behavioral abnormalities) report higher levels of distress than caregivers of individuals with AD (De Vugt et al., 2006). For FTD caregivers, the greatest source of distress is psychosis and agitation; compared to AD caregivers, they tend to be dissatisfied with information about the disease and counseling/support they receive (Mourik et al., 2004; Rosness, Haugen, & Engedal, 2008). Individuals with FTD may encounter similar problems as those faced by families with early-onset AD, because the mean age of onset of FTD is in the 50s. Early behavior problems specific to LBD (e.g., hallucinations, delusions, sleep disturbance) are strongly related to caregiver strain (Leggett, Zarit, Taylor, & Galvin, 2011). Overall, early-onset AD and non-Alzheimer's dementias are associated with unique challenges, and these caregivers need detailed information about the disease as well as tailored interventions to assist with coping.

Positive Aspects of Caregiving

Most research focuses on the negative consequences of dementia caregiving. However, there has been recent attention paid to the positive aspects of providing care. Not all caregivers experience distress and burden, especially very early in the caregiving process (Hirst, 2005). Length of caregiving may result in stability or decreases in burden and may increase time to nursing home placement, suggesting adaptation to the caregiving role (Gaugler, Kane, Kane, & Newcomer, 2005b). Many caregivers report some degree of satisfaction with providing care, including feeling needed and useful, feeling good about oneself, learning new skills, developing a positive attitude and appreciation for life, and strengthening relationships with others (Tarlow et al., 2004). Positive aspects of caregiving are inversely related to burden and depression and have the potential to buffer against negative consequences of caregiving (Hilgeman, Allen, DeCoster, & Burgio, 2007). Caregiver personality characteristics such as extroversion and agreeableness along with social support (especially from one's spouse/partner) are associated with higher reports of positive aspects of caregiving (Silverberg Koerner, Baete Kenyon, & Shirai, 2009). Caregiver resilience, defined as lower levels of perceived burden in the face of high care demands, is associated with less-frequent institutionalization (Gaugler, Kane, & Newcomer, 2007). When working with caregivers, it can be extremely beneficial to assist them in recognizing and acknowledging the benefits they gain from providing care. Table 18.2 provides some useful questions for eliciting positive aspects of care. There are also questionnaires available that measure positive aspects of caregiving.

Community Resource Use in Dementia Caregivers

Caregivers face increasing political, social, and financial pressures to maintain the care recipient in the home rather than place the individual in long-term care. There are a variety of community-based resources to assist dementia caregivers. Many of these are considered respite services, such as in-home care, support services, adult day care centers, and temporary institutional placement. Caregivers can become easily overwhelmed with the task of identifying and accessing these resources, determining eligibility for the service, and arranging for the service. There is even a suggestion that formal services may produce stress rather than reduce it (Ducharme et al., 2007). Although some limited services may be available through state agencies, health charity associations, and private insurance, many programs involve a cost, thereby limiting access. Dementia caregivers tend to be resistant to accessing services and may connect with services late in the caregiving process (Gottlieb & Johnson, 2000). Most of the limited research on the impact of respite service use on caregiver

TABLE 18.2 Prompts for Eliciting Positive Aspects of Caregiving

Does caregiving for your loved one:
 Make you feel more useful?
 Make you feel good about yourself?
 Make you feel important?
 Make you feel strong and confident?
 Enable you to develop a more positive attitude toward life?
 Give more meaning to your life?
 Enable you to learn new skills?
 Enable you to appreciate life?
 Strengthen your relationship with others?

burden and distress shows high levels of satisfaction with the services, but there are mixed findings about benefits in terms of caregiver burden (Sussman & Regehr, 2009). The inconsistent findings may be related to when caregivers use services and which services they select. There is evidence that caregivers who use in-home care early in the caregiving process are more likely to delay institutionalization; in addition, more consistent and frequent use of these services is associated with reduced stress, role overload, and caregiver depression (Gaugler, Kane, Kane, & Newcomer, 2005a; Gaugler, Zarit, Townsend, Stephens, & Greene, 2003). Recent work also suggests that day care may be particularly helpful in reducing caregiver burden, possibly because it provides respite for the caregiver and opportunities for social interaction for the care recipient (Sussman & Regehr, 2009). Many caregivers remain dissatisfied with their use of time during respite, so careful planning of desired activities is important (Lund, Utz, Caserta, & Wright, 2008). As is seen in caregiving intervention research, use of multiple services (e.g., day care, support group, in-home care) that are tailored for the specific needs of the caregiver may have the greatest impact (Gaugler, Kane, & Newcomer, 2007). Overall, caregivers need to access multiple community resources early in their caregiving careers to potentially reduce stress and to have long-term effects on the caregiving process.

LONG-TERM CARE PLACEMENT

Primary caregivers are typically integral in making the decision to place the care recipient into long-term care. Currently, assisted-living and nursing home facilities are options for long-term placement of individuals with dementia. Assisted-living residences are the fastest growing residential care option for older adults who are not yet in need of full nursing home care. Many facilities offer levels of support within the same facility, offering a range of independent living through nursing home care. This is a nice benefit for caregivers and other family members as they anticipate needing increasing levels of care with dementia progression. The placement rate for individuals with AD is estimated to be 33% at 2 years postdiagnosis and 75% at 7 years postdiagnosis, with an average time from diagnosis to placement ranging from 2 to 6 years (Smith, O'Brien, Ivnik, Kokmen, & Tangalos, 2001). There are important ethnic differences in time from diagnosis until placement. For example, Caucasians tend to place earlier when compared to Latino caregivers (Mausbach et al., 2004).

Despite the fact that nursing home placement is a common event in that it occurs in the natural trajectory of AD, the decision to place is unplanned for many caregivers. One of the most frequent reasons for placement is a serious health event resulting in an unexpected placement in a hospital stay or rehabilitation facility. The majority of other caregivers seek placement when they have exceeded their emotional resources for caregiving, and this appears strongly linked to disease progression and persistent behavioral problems (Gaugler et al., 2010). Caregivers' desire to institutionalize is closely related to their emotional burden, more knowledge about dementia, greater family dysfunction, and decreased social support compared to caregivers expressing minimal desire for placement (Spitznagel, Tremont, Davis, & Foster, 2006). Typically, placement occurs about 3 months after the caregiver begins investigating placement options (McLennon, Habermann, & Davis, 2010). For those planned admissions, the most consistently identified predictors of nursing home placement of individuals with dementia are severity of cognitive impairment; dependency in basic daily activities (i.e., toileting, bathing); behavioral symptoms; and depression. Caregiver variables are also important to consider. Caregivers experiencing higher levels of emotional distress and feeling trapped in their care responsibilities are most likely to place their care recipient (Gaugler, Yu, Krichbaum, & Wyman, 2009). Interestingly, risk of nursing home placement increased significantly with the number of days of adult day care attendance, above and beyond the effects of burden and disease severity, suggesting that the relationship between respite service use and tendency to institutionalize is complex (McCann et al., 2005). There is some evidence that supportive counseling for caregivers while they are providing care at home may actually delay nursing home placement by a little more than 1 year when compared to caregivers receiving usual care (Mittelman, Haley, Clay, & Roth, 2006). It should be emphasized, however, that nursing home placement should not be considered a negative outcome or event, as placement is often necessary for meeting the needs of the family and care recipient. Rather, it is important for professionals who are working with caregivers to be aware of the factors that may be associated with premature or inappropriate placement.

NURSING HOME: FAMILY CAREGIVER BURDEN

Following nursing home placement, the majority of caregivers do not abandon their family member to the care of others. Rather, most caregivers continue to be actively involved in their care. Caregivers tend to perform similar tasks of daily care that they carried out when their family member was living at home, including basic activities of daily living (ADL), managing finances, completing small errands, transportation to appointments, and other activities. Most caregivers also continue to visit routinely, with more than half of spouses visiting daily (Schulz et al., 2004). While family members can play an essential role in caregiving, and regular visitation has been associated with increased staff satisfaction (Karner, Montgomery, Dobbs, & Wittmaier, 1998), striking a balance between the care provided by the family and the nursing home staff is a unique challenge that can cause stress among both family caregivers and staff.

Immediately following nursing home placement, many caregivers experience a sense of relief (Zarit & Whitlatch, 1992), but longitudinal studies suggest that this sense of relief is replaced with new stresses and challenges associated with nursing home placement (Gaugler, Kane, Kane, Clay, & Newcomer, 2005; Gaugler, Pot, & Zarit, 2007; Gaugler, Roth, Haley, & Mittelman, 2008). In fact, levels of depression and anxiety have been reported to be comparable to preplacement levels in longitudinal studies (Schulz et al., 2004) and cross-sectional studies comparing nursing home caregivers to home caregivers (Bowman, Mukherjee, & Fortinsky, 1998). Furthermore, family nursing home caregivers report poorer health and higher burden levels compared to family members of dementia patients in residential care or assisted-living centers (Port et al., 2005). The effect of stress and depression subsequently affects the physical health of caregivers. For example, health and well-being of family caregivers failed to improve even 2 years after placement (Lieberman & Fisher, 2001). In a longitudinal study of caregiver adaptation, Gaugler, Pot, and Zarit (2007) evaluated caregivers 1 to 4 years following placement. As a group, caregivers adapted to nursing home placement, reporting lower stress levels and negative mood. However, there was significant variability in many outcomes, particularly at 3 and 4 years post-placement, suggesting that a subset of caregivers is at risk of negative mental health outcomes.

Persistent burden and depressive symptoms following placement are likely related to multiple factors, including the practicalities of visitation, readjusting their expectations about care, relinquishing control over aspects of their family members' care, and taking on new responsibilities in care coordination and monitoring.

On average, dementia caregivers will have provided home care for 5 years prior to placement, and at the time of placement they may view themselves as experts in their family member's care. Turning over care to professionals and balancing expectations of care between the family and staff are challenging and a source of stress. Caregivers report difficulty relinquishing caregiving duties to the staff, being highly critical of staff, and frustration about not being involved in care decisions. Consequently, successful renegotiation of their role following placement is vital to healthy adaptation (Gaugler et al., 2005b). In fact, the quality of the family–staff relationship is associated with caregiver depression (Chen, Sabir, Zimmerman, Suitor, & Pillemer, 2007; Whitlatch, Schur, Noelker, Ejaz, & Looman, 2001) and burnout (Almberg, Grafström, Krichbaum, & Winblad, 2000).

In addition to role adjustment, cultural and personal expectations about the acceptability of institutionalization may contribute to the continued high level of depressive symptoms. Many dementia caregivers report significant emotional conflict related to guilt about the decision to place (Bern-Klug, 2008; Garity, 2006; Nolan & Dellasega, 1999, 2000; Ryan & Scullion, 2000; Zarit & Whitlatch, 1992). In particular, caregivers describe guilt related to breaking a promise or direct betrayal of a loved one's wishes, as well as guilt about not being able to continue fulfilling their duty to provide care. In fact, guilt around the placement decision has been shown to directly affect caregivers' coping with the burden of post–nursing home placement (Garity, 2006). Caregivers also report perceived failure as a caregiver, and concern about worsening cognitive and behavioral problems in their family member, financial challenges, and family conflict about the family member's care (Garity, 2006) as significant post-placement stressors.

Given the variability of caregiver health outcomes and the multiple factors associated with depression and anxiety in caregivers following placement, it is important to identify those caregivers who are at increased risk of poor adjustment. Postplacement stress appears particularly heightened for spouses, caregivers who visit more frequently, caregivers with poor social support networks, and caregivers who are less satisfied with the help they receive from others (Schulz et al., 2004). Similarly, older caregiver age, poor physical health, and low income are significant predictors of caregiver depression following placement, regardless of whether the individual has a diagnosis of dementia; burden is even greater if the person has cognitive impairment (Majerovitz, 2007). As would be expected, preplacement levels of depression and burden appear to be risk factors for poor adjustment (Gaugler, Mittelman, Hepburn, & Newcomer, 2009).

NURSING HOME: PROFESSIONAL CAREGIVER BURDEN

Professional caregivers (i.e., nurses, certified nursing aides, etc.) may experience the same burden and emotional difficulties as family caregivers, but to a lesser extent (Takahashi, Tanaka, & Miyoaka, 2010). Similar to family caregivers, professional caregivers are faced with managing many of the challenging behaviors and functional dependence associated with advanced dementia. The professional group reporting the highest level of burnout, depressive symptoms, and reduced quality of life is certified nursing assistants (CNAs) compared to registered nurses (RNs) and licensed practical nurses (LPNs; Aström, Nilsson, Norberg, & Winblad, 1990). This is not surprising, given that the majority of day-to-day care for persons with dementia is provided by CNAs, and these workers typically work long hours and receive low pay and minimal benefits for their work. Furthermore, this is the group with whom family members are typically interacting, placing both groups at high risk of conflict and stressful interactions. In a state-wide survey examining turn-over and job satisfaction among CNAs, CNA turnover was linked to job satisfaction and 40% of the respondents were either neutral or dissatisfied with their position. Respondents were most satisfied with their closeness to residents and their effect on residents' care, and dissatisfied with limited decision making, pay, and employee benefits. The CNAs identified their relationship with the residents and coworkers as the most important work issue. Even residents' physical assaults or disruptive behavior were not seen negatively. Conceptually, the experience of professional caregivers is not so dissimilar from the experience of the family caregiver who also may experience lost income and may feel unappreciated for his or her efforts by other family members and medical professionals. Due to the high levels of staff burden and minimal professional benefits offered to CNAs, turnover rates among CNAs are the highest when compared with other health professionals, including RNs and LPNs. Unfortunately, high turnover rates directly adversely affect quality of care in the nursing home setting.

Although caregiver burden has been studied extensively in family caregivers, the studies of professional burden are more limited. Nonetheless, the concept of burn-out for professional caregivers was introduced into the literature 30 years ago and has been used to describe a syndrome of emotional exhaustion, depersonalization, and reduced personal accomplishment, which occurs in persons who provide direct patient care (Maslach & Jackson, 1981). The consequences of professional caregiver burden are significant as they impact the quality of care provided in the nursing home setting, the relationship with the family and patient, and the professional caregivers' emotional and physical well-being. In addition to the low pay, minimal professional rewards, and lack of autonomy inherent to the CNA worker, resident and family factors also contribute to burnout in CNAs. For example, residents' aggressive behavior and the number of hours worked weekly are associated with emotional exhaustion among staff in long-term care (Evers, Brouwers, & Tomic, 2002). Behavioral issues among residents with dementia are common. Professional caregivers spend approximately 40% of their time managing disruptive behaviors while providing complex physical care to residents with dementia (Cassidy & Sheikh, 2002). Residents with more behavioral symptoms create more distress for nursing staff. In addition, conflict with family members is a strong predictor of nursing home staff's feelings of burnout and low job satisfaction (Abrahamson, Jill Suitor, & Pillemer, 2009). Often nursing home staff experience conflict when they attempt to meet the expectations of family members in providing individualized care within a system that values efficiency, uniformity, and cost containment. Staff–family conflict frequently centers on role conflict and ambiguity in providing care and responding to disruptive behaviors. Administrative support is limited regarding how to best develop and maintain trusting relationships and open communication (Abrahamson et al., 2009). Overall, nursing home staffs face significant burnout linked to low pay, minimal benefits, challenges related to managing residents' behavioral symptoms, and the complexities of coordinating care with families.

INTERVENTIONS FOR DEMENTIA CAREGIVERS

There is an extensive literature on interventions for dementia caregivers. In this section, we will briefly review outcome research for home-based caregivers and for caregivers of individuals in a nursing home. We will describe details of these intervention approaches to highlight strategies that may be effective when working with dementia caregivers.

Home Caregiver Interventions

Accumulating evidence shows that psychosocial interventions can reduce the negative consequences for family caregivers of individuals with dementia (Belle et al., 2006). There are varieties of approaches that are used with dementia caregivers. Table 18.3 lists the different types of interventions and a brief description. In addition to these direct caregiver interventions, pharmacological and nonpharmacological approaches with the dementia patient can also indirectly improve caregiver burden and distress by reducing memory and behavior problems in the patient. Similarly, caregiver interventions can positively impact patient mortality and institutional placement (McClendon, Smyth, & Neundorfer, 2004; Mittelman, Roth, Coon, & Haley, 2004). Many intervention studies are plagued by methodological problems, such as small sample sizes and inclusion of nondistressed caregivers. The latter issue is of significant concern because effective interventions may be deemed ineffective if caregivers are not selected based on the expected outcome from the intervention. For example, if a caregiver intervention is developed to reduce anxiety, it would be important to select caregivers who are experiencing high levels of anxiety rather than assuming that all dementia caregivers require treatment for anxiety.

Interventions that have more generic educational components tend to increase caregivers' knowledge about dementia, although they have less significant impact on caregiver distress and burden (Brodaty, Green, & Koschera, 2003). Interestingly, inclusion of an active component (i.e., skill building) rather than education alone is necessary to have any effect on caregiver distress, burden, and satisfaction (Pinquart & Sörensen, 2006b). Consultation and case management can improve caregiver skills and help caregivers identify resources, but have less of an effect on the subjective

TABLE 18.3 List of Commonly Used Intervention Approaches for Dementia Caregivers

INTERVENTION TYPE	DESCRIPTION
Consultation/case management	Provide practical advice and information about dementia and caregiving. Makes referrals to community agencies, programs, and services.
Counseling/psychotherapy	Individual or group-based therapy. Most approaches are based in cognitive behavioral therapy that focuses on identifying and restructuring negative beliefs and behaviors about the care recipient or caregiving.
Psychoeducation/skills training	Increase caregiver knowledge of dementia, dementia care, and risks for caregiving. Some approaches teach specific skills, such as problem solving, modifying home environment, managing dementia behaviors, or stress management.
Support groups	Provide the opportunity for caregivers to meet and share their feelings, strategies for managing care, and to reduce feelings of isolation. These may be facilitated by dementia care professionals.
Respite care	Provides alternate care for the dementia patient, so that the caregiver can work, run errands, rest, vacation, or engage in other activities. This can involve adult day care, in-home care, or temporary nursing home stays.
Multicomponent	Combines components from different interventions or strategies. For example, a multicomponent intervention might combine family counseling, telephone support, and respite care. Some interventions involve delivery of all components, whereas others may be tailored to the specific needs of the caregiver.

experience of burden. Cognitive behavioral therapy (CBT) can be effective for reducing depression and anxiety in caregivers, although it may have less of an impact on increasing knowledge and managing the dementia care (Pinquart & Sörensen, 2006b). As previously noted, respite care appears to have mixed effects on caregiver distress. Data from clinical trials testing pharmacological approaches for dementia patients show small improvements in caregiver burden as well as mild reductions in the amount of time a caregiver spends on caregiving tasks (Lingler, Martire, & Schulz, 2005). However, the combination of a psychosocial intervention and anti-dementia medication significantly reduces caregiver depression compared to medication alone (Mittelman, Brodaty, Wallen, & Burns, 2008). Adding a psychotherapeutic component may help caregivers apply strategies learned in the intervention and/or address barriers to making changes. Overall, various intervention types tend to have domain-specific effects, which has led to the study and use of multicomponent interventions.

Because caregiver burden and distress is a complex, multifaceted construct, it is no surprise that multicomponent interventions seem to be more effective than interventions targeting one aspect of caregiver functioning (Brodaty et al., 2003). Multicomponent interventions involve use of two or more conceptually different strategies to help caregivers. Two of the largest and best-controlled multicomponent studies are the Resources for Enhancing Alzheimer's Caregiver Health studies (REACH & REACH-II) and the New York University (NYU) Caregiver studies. In the large, multisite REACH-II study, the following strategies were used during home visits and telephone contacts: psychoeducation, didactic instruction, role-playing, problem solving, skill training, stress management techniques, and telephone support groups (Belle et al., 2006). For the NYU caregiver study, caregivers received family counseling, individual counseling, weekly support groups, and ad hoc telephone counseling (Mittelman, Ferris, Shulman, Steinberg, & Levin, 1996). Multicomponent interventions can be fixed, in which all caregivers receive all components of the intervention or ones that are tailored to the specific needs of the caregiver or caregiving situation. In general, tailored approaches are more effective than fixed ones. The REACH-II study used a tailored approach in which caregivers completed a risk appraisal measure to assess domains related to poor caregiver outcomes (i.e., depression, burden, self-care, health behaviors, social support, safety, and patient problem behaviors) and to guide intervention implementation (Belle et al., 2006). Meta-analytic studies have also shown that interventions of 6 months or greater are more effective than briefer interventions (Sörensen, Pinquart, & Duberstein, 2002). In addition to caregiver burden, distress, and depression, several multicomponent interventions have shown effects on physical health, service utilization, and delayed institutionalization (Mittelman, Roth, Haley, & Zarit, 2004).

Similar to multicomponent interventions, collaborative care models have also shown efficacy in improving dementia patient behaviors and decreasing caregiver burden and distress. In one study, care recipients and their caregivers received 1 year of integrated care involving their primary care physician and a geriatric nurse practitioner. They received case management, education on communication skills, coping skills, legal and financial advice, patient exercise guidelines, and a caregiver guide (Callahan et al., 2006). Taken together, individually tailored, multicomponent interventions or integrated collaborative care models seem to be the best approaches for treating the distress associated with dementia caregiving. Very few studies have addressed long-term outcomes of interventions, although there is limited evidence that positive effects of a caregiver intervention can be sustained (Mittelman, Roth, Coon, & Haley, 2004). The next step is to determine whether these effective interventions can be used in real-world settings. Initial attempts at studying effectiveness of the REACH intervention in a community agency have shown good feasibility and positive outcomes (Burgio et al., 2009).

Limited data are available about factors that moderate the response to interventions. Caregivers with high levels of self-efficacy may require less-intensive interventions to respond (Rabinowitz et al., 2006). Racial and ethnic minorities show a differential response to intervention approaches, although this issue has received only limited investigation. In the REACH-II study involving equal numbers of Caucasian, Latino, and African-American caregivers, intervention effects were seen for Caucasian and Latino caregivers, but not for African Americans (Belle et al., 2006). Spouses who receive interventions exhibit stronger effects on care-recipient behavior problems and delayed nursing home placement than adult children caregivers (Pinquart & Sörensen, 2006a). Preliminary findings also show that women seem to improve more than men in depression and dementia knowledge but less in subjective well-being (Pinquart & Sörensen, 2006b). Clearly, much more work needs to be done to match caregiver characteristics or situational variables with the most effective treatment strategies.

In response to the need for cost-effective and highly accessible dementia caregiver interventions, our group developed a telephone-based, psychosocial intervention for dementia caregivers that is theoretically driven by a model of family functioning and the traditional stress-coping model (Family Intervention: Telephone Tracking—Caregiver; FITT-C). The FITT-C involves 16 telephone contacts over a 6-month period. Each call involves an assessment of key areas (i.e., social support, mood, family functioning, health) to allow therapists to set treatment priorities and to select the most appropriate intervention strategies. The therapist selects from a menu of directive and supportive intervention strategies (see Table 18.4) to address the most pressing issues. In a preliminary study of an earlier version of intervention, we found that dementia caregivers who received the FITT-C showed greater reductions in perceived burden and less-severe reactions to memory and behavior problems than individuals under standard care conditions (Tremont, Davis, Bishop, & Fortinsky, 2008). We are currently conducting a large-scale, randomized controlled study comparing the FITT-C to an active control condition involving nondirective support for caregivers through empathic and reflective listening and open-ended questioning.

The future of caregiver interventions may lie in technology-based approaches. Thus far, there have been limited studies of computer-based interventions or automated telephone systems, which have met with mixed results (e.g., Mahoney, Tarlow, & Jones, 2003). One possible explanation of the modest findings may be that the current cohort of caregivers (particularly spouses) is not comfortable with technology.

Nursing Home Interventions

The majority of nursing homes have support programs for care recipients, but only a small minority offers support groups for family members (Alzheimer's Association, 2009). Although caregiving support groups may be of value, there are no empirically validated intervention programs available for caregivers at risk of depression, persistent burden, and physical health declines. As discussed earlier, psychosocial interventions that are comprised of multiple components (e.g., education, problem solving, and family approaches) are effective in reducing burden and depressive symptoms in family caregivers who are caring for their family member at home. Far fewer interventions have been studied for nursing home caregivers, and the

TABLE 18.4 Intervention Strategies Used in the Family Intervention: Telephone Tracking—Caregiver (FITT-C)

	DESCRIPTION
Supportive Strategies	
Empathy	Providing caregivers nonjudgmental support as they discuss issues
Giving permission	Encouraging caregivers to do something they feel hesitant about, including prioritizing their own well-being
Normalizing	Reconceptualizing a caregiver's stress, anger, or other emotions as a normal part of the caregiving process
Provision of information/education	Providing the caregiver with specific information about a dementia- or caregiver-related issue (e.g., diagnosis, treatment, course of illness)
Validation	Providing support for a caregiver's beliefs or thoughts about a problem or situation
Venting	Allowing caregivers to express their feelings about caregiving or the care recipient; these typically involve anger or frustration
Active Strategies	
Bibliotherapy	Referring the caregiver to specific reading material about an important issue; these may involve brochures from a local Alzheimer's Association chapter or a book about dementia caregiving (e.g., *The 36-hour day*, *Learning to Speak Alzheimer's*)
Interpretation	Formulating a psychological cause for a caregiver's behavior
Positive reframing	Restating a caregiver's thoughts in a positive manner
Problem solving	Helping the caregiver to generate solutions to caregiving problems
Reference to resource binder	Directing the caregiver to specific educational material to illustrate a possible solution to a problem
Referral	Referring caregivers to a psychotherapist, psychiatrist, or other mental health professional if issues are beyond the scope of intervention
Review of case with senior research staff	Discuss issues that arise in session with staff to determine if additional referral is needed or assist with direction of intervention
Set task directive and follow-up	Assign caregiver a specific task to be completed before next contact; therapist reviews barriers to completion or outcome if task completed

majority focus on either educating staff or on the interaction between family caregivers and staff. Several intervention programs show promise for improving the relationship between family and nursing home staff and reducing behavioral problems in the patient, but far fewer intervention programs impact caregiver mental health outcomes specifically. As previously discussed, the NYU caregiver intervention program provided ongoing support to spousal caregivers and compared mental health outcomes to those caregivers receiving no intervention. After following these caregivers through placement, results indicated that caregivers receiving counseling showed fewer depressive symptoms and lower levels of burden following nursing home placement compared to those caregivers receiving no intervention (Gaugler, Roth, Haley, & Mittelman, 2008). This is not surprising, given that higher burden levels at the time of admission are associated with poorer caregiver adjustment in other studies (Gaugler, Pot, & Zarit, 2007). The NYU program worked with caregivers only and did not address resident outcomes. Similarly, our group designed the FITT—Nursing Home (FITT-NH) to facilitate caregiver adjustment within the first

6 months of nursing home placement. The intervention was delivered entirely by telephone. Interventions were based on a risk assessment approach, evaluating key areas of caregiver emotional adjustment, caregiver–staff interactions, family functioning, caregiver health, and social support. This assessment approach is consistent with home caregiver interventions, such as the REACH and FITT-C protocols, which have shown positive effects on caregiver emotional health. For the FITT-NH intervention, caregivers who received the intervention showed a significant reduction in feelings of guilt related to placement and reported more positive perceptions of interactions with staff compared to a noncontact control group (Davis, Tremont, Bishop, & Fortinsky, 2011). Another intervention, the Family Intervention Education Program, took a slightly different approach and specifically targeted verbal and nonverbal communication between family caregivers and residents with Alzheimer's dementia. The intervention was associated with positive outcomes in patient mood and behavior and caregiver communication with the patient (McCallion, Toseland, & Freeman, 1999). Similarly, Bakker et al. used a multidisciplinary team to deliver an integrated psychotherapy program to the caregiver and patient. Results were compared to a group randomized to usual care. The 13-week randomized, controlled trial was associated with caregiver report of reduced behavioral symptoms in the care recipient and reduced caregiver burden, but there was no impact of the intervention on staff's perception of patient behavior (Bakker et al., 2011). Taken together, psychosocial interventions that target patient and caregiver adjustment to nursing home placement are minimal. More work is needed in this area given that family caregivers experience a great deal of stress and are at risk of declines in their mental and physical health.

Innovative intervention programs have also been developed to retain nursing home staff and decrease the level of stress in caring for residents with dementia. Intervention strategies include specialized care units (Middleton, Stewart, & Richardson, 1999); self-managed and CNA-empowered work teams (Yeatts & Cready, 2007); peer support (Davison et al., 2007; Hegeman, Hoskinson, Munro, Maiden, & Pillemer, 2007); and direct training in managing behavioral symptoms (Noel, Pearce, & Metcalf, 2000; Visser et al., 2008). Intervention programs have also been tested in the assisted-living environment. For example, the Staff Training in Assisted living Residences program (STAR) is an education program for direct care staff. The intervention was associated with lower levels of mood disturbance and behavioral disturbance in the resident, and the staff reported less of an impact and reaction to residents' behavior problems, as well as greater job satisfaction (Teri, Huda, Gibbons, Young, & van Leynseele, 2005). In general, extensive interventions with ongoing support show positive effects, mostly in the area of new knowledge, but effects on staff burden and quality of resident care are generally modest (Kuske et al., 2007).

Individual intervention programs that target caregivers and staff individually are certainly important. However, many stressors described by both family and professional caregivers directly relate to perceptions and interactions between staff and family. These issues include role allocation for certain tasks (Stephens, Ogrocki, & Kinney, 1991); barriers to communication (e.g., language, barriers, lack of time); and negative attitudes and stereotypes that families and staff have of each other (Duncan & Morgan, 1994). Given the unique nature of the nursing home where collaboration of care between professional staff and family is critical to positive outcomes for the care recipient, interventions that target the family–staff relationship may be the most effective. This is particularly important because caregivers and family members are typically interacting most frequently with CNAs, the group that may be experiencing the greatest amount of their own stress and burnout. Several intervention strategies show promise for improving caregiver well-being and staff–family interactions. Pillemer et al. (2003) attempted to increase cooperation and effective communication among nursing home family caregivers and staff through the Partners in Caregiving program. Participants were taught communication and conflict-resolution techniques. The intervention was associated with improved attitudes toward each other and no increase in staff–family conflicts. In addition, participants showed a reduction in depressive symptoms, but not burden, compared to a control condition. This approach was modified for and evaluated in dementia special care units (Robison et al., 2007). Results of a randomized trial showed significant improvements in family caregivers' communication with staff and increased care involvement in spouse caregivers. Staff reported reduced conflict with families, and reduced depression and staff behavior toward family was improved. Staff burnout increased in the control group. Similarly, Maas et al. (2004) showed that a family–staff written negotiation of the extent and nature of family involvement in care (Family Involvement in Care Intervention) improved both caregiver and staff attitudes of caregiving, although minimal effects were identified for perceived conflicts between family and staff. Technology-based education programs have also been used with nursing home caregivers. A Web-based system of interactive training and interactive communication with the facilities was associated with increased knowledge of dementia care, although a small sample size and lack of a control group limit the interpretation of these findings (Rosen et al., 2003). Currently, results based on smaller, pilot intervention programs offer promise for psychosocial treatment for caregivers and staff in long-term care facilities, but effectiveness trials need to be conducted to determine sustainability and feasibility of including these types of programs within long-term care facilities. The most effective approach may be to develop interventions that include both staff and family caregivers. Ideally, integrated care with family and staff will result in reduced staff turnover and burden, improved care for the resident, and better quality of life for family caregivers.

DEATH AND BEREAVEMENT

The process of loss in AD is slow and progressive, reflecting losses of both cognitive capacity and functional abilities. Given the progressive course of deterioration, both anticipatory grief and death-related grief are two very important emotional experiences for dementia caregivers. Anticipatory grief, or the experience of current and predicted loss, is one aspect of emotional caregiver burden (Holley & Mast, 2009). Caregivers with greater depression and burden leading up to and during the end-of-life period are at increased risk of complicated grief (Schulz, Boerner, Shear, Zhang, & Gitlin, 2006). The vast majority of caregivers show resilience following the care recipients' death. Some may experience a sense of relief, and symptoms of depression and grief typically decline rapidly following death and usually return to normal levels within 1 year (Schulz et al., 2003). A minority of bereaved caregivers, approximately 20%, experience the syndrome of complicated grief following the death of their family member. Complicated grief is distinct from the typical grief experience and is characterized by grief symptoms lasting for 6 months or longer. Symptoms often involve intense longing and yearning for the person who has died and recurrent intrusive thoughts of mourning that interfere with daily functioning and other social relationships (Zhang, El-Jawahri, & Prigerson, 2006). There is some evidence that supportive and educational counseling prior to the death of their loved one can help caregivers grieve in a healthier manner and minimize the risk of prolonged grief symptoms and depression (Haley et al., 2008; Holland,

Currier, & Gallagher-Thompson, 2009; Schulz et al., 2006). It is important to direct caregivers to supportive resources if it is evident that they are struggling with anticipatory grief symptoms and to encourage the active use of resources in the end-of-life period. At the end of life, patients with AD and their caregivers are entitled to hospice care to facilitate the dying process and bereavement. Hospice care can serve an important role for caregivers, and one survey of hospice and non-hospice palliative care programs indicated that assistance with caregiver burden was one of the most highly rated needs among family members (Torke et al., 2010). In sum, professionals working with caregivers of patients with dementia need to identify caregivers who may be experiencing anticipatory grief as a central feature of their emotional burden and to ensure that caregivers receive support during the end-of-life process (e.g., hospice services) and possibly enhanced bereavement counseling following the death of their family member.

SUMMARY

In this chapter, we highlighted the significant role that family and professional caregivers play in the management of dementia across multiple transition points and health care systems. Models of chronic stress on mental and physical health serve as a framework to understand the significant consequences of dementia caregiving, which may be ameliorated by education, support, and community-based resources. It is important to address caregiver needs immediately on diagnosis of dementia to possibly reduce the likelihood of future distress. At these early stages, education about the diagnosis and working toward acceptance are critical, especially given the high frequency of anosognosia. The literature clearly indicates that cumulative stress experienced by these caregivers has far-reaching implications on their own physical and mental health and family functioning. Poor adaptation to the caregiving process can lead to continued health declines even after nursing home placement and the death of the care recipient. As the disease progresses, each time the patient is seen, the caregiver should also be assessed for overall adjustment and functioning to identify those at risk of poor adaptation. Current pharmacological treatments for dementia can reduce burden and stress for caregivers, but there is considerable additive benefit of a psychosocial caregiver intervention. Caregivers benefit from tailored approaches to address their specific needs based on their characteristics, situation, and transition point. Skill building for symptom and behavioral management may serve caregivers well as they proceed through the unpredictable course of a dementing illness. Caregiver interventions can be enhanced by including a psychotherapeutic component to address emotional distress. Multicomponent interventions and approaches that make use of integrated care models seem to hold the most promise and can include conceptually different strategies to help caregivers. This approach appears to work for caregivers in multiple contexts, including home care and long-term care. These interventions need at least 6 months to be effective, and ongoing support is associated with long-term mental health benefits as well as public health implications, such as delayed nursing home placement. If nursing home placement does occur, caregivers who have received psychosocial interventions at some point in their caregiving career adjust better to placement. Caregivers who experience high levels of burden and distress prior to placement are likely to continue to experience distress following placement, suggesting that the earlier the interventions can be provided, the better the caregivers will adjust during the latter part of the disease. The current challenge is integrating these approaches in community and long-term care settings, so that all who need it can have access. The future of caregiver interventions may lie in technology-based approaches, such as the telephone or videoconferencing. Such approaches may be used to reach rural or homebound caregivers and/or integrate families in the caregiving process who may not reside near each other. In sum, caregivers are integral to the treatment of patients with dementia. They often make decisions about the care recipient's care and interact directly with health care professionals, respite services, and nursing home staff. AD and related dementias directly impact the caregiver, and the consequences can be negative. Caregivers will benefit from intervention programs as part of an integrated treatment approach for dementia.

REFERENCES

Abrahamson, K., Jill Suitor, J., & Pillemer, K. (2009). Conflict between nursing home staff and residents' families: Does it increase burnout? *Journal of Aging and Health, 21*(6), 895–912.

Almberg, B., Grafström, M., Krichbaum, K., & Winblad, B. (2000). The interplay of institution and family caregiving: Relations between patient hassles, nursing home hassles and caregivers' burnout. *International Journal of Geriatric Psychiatry, 15*(10), 931–939.

Alzheimer's Association. (2009). 2009 Alzheimer's disease facts and figures. *Alzheimer's and Dementia, 5*, 234–270.

Aminzadeh, F., Byszewski, A., Molnar, F. J., & Eisner, M. (2007). Emotional impact of dementia diagnosis: Exploring persons with dementia and caregivers' perspectives. *Aging & Mental Health, 11*(3), 281–290.

Amirkhanyan, A. A., & Wolf, D. A. (2003). Caregiver stress and noncaregiver stress: Exploring the pathways of psychiatric morbidity. *The Gerontologist, 43*(6), 817–827.

Aneshensel, C., Pearlin, L. I., Mullan, J., Zarit, S., & Whitlach, C. (1995). *Profiles in caregiving: The unexpected career.* New York, NY: Academic Press.

Ankri, J., Andrieu, S., Beaufils, B., Grand, A., & Henrard, J. C. (2005). Beyond the global score of the Zarit Burden Interview: Useful dimensions for clinicians. *International Journal of Geriatric Psychiatry, 20*(3), 254–260.

Aström, S., Nilsson, M., Norberg, A., & Winblad, B. (1990). Empathy, experience of burnout and attitudes towards demented patients among nursing staff in geriatric care. *Journal of Advanced Nursing, 15*(11), 1236–1244.

Baker, L. D., Frank, L. L., Foster-Schubert, K., Green, P. S., Wilkinson, C. W., McTiernan, A.,... Craft, S. (2010). Effects of aerobic exercise on mild cognitive impairment: A controlled trial. *Archives of Neurology, 67*(1), 71–79.

Bakker, T. J., Duivenvoorden, H. J., van der Lee, J., Olde Rikkert, M. G., Beekman, A. T., & Ribbe, M. W. (2011). Integrative psychotherapeutic nursing home program to reduce multiple psychiatric symptoms of cognitively impaired patients and caregiver burden: Randomized controlled trial. *American Journal of Geriatric Psychiatry, 19*(6), 507–520.

Ball, V., Snow, A. L., Steele, A. B., Morgan, R. O., Davila, J. A., Wilson, N., & Kunik, M. E. (2010). Quality of relationships as a predictor of psychosocial functioning in patients with dementia. *Journal of Geriatric Psychiatry and Neurology, 23*(2), 109–114.

Bamford, C., Lamont, S., Eccles, M., Robinson, L., May, C., & Bond, J. (2004). Disclosing a diagnosis of dementia: A systematic review. *International Journal of Geriatric Psychiatry, 19*(2), 151–169.

Bandura, A. (1997). *Self-efficacy: The exercise of control.* New York, NY: W.H. Freeman.

Beisecker, A., Chrisman, S., & Wright, L. (1997). Perceptions of family caregivers of persons with Alzheimer's disease: Communication with physicians. *American Journal of Alzheimer's Disease and Other Dementias, 12*, 73–83.

Belle, S. H., Burgio, L., Burns, R., Coon, D., Czaja, S. J., Gallagher-Thompson, D.,... Zhang, S.; Resources for Enhancing Alzheimer's Caregiver Health (REACH) II Investigators. (2006). Enhancing the quality of life of dementia caregivers from different ethnic or racial groups: A randomized, controlled trial. *Annals of Internal Medicine, 145*(10), 727–738.

Bern-Klug, M. (2008). The emotional context facing nursing home residents' families: A call for role reinforcement strategies from nursing homes and the community. *Journal of the American Medical Directors Association, 9*(1), 36–44.

Bowman, K. F., Mukherjee, S., & Fortinsky, R. H. (1998). Exploring strain in community and nursing home family caregivers. *The Journal of Applied Gerontology, 17*, 371–392.

Brodaty, H., Green, A., & Koschera, A. (2003). Meta-analysis of psychosocial interventions for caregivers of people with dementia. *Journal of the American Geriatrics Society, 51*(5), 657–664.

Bruce, J. M., McQuiggan, M., Williams, V., Westervelt, H., & Tremont, G. (2008). Burden among spousal and child caregivers of patients with mild cognitive impairment. *Dementia and Geriatric Cognitive Disorders, 25*(4), 385–390.

Burgio, L. D., Collins, I. B., Schmid, B., Wharton, T., McCallum, D., & Decoster, J. (2009). Translating the REACH caregiver intervention for use by area agency on aging personnel: The REACH OUT program. *The Gerontologist, 49*(1), 103–116.

Callahan, C. M., Boustani, M. A., Unverzagt, F. W., Austrom, M. G., Damush, T. M., Perkins, A. J.,... Hendrie, H. C. (2006). Effectiveness of collaborative care for older adults with Alzheimer disease in primary care: A randomized controlled trial. *The Journal of the American Medical Association, 295*(18), 2148–2157.

Cassidy, E. L., & Sheikh, J. I. (2002). Pre-intervention assessment for disruptive behavior problems: A focus on staff needs. *Aging & Mental Health, 6*(2), 166–171.

Chen, C. K., Sabir, M., Zimmerman, S., Suitor, J., & Pillemer, K. (2007). The importance of family relationships with nursing facility staff for family caregiver burden and depression. *The Journals of Gerontology, 62*(5), P253–P260.

Christakis, N. A., & Allison, P. D. (2006). Mortality after the hospitalization of a spouse. *The New England Journal of Medicine, 354*(7), 719–730.

Connell, C. M., Boise, L., Stuckey, J. C., Holmes, S. B., & Hudson, M. L. (2004). Attitudes toward the diagnosis and disclosure of dementia among family caregivers and primary care physicians. *The Gerontologist, 44*(4), 500–507.

Cooney, C., Howard, R., & Lawlor, B. (2006). Abuse of vulnerable people with dementia by their carers: Can we identify those most at risk? *International Journal of Geriatric Psychiatry, 21*(6), 564–571.

Craig, D., Mirakhur, A., Hart, D. J., McIlroy, S. P., & Passmore, A. P. (2005). A cross-sectional study of neuropsychiatric symptoms in 435 patients with Alzheimer's disease. *The American Journal of Geriatric Psychiatry, 13*(6), 460–468.

Damjanovic, A. K., Yang, Y., Glaser, R., Kiecolt-Glaser, J. K., Nguyen, H., Laskowski, B.,... Weng, N. P. (2007). Accelerated telomere erosion is associated with a declining immune function of caregivers of Alzheimer's disease patients. *Journal of Immunology, 179*(6), 4249–4254.

Davis, J. D., & Tremont, G. (2007). Impact of frontal systems behavioral functioning in dementia on caregiver burden. *The Journal of Neuropsychiatry and Clinical Neurosciences, 19*(1), 43–49.

Davis, J. D., Tremont, G., Bishop, D. S., & Fortinsky, R. H. (2011). A telephone-delivered psychosocial intervention improves dementia caregiver adjustment following nursing home placement. *International Journal of Geriatric Psychiatry, 26*(4), 380–387. doi: 10.1002/gps.2537

Davison, T. E., McCabe, M. P., Visser, S., Hudgson, C., Buchanan, G., & George, K. (2007). Controlled trial of dementia training with a peer support group for aged care staff. *International Journal of Geriatric Psychiatry, 22*(9), 868–873.

De Vugt, M., Riedijik, S., Aalten, P., Tibben, A., van Swieten, J., & Verhey, F. (2006). Impact of behavioural problems on spousal caregivers: A comparison between Alzheimer's disease and frontotemporal dementia. *Dementia and Geriatric Cognitive Disorders, 22,* 35–41.

Ducharme, F., Levesque, L., Lachance, L., Gangbe, M., Zarit, S., Vezina, J., & Caron, C. D. (2007). Older husbands as caregivers. Factors associated with health and the intention to end caregiving. *Research on Aging, 29,* 3–31.

Duncan, M. T., & Morgan, D. L. (1994). Sharing the caring: Family caregivers' views of their relationships with nursing home staff. *The Gerontologist, 34*(2), 235–244.

Epstein-Lubow, G., Davis, J. D., Miller, I. W., & Tremont, G. (2008). Persisting burden predicts depressive symptoms in dementia caregivers. *Journal of Geriatric Psychiatry and Neurology, 21*(3), 198–203.

Evers, W. J., Brouwers, A., & Tomic, W. (2002). Burnout and self-efficacy: A study on teachers' beliefs when implementing an innovative educational system in the Netherlands. *The British Journal of Educational Psychology, 72*(Pt 2), 227–243. doi: 10.1348/000709902158865

Fortinsky, R. H., Kercher, K., & Burant, C. J. (2002). Measurement and correlates of family caregiver self-efficacy for managing dementia. *Aging & Mental Health, 6*(2), 153–160.

Freyne, A., Kidd, N., Coen, R., & Lawlor, B. A. (1999). Burden in carers of dementia patients: Higher levels in carers of younger sufferers. *International Journal of Geriatric Psychiatry, 14*(9), 784–788.

Galvin, J. E., Duda, J. E., Kaufer, D. I., Lippa, C. F., Taylor, A., & Zarit, S. H. (2010). Lewy body dementia: The caregiver experience of clinical care. *Parkinsonism & Related Disorders, 16*(6), 388–392.

Garity, J. (2006). Caring for a family member with Alzheimer's disease: Coping with caregiver burden post-nursing home placement. *Journal of Gerontological Nursing, 32*(6), 39–48.

Gaugler, J. E., Kane, R. L., Kane, R. A., Clay, T., & Newcomer, R. C. (2005). The effects of duration of caregiving on institutionalization. *The Gerontologist, 45*(1), 78–89.

Gaugler, J. E., Kane, R. L., Kane, R. A., & Newcomer, R. (2005a). Early community-based service utilization and its effects on institutionalization in dementia caregiving. *The Gerontologist, 45*(2), 177–185.

Gaugler, J. E., Kane, R. L., Kane, R. A., & Newcomer, R. (2005b). The longitudinal effects of early behavior problems in the dementia caregiving career. *Psychology and Aging, 20*(1), 100–116.

Gaugler, J. E., Kane, R., & Newcomer, R. (2007). Resilence and transitions from dementia caregiving. *Journal of Gerontology: Psychological Sciences, 62B,* 38–44.

Gaugler, J. E., Mittelman, M. S., Hepburn, K., & Newcomer, R. (2009). Predictors of change in caregiver burden and depressive symptoms following nursing home admission. *Psychology and Aging, 24*(2), 385–396.

Gaugler, J. E., Pot, A. M., & Zarit, S. H. (2007). Long-term adaptation to institutionalization in dementia caregivers. *The Gerontologist, 47*(6), 730–740.

Gaugler, J. E., Roth, D. L., Haley, W. E., & Mittelman, M. S. (2008). Can counseling and support reduce burden and depressive symptoms in caregivers of people with Alzheimer's disease during the transition to institutionalization? Results from the New York University caregiver intervention study. *Journal of the American Geriatrics Society, 56*(3), 421–428.

Gaugler, J. E., Wall, M. M., Kane, R. L., Menk, J. S., Sarsour, K., Johnston, J. A.,...Newcomer, R. (2010). The effects of incident and persistent behavioral problems on change in caregiver burden and nursing home admission of persons with dementia. *Medical Care, 48*(10), 875–883.

Gaugler, J. E., Yu, F., Krichbaum, K., & Wyman, J. F. (2009). Predictors of nursing home admission for persons with dementia. *Medical Care, 47*(2), 191–198.

Gaugler, J., Zarit, S., Townsend, A. L., Stephens, M. A. P., & Greene, R. (2003). Evaluating community-based programs for dementia caregivers: The cost implications of adult day services. *Journal of Applied Gerontology, 22*, 118–133.

Gottlieb, B., & Johnson, J. (2000). Respite programs for caregivers of persons with dementia: A review with practice implications. *Aging and Mental Health, 4*, 119–129.

Graham, C., Ballard, C., & Sham, P. (1997). Carers' knowledge of dementia and their expressed concerns. *International Journal of Geriatric Psychiatry, 12*(4), 470–473.

Gray, H. L., Jimenez, D. E., Cucciare, M. A., Tong, H. Q., & Gallagher-Thompson, D. (2009). Ethnic differences in beliefs regarding Alzheimer disease among dementia family caregivers. *The American Journal of Geriatric Psychiatry, 17*(11), 925–933.

Haley, W. E., Bergman, E. J., Roth, D. L., McVie, T., Gaugler, J. E., & Mittelman, M. S. (2008). Long-term effects of bereavement and caregiver intervention on dementia caregiver depressive symptoms. *The Gerontologist, 48*(6), 732–740.

Hegeman, C., Hoskinson, D., Munro, H., Maiden, P., & Pillemer, K. (2007). Peer mentoring in long-term care: Rationale, design, and retention. *Gerontology & Geriatrics Education, 28*(2), 77–90.

Hilgeman, M. M., Allen, R. S., DeCoster, J., & Burgio, L. D. (2007). Positive aspects of caregiving as a moderator of treatment outcome over 12 months. *Psychology and Aging, 22*(2), 361–371.

Hirst, M. (2005). Carer distress: A prospective, population-based study. *Social Science & Medicine, 61*(3), 697–708.

Holland, J., Currier, J., & Gallagher-Thompson, D. (2009). Outcomes from the Resources for Enhancing Alzheimer's Caregiver Health (REACH) program for bereaved caregivers. *Psychology and Aging, 24*(1), 190–202.

Holley, C. K., & Mast, B. T. (2009). The impact of anticipatory grief on caregiver burden in dementia caregivers. *The Gerontologist, 49*(3), 388–396.

Karner, T. X., Montgomery, R. J., Dobbs, D., & Wittmaier, C. (1998). Increasing staff satisfaction. The impact of SCUs and family involvement. *Journal of Gerontological Nursing, 24*(2), 39–44.

Keady, J., Nolan, M. R., & Gilliard, J. (1995). Listen to the voices of experience. *Journal of Dementia Care, 13*, 15–17.

Kiecolt-Glaser, J. K., Glaser, R., Gravenstein, S., Malarkey, W. B., & Sheridan, J. (1996). Chronic stress alters the immune response to influenza virus vaccine in older adults. *Proceedings of the National Academy of Sciences of the United States of America, 93*(7), 3043–3047.

Kiecolt-Glaser, J. K., Preacher, K. J., MacCallum, R. C., Atkinson, C., Malarkey, W. B., & Glaser, R. (2003). Chronic stress and age-related increases in the proinflammatory cytokine IL-6. *Proceedings of the National Academy of Sciences of the United States of America, 100*(15), 9090–9095.

Kolanowski, A. M., Fick, D., Waller, J. L., & Shea, D. (2004). Spouses of persons with dementia: Their healthcare problems, utilization, and costs. *Research in Nursing & Health, 27*(5), 296–306.

Kuske, B., Hanns, S., Luck, T., Angermeyer, M. C., Behrens, J., & Riedel-Heller, S. G. (2007). Nursing home staff training in dementia care: A systematic review of evaluated programs. *International Psychogeriatrics/IPA, 19*(5), 818–841.

Lazarus, R., & Folkman, S. (1984). *Stress, appraisal, and coping.* New York, NY: Springer.

Lee, S., Colditz, G. A., Berkman, L. F., & Kawachi, I. (2003). Caregiving and risk of coronary heart disease in U.S. women: A prospective study. *American Journal of Preventive Medicine, 24*(2), 113–119.

Leggett, A. N., Zarit, S., Taylor, A., & Galvin, J. E. (2011). Stress and burden among caregivers of patients with Lewy body dementia. *The Gerontologist, 51*(1), 76–85.

Lieberman, M. A., & Fisher, L. (2001). The effects of nursing home placement on family caregivers of patients with Alzheimer's disease. *The Gerontologist, 41*(6), 819–826.

Lingler, J. H., Martire, L. M., & Schulz, R. (2005). Caregiver-specific outcomes in antidementia clinical drug trials: A systematic review and meta-analysis. *Journal of the American Geriatrics Society, 53*(6), 983–990.

Lund, D., Utz, R., Caserta, M., & Wright, S. (2008). Examining what caregivers do during respite time to make respite more effective. *Journal of Applied Gerontology, 28,* 109–131.

Lussignoli, R., Sabbatine, F., Chiappa, A., Cesare, S., Lamanna, L., & Zanetti, O. (2010). Needs of caregivers of the patient with dementia. *Archives of Gerontological Geriatrics, 51,* 54–58.

Maas, M. L., Reed, D., Park, M., Specht, J. P., Schutte, D., Kelley, L. S.,…Buckwalte, K. C. (2004). Outcomes of family involvement in care intervention for caregivers of individuals with dementia. *Nursing Research, 53*(2), 76–86.

Mahoney, D. F., Tarlow, B. J., & Jones, R. N. (2003). Effects of an automated telephone support system on caregiver burden and anxiety: Findings from the REACH for TLC intervention study. *The Gerontologist, 43*(4), 556–567.

Majerovitz, S. D. (2007). Predictors of burden and depression among nursing home family caregivers. *Aging & Mental Health, 11*(3), 323–329.

Maslach, C., & Jackson, S. E. (1981). The measurement of experienced burnout. *Journal of Occupational Behavior, 2,* 99–113.

Mausbach, B. T., Coon, D. W., Depp, C., Rabinowitz, Y. G., Wilson-Arias, E., Kraemer, H. C.,… Gallagher-Thompson, D. (2004). Ethnicity and time to institutionalization of dementia patients: A comparison of Latina and Caucasian female family caregivers. *Journal of the American Geriatrics Society, 52*(7), 1077–1084.

McCallion, P., Toseland, R. W., & Freeman, K. (1999). An evaluation of a family visit education program. *Journal of the American Geriatrics Society, 47*(2), 203–214.

McCann, J. J., Hebert, L. E., Li, Y., Wolinsky, F. D., Gilley, D. W., Aggarwal, N. T.,…Evans, D. A. (2005). The effect of adult day care services on time to nursing home placement in older adults with Alzheimer's disease. *The Gerontologist, 45*(6), 754–763.

McClendon, M. J., Smyth, K. A., & Neundorfer, M. M. (2004). Survival of persons with Alzheimer's disease: Caregiver coping matters. *The Gerontologist, 44*(4), 508–519.

McLennon, S. M., Habermann, B., & Davis, L. L. (2010). Deciding to institutionalize: Why do family members cease caregiving at home? *The Journal of Neuroscience Nursing, 42*(2), 95–103.

Middleton, J. I., Stewart, N. J., & Richardson, J. S. (1999). Caregiver distress. Related to disruptive behaviors on special care units versus traditional long-term care units. *Journal of Gerontological Nursing, 25*(3), 11–19.

Mittelman, M. S., Brodaty, H., Wallen, A. S., & Burns, A. (2008). A three-country randomized controlled trial of a psychosocial intervention for caregivers combined with pharmacological treatment for patients with Alzheimer disease: Effects on caregiver depression. *The American Journal of Geriatric Psychiatry, 16*(11), 893–904.

Mittelman, M. S., Ferris, S. H., Shulman, E., Steinberg, G., & Levin, B. (1996). A family intervention to delay nursing home placement of patients with Alzheimer disease. A randomized controlled trial. *The Journal of the American Medical Association, 276*(21), 1725–1731.

Mittelman, M. S., Haley, W. E., Clay, O. J., & Roth, D. L. (2006). Improving caregiver well-being delays nursing home placement of patients with Alzheimer disease. *Neurology, 67*(9), 1592–1599.

Mittelman, M. S., Roth, D. L., Coon, D. W., & Haley, W. E. (2004). Sustained benefit of supportive intervention for depressive symptoms in caregivers of patients with Alzheimer's disease. *The American Journal of Psychiatry, 161*(5), 850–856.

Mittelman, M. S., Roth, D. L., Haley, W. E., & Zarit, S. H. (2004). Effects of a caregiver intervention on negative caregiver appraisals of behavior problems in patients with Alzheimer's disease: Results of a randomized trial. *The Journals of Gerontology, 59*(1), P27–P34.

Mourik, J. C., Rosso, S. M., Niermeijer, M. F., Duivenvoorden, H. J., Van Swieten, J. C., & Tibben, A. (2004). Frontotemporal dementia: Behavioral symptoms and caregiver distress. *Dementia and Geriatric Cognitive Disorders, 18*(3–4), 299–306.

Noel, M. A., Pearce, G. L., & Metcalf, R. (2000). Front line workers in long-term care: The effect of educational interventions and stabilization of staffing ratios on turnover and absenteeism. *Journal of the American Medical Directors Association, 1*(6), 241–247.

Nolan, M., & Dellasega, C. (1999). "It's not the same as him being at home": Creating caring partnerships following nursing home placement. *Journal of Clinical Nursing, 8*(6), 723–730.

Nolan, M., & Dellasega, C. (2000). "I really feel I've let him down": Supporting family carers during long-term care placement for elders. *Journal of Advanced Nursing, 31*(4), 759–767.

Norton, M. C., Smith, K. R., Østbye, T., Tschanz, J. T., Corcoran, C., Schwartz, S.,...Welsh-Bohmer, K. A.; Cache County Investigators. (2010). Greater risk of dementia when spouse has dementia? The Cache County study. *Journal of the American Geriatrics Society, 58*(5), 895–900.

Oremus, M., Wolfson, C., Vandal, A. C., Bergman, H., & Xie, Q. (2007). Caregiver acceptance of adverse effects and use of cholinesterase inhibitors in Alzheimer's disease. *Canadian Journal on Aging, 26*(3), 205–212.

Ory, M. G., Hoffman, R. R., Yee, J. L., Tennstedt, S., & Schulz, R. (1999). Prevalence and impact of caregiving: A detailed comparison between dementia and nondementia caregivers. *The Gerontologist, 39*(2), 177–185.

Pillemer, K., Suitor, J. J., Henderson, C. R., Meador, R., Schultz, L., Robison, J., & Hegeman, C. (2003). A cooperative communication intervention for nursing home staff and family members of residents. *The Gerontologist, 43*(Suppl 2), 96–106. doi: 10.1093/geront/43.suppl_2.96

Pinquart, M., & Sörensen, S. (2003a). Associations of stressors and uplifts of caregiving with caregiver burden and depressive mood: A meta-analysis. *The Journals of Gerontology. Series B, Psychological Sciences and Social Sciences, 58*(2), P112–P128.

Pinquart, M., & Sörensen, S. (2003b). Differences between caregivers and noncaregivers in psychological health and physical health: A meta-analysis. *Psychology and Aging, 18*(2), 250–267.

Pinquart, M., & Sörensen, S. (2005). Ethnic differences in stressors, resources, and psychological outcomes of family caregiving: A meta-analysis. *The Gerontologist, 45*(1), 90–106.

Pinquart, M., & Sörensen, S. (2006a). Gender differences in caregiver stressors, social resources, and health: An updated meta-analysis. *The Journals of Gerontology, 61*(1), P33–P45.

Pinquart, M., & Sörensen, S. (2006b). Helping caregivers of persons with dementia: Which interventions work and how large are their effects? *International Psychogeriatrics/IPA, 18*(4), 577–595.

Pinquart, M., & Sörensen, S. (2007). Correlates of physical health of informal caregivers: A meta-analysis. *The Journals of Gerontology, 62*(2), P126–P137.

Port, C. L., Zimmerman, S., Williams, C. S., Dobbs, D., Preisser, J. S., & Williams, S. W. (2005). Families filling the gap: Comparing family involvement for assisted living and nursing home residents with dementia. *The Gerontologist, 45 Spec No 1*(1), 87–95.

Rabinowitz, Y. G., Mausbach, B. T., Coon, D. W., Depp, C., Thompson, L. W., & Gallagher-Thompson, D. (2006). The moderating effect of self-efficacy on intervention response in women family caregivers of older adults with dementia. *The American Journal of Geriatric Psychiatry, 14*(8), 642–649.

Reed, B. R., Jagust, W. J., & Coulter, L. (1993). Anosognosia in Alzheimer's disease: Relationships to depression, cognitive function, and cerebral perfusion. *Journal of Clinical and Experimental Neuropsychology, 15*(2), 231–244.

Robinson, L., Clare, L., & Evans, K. (2005). Making sense of dementia and adjusting to loss: Psychological reactions to a diagnosis of dementia in couples. *Aging & Mental Health, 9*(4), 337–347.

Robison, J., Curry, L., Gruman, C., Porter, M., Henderson, C. R., & Pillemer, K. (2007). Partners in caregiving in a special care environment: Cooperative communication between staff and families on dementia units. *The Gerontologist, 47*(4), 504–515.

Romero-Moreno, R., Losada, A., Mausbach, B. T., Márquez-González, M., Patterson, T. L., & López, J. (2011). Analysis of the moderating effect of self-efficacy domains in different points of the dementia caregiving process. *Aging & Mental Health, 15*(2), 221–231.

Rosen, J., Mittal, V., Mulsant, B. H., Degenholtz, H., Castle, N., & Fox, D. (2003). Educating the families of nursing home residents: A pilot study using a computer-based system. *Journal of the American Medical Directors Association, 4*, 128–134.

Rosness, T. A., Haugen, P. K., & Engedal, K. (2008). Support to family carers of patients with frontotemporal dementia. *Aging & Mental Health, 12*(4), 462–466.

Ryan, A. A., & Scullion, H. F. (2000). Nursing home placement: An exploration of the experiences of family carers. *Journal of Advanced Nursing, 32*(5), 1187–1195.

Scarmeas, N., Stern, Y., Mayeux, R., Manly, J. J., Schupf, N., & Luchsinger, J. A. (2009). Mediterranean diet and mild cognitive impairment. *Archives of Neurology, 66*(2), 216–225.

Schulz, R., & Beach, S. R. (1999). Caregiving as a risk factor for mortality: The Caregiver Health Effects Study. *The Journal of the American Medical Association, 282*(23), 2215–2219.

Schulz, R., Belle, S. H., Czaja, S. J., McGinnis, K. A., Stevens, A., & Zhang, S. (2004). Long-term care placement of dementia patients and caregiver health and well-being. *The Journal of the American Medical Association, 292*(8), 961–967.

Schulz, R., Boerner, K., Shear, K., Zhang, S., & Gitlin, L. N. (2006). Predictors of complicated grief among dementia caregivers: A prospective study of bereavement. *The American Journal of Geriatric Psychiatry, 14*(8), 650–658.

Schulz, R., & Martire, L. M. (2004). Family caregiving of persons with dementia: Prevalence, health effects, and support strategies. *The American Journal of Geriatric Psychiatry, 12*(3), 240–249.

Schulz, R., McGinnis, K. A., Zhang, S., Martire, L. M., Hebert, R. S., Beach, S. R.,...Belle, S. H. (2008). Dementia patient suffering and caregiver depression. *Alzheimer Disease and Associated Disorders, 22*(2), 170–176.

Schulz, R., Mendelsohn, A. B., Haley, W. E., Mahoney, D., Allen, R. S., Zhang, S.,...Belle, S. H.; Resources for Enhancing Alzheimer's Caregiver Health Investigators. (2003). End-of-life care and the effects of bereavement on family caregivers of persons with dementia. *The New England Journal of Medicine, 349*(20), 1936–1942.

Segerstrom, S. C., Schipper, L. J., & Greenberg, R. N. (2008). Caregiving, repetitive thought, and immune response to vaccination in older adults. *Brain, Behavior, and Immunity, 22*(5), 744–752.

Silverberg Koerner, S., Baete Kenyon, D., & Shirai, Y. (2009). Caregiving for elder relatives: Which caregivers experience personal benefits/gains? *Archives of Gerontological Geriatrics, 48*, 238–245.

Smith, G. E., O'Brien, P. C., Ivnik, R. J., Kokmen, E., & Tangalos, E. G. (2001). Prospective analysis of risk factors for nursing home placement of dementia patients. *Neurology, 57*(8), 1467–1473.

Sörensen, S., Pinquart, M., & Duberstein, P. (2002). How effective are interventions with caregivers? An updated meta-analysis. *The Gerontologist, 42*(3), 356–372.

Spitznagel, M. B., Tremont, G., Davis, J. D., & Foster, S. M. (2006). Psychosocial predictors of dementia caregiver desire to institutionalize: Caregiver, care recipient, and family relationship factors. *Journal of Geriatric Psychiatry and Neurology, 19*(1), 16–20.

Steadman, P. L., Tremont, G., & Davis, J. D. (2007). Premorbid relationship satisfaction and caregiver burden in dementia caregivers. *Journal of Geriatric Psychiatry and Neurology, 20*(2), 115–119.

Steffen, A. M., McKibbin, C., Zeiss, A. M., Gallagher-Thompson, D., & Bandura, A. (2002). The revised scale for caregiving self-efficacy: Reliability and validity studies. *The Journals of Gerontology, 57*(1), P74–P86.

Stephens, M. A., Ogrocki, P. K., & Kinney, J. M. (1991). Sources of stress for family caregivers of institutionalized dementia patients. *Journal of Applied Gerontology, 10*(3), 328–342.

Sussman, T., & Regehr, C. (2009). The influence of community-based services on the burden of spouses caring for their partners with dementia. *Health & Social Work, 34*(1), 29–39.

Szinovacz, M. (2003). Caring for a demented relative at home: Effects on parent-adolescent relationships and family dynamics. *Journal of Aging Studies, 17*, 445–472.

Takahashi, M., Tanaka, K., & Miyoaka, H. (2005). Depression and associated factors of informal caregivers versus professional caregivers of demented patients. *Psychiatry and Clinical Neurosciences, 59*(4), 473–480.

Tarlow, B. J., Wisniewski, S. R., Belle, S. H., Rubert, M., Ory, M. G., & Gallagher-Thompson, D. (2004). Positive aspects of caregiving. *Research on Aging, 26*, 429–453.

Teri, L., Huda, P., Gibbons, L., Young, H., & van Leynseele, J. (2005). STAR: A dementia-specific training program for staff in assisted living residences. *The Gerontologist, 45*(5), 686–693.

Torke, A. M., Holtz, L. R., Hui, S., Castelluccio, P., Connor, S., Eaton, M. A., & Sachs, G. A. (2010). Palliative care for patients with dementia: A national survey. *Journal of the American Geriatrics Society, 58*(11), 2114–2121.

Tremont, G., Davis, J. D., & Bishop, D. S. (2006). Unique contribution of family functioning in caregivers of patients with mild to moderate dementia. *Dementia and Geriatric Cognitive Disorders, 21*(3), 170–174.

Tremont, G., Davis, J. D., Bishop, D. S., & Fortinsky, R. H. (2008). Telephone-delivered psychosocial intervention reduces burden in dementia caregivers. *Dementia, 7*(4), 503–520.

Visser, S. M., McCabe, M. P., Hudgson, C., Buchanan, G., Davison, T. E., & George, K. (2008). Managing behavioural symptoms of dementia: Effectiveness of staff education and peer support. *Aging & Mental Health, 12*(1), 47–55.

Vitaliano, P. P., Scanlan, J. M., Zhang, J., Savage, M. V., Hirsch, I. B., & Siegler, I. C. (2002). A path model of chronic stress, the metabolic syndrome, and coronary heart disease. *Psychosomatic Medicine, 64*(3), 418–435.

Vitaliano, P. P., Zhang, J., & Scanlan, J. M. (2003). Is caregiving hazardous to one's physical health? A meta-analysis. *Psychological Bulletin, 129*(6), 946–972.

Wagner, A. W., Logsdon, R. G., Pearson, J. L., & Teri, L. (1997). Caregiver expressed emotion and depression in Alzheimer's disease. *Aging & Mental Health, 1*(2) 132–139.

Wald, C., Fahy, M., Walker, Z., & Livingston, G. (2003). What to tell dementia caregivers—the rule of threes. *International Journal of Geriatric Psychiatry, 18*(4), 313–317.

Werner, P. (2001). Correlates of family caregivers' knowledge about Alzheimer's disease. *International Journal of Geriatric Psychiatry, 16*(1), 32–38.

Whitlatch, C. J., Schur, D., Noelker, L. S., Ejaz, F. K., & Looman, W. J. (2001). The stress process of family caregiving in institutional settings. *The Gerontologist, 41*(4), 462–473.

Wilson, R. S., Barnes, L. L., Aggarwal, N. T., Boyle, P. A., Hebert, L. E., Mendes de Leon, C. F., & Evans, D. A. (2010). Cognitive activity and the cognitive morbidity of Alzheimer disease. *Neurology, 75*(11), 990–996.

Yeatts, D. E., & Cready, C. M. (2007). Consequences of empowered CNA teams in nursing home settings: A longitudinal assessment. *The Gerontologist, 47*(3), 323–339.

Zarit, S. H., & Whitlatch, C. J. (1992). Institutional placement: Phases of the transition. *The Gerontologist, 32*(5), 665–672.

Zarit, S. H., Reever, K. E., & Bach-Peterson, J. (1980). Relatives of the impaired elderly: Correlates of feelings of burden. *The Gerontologist, 20*(6), 649–655.

Zhang, B., El-Jawahri, A., & Prigerson, H. G. (2006). Update on bereavement research: Evidence-based guidelines for the diagnosis and treatment of complicated bereavement. *Journal of Palliative Medicine, 9*(5), 1188–1203.

CHAPTER 19

Comorbid Manifestations and Secondary Complications of Dementia

Julie Sheffler and Chad A. Noggle

Two types of secondary complications can be analyzed in relation to dementia: conditions that arise outside of the dementia and then conditions that appear to develop due to the neurological degeneration inherent in dementia. Conditions can then be classified within these two categories as psychiatric or medical issues. Examples of psychiatric complications include depression, anxiety, and psychosis. Medical problems consist of issues such as stroke, cardiovascular problems, cancer, infections, orthopedic issues, diabetes, nutritional disorders, vision and hearing problems, as well as general pain. These comorbid conditions and complications have numerous potential ramifications for patients, physicians, caregivers, screening methods, and treatment plans.

The high comorbidity of dementias with other psychiatric and medical issues can seriously complicate the diagnosis and treatment of patients with dementia. Many people misinterpret the complications that arise following the diagnosis of dementia as symptoms of dementia when in reality those issues may need to be treated as a separate entity or may alter the treatment of the dementia entirely. Estimates of overall prevalence rates of dementia with other medical and psychiatric conditions are very high. In one study, 61% of patients with dementia had three or more medical conditions, and medical comorbidity continued to increase as the severity of cognitive impairment increased (Doraiswamy, Leon, Cummings, Marin, & Neumann, 2002). Another study found that on average, patients with dementia in primary care have 2.4 chronic medical conditions (Schubert et al., 2006). However, these numbers do not account for psychiatric comorbidity. As high as 75% of patients with dementia demonstrate symptoms such as depression, irritability, and apathy, while 20% to 40% of dementia patients qualify for the diagnosis of depression (DesRosiers, 2000). Schubert et al. (2006) explain that "comorbid conditions are not the exception, but rather the rule, among older patients with dementia in primary care." The degenerative nature of dementia causes physiological and mental hardships, and the already burdensome symptoms of dementia are only exacerbated by comorbid conditions. Still, these conditions are far too often overlooked or ignored.

Either due to the patients' inability to articulate their experience, remember their symptoms, or even due to practitioner carelessness and oversight, many medical illnesses are not considered separately in patients with dementia. Even with such high estimates of comorbidity, actual comorbid conditions may be more numerous than previously hypothesized. A postmortem study of 51 patients with dementia revealed cases of comorbidity in almost every patient examined, none of which had been diagnosed during their lifetime. Had some of these conditions been found antemortem, treatment and care of the patients would likely have been altered (Fu et al., 2004). Because dementia is associated with an overall loss of functioning, secondary conditions and symptoms are often ignored. Yet comorbidity in older adults can seriously impact mortality. In fact, according to Zekry et al. (2009), the best predictor of a patient's likelihood to die or have an extensive hospital stay is higher comorbidity with dementia, regardless of the patient's cognitive status. Changing the management of patients to correspond to the unique medical and psychiatric conditions that often arise alongside dementia can improve the quality of life and longevity of the patients.

Comorbidity is not the only issue to complicate the treatment and diagnosis of dementia. Certain symptoms such as forgetfulness, paranoia, hallucinations, sleep loss, and depression disturb the patient's ability to care for his or her physical well-being. As memory deteriorates, patients forget to take medications, to eat healthily or to eat at all, and often lapse in taking care of personal hygiene. All of these simple lapses in memory can ultimately lead to much more serious medical conditions. Because effective management of dementia is determinant on so many factors, it is necessary for care providers to understand the complex interactions between these complications.

PSYCHIATRIC ISSUES IN DEMENTIA

Psychiatric disturbances can be some of the most problematic issues to treat due to their complex relationship with dementia. In some cases, it can be extremely difficult to determine whether the psychiatric illness began prior to or following the diagnosis of dementia. Self-reports of well-being and symptoms in the demented are frequently inaccurate or misleading. Because psychiatric conditions comorbid with dementia are associated with "poorer outcomes, decreased quality of life, increased institutionalization, and caregiver distress" (Weintraub & Porsteinsson, 2006), it is necessary for patients, caregivers, and physicians to fully understand the etiology and treatment of these problems. Depression and anxiety are the most common syndromes associated with dementia (Fichter, Meller, Schröppel, & Steinkirchner, 1995). Additionally, psychosis, both preexisting and postdiagnosis, can deter proper treatment.

Depression is frequently associated with old age and perhaps even more so in the context of dementia. In fact, in some cases, depression can even cause reversible cognitive decline in what has been traditionally called pseudodementia. However, the relationship between true dementia and depression is still not well understood. One study looking at possible biological influences that depression may have on dementia found that patients with depression and diabetes were three times as likely to develop dementia than patients with diabetes alone (Katon et al., 2010). A meta-analysis of the association determined three possible explanations for the relationship: (a) Depression may actually be the early stages of dementia; (b) depression may directly cause the manifestation of dementia; or (c) "Depression leads to damage to the hippocampus through a glucocorticoid cascade" (Jorm, 2001). Others like Jorm have looked at the biological similarities in the presentation of the two disorders.

Changes in white matter as well as neurotransmitter loss are characteristic of both depression and Alzheimer's disease (AD) (Korczyn & Halperin, 2009). Although none of the studies was able to determine the true interaction, it is clear that depression is an important component to consider when dealing with dementia.

In the case of pseudodementia, effectively treating the depressive symptoms can reverse the apparent cognitive decline of patients. Even in true dementia, some studies have found that treating depression can alleviate some of the symptoms of cognitive decline. Greenwald et al. (1989) found that when patients with comorbid dementia and depression were treated for depression, their performance on cognitive tasks improved, although still remaining within a demented range. Some may be discouraged to treat depression in patients due to the structural changes that occur in dementia. However, clinical trials have found that depression in patients with AD responds to both psychopharmacological and psychosocial treatments (Katz, 1998). This finding suggests that regardless of its cause-and-effect relationship with dementia, treating depression alone can improve the quality of life and cognizance of people already dealing with cognitive diminution.

Another psychiatric condition, which is exceedingly common in elderly with dementia, is anxiety. It is estimated that 60% of persons with dementia will also present with symptoms of generalized anxiety disorder (GAD; Mintzer & Brawman-Mintzer, 1996). Yet again, however, too little is known about the relationship between anxiety and dementia. Anxiety is also highly comorbid with depression, complicating the etiology and treatment even more. Studies show that much like depression, anxiety symptoms increase in the early stages of cognitive decline and then decrease in the latest stages due to loss of insight (Bierman, Comijs, Jonker, & Beekman, 2007). One might assume that the anxiety is tied to depression rather than the dementia; however, anxiety often appears regardless of depressive symptoms and is treated much differently. Even after controlling for depression, anxiety in dementia is related to "poor quality of life and behavioral disturbances" (Seignourel, Kunik, Snow, Wilson, & Stanley, 2008). The destructive effects anxiety can have on the demented person can cause caregivers stress in dealing with the patient as well as negative physiological reactions to the stress in the patient.

Old age, the diagnosis of a degenerative illness, and numerous other factors can contribute to normal anxious symptoms in old age. One example of an anxious presentation has been coined *sundowning*. According to Burney-Puckett (1996), sundowning can be described as increased agitation and confusion occurring in late afternoon in patients with dementia. Sundown syndrome is considered a type of anxiety directly related to dementia. However, symptoms like sundowning and the similarity of symptoms in anxiety, depression, and dementia can severely complicate the diagnosis of GAD. Considering the high overlap in symptoms along with understandable amounts of normal anxiety, special considerations must be used when GAD is a possibility in a demented patient. Starkstein, Jorge, Petracca, and Robinson (2007) validated "irritability, muscle tension, fears, and respiratory symptoms in the context of excessive anxiety and worry" as the criteria necessary to diagnose an Alzheimer's patient with GAD. Differentiating between GAD and dementia-induced anxiety is important in determining the most efficacious treatment methods. Flint (2005) determined that GAD in the elderly is best treated using antidepressants, while maintaining that cognitive behavioral therapy (CBT) is also beneficial. Other researchers have found that structuring the environment of the patient in addition to CBT can improve patients' self-esteem, independence, and reduce the chance of hospitalization (Koder, 1998). Making subtle differentiations in patients with anxious presentations in dementia can make all the difference in their outcomes.

Psychosis can be one of the most difficult complications of dementia for the patient, loved ones, and caregivers to understand. The delusions and hallucinations can be troublesome to the patient and family, and the psychoses' origins can sometimes be difficult to determine for health care providers. As Ballard, Bannister, Solis, Oyebode, and Wilcock (1996) explain, psychotic symptoms in relation to dementia have previously been lumped into a single category, masking necessary distinctions and associations. Additionally, psychosis may occur in patients with dementia due to a variety of origins not related to the dementia. In late life, psychosis can arise due to depression, medical problems (toxicity of medications, brain tumors, etc.), schizophrenia, bipolar disorder, and delirium, to name a few (Webster & Grossberg, 1998). Because dementias are the leading cause of late-life psychosis (Webster & Grossberg, 1998), the search for other causes and treatments of hallucinations and delusions in the elderly is sometimes neglected. This neglect can cause problems if, for example, a patient is treated with antipsychotics when the cause of his or her delusions is actually a major depressive episode that should be treated with antidepressants. However, if the psychosis is determined to be brought on by dementia, then it is also necessary to determine the underlying form of dementia (e.g., AD, vascular dementia [VaD], Lewy-body dementia [LBD]).

All forms of dementia can present with psychotic symptoms. Weintraub and Porsteinsson (2006) report that up to one half of AD and VaD patients present with psychotic symptoms, whereas psychotic symptoms are rather uncommon in frontotemporal dementia (FTD). Psychosis, especially in the form of visual hallucinations, is most common and persistent in patients with LBD (Ballard et al., 2001). This is an example of a case in which the underlying disease course is important to know so that medicinal intervention is properly directed. While a patient with AD may respond to an atypical antipsychotic to control psychoses and even agitation, if used in a patient with LBD, significant exacerbation of motor symptoms (e.g., rigidity) may occur due to the effect the agent has on dopamine levels.

Understanding the stages of each dementia and the presentation of the psychosis is vital in providing proper treatment. For example, the complex and recurrent visual and audio hallucinations in LBD can be extremely useful in differentiating it from AD and Parkinson's disease (Latoo & Jan, 2008), which share a similar diagnosis criteria. Because diseases like AD cannot be definitively diagnosed until after death, ruling out other causes of patients' symptoms can aid in treatment. With so many different origins, psychosis can become both a complication and an aid in diagnosis. The time of onset and presentation of the symptoms can lead researchers and practitioners to better understand the diseases and determine diagnoses.

Other complications that arise predominantly as symptoms rather than possible comorbid disorders, such as aggression, irritability, apathy, and changes in personality, can also be problematic for patients and caregivers. Although these changes can certainly be troublesome for the patients, they can be especially wearing on family and health care providers. Apathy in a patient may help lead to a more accurate diagnosis of FTD over AD (Weintraub & Porsteinsson, 2006), yet pushing a highly apathetic patient to take his or her medications may be much more difficult. Conversely, a patient who is consistently fighting and irritable with his or her caregivers can cause stress, burnout, and may even lead the caregiver to induce an almost catatonic state through medications. Psychosis, depression, anxiety, and all of the psychiatric symptoms discussed must be considered on a case-by-case basis. They can complicate treatment or possibly aid in diagnosis; either way, every psychiatric issue should be carefully examined.

MEDICAL COMPLICATIONS

Old age commonly corresponds to various medical conditions such as pain, incontinence, loss of vision and hearing, and coronary issues, as well as joint and muscle problems. The presence of dementia can often cause physicians to overlook these conditions as well as more serious problems due to the assumption that they are part of the degenerative disease. In this way, medical conditions can be just as difficult to differentiate as psychiatric illnesses. The deleterious effects of dementia do not stay confined to the mind; over time, they cause the body's functioning to deteriorate as well. Just as dementia can complicate the diagnosis of these more prevalent ailments, the common treatments for those issues can adversely interact with the effectiveness of dementia medications. According to Schubert et al. (2006), pharmacological complications of medications used to treat conventional symptoms of old age can antagonistically interact with cholinesterase inhibitors often used in the treatment of dementia, rendering them useless. In such a scenario, physicians may be forced to choose less effective treatments or must make the difficult decision to only focus treatment on one condition.

The amount of medical issues that interact with dementia is extensive. Stroke, cancer, infections, orthopedic issues, diabetes, cardiovascular conditions, nutritional disorders, pain, and loss of vision and hearing are some of the most prominent complications occurring with mental deterioration. Some patients may even have multiple comorbid medical conditions in addition to dementia and other psychiatric problems. Much like many of the psychiatric conditions, medical issues can have a complicated and confusing cause-and-effect relationship with dementia. The treatment of these conditions has the potential to improve the patients' quality of life; however, many patients' dementias are not taken into consideration for treatment plans. One study found that as high as 50% of older adults with dementia are using medications with anticholinergic activity, a reaction that prevents many dementia medications from working effectively (Schubert et al., 2006). In these instances, physicians treat one condition while unknowingly antagonizing another. Carefully considering dementia when treating medical conditions can reduce the likelihood of this negative reaction occurring.

Central Nervous System

Issues in the central nervous system (CNS) have long been looked at as possible predictors of dementia. Moroney et al. (1996) followed 185 nondemented patients (who had experienced hypoxic-ischemic disorders, mainly ischemic stroke) for 52.8 months and found that $78.2 \pm 4.3\%$ of patients developed dementia. These findings indicate CNS problems as independent risk factors for dementia; yet dementia is also known to alter the CNS on its own. For example, Buée, Hof, and Delacourte (1997) demonstrate the decrease in vascular density, atrophy, glomerular loop formations, and coiling structures associated with AD. These complexities are only intensified in VaD, where hypoxic-ischemic strokes are part of the diagnosis and commonly occur throughout the disease's progression.

As with many medical conditions, stroke can have a significant impact on any person's mood and affect. In the elderly, these mood disorders can often share a confusing association with dementia. Depression is especially prevalent in stroke survivors, but even higher in people with dementia. One study determined that as high as 50% of patients with comorbid dementia demonstrate depressive symptoms as well as "slowness, psychic slowness, lack of energy, and concentration difficulties"

3 years after the stroke (Verdelho , Henon, Lebert, Pasquier, & Leys, 2004). Poststroke depression then in turn may be implicated in even more complications. Schiffer and Pope (2005) discuss the frequency of pseudobulbar affect (emotional lability) in patients after stroke and how it may be exacerbated by the high prevalence of depression in this population. This evidence might imply that stroke increases the likelihood of developing dementia, and dementia intensifies the negative poststroke symptoms.

Cardiovascular Problems

Increasingly, research is showing a link between cardiovascular risk factors and likelihood of developing dementia later in life. Risk factors include high cholesterol, diabetes, hypertension, obesity, and substance abuse, most commonly associated with cigarette smoking. In a retrospective cohort study, Whitmer, Sidney, Selby, Johnston, and Yaffe (2005) evaluated 8,845 participants' medical records in midlife (ages: 40–45 years) compared to late life and found a 20% to 40% increased risk of dementia in participants who had cardiovascular risk factors earlier in life. Some studies have found that certain factors may be greater risks than others. Another study by Whitmer, Gunderson, Barrett-Connor, Quesenberry, and Yaffe (2005) used longitudinal data collected from 10,276 participants to determine the relationship between weight and dementia. Obesity was shown to be the single highest predictor, increasing the risk of dementia by 74%, while simply being overweight increased dementia risk by 35% compared to people with a healthy body mass index (Whitmer, Gunderson, et al., 2005). These studies demonstrate the importance of considering cardiovascular risk factors, both combined and individually, as dual risks for developing dementia.

Because cardiovascular risk factors such as obesity and high cholesterol are also risk factors for diabetes, it is unsurprising that diabetes may significantly increase the risk of dementia as well. Diabetes seems to have an extremely complicated relationship with dementia. Through many of the complications that can occur with diabetes, the depression risk is increased; and in those with a dual diagnosis of depression and diabetes, the likelihood of dementia developing is increased two- to threefold (Katon et al., 2010). Type 2 diabetes is also commonly comorbid with hypertension, and Hassing et al. (2004) found that type 2 diabetes was implicated with more pronounced cognitive decline with aging, and when the diabetes is comorbid with hypertension in a demented person, the decline is even greater. With diabetes and hypertension becoming so prevalent in the elderly, managing these conditions may be essential for effectively treating dementia.

Myocardial infarction (MI) and heart failure can lead to functional decline, especially in older adults. One study found that unrecognized MI in men nearly doubles the risk of developing dementia later in life, but not for women (Ikram et al., 2008). These results demonstrate the importance of treating and screening for MI in late adulthood. Alternately, problems also seem to be arising from the treatment of dementias. Wooltorton (2004) found that olanzapine (Zyprexa), an antipsychotic medication used to treat behavioral problems associated with dementia, may increase the risk of cerebrovascular events. Such findings indicate the importance of considering side effects and alternatives to drug treatments when dementia is involved. There is building evidence that improved self-efficacy can lead to better physical and psychological functioning, especially in relation to major medical events. Kempen Sanderman, Miedena, Meyboom-de Jong, and Ormel, J. (2000) found that the amount of functional decline after an MI was often dependent on a person's psychological attributes, specifically neuroticism, mastery, and self-efficacy expectancy. However, considering that dementia is associated with a decline in many of these attributes, complications can become unavoidable.

Cancer

Two of the most feared disorders that come with old age are cancer and dementia; when these conditions co-occur, the result can be overwhelming for the patient and care providers. The combination of these disorders is yet another example of the ways in which treatment of one condition conflicts or may even induce the other. Mounting evidence points to a link between chemotherapy and the development of AD or some form of cognitive impairment due to its "potential to interfere with the maintenance of genomic integrity" (Backon, 1991; Davis et al., 2011). Because chemotherapy is such a common treatment for so many types of cancers, understanding the potential for such devastating side effects in the elderly should be strongly considered by physicians and patients alike. Yet there is also the issue of elderly patients with comorbid illnesses failing to seek treatment at all. One study found that decreased mental status was one of the strongest predictors of whether a person failed to seek treatment, even more so than lack of transportation or physical ability (Goodwin, Hunt, & Samet, 1993). Of course, the decision to seek treatment lies on the patient; however, if quality of life can be improved through treatment, these options should be provided.

General Pain

Medical conditions and even some treatments for those conditions can cause a great deal of physical pain and distress, especially in the elderly. Dementia complicates the treatment of pain in a variety of ways. Elderly in the more advanced stages of the disease are often unable to articulate or even demonstrate their feelings of pain, which leads to undertreatment. Studies suggest that as few as 33% of dementia patients receive proper treatment for postsurgery-related pains even though physicians estimate the need for pain relief to be equivalent to other patients (Scherder et al., 2009). Another study comparing cognitively intact and demented patients with hip fractures pre- and postoperatively found that the cognitively intact patients were not receiving sufficient pain treatment; yet dementia patients received only one third of the amount of analgesics as the cognitively intact group (Morrison & Siu, 1999). These results demonstrate the need for new pain evaluation methods in demented elderly. Because of their inability to express pain verbally or even behaviorally, many patients with dementia may be suffering from severe, untreated pain, which may further reduce cognitive integrity due to greater reductions in attention. Many health workers assume that a non-expression of pain means that pain is nonexistent; however, as Scherder et al. (2009) explains, pain is likely just as frequent and intense, even if it is no longer reported due to cognitive impairment.

Orthopedic Issues

Orthopedic issues such as hip and knee replacements, tendonitis, arthritis, and fractured bones are some of the most common problems associated with old age. Because so many orthopedic issues require serious surgeries, it is important to consider the effects of anesthetics and the recovery process in relation to dementia. Dodds and Allison (1998) found an increase in the occurrence of postoperative cognitive deficits in the elderly with dementia, and surprisingly found that an even larger percentage of patients experienced cognitive deficits postsurgery when no prior deficit was present. Older populations should receive special consideration when presenting surgery as a treatment option due to the increased potential for cognitive complications following surgery. In a study of cognitively unimpaired elderly participants, one major indicator that surgery may lead to more serious cognitive decline, and possibly dementia, is the presence of delirium after operations (Wacker, Nunes, Cabrita, & Forlenza, 2006). Assessing a patient's history for occurrences of postoperative delirium may be a useful tool in estimating an elderly patient's potential to develop cognitive complications.

Dementia, although a cognitive disorder, can cause many physical problems as well due to falls and the degeneration of the nervous system. Buchner and Larson (1987) found that the fracture rate of patients with AD was more than three times that of the general population, even when adjusting for age and sex. In the study, AD patients were at substantially greater risk of falls and fractures when they experienced toxic reactions to medications, and when wandering was a feature of their dementia (Buchner & Larson, 1987). Another study demonstrated that strength and flexibility training can be successfully carried out and cause musculoskeletal improvements in the elderly with dementia (Brill, Drimmer, Morgan, & Gordon, 1995). Prevention is therefore key in assisting demented persons from incurring fractures and physical problems.

Nutritional Disorders

Nutrition plays one of the most significant roles in the maintenance of positive health in old age; so it is unsurprising that it might interact with the development, treatment, and symptom presentation of dementia. Nutrition may be a contributing factor to the development of dementia; conversely, nutritional deficiencies may result from the dementia. Although caretakers cannot generally control nutritional intake at pre-dementia, the necessity for a balanced healthy diet remains imperative post-diagnosis. As Kerstetter, Holthausen, and Fitz (1992) point out, depression, medical conditions, and medications can all lead to poor appetite and malnutrition. When these issues are combined with a person's cognitive decline and possible apathy, the ability or desire to make healthy choices is often no longer present. Gillette-Guyonnet et al. (2000) found that high caregiver burden also increases the risk of malnutrition in AD patients, because caregivers may not be willing to invest in healthier diets for the patient to properly nourish themselves. The importance of good nutrition in preventing further disability and burden must therefore be stressed with regard to caregivers.

Loss of Abilities

Possibly, the most difficult and definite feature dementia patients and caregivers face is the loss of the ability to live alone and care for themselves. Although the loss of functioning progresses differently across the various forms of dementia, the ultimate loss of ability to perform activities of daily living (ADL) is seemingly inevitable. A study of 243 elderly women found that poor health, regardless of age or other factors, was the most pronounced indicator of more depression and anxiety and lower levels of positive relationships and autonomy (Heidrich, 2007). Changes in functioning and health can negatively affect people of all ages and often decreases psychological well-being. In fact, Andersen, Wittrup-Jensen, Lolk, Andersen, & Kragh-Sørensen (2004) found that a person's loss of ability to perform ADLs and the necessity to rely on others were the largest factors contributing to patients' self-rated quality of life. Clearly, the loss of physical abilities can have a profound impact on a person's mood, affect, and overall well-being. These findings must especially be considered by caretakers.

Nursing homes can often be decision-free environments, leading many residents to feel as though even the smallest choices are out of their control. One field experiment emphasizes the importance of giving patients some independence and free choice. The nursing home was divided into a group where the individual's ability to make decisions about his or her care was emphasized and a group where the nursing staff's role was emphasized; the results found a lower morbidity rate and "improved alertness, active participation, and a general sense of well-being" in the experimental group (Langer & Rodin, 1976). These findings highlight the importance of emphasizing the patient's own active role in his or her life, regardless of disability.

SUMMARY

Old age brings with it unique challenges in diagnosis, treatment, and care; dementia complicates these issues even more. Improving the management and care of persons with dementia has positive implications for patients, caregivers, and physicians alike. The complicated interactions among psychiatric disorders, medical conditions, their methods of treatment, and the different types of dementia demonstrate the importance of close case-by-case consideration. Because many demented patients become unable to recall symptoms or explain the side effects they experience, caregivers and physicians must keep very detailed medical and psychiatric records, and remain constantly on the lookout for complications.

Slowing the onset of the more debilitating features of dementia while making the inevitable problems more manageable can reduce the burden of all parties involved. Patients and caregivers alike often become hopeless when faced with the diagnosis of an incurable degenerative disorder. However daunting such a diagnosis might be, focusing on maintaining the best quality of life and reducing caregiver and patient stress remains key in effectively working through the progression of the illness and its secondary complications.

REFERENCES

Andersen, C. K., Wittrup-Jensen, K. U., Lolk, A., Andersen, K., & Kragh-Sørensen, P. (2004). Ability to perform activities of daily living is the main factor affecting quality of life in patients with dementia. *Health and Quality of Life Outcomes, 2,* 52. doi:10.1186/1477-7525-2-52

Backon, J. (1991). Dementia in cancer patients undergoing chemotherapy: Implication of free radical injury and relevance to Alzheimer disease. *Medical Hypotheses, 35*(2), 146–147. doi:10.1016/0306-9877(91)90038-Z

Ballard, C., Bannister, C., Solis, M., Oyebode, F., & Wilcock, G. (1996). The prevalence, associations, and symptoms of depression amongst dementia sufferers. *Journal of Affective Disorders, 36*(3–4), 135–144.

Ballard, C. G., O'Brien, J. T., Swann, A. G., Thompson, P., Neill, D., & McKeith, I. G. (2001). The natural history of psychosis and depression in dementia with Lewy bodies and Alzheimer's disease: Persistence and new cases over 1 year of follow-up. *The Journal of Clinical Psychiatry, 62*(1), 46–49.

Bierman, E. J., Comijs, H. C., Jonker, C., & Beekman, A. T. (2007). Symptoms of anxiety and depression in the course of cognitive decline. *Dementia and Geriatric Cognitive Disorders, 24*(3), 213–219.

Brill, P. A., Drimmer, A. M., Morgan, L. A., & Gordon, N. F. (1995). The feasibility of conducting strength and flexibility programs for elderly nursing home residents with dementia. *The Gerontologist, 35*(2), 263–266. doi: 10.1093/geront/35.2.263

Buchner, D. M., & Larson, E. B. (1987). Falls and fractures in patients with Alzheimer-type dementia. *The Journal of the American Medical Association, 257*(11), 1492–1495. doi: 10.1001/jama.1987.03390110068028

Buée, L., Hof, P. R., & Delacourte, A. (1997). Brain microvascular changes in Alzheimer's disease and other dementias. *Annals of the New York Academy of Sciences, 826*, 7–24. doi: 10.1111/j.1749-6632.1997.tb48457.x

Burney-Puckett, M. (1996). Sundown syndrome: Etiology and management. *Journal of Psychosocial Nursing and Mental Health Services, 34*(5), 40–43.

Davis, B., Fernandez, F., Adams, F., Holmes, V., Levy, J., Lewis, D., & Neidhart, J. (2011). Diagnosis of dementia in cancer patients: Cognitive impairment in these patients can go unrecognized. *Psychosomatics, 28*(4), 175–179. doi: 10.1016/S0033-3182(87)72542-0

DesRosiers, G. (2000). Depressive pseudodementia. In G. E. Berrios & J. R. Hodges (Eds.), *Memory disorders in psychiatric practice* (pp. 268–290). New York, NY: Cambridge.

Dodds, C., & Allison, J. (1998). Postoperative cognitive deficit in the elderly surgical patient. *British Journal of Anaesthesia, 81*(3), 449–462.

Doraiswamy, P. M., Leon, J., Cummings, J. L., Marin, D., & Neumann, P. J. (2002). Prevalence and impact of medical comorbidity in Alzheimer's disease. *The Journals of Gerontology, 57*(3), M173–M177. doi: 10.1093/gerona/57.3.M173

Fichter, M. M., Meller, I., Schröppel, H., & Steinkirchner, R. (1995). Dementia and cognitive impairment in the oldest old in the community. Prevalence and comorbidity. *The British Journal of Psychiatry, 166*(5), 621–629.

Flint, A. J. (2005). Generalised anxiety disorder in elderly patients: Epidemiology, diagnosis and treatment options. *Drugs & Aging, 22*(2), 101–114.

Fu, C., Chute, D. J., Farag, E. S., Garakian, J., Cummings, J. L., & Vinters, H. V. (2004). Comorbidity in dementia: An autopsy study. *Archives of Pathology & Laboratory Medicine, 128*(1), 32–38.

Gillette-Guyonnet, S., Nourhashemi, F., Andrieu, S., de Glisezinski, I., Ousset, P. J., Riviere, D., . . . & Vellas, B. (2000). Weight loss in Alzheimer disease. *The American Journal of Clinical Nutrition, 71*(2), 637S–642S.

Goodwin, J. S., Hunt, W. C., & Samet, J. M. (1993). Determinants of cancer therapy in elderly patients. *Cancer, 72*(2), 594–601. doi: 10.1002/1097-0142(19930715)

Greenwald, B. S., Kramer-Ginsberg, E., Marin, D. B., Laitman, L. B., Hermann, C. K., Mohs, R. C., & Davis, K. L. (1989). Dementia with coexistent major depression. *The American Journal of Psychiatry, 146*(11), 1472–1478.

Hassing, L. B., Hofer, S. M., Nilsson, S. E., Berg, S., Pedersen, N. L., McClearn, G., & Johansson, B. (2004). Comorbid type 2 diabetes mellitus and hypertension exacerbates cognitive decline: Evidence from a longitudinal study. *Age and Ageing, 33*(4), 355–361. doi: 10.1093/ageing/afh100

Heidrich, S. M. (2007). The relationship between physical health and psychological well-being in elderly women: A developmental perspective. *Research in Nursing & Health, 16*(2), 123–130. doi: 10.1002/nur.4770160207

Ikram, A., Oijen, M., Jan de Jong, F., Kors, J., Koudstaal, P., Hofman, A., . . . Breteler, M. (2008). Unrecognized myocardial infarction in relation to risk of dementia and cerebral small vessel disease. *Stroke, 39*, 1421–1426.

Jorm, A. F. (2001). History of depression as a risk factor for dementia: An updated review. *The Australian and New Zealand Journal of Psychiatry, 35*(6), 776–781. doi: 10.1046/j.1440-1614.2001.00967.x

Katon, W. J., Lin, E. H., Williams, L. H., Ciechanowski, P., Heckbert, S. R., Ludman, E., Rutter, C., . . . Von Korff, M. (2010). Comorbid depression is associated with an increased risk of dementia diagnosis in patients with diabetes: A prospective cohort study. *Journal of General Internal Medicine, 25*(5), 423--429.

Katz, I. R. (1998). New strategies for treating Alzheimer's disease. *The Journal of Clinical Psychiatry, 59*(9), 38–44.

Kempen, G. I. J. M., Sanderman, R., Miedena, I., Meyboom-de Jong, B., & Ormel, J. (2000). Functional decline after congestive heart failure and acute myocardial infarction and the impact of psychological attributes: A prospective study. *Quality of Life Research, 9*(4), 439–450.

Kerstetter, J. E., Holthausen, B. A., & Fitz, P. A. (1992). Malnutrition in the institutionalized older adult. *Journal of the American Dietetic Association, 92*(9), 1109–1116.

Koder, D. A. (1998). Treatment of anxiety in the cognitively impaired elderly: Can cognitive-behavior therapy help? *International Psychogeriatrics, 10*(2), 173–182.

Korczyn, A. D., & Halperin, I. (2009). Depression and dementia. *Journal of the Neurological Sciences, 283*(1–2), 139–142. doi: 10.1016/j.jns.2009.02.346)

Langer, E. J., & Rodin, J. (1976). The effects of choice and enhanced personal responsibility for the aged: A field experiment in an institutional setting. *Journal of Personality and Social Psychology, 34*(2), 191–198. doi: 10.1037/0022–3514.34.2.191

Latoo, J., & Jan, F. (2008). Dementia with Lewy bodies: Clinical review. *British Journal of Medical Practitioners, 1*(1), 10–14.

Mintzer, J. E., & Brawman-Mintzer, O. (1996). Agitation as a possible expression of generalized anxiety disorder in demented elderly patients: Toward a treatment approach. *The Journal of Clinical Psychiatry, 57* (Suppl 7), 55–63; discussion 73.

Moroney, J. T., Bagiella, E., Desmond, D. W., Paik, M. C., Stern, Y., & Tatemichi, T. K. (1996). Risk factors for incident dementia after stroke: Role of hypoxic and ischemic disorders. *Stroke, 27,* 1283–1289.

Morrison, R. S., & Siu, A. L. (1999). A comparison of pain and its treatment in advanced dementia and cognitively intact patients with hip fracture. *Journal of Pain and Symptom Management, 19*(4), 240–248. doi: 10.1016/S0885–3924(00)00113–5

Scherder, E., Herr, K., Pickering, G., Gibson, S., Benedetti, F., & Lautenbacher, S. (2009). Pain in dementia. *Pain, 145*(3), 276–278. doi: 10.1016/j.pain.2009.04.007

Schiffer, R. & Pope, L. E. (2005). Review of Pseudobulbar affect including a novel and potential therapy. *The Journal of Neuropsychiatry and Clinical Neurosciences, 17*(4), 447–454.

Schubert, C. C., Boustani, M., Callahan, C. M., Perkins, A. J., Carney, C. P., Fox, C.,…& Hendrie, H. C. (2006). Comorbidity profile of dementia patients in primary care: Are they sicker? *Journal of the American Geriatrics Society, 54*(1), 104–109. doi: 10.1111/j.1532–5415.2005.00543

Seignourel, P. J., Kunik, M. E., Snow, L., Wilson, N., & Stanley, M. (2008). Anxiety in dementia: A critical review. *Clinical Psychology Review, 28*(7), 1071–1082. doi:10.1016/j.cpr.2008.02.008

Starkstein, S. E., Jorge, R., Petracca, G., & Robinson, R. G. (2007). The construct of generalized anxiety disorder in Alzheimer disease. *The American Journal of Geriatric Psychiatry, 15*(1), 42–49. doi: 10.1097/01.JGP.0000229664.11306.b9

Verdelho, A., Henon, H., Lebert, F., Pasquier, F., & Leys, D. (2004). Depressive symptoms after stroke and relationship with dementia: A three year follow-up study. *Neurology, 62*(6), 905–911.

Wacker, P., Nunes, P. V., Cabrita, H., & Forlenza, O. V. (2006). Post-operative delirium is associated with poor cognitive outcome and dementia. *Dementia and Geriatric Cognitive Disorders, 21*(4), 221–227. doi: 10.1159/000091022

Webster, J., & Grossberg, G. T. (1998). Late-life onset of psychotic symptoms. *The American Journal of Geriatric Psychiatry, 6*(3), 196–202.

Weintraub, D., & Porsteinsson, A. (2006). Psychiatric complications in dementia. *Current Clinical Neurology, 4*, 125–136. doi: 10.1007/978–1-59259–960-8_11

Whitmer, R. A., Gunderson, E. P., Barrett-Connor, E., Quesenberry, C. P., & Yaffe, K. (2005). Obesity in middle age and future risk of dementia: A 27 year longitudinal population based study. *British Medical Journal, 330*(7504), 1360. doi: 10.1136/bmj.38446.466238.E0

Whitmer, R. A., Sidney, S., Selby, J., Johnston, S. C., & Yaffe, K. (2005). Midlife cardiovascular risk factors and risk of dementia in late life. *Neurology, 64*(2), 277–281. doi: 10.1212/01. WNL.0000149519.47454.F2

Wooltorton, E. (2004). Olanzapine (Zyprexa): Increased incidence of cerebrovascular events in dementia trials. *Canadian Medical Association Journal, 170*(9), 1395. doi:10.1503/cmaj 0.1040539.

Zekry, D., Herrmann, F. R., Grandjean, R., Vitale, A. M., De Pinho, M. F., Michel, J. P.,...Krause, K. H. (2009). Does dementia predict adverse hospitalization outcomes? A prospective study in aged inpatients. *International Journal of Geriatric Psychiatry, 24*(3), 283–291.

CHAPTER 20

Determination of Capacity: Pragmatic, Legal, and Ethical Considerations

Stacey Wood and Daniel Krauss

CASE EXAMPLE

A probate attorney calls you with a potential referral related to an 80-year-old client with a history of memory loss and falls, but no definitive diagnosis of dementia. Per the attorney, the client has started to demonstrate some inconsistencies in her presentation and some minor memory lapses in her conversations. The attorney reports a long history with the client and her family. The client was widowed 5 to 6 years ago and has adult children. Approximately 6 months earlier, she came to the office with a new partner and made some modifications to her estate plans to include her new partner among her beneficiaries. Now, the client is expressing an interest in modifying her estate, planning to only benefit her new partner. The attorney wants to know if the client "has capacity" to change her will, and if not, at what point in time she lacked capacity. This chapter describes an overview of the procedures that a neuropsychologist may apply to a range of similar referrals in the area of civil capacities. It will begin with the presentation of a framework developed by the American Bar Association/American Psychological Association (ABA/APA) working group on capacity issues and will next provide more specific guidance regarding assessment tools.

NEUROPSYCHOLOGISTS AND CAPACITY ASSESSMENTS: AN OVERVIEW

Neuropsychologists bring a number of critical skills to questions related to decisional capacity. As the *American Psychological Association Guidelines for the Evaluation of Dementia and Age-Related Cognitive Change* notes, "Psychologists are uniquely equipped by training, expertise, and the use of specialized neuropsychological tests to assess changes in memory and cognitive functioning and to distinguish normal changes from early signs of pathology" (APA, Presidential Task Force on the Assessment of Age-Consistent Memory Decline and Dementia, 1998, p. 1298). Neuropsychologists have extensive training in standardized assessment so they can develop objective data relevant to the legal questions being asked. This is important because research in the area has revealed poor quality in clinical data that is proffered in many of these legal hearings (Moye et al., 2007). Neuropsychologists, especially those who work in rehabilitation, are also familiar with the importance and nature of functional assessments. Therefore, they can describe how certain conditions will affect an individual's ability to perform specific functions (e.g., balance a checkbook, drive, or understand the language in a complex will or trust). In addition, neuropsychologists are able to explain complex medical disorders to patients and families, and these skills are useful when working with attorneys and judges who may similarly lack basic knowledge of many of these disorders. Taken together, neuropsychologists bring a number of strengths to questions of decisional capacity.

However, there are some key differences between a standard clinical assessment and an assessment of legal capacity. Generally, any type of forensic assessment differs from the typical clinical or neuropsychological assessment on a number of dimensions, including scope (i.e., legal assessments call for a narrower focus on the legal standard); importance of the client's perspective (i.e., in legal assessments the well-being of the examinee is often secondary to answering the legal question); voluntariness (i.e., oftentimes an examinee in a legal assessment has been ordered to undergo it); threats to validity (i.e., legal assessments often call for the evaluation of intentional or unintentional distortion of information); relationship and dynamics (i.e., legal assessments often require more emotional distance from the examinee); and pace and setting (i.e., legal assessments are often constrained by time and opportunities to have contact with the examinee) (Melton, Petrila, Poythress, & Slobogin, 2007). More specifically, legal capacity referrals have a more extensive pre-assessment phase (Moye, 1999). Psychologists must know relevant legal standards, and because these standards are often functional in nature, a functional assessment may be part of the assessment. Finally, the legal system will often ask for the examiner to offer a clear clinical opinion regarding the client's ability to make a decision, either contemporaneously or retrospectively. There is considerable controversy within the legal and forensic fields about whether a clinician should attempt to answer this question, commonly referred to as *ultimate opinion testimony*. Some commentators (Melton et al., 2007) suggest that it is inappropriate for a clinician to ever answer what is fundamentally a legal question, while others argue that proffering an opinion is appropriate and useful as long as the clinician can adequately justify his or her conclusions based on sound psychological practice (Goldstein, 2006). In summary, neuropsychologists will use similar tools and approaches in these cases, but they will need to know the relevant legal standards, understand the different constraints of the legal context, often add a more extensive functional assessment, and be prepared to voice or not voice an opinion regarding the specific legal capacities in question.

General Conceptual Framework for Capacity Assessments

In 2003, under the auspices of the interdisciplinary task force on facilitating ABA–APA relations, a working group was formed comprising both psychologists and attorneys. The working group has produced a series of three handbooks to provide guidance in capacity issues for attorneys, judges, and psychologists (ABA/APA Assessment of Capacity in Older Adults Project Working Group, 2008; ABA Commission on Law and Aging & APA, 2005; ABA, APA, & NCPJ, 2006). One product of this collaborative venture has been the development of a conceptual framework for capacity assessments. Because of the nature of capacity referrals that can address a wide range of behaviors from capacity to drive, marry, vote, manage finances, make a will, give a gift, make medical decisions, or consent to research, a one-size-fits-all neuropsychological battery is not appropriate. The ABA/APA conceptual framework can serve to help clinicians design more relevant batteries and make certain that they have gathered the information necessary to address the legal question.

Current theoretical conceptualizations of clinical assessments of capacity draw heavily from the seminal work of Thomas Grisso (Grisso, 1986, 2003). The Grisso model included a causal component (e.g., medical diagnosis), a functional component, a contextual component, and an interactive component. The ABA/APA framework begins with this framework and expands the model by setting out nine components necessary for clinical capacity assessment of older adults: (a) legal standard; (b) functional elements; (c) diagnosis; (d) cognitive underpinnings; (e) psychiatric or emotional factors; (f) values; (g) risk considerations; (h) steps to enhance capacity; and (i) clinical judgment of capacity. These relationships have been the main focus of empirical efforts to understand the underpinnings of capacity and to guide recommendations for assessment. This conceptual model has been described in detail elsewhere, and those interested should see the ABA/APA handbook for a complete discussion of these concepts (www.apa.org/pi/aging/programs/assessment/index.aspx).

How Do Neuropsychological Constructs Relate to Legal Standards?

Legal standards refer to the legal question, relevant legal statutes, and case law necessary for completing an assessment. Legal definitions of capacity vary from state to state; therefore, it is important to become familiar with the specific language that is being used in your jurisdiction and how these standards and language have been interpreted in legal decisions. Legal standards also vary by type of capacity. In a capacity assessment, you will be asked to answer a concrete legal question, such as, "Does this individual have the capacity to manage his or her finances?" Because the clinical assessment will be used to help determine the legal rights of the alleged incapacitated person to specifically make financial decisions, the clinician must be familiar with the specific legal standards of financial capacity in his or her state to provide guidance for the assessment. Next, the clinician should ascertain the legal setting involved. For example, many capacity assessments are completed to assist in conservatorship/guardianship matters that are handled in probate courts. Cases of elder abuse and neglect may be handled in criminal courts that follow criminal legal standards. Some questions of capacity, such as the capacity to make medical decisions and participate in research, are often handled outside the legal context. In order to determine the specific legal standards in your practice jurisdiction, there are a number of resources available to you. For example, the referring attorney can usually provide you with that information as well as clarify any legal questions that may emerge. Reference books, such as the *Law and Mental Health Professional Health* series, offer compilations of relevant legal statutes by state. In addition, each state may have similar compilations of legal statutes, such as the *California Department of Mental Health Laws and Regulations* (2010), to provide much of the needed information. Many states (including California) have probate (conservatorship) related code posted online as well (e.g., see law.onecle.com/california/probate/811 .html). Before completing the evaluation, however, it is useful to communicate with an attorney about how the explicit language used in the statutes has been interpreted by courts in your jurisdiction. For example, a word as simple as *impairment* may exist in many jurisdiction statutes but has been interpreted in widely divergent ways by separate jurisdiction courts.

Probate courts are usually open to the public and allow for observations during some matters. Once familiar with the legal standards, the neuropsychologist can build a test battery that will provide data that better fit the relevant legal standards. Some states have forms that must be completed as part of a capacity assessment that specifically ask about different cognitive domains and are used in court to guide legal decision making.

A common referral question relates to the potential need for a guardianship over person and estate (or conservatorships, in some jurisdictions). More specifically, some states (e.g., Alabama, Colorado, Hawaii, Minnesota, and Montana) have adopted laws similar to the model law, the Uniform Guardianship and Protective Proceedings Act (UGPPA, 1997), regarding guardianship proceedings. The UGPPA emphasized the need for domain-specific recommendations versus an all-or-none determination of capacity. The Act defines an incapacitated person as "an individual that lacks the ability to meet essential requirements for physical health, safety, or self-care, even with appropriate technological assistance" (UGPPA, 1997, pp. 45–102). In contrast, the California Probate Code 1801a defines an incapacitated person as one who is "unable to provide properly for his or her personal needs for physical health, food, clothing, or shelter" (CAL Probate Code §1801a, 2009). Note that the Act language expressly incorporates a number of elements, including a cognitive component and a functional component, whereas California's statute language does not. However, the California statute is further defined by additional statutes (see CAL Probate Code §810–813, 2009) and decisions that implicitly acknowledge an ability component to this standard. In order to provide optimal clinical evidence, an assessment must include both aspects.

Additionally, some jurisdictions (e.g., Kentucky) require that guardianship assessments be performed by an "interdisciplinary evaluation team" consisting of a physician, a psychologist, and a social worker (Drogin & Barrett, 2010). Furthermore, one member of the team must have specialized knowledge in the area of the disability that is alleged in the petition for evaluation. As a result, each member of the team would necessarily have to focus on different aspects of the evaluation, but one would expect in such an assessment for a neuropsychologist to draw a link between the medical disorder and specific functional impairment. In summary, neuropsychological constructs are relevant to legal standards but do not map on perfectly. The neuropsychologist should make an effort to become familiar with the relevant legal standards and design his or her test battery explicitly to be able to address relevant questions.

HOW DO CORTICAL DEMENTIAS IMPACT DECISION MAKING?

Decision making is complex and involves multiple cortical and subcortical brain regions. Cognitive underpinnings of capacity are also varied, depending on the specific issue in question. As such, there is no specific test instrument or even classic neuropsychological domain that can capture "decision making" as understood by the legal community. The following sections review what is known regarding the cognitive underpinnings of different, legally relevant domains. Injuries to the prefrontal cortex are common in dementia and are often linked to changes in decision-making abilities. Three subregions, the dorsolateral prefrontal cortex (DLPFC), the ventromedial prefrontal cortex (VMF), and the anterior cingulate, contribute to decision making in various ways, primarily impacting judgment. However, as reviewed in the following text, verbal memory, calculation abilities, and literacy may all impact decisional capacity.

Understanding the Cognitive Underpinnings of Decision Making

Decision making is a complex cognitive process that involves multiple brain regions and brain systems. Specific capacities (e.g., capacity to drive, make medical decisions, draft a will) differ in their cognitive underpinnings. While research relating neuropsychological constructs to specific legal constructs of decision making in dementia is uneven, there are some decisional domains for which we can provide some empirical guidance. These include medical decision making, financial capacity, testamentary capacity, and independent living. We will also note those areas for which more research is necessary regarding these relationships in dementia populations. Where data do exist for cortical dementia populations, they almost exclusively come from Alzheimer's disease (AD) and related disorders.

Medical Decision Making

The relationship between cognitive functions and medical consent abilities has been one of the better-studied areas in the decisional capacity literature in dementia patients (ABA/APA, 2008; Gurrera, Moye, Karel, Azar, & Armesto, 2006). In general, in order to ascertain medical consent capacity, three subabilities must be intact: understanding (e.g., comprehension of relevant information); appreciation (e.g., the ability to integrate relevant information with one's current situation); and expressing a choice (e.g., the ability to communicate a choice; Moye, Karel, Azar, & Gurrera, 2004). However, it should be noted that jurisdictions differ regarding the requirement that all four elements are required.

In terms of assessment tools, tasks of verbal memory, comprehension, abstract reasoning, confrontational naming, and executive functioning have all been significantly linked to medical consent abilities among dementia patients (ABA/APA, 2008; Marson, Chatterjee, Ingram, & Harrell, 1996). However, it should be noted that the relationships between individual neuropsychological tasks and all four abilities show considerable variance (ranging from about 10% in expressing a choice to 78% of understanding; Gurrera et al., 2006; Wood, 2007). As such, it is recommended that neuropsychologists augment their test battery with a specific tool for medical consent capacity (such as the MacCAT-T; MacArthur Competence Assessment Tool-Treatment), and interview questions to assess the specifics of the patient's health.

Financial Capacity

Financial capacity is perhaps the decisional capacity with the highest cognitive component. A conceptual framework developed suggests that financial capacity is comprised of three types of knowledge, including declarative knowledge; skills (e.g., checkbook balancing); and judgment. Based on a series of studies in patients with mild cognitive impairment (MCI) and moderate dementia, the following neuropsychological measures have been linked to financial capacity: arithmetic abilities (assessed with the Wide Range Achievement Test [WRAT]), executive functioning, and memory. Decline in arithmetic skills was linked with impairment in financial capacity even in early stages of AD and suggests that financial capacity may be impacted earlier than other types of decisional capacities (Griffith et al., 2003; Marson, Earnst, Jamil, Bartolucci, & Harrell, 2000; Marson, Sawrie, et al., 2000; Marson & Hebert, 2008). Related research on financial decision making has found that numeracy, working memory, and speed of processing are related to optimal decision making in the area of financial decision making in healthy adults (Wood et al., 2011). Neuropsychological measures help to ascertain an individual's cognitive functioning and risk, but in order to assess all three core areas of knowledge, skills, and judgment, it is recommended that neuropsychologists include a measure of financial capacity (Independent Living Scales, Financial Capacity Instrument) and interview questions that relate to the individual's situation.

Testamentary Capacity and Undue Influence

Testamentary capacity represents the legal ability to execute a will. While testamentary capacity is clearly related to the broader construct of financial capacity, it is often described as having a lower legal standard (Melton et al., 2007) and is related to four specific elements (i.e., [a] knowledge of what a will is; [b] knowledge of potential heirs [natural objects of bounty]; [c] knowledge of nature and extent of assets; and [d] plan for distribution of assets). At present, there is limited work linking specific neuropsychological constructs and diagnosis to testamentary capacity, although Marson, Huthwaite, and Hebert have provided a preliminary framework integrating the legal elements to assessment issues (Marson et al., 2004). An additional challenge is that often, these referrals relate to a time in the past. The first element of testamentary capacity is understanding the nature of a will. In order to meet this standard, a client must be able to state the purpose of a will and consequences of a will. This element may be compromised by aphasia, verbal abstraction, and low levels of sophistication. The second element is related to the knowledge and extent of property (bounty). In order to assess this construct, the assessor must have accurate knowledge himself or herself from a collateral source regarding property, investments, 401ks, savings accounts, pensions, and other sources of assets. Neurocognitive domains relevant to this element may include explicit memory, language functioning, and executive functioning. The third element is related to knowing the objects of one's bounty, or heirs. Retrograde amnesia, as can occur in Alzheimer's, may impair the ability to recognize one's heirs, especially "newer" family members such as grandchildren. If, during an interview, a client does not name a natural heir (e.g., a son), it can be important to ask why. If the client simply forgot and overlooked the heir, it may be secondary to a dementia process. However, if the client can give a cogent explanation for his or her absence (e.g., substance use), it helps to support a finding of testamentary capacity. The final element relates to the client's ability to specify a plan for distribution of assets. This element requires the client to state specific allocations per heir. In recent times, it has been difficult to accurately assess property values on any given day as these have fluctuated quite dramatically in some regions. In some cases, rather than asking a client to express a plan based on an exact dollar amount of worth, it may be reasonable to ask the client to allocate resources based on percent of assets to heirs. This element requires calculation abilities and executive functioning. A further consideration is related to the presence of psychiatric and neuropsychiatric symptoms. If an individual possesses the cognitive abilities related to testamentary capacity, he or she must also be demonstrated to be free of delusions that may impact his or her estate planning (e.g., son is stealing from him or her, daughter is trying to harm her). This type of delusion is common in AD and is often accompanied by memory impairment that would impair other elements as well. However, in a frontotemporal lobular disease, psychotic symptoms, including paranoia, can emerge prior to cognitive symptoms and may impair judgment to a degree that this element cannot be met.

Finally, in order for a will to be considered valid, the testator must be found to be free of "undue" influence. Undue influence refers to a dynamic between two individuals where the stronger bends the weaker to his or her will (ABA/APA, 2008). Undue influence can occur either in the absence or presence of cognitive impairment. Cognitive impairment increases the susceptibility of the older adult to undue influence, as does the presence of psychological disorders, medical conditions, dependency, and isolation. In terms of assessment, there is no empirically validated tool at this point in time for either testamentary capacity or undue influence. It may be prudent to include a measure of financial capacity (i.e., Financial Capacity Inventory [FCI], Independent Living Scales [ILS]) in addition to drawing up specific questions relevant to the estate planning and completing a dementia battery.

In many cases, requests for assessments of testamentary capacity will be retrospective, meaning that the clinician will be asked to opine on a date in the past. In some cases, the testator may still be living and can be assessed. However, in other situations, the evaluation must be completed based on a review of medical records and other evidence. In cases of AD, it may be possible to trace past Mini-Mental State Examination (MMSE) scores available in medical records to help gauge the stage of the illness at the time of the drafting of the will. For many dementia processes, MMSE scores will probably not possess enough sensitivity to gauge functional ability, except at extremes. Other evidence that may be useful includes videotapes; collateral interviews (e.g., of family members, neighbors, health care providers, and adult protective services); court transcripts; banking statements (e.g., changes in financial habits); driving records; legal records; psychological records; and personal diaries/letters, if available. There are other resources to assist the clinician in performing a retrospective evaluation (e.g., see ABA/APA, 2008). For the purposes of this chapter, the clinician needs to bring to these assessments an understanding of the course of the dementia process and construct a timeline with regard to the events in question, etiology of cognitive impairment, and expected course of the dementia.

Independent Living

One of the key distinctions between a traditional neuropsychological assessment and an assessment of decisional capacity is the added emphasis on functional assessments. Legal standards often combine cognitive and functional elements; as such, clinicians completing these assessments need to be able to explicitly discuss how the client is performing at a functional level. Most commonly, clinicians will use their typical neuropsychological battery and add a section for the "functional" domain in question. Three of the most common referral questions are the capacity to manage person, manage estate, and to make medical decisions. An assessment of functional elements may then include a home visit, an explicit assessment of activities of daily living (ADL) and instrumental ADL (IADL; ideally in the home), the use of functional test instruments to assess medical decision making and financial capacity, or some combination of these (i.e., Hopemont, Independent Living Scales, Financial Capacity Instrument; Griffith et al, 2003; Loeb, 1996; Staats & Edelstein, 1995). In addition to the instruments that tend to provide hypothetical situations, it is extremely helpful to ask questions regarding the specific incidents in question. For example, if the client seems to be making poor medical decisions, questions designed to assess his or her knowledge of the issues at hand will be critical to your assessment. In cases of financial decision making, specific questions regarding their financial situation (based on collateral information) will allow you to ascertain their practical day-to-day knowledge. It would be difficult to overstate the importance of collecting valid functional data to augment the traditional neuropsychological battery.

Putting Together a Test Battery for a Capacity Assessment

Because of the diversity of capacity questions (e.g., testamentary, financial, independent living, medical decision making) that may arise, there is not one standard neuropsychological battery that will be appropriate for all capacity referrals. The first step will be to determine the capacity in question and the relevant legal standards. In general, a capacity assessment will include an extended clinical interview, collateral interviews, a complete cognitive battery assessing all major domains, and a functional assessment.

As such, begin with a test battery that will allow for differential diagnosis in a potential dementia population, including delirium and depression screens where relevant as per the APA *Guidelines for the Evaluation of Dementia and Age-Related Cognitive Change* (APA, Presidential Task Force on the Assessment of Age-Consistent Memory Decline and Dementia, 1998). In order to tap into domains that have been linked to decisional capacity, include an explicit measure of calculation abilities and literacy, such as the WRAT-III. Just as in clinical cases, a neuropsychologist will use these tests to determine strengths and weaknesses, differential diagnosis, and prognosis. Add some type of functional assessment using direct observation, a standardized measure (e.g., Independent Living Scales), interview questions, or some combination of these approaches.

Writing an Opinion

In the conclusion of the report, begin with a section that details the neuropsychological findings, differential diagnosis, and prognosis. As much as possible, write the report to be accessible to legal professionals. Next, draft a section that addresses the specific legal question in the referral. In this section, integrate the cognitive and functional aspects to make clear how you derived your opinion.

CASE EXAMPLE 1

Neuropsychological Findings

From the clinical interview and neuropsychological test battery, as well as a review of medical records, it is the examiner's opinion that Mrs. K presents with a moderate dementia syndrome. At this time, she has significant deficits in verbal memory, language skills, executive functioning, and visual-spatial skills. In terms of etiology, her preserved social skills, pattern of gradual decline, and, especially, poor memory are consistent with a diagnosis of possible AD. However, her history of diabetes puts her at some increased risk for a vascular process or some type of mixed etiology. A full neurological work-up, including neuroimaging, is recommended to assist in the differential diagnosis.

Capacity Findings

Financial Capacity

It is the examiner's opinion that Mrs. K did not have the capacity to manage her simple and complex finances independently, and she was not able to perform these financial tasks in January 2007. Her current presentation (moderate dementia) suggests that her memory loss has been present for 2 to 3 years. Additionally, it is the examiner's opinion that Mrs. K is not able to make small purchases, write checks, or read or understand her bank statements without assistance at present based on her test performance. Further, she is not able to manage her complex finances, balance her checkbook, or sign real-estate agreements secondary to her moderate to severely impaired verbal memory, executive functioning, and calculation abilities. In summary, Mrs. K will benefit from formal protections to manage her estate.

Capacity to Manage Her Person

It is the examiner's opinion that Mrs. K is currently able to take care of herself independently with the current assistance that she has in place. Mrs. K has lived in the same home for almost 40 years and compensates functionally. If she progresses or moves, she will need more structure and, at that time, may need a more formal mechanism to manage her person.

CASE EXAMPLE 2

Neuropsychological Findings

The results of the clinical interview and neuropsychological test battery, as well as a review of available records, revealed that Mrs. C presented with neurocognitive patterns much more impaired than one would predict by age alone. Although she is 89 years old and she presents well in terms of her language skills and immediate memory, her long-term memory and ability to learn are severely impaired. Similarly, she demonstrated difficulty with executive functioning, calculation, and financial management. These deficits could be caused by a number of etiologies including that secondary to a head injury as a result of one of her numerous falls or some type of vascular dementia related to hypertension. Furthermore, it is possible that she is suffering from an Alzheimer's-like dementia. Neuroimaging is highly recommended in order to determine etiology. Mrs. C discontinued the Geriatric Depression Scale. However, there was evidence within the clinical interview that is consistent with the presence of some depression symptoms. In any case, cognitive impairment present at the interview and evaluation would make it difficult for Mrs. C to complete her financial management herself.

In summary, Mrs. C currently has severely impaired memory and has difficulty learning new information. Beginning in 2006, she was discovered as incapacitated at her home by her family and hospitalized for over 3 months. At that point, the family stepped in and began assisting her with her ADL and financial management. They withdrew somewhat as she recovered, but again discovered her in less than 1 year's time in the same poor condition in a disheveled home and needed to step in again to have her hospitalized. At present, she requires 24-hour, 7-day-a-week assistance to manage and stay in her home. Fortunately, she has the assets to support that level of care.

Capacity Findings

Financial Capacity

It is the examiner's opinion with a reasonable degree of certainty that Mrs. C does not have capacity to manage her finances. She demonstrated impaired verbal memory, executive functioning, and calculation skills during the cognitive assessment and performed poorly on functional tasks of financial management. She had difficulty stating her current income. She has no memory for signing the checks or the financial transactions of interest. At this time, she will have difficulty managing her simple and complex affairs, writing checks, running errands, doing shopping, or managing real-estate transactions. The current plan with her sister and brother-in-law as financial conservators and a living trust appears to be adequate for her protection.

Capacity to Manage Her Person

It is the examiner's opinion with a reasonable degree of certainty that Mrs. C does not have the capacity to manage her person. At present, Mrs. C has 24-hour assistance, 7 days a week to assist with ADL. Because of cognitive impairment, she is unable to direct her care staff independently. As such, she would benefit from a formal mechanism for the management of person. Her sister and brother-in-law are willing to take on this additional role.

Legal and Ethical Issues

Beyond the appropriate legal standard to address in an evaluation and whether the examiner should offer an ultimate opinion as to whether the examinee meets it, there is a host of other legal and ethical issues that a neuropsychologist might face in performing legal capacity evaluations. There is a growing literature of articles from the APA as well as other professional organizations available that will aid the practitioner in navigating everything from how to respond to a subpoena (Committee on Legal Issues, 2006) to whether to allow a third party to be present during an evaluation (American Academy of Clinical Neuropsychology, 2001; Committee on Psychological Tests and Assessment, APA (CPTA), 2007; National Academy of Neuropsychology, 2000; Otto & Krauss, 2009). It is beyond the scope of the chapter, however, to address all the issues that might arise in these assessments.

Instead, three ethical and legal issues that are central to capacity evaluations will be examined. They are: (a) determining who is the client in a capacity evaluation; (b) how to contemplate informed consent with a potentially incapacitated client; and (c) what are the evidentiary admissibility standards that are relevant to whether the court will allow the examiner to offer expert testimony on any legal capacity issue? In addition to the APA ethics code (APA, 2002), there are a number of important guidelines, including the *Guidelines for the Evaluation of Dementia and Age-Related Cognitive Decline* (APA, Presidential Task Force on the Assessment of Age-Consistent Memory Decline and Dementia [1998], and currently in the last stages of revision) and the *Specialty Guidelines for Forensic Psychologists* (Committee on Ethical Guidelines for Forensic Psychologists [1991] also in the last stages of revision) that are not only relevant but helpful in responding to these dilemmas. It is important to recognize that these guidelines are intended as aspirational in nature and are not specifically designed to create a standard of care for the practitioner. The practitioner would be well advised, however, to be at least aware of the guidance these sources offer with regard to these and other ethical issues. The APA Ethics Code requires, and the two guidelines strongly suggest, that any practitioner taking on the role of a forensic evaluator, which a legal capacity assessment clearly requires, be reasonably familiar with the legal rules and procedures that govern these evaluations (Drogin & Barrett, 2010).

Unlike a normal neuropsychological assessment situation in which the examinee is most often your client, a legal capacity evaluation can produce instances where this is not the case. For example, in the opening vignette to this chapter it is the probate attorney rather than the examinee who is contacting you for your services. As a result, it is possible that the attorney will contract and pay for your services rather than an 80-year-old individual. If this is the case, it is important that you as the examiner discuss the limits of confidentiality with both the probate attorney and the examinee as well as express the advantages and disadvantages of performing the evaluation to both parties. Even though the attorney is your primary client, you would have secondary obligations to the examinee. From the examinee's perspective, a finding of incapacity to change her will may lead to loss of freedom to make testamentary decisions and could be used by other family members who became aware of this finding to contest her current ability to care for herself or make other important financial or life decisions. The examinee would also likely have control over release of the evaluation beyond the probate attorney. Therefore, in the end, a discussion of the lack of confidentiality between the probate attorney and examinee would be necessary as well as instruction on the possible benefits and costs of the evaluation.

Similarly, a guardianship evaluation that is court ordered would place the court rather than the examinee in the role of the client. The examinee may have limited ability to refuse to participate and no confidentiality with regard to the evaluation being used in the court proceeding. During a limited informed consent procedure, it would be incumbent on the examiner to accurately express these limitations to the examinee. As a result of the court order, the examinee may also have little ability to refuse to participate in the proceedings without judicial sanction.

The informed consent procedure for some legal capacity evaluations may also provide a significant dilemma for the examiner. This issue brings to mind a Catch-22 as one tries to imagine an examiner seeking informed consent from an examinee to perform an evaluation that may show that the examinee lacks the capacity to offer informed consent. The APA Ethics Code in Rule 903 recognizes this conundrum and allows an exception from informed consent "when the purpose of testing is to evaluate decisional capacity" (APA, 2002, p. 1071). Alternatively, the code suggests that the psychologist: (a) provide individuals with questionable capacity an appropriate explanation of the services being offered; (b) seek the individual's assent; (c) consider such person's interests and preference; and (d) obtain permission for a legal authorized person if such authorization is allowed by law. In the event that this last element is not required, the psychologist should act in the patient's best interest (APA, 2002). This mandate is unclear how the examiner would find a legally authorized person if the examinee has not been adjudicated incompetent, nor does it explain how the examiner should infer what is in the patient's best interest. For example, is completing an examination of an examinee who is incompetent to care for himself or herself and offer informed consent in the patient's best interest, when the results may lead to a significant deprivation of that individual's autonomy? The latest revision of the Forensic Specialty Guidelines offers a similarly perplexing response in Rule 8.03.03, *Person's lacking capacity to provide informed consent*:

> For examinees adjudicated or presumed by law to lack the capacity to provide informed consent for the anticipated forensic service, the forensic practitioner nevertheless provides an appropriate explanation, seeks the examinee's assent, and obtains appropriate permission from a legally authorized person, as permitted or required by law (EPPCC Sections 3.10, 9.03).
> For examinees whom the forensic practitioner has concluded to be with lack capacity to provide informed consent to a proposed, non-court-ordered service, but who have not been adjudicated as lacking such capacity, the forensic practitioner strives to take reasonable steps to protect their rights and welfare (EPPCC

Section 3.10). This may be accomplished by suspending the proposed service or notifying the examinee's attorney or the retaining party (Committee on Ethical Guidelines for Forensic Psychologists, 2010, revision, p. 11).

Although this guideline appears to offer more concrete guidance to the practitioner, the first paragraph simply tracks the requirements of the APA Ethics Code rule. Furthermore, the guideline's advice in the second paragraph is also difficult to fully implement. It is not clear how the concrete advice offered of "suspending the proposed service" or "notifying the examinee's attorney or the retaining party" will protect the client's welfare, nor is it clear what the next step would be once you have suspended the evaluation or notified the attorney. Perhaps, the most reasonable course of action would be to seek a court order to complete the evaluation because then the informed consent requirement for the examinee would be much more limited.

Finally, the latest revision of the *Guidelines for the Evaluation of Dementia and Age-Related Cognitive Decline* (APA, Presidential Task Force on the Assessment of Age-Consistent Memory Decline and Dementia, 2010 revision) defers to the ABA/APA handbook on this issue. The handbook offers the most concrete and reasonable statement for handling this ethical issue, stating that:

> The person may have capacity to consent to the evaluation, and either agrees or refuses. In this case, the person has provided a valid agreement or refusal, and this can be documented. Alternatively, the person may not have the capacity to consent to the evaluation, and either agrees or refuses. If the person agrees, he or she is generally said to have "assented" and the assessment process goes forward. If the person disagrees, and refuses to comply with an interview, then the psychologist must document why the person is believed to lack the capacity to refuse the evaluation. In some situations, the capacity evaluation stops there. In other situations, where a capacity evaluation is court ordered, the psychologist may be asked to provide an opinion based on his or her observations of the person.

Taken together, all these sources appear to agree that it is necessary to provide a potentially incapacitated examinee with relevant information concerning the evaluation and seek their assent. In situations where the individual refuses to provide his or her assent, the psychologist should document that refusal, notify relevant parties, and possibly seek a court order to complete the evaluation. Regardless of the existence of a court order, the examinee may still refuse to participate in the assessment and evaluation, in which case the examiner should document the patient's continued refusal. If the examiner is asked to testify concerning a legal capacity without completing a thorough assessment, he or she should acknowledge the limitations of the data and observations and be cautious in offering any opinion on legal capacity.

Finally, neuropsychologists should be aware of the evidentiary rules that govern the admissibility of expert evidence in courts where they are testifying. In most cases, when a neuropsychologist offers evidence concerning a legal capacity, he or she will be offering expert testimony, and this testimony is subject to specific admissibility procedures by the court. Almost all jurisdictions have adopted language in their evidentiary rules similar to that of the Federal Rules of Evidence (Sales & Shuman, 2007). These rules allow any expert to offer expert testimony when his or her specialized knowledge will assist the trier of fact (i.e., the jury or the judge in a bench trial) to understand an important issue at trial. However, this general rule has been interpreted differently by the federal courts and individual state jurisdictions. The federal courts and the majority of state jurisdictions follow the *Daubert* rule, based on *Daubert v. Merrell Dow Pharmaceutical* (1993), *General Electric v. Joiner* (1997), and

Kumho v. Carmichael (1999), sometimes referred to as the *Daubert* trilogy. The *Daubert* rule bases evidentiary admissibility decisions on the scientific validity of expert testimony being offered. The *Daubert* trilogy cases suggest a nonexhaustive list of flexible criteria that courts could use in evaluating expert testimony's scientific validity, including the falsifiability, peer review, error rate, and general acceptance of that testimony. If applied appropriately, the *Daubert* standard could potentially prohibit less than scientific or inappropriately applied expert testimony from reaching the jury.

In contrast, a significant minority of state jurisdictions (e.g., Arizona, California, Illinois, Kansas, Maryland, Michigan, Minnesota, New Jersey, New York, Pennsylvania, and Washington) follows the *Frye* standard, which is based on the case of *Frye v. United States* (1923), for the admissibility of expert testimony. The central requirement of the *Frye* standard is that admissible expert testimony is evidence that is generally accepted in the field from which it originates. There has been considerable dispute about whether these different evidentiary admissibility standards should and do affect the admissibility of different types of expert testimony across psychology, with many arguing that the *Daubert* rule creates a higher threshold for the admissibility of psychological expert testimony (e.g., Sales & Shuman, 2007). In fact, in the neuropsychological field there has been a significant controversy over whether flexible batteries in contrast to fixed batteries meet the requirements of the *Daubert* rule (e.g., Bigler, 2007; Reed, 1996). Yet, most legal commentators agree that while *Daubert* could, in theory, raise the threshold for admissibility of expert testimony, in practice this has not often occurred (e.g., Sales & Shuman, 2007).

Most importantly, for neuropsychologists who are completing a legal capacity evaluation, it is necessary that they know the evidentiary admissibility standard that is used in their jurisdiction (e.g., *Frye* or *Daubert*), and be able to answer questions about the expert testimony they will offer that is appropriate to that standard. For example, in a *Frye* jurisdiction, neuropsychological experts should know whether the methods they used to collect data for their evaluations are generally accepted within their field. Likewise, in a *Daubert* jurisdiction, the neuropsychologist should be able to provide evidence concerning the scientific validity of the techniques and tests that were used to reach an opinion. In the end, it is important to remember that it is left to the court to decide if the testimony presented by neuropsychologists is sufficiently valid or reliable for it to be used by the court, but that should not stop neuropsychologists from being strong advocates for the scientific quality of their evaluation.

SUMMARY

In summary, neuropsychologists have the potential to bring important skills to the assessment of decisional capacity in cases of dementia. Key differences between clinical assessments and those for capacity evaluations include knowledge of relevant legal and ethical issues, a functional assessment, and an ability to present neuropsychological data to lay readers. Research on medical consent capacity and financial capacity highlight the importance of the assessment of calculation, executive function, and verbal memory as part of any test battery, but note the limitations of solely relying on neuropsychological tools. A strong assessment will include some type of functional assessment, ideally designed to address the specific legal questions. Research on the neuropsychological underpinnings of testamentary capacity is somewhat underdeveloped and should be an area of growth in the near future.

REFERENCES

American Academy of Clinical Neuropsychology. (2001). Policy statement on the presence of third party observers in neuropsychological assessments. *The Clinical Neuropsychologist, 15*, 433–439.

American Bar Association (ABA) Commission on Law and Aging & American Psychological Association (APA). (2005). *Assessment of older adults with diminished capacity: A handbook for lawyers*. Washington, DC: American Bar Association and American Psychological Association.

American Bar Association (ABA), American Psychological Association (APA), & National College of Probate Judges (NCPJ). (2006). *Judicial determination of capacity of older adults in guardianship proceedings*. Washington, DC: ABA and APA.

American Bar Association/American Psychological Association Assessment of Capacity (ABA/APA) in Older Adults Project Working Group. (2008). *Assessment of older adults with diminished capacity: A handbook for psychologists*. Washington, DC: ABA and APA.

American Psychological Association (APA). (2002). Ethical principles of psychologists and code of conduct. Washington, DC: Author.

American Psychological Association (APA), Presidential Task Force on the Assessment of Age-Consistent Memory Decline and Dementia. (1998). *Guidelines for the evaluation of dementia and age-related cognitive decline*. Washington, DC: American Psychological Association.

American Psychological Association, Presidential Task Force on the Assessment of Age-Consistent Memory Decline and Dementia. (2010, revision). *Guidelines for the evaluation of dementia and age-related cognitive decline*. Washington, DC: American Psychological Association. Retrieved October 5, 2010, from http://apaoutside.apa.org/PubIntCSS/ Public/

Bigler, E. D. (2007). A motion to exclude and the "fixed" versus "flexible" battery in "forensic" neuropsychology: Challenges to the practice of clinical neuropsychology. *Archives of Clinical Neuropsychology, 22*(1), 45–51.

California Department of Mental Health. (2010). *California Department of Mental Health Laws and Regulations*. San Francisco, CA: Barclays Official California Code of Regulations.

California Probate Code §1801a. (2009).

California Probate Code §810–813. (2009).

Committee on Ethical Guidelines for Forensic Psychologists. (1991). Specialty guidelines for forensic psychologists. *Law and Human Behavior, 15*, 655–665.

Committee on Ethical Guidelines for Forensic Psychologists. (2010). *Specialty guidelines for forensic psychologists*. Retrieved December 17, 2010, from http://www.ap-ls.org/ aboutpsychlaw/080110sgfpdraft.pdf

Committee on Legal Issues. (2006). Strategies for private practitioners coping with subpoenas or compelled testimony for client records or test data. *Professional Psychology: Research and Practice, 37*, 215–222.

Committee on Psychological Tests and Assessment, American Psychological Association. (2007). *Statement on third party observers in psychological testing and assessment: A framework for decision making*. Washington, DC: Author.

Daubert v. Merrell Dow Pharmaceuticals, 509 U.S. 579 (1997).

Drogin, E. Y., & Barrett, C. L. (2010). *Evaluations for guardianship*. Part of the Best Practices in Forensic Mental Health Assessment series. Oxford: Oxford University Press.

Frye v. United States, 292 F. 1013 (D.C. Cir. 1923).

General Electric v. Joiner, 522 U.S. 136 (1997).

Goldstein, A. M. (2006). *Forensic psychology: Emerging topics and expanding roles.* Hoboken, NJ: John Wiley & Sons, Inc.

Griffith, H. R., Belue, K., Sicola, A., Krzywanski, S., Zamrini, E., Harrell, L., & Marson, D. C. (2003). Impaired financial abilities in mild cognitive impairment: A direct assessment approach. *Neurology, 60*(3), 449–457.

Grisso, T. (1986). *Evaluating competencies.* New York: Plenum.

Grisso, T. (2003). *Evaluating competencies: Forensic assessments and instruments* (2nd ed.). New York: Kluwer Academic.

Gurrera, R. J., Moye, J., Karel, M. J., Azar, A. R., & Armesto, J. C. (2006). Cognitive performance predicts treatment decisional abilities in mild to moderate dementia. *Neurology, 66*(9), 1367–1372.

Kumho Tire v. Carmichael 526 U.S. 137 (S.Ct. 1999).

Loeb, P. A. (1996). *ILS: Independent living scales manual.* San Antonio, TX: Psychological Corp, Harcourt Brace Jovanovich.

Marson, D. C., Chatterjee, A., Ingram, K. K., & Harrell, L. E. (1996). Toward a neurologic model of competency: Cognitive predictors of capacity to consent in Alzheimer's disease using three different legal standards. *Neurology, 46*(3), 666–672.

Marson, D. C., Earnst, K. S., Jamil, F., Bartolucci, A., & Harrell, L. E. (2000). Consistency of physicians' legal standard and personal judgments of competency in patients with Alzheimer's disease. *Journal of the American Geriatrics Society, 48*(8), 911–918.

Marson, D. C., & Hebert, T. (2008). Financial capacity. In B. L. Cutler (Ed.), *Encyclopedia of psychology and the law* (Vol. 1, pp. 313–316). Thousand Oaks, CA: Sage Publications.

Marson, D., Huthwaite, J., & Hebert, K. (2004). Testamentary capacity and undue influence in the elderly: A jurisprudent therapy perspective. *Law & Psychology Review, 28*, 71–96.

Marson, D. C., Sawrie, S. M., Snyder, S., McInturff, B., Stalvey, T., Boothe, A.,... Harrell, L. E. (2000). Assessing financial capacity in patients with Alzheimer disease: A conceptual model and prototype instrument. *Archives of Neurology, 57*(6), 877–884.

Melton, G. B., Petrila, J., Poythress, N. G., & Slobogin, C. (2007). *Psychological evaluations for the courts: A handbook for mental health professionals and lawyers.* New York, NY: The Guilford Press.

Moye, J. (1999). Assessment of competency and decision making capacity. In P. A. Lichtenberg (Ed.), *Handbook of assessment in clinical gerontology* (pp. 488–528). New York, NY: Wiley.

Moye, J., Karel, M. J., Azar, A. R., & Gurrera, R. J. (2004). Capacity to consent to treatment: Empirical comparison of three instruments in older adults with and without dementia. *The Gerontologist, 44*(2), 166–175.

Moye, J., Wood, E., Edelstein, B., Wood, S., Bower, E. H., Harrison, J. A., & Armesto, J. C. (2007). Statutory reform is associated with improved court practice: Results of a tri-state comparison. *Behavioral Sciences & the Law, 25*(3), 425–436.

National Academy of Neuropsychology. (2000). Presence of third party observers during neuropsychological testing. *Archives of Clinical Neuropsychology, 15*, 379–380.

Otto, R. K., & Krauss, D. A. (2009). Contemplating the presence of third party observers and facilitators in psychological evaluations. *Assessment, 16*(4), 362–372.

Reed, J. E. (1996). Fixed vs. flexible neuropsychological test batteries under the Daubert standard for the admissibility of scientific evidence. *Behavioral Sciences & the Law, 14*(3), 315–322.

Sales, B., & Shuman, D. (2007). Science, experts, and the law: Reflections on the past and the future. In M. Costanzo, D. Krauss, & K. Pezdek (Eds.), *Expert psychological testimony for the courts* (pp. 9–31). Mahwah, NJ: Lawrence Erlbaum.

Staats, N., & Edelstein, B. (1995). *Cognitive changes associated with the declining competency of older adults.* Paper presented at the Gerontological Society of America, Los Angeles, CA.

Uniform Guardianship and Protective Proceedings Act (UGPPA). (1997).

Wood, S. (2007). Assessment of decisional capacity from a neuropsychological perspective. In S. H. Qualls & M. A. Smyer (Eds.), *Aging and decision-making capacity: Clinical family, and legal issues* (pp. 191–205). Hoboken, NJ: John Wiley & Sons Inc.

Wood, S., Hanoch, Y., Barnes, A., Liu, P.-J., Cummings, J., Bhattacharya, C., & Rice, T. (2011). Numeracy and Medicare Part D: The importance of choice & literacy for numbers in optimizing decision making for Medicare's prescription drug program. *Psychology and Aging, 26*(2), 295–307. doi: 10.1037/a0022028

Index

abilities, loss of, 430–431
acetylcholine, 9
acetylcholinesterase inhibitors (AChIs),
    9, 369–372, 379
  for behavioral variant FTD, 227
  for CADASIL, 135
  comparison of drugs, 371–372
actin, 101
Aesop's Fables subtest of BDAE-3, 268–269
aging
  and Alzheimer's disease, 101–102
  -associated cognitive decline, diagnostic
    criteria for, 329
  dementia risk from, 315–316
alcohol withdrawal, 201–202
alcoholism, 199–200
  alcohol detoxification/abstinence, 201–202
    attention during, 203
    executive functioning and problem
      solving, 205–206
    intelligence during, 202–203
    learning and memory during, 203–205
    sensorimotor functioning, 206
    visuospatial and perceptual–motor
      functioning, 205
  and dementia, 206
  Korsakoff's syndrome, 208–211
  and neuropathological changes, 200–201
  Wernicke–Korsakoff's syndrome, 206
  Wernicke's encephalopathy, 206–208
Ali, Muhammad (DP case report), 308
alpha 2 agonist dexmedetomidine
  for delirium, 357
alpha-synuclein, 96, 179, 184
Alzheimer, Alois, 93, 94, 127
Alzheimer's disease (AD), 4–5, 69, 93–94,
    124, 315–316, 367–368
  and age, 101–102

amyloid plaques, 95–96
attentional abilities deficits, 9–10
atypical profiles, 107–108
behavioral symptoms, 70
biomarkers/genetics, 71, 102–103, 109–110
cell loss, 97–99
cerebral amyloid angiopathy, 100
clinical interview, 70
and cognitive reserve, 104–105
cognitive symptoms, 69–70
comparison
  with behavioral variant FTD, 16–17
  with semantic dementia, 18
  with vascular dementia, 21–22
cortico-cortical disconnectivity
  hypothesis of, 8–9
course of dementia, 23, 106–107
dementia due to, 3
dementia with Lewy bodies,
  distinguishing from, 11–12, 14
diagnosis and assessment, 108–111
differential diagnosis, 71
early stage, 105–106
episodic memory loss, 5–6
executive dysfunction, 9–10, 169
functional deficits in, 105–108
granulovacuolar degeneration (GVD),
  100–101
Hirano bodies in, 101
intervention, 111–112
mental set and inhibitory control, 169
neurocognition, 23
neurofibrillary tangles (NFT), 96–97
neuroimaging, 23, 36–39, 71, 109
neuropathology, 23, 94–101
neuropil and synapse loss, 99–100
neuropsychological assessment, 71,
  110–111